MIND, MODERNITY, MADNESS

MIND, MODERNITY, MADNESS

The Impact of Culture on Human Experience

LIAH GREENFELD

HARVARD UNIVERSITY PRESS

Cambridge, Massachusetts, and London, England

2013

Library of Congress Cataloging-in-Publication Data

Greenfeld, Liah.
  Mind, modernity, madness : the impact of culture on human experience / Liah Greenfeld.
      p. cm.
  Includes bibliographical references and index.
  ISBN 978-0-674-07276-3
  1. Mental illness—Social aspects—History. 2. Cultural psychiatry—History.
3. Nationalism—Psychological aspects. I. Title.
  RC455.G726 2013
  616.89—dc23   2012035113

To Gil and Natan Press
and to Dr. Victoria Kirshenblatt

Contents

Acknowledgments

This book is dedicated to my son, my mother, and my husband.

My son accompanied me on the exploration of medical libraries—spending hours at the copying machine in the freezing lower floor of Boston Countway Library while I read, and making sure I didn't expire in the heat of Bethesda in August as I walked between the National Library of Medicine and the motel in which we bivouacked for the purpose of researching the rarest gems of literature on madness. He also served as my guide to the confused world of American young adulthood, ravaged by this modern disease. In many ways he inspired this project and helped me think through it. In particular, he helped me to arrive at the definition of love.

My mother, a person of most powerful intelligence and iron will, a questioner and a doubter, has been a lifelong example for me of truly independent mind. She dreamt of becoming a physicist, but was forced by the circumstances to become a physician, wanted to be a psychiatrist, but was forced by the circumstances to spend the first two decades of her medical career as a tuberculosis specialist and the last three as a pediatrician. She shared with me her exceptionally broad knowledge of medicine and of Russian and world literature, specifically attracting my attention to the depictions of mental disease. Working on this book, I felt that I was in some way going in the direction in which she might have wished to go, were her circumstances different, and it has been of tremendous importance for me to finish this work while she is still here to know that.

Without my husband this book could not be written simply because I would not be, which says it all.

In the twenty years that passed between the publication of the first book in this trilogy and the third, this, one, I have been fortunate to meet and acquire the friendship of colleagues and students—increasingly students who became colleagues—from many countries and a wide range of disciplines. Together, they now form a vibrant intellectual community (a sort of "invisible college"), truly sustaining for me. In the time that it took this book to gestate, they patiently listened to my first attempts to formulate its argument, read drafts of chapters, asked probing questions, offered critical comments. They include, in alphabetical order, Mike Aronson (my caring Harvard University Press editor), Peter Baehr, Darius Barron, Oliver Benoit, Harold Bursztajn, Katrina Demulling, Francesco Duina, Jonathan Eastwood, Edward Gormbley, George Liber, Charles Lindholm, Eric Malczewski, Dmitri Panchenko, David Phillippi, Nikolas Prevelakis, Nathalie Richard, Chandler Rosenberger, Mark Simes, James Stergios, John Stone, and Chikako Takeishi. I thank them all. I am in particular obliged to Nikolas Prevelakis for the help with the annotation of the first chapter, and to David Phillippi, who read the entire book several times and started a blog to popularize its ideas, and Mark Simes, my official and most excellent assistant, who followed their development from day one, kept me abreast of every piece of news in neuroscience, and helped me to prepare the text for publication. I cannot stress enough how important the belief of all these people in my work has been for me.

MIND, MODERNITY, MADNESS

Introduction

The purpose of this book is to make evident that culture is an empirical reality of the first order in human life—that it, in the most profound sense of the word *makes* us human and *defines* human experience. Its empirical focus, the area of experience chosen to drive this point home, is the phenomenon for a long time called simply "madness," but today regarded either as three mental diseases—"the big three of contemporary psychiatry":[1] schizophrenia, bipolar disorder, and major depression—or as the two varieties of psychotic disorder with unknown organic basis: schizophrenia and manic-depressive affective illness (which includes major depression). There are very good reasons for this choice. Schizophrenia and manic-depressive illness are the most severe mental diseases whose biological reality and life-threatening effects are undeniable. Schizophrenia is referred to as "the cancer of the mind," and suicide in the Western world in the vast majority of cases is believed to result from depression. Proving that these biologically real diseases are culturally caused, that they are products of culture—which is what the book argues—would demonstrate the impact of culture on human experience in the seemingly most unlikely case and make self-evident its influence in other spheres of life, such as economics and politics, for instance, in which, though largely disputed, it has been arguable.

Being, generally speaking, a book about the impact of culture on the human mind, it is, more specifically, one about the ways *modern* culture shapes the mind. Even more specifically, it is a book about the role of national consciousness—which forms the framework of modern culture—in causing psychiatry's "big three." Thus, though it stands on its own, it forms the concluding volume of the trilogy on nationalism, the first two volumes of which are *Nationalism: Five Roads to Modernity* and *The Spirit of Capitalism: Nationalism and Economic Growth*.[2]

In addition to extending the discussion of the effects of nationalism from the public sphere, in which political and economic activities take place, into the most personal corners of existential experience, this concluding volume spells out the philosophical and theoretical principles underlying the argument of the entire trilogy and, in particular, explains what makes historical evidence empirical in precisely the sense in which evidence drawn upon in biology and physics is empirical, allowing one to place historical and sociological accounts of human affairs in the same epistemic category: i.e., within science. It explains, in other words, why historical phenomena, while being different in kind, lend themselves no less than biological and physical phenomena (which are also different in kind from each other) to empirical and logical analysis, which, like such analysis in other areas of study, can lead to the accumulation of objective knowledge.

The Argument and Its Provenance

The central argument of this book connects in a causal relationship the cultural phenomenon of nationalism and psychiatric diseases of unknown etiology: schizophrenia, manic depression, and major unipolar depression. These diseases are the *explanans*, the effect, and nationalism is the *explanandum*, the cause. Nationalism is understood in the terms developed in *Nationalism: Five Roads to Modernity* and applied in *The Spirit of Capitalism*. It is a form of consciousness, an essentially secular view of reality, whose socio-political component rests on the principles of fundamental equality of membership in a community and popular sovereignty. As I hope I have demonstrated in *Nationalism* and *The Spirit of Capitalism*, this consciousness forms the cultural framework of modern society: the vision of reality it implies represents the very core of modern culture and is reflected in all the characteristic institutions of modernity, including the open system of stratification, the impersonal—state—form of government, and the economy oriented to sustained growth. Indeed, it is called "nationalism" because the ideal of society it presupposes was named by the sixteenth-century Englishmen, who first conceived of it, "nation." The essence of this ideal is the demand for the embodiment of two principles: the principles of fundamental equality of membership and of popular sovereignty; the nation, in other words, is defined as a community of equals and as sovereign. Equality in shared sovereignty may be interpreted as individual liberty, and was so interpreted in England as well as in societies that closely modeled their nationalism on its example later. But equality could also be interpreted as collective independence from foreign domination. In either case, equality changes the nature of the individual identity, specifically endowing identity with dignity irrespective of personal circumstances, changes, therefore, the nature of social hierarchy, and at least to some extent makes one's position in it a matter of individual choice. At the same time, popular sovereignty, which makes an earthly community the source of all law, drastically diminishes the importance of transcendental forces—of God, above all—in human life. The importance of human life grows proportionately, and before long the transcendental sphere fades from view and man (and eventually woman too) emerges as one's own maker. It is in this broad and historically accurate sense that the term "nationalism" is used in this book, not in the popular connotation of a variety of xenophobia, which is but an aspect of certain nationalisms. Please keep this in mind.

It is obvious that this dramatic transformation in the image of reality, i.e., in how one thinks about it, must significantly affect the nature of existential experience—the very way life is lived and felt. This is what happened in fact. Already in its early days, nationalism contributed greatly to the human emotional repertoire, adding to it such heretofore- unknown emotions as ambition, aspiration, and, remarkably, happiness and romantic love. With this it changed both the reasons for and the experience of suffering.[3] Of course, its effects, positive and negative, were at first limited to England. There a new malaise emerged in the early sixteenth century. It was recognized as a mental disease, but appeared so different from all the known mental diseases that none of the terms of the extensive existing vocabulary (medical or general) were judged adequate to capture it. By the 1530s new words were invented, the strange ailment was named "madness" or "lunacy"; four centuries later German psychiatrists would divide it into two separate diseases, naming them "schizophrenia" and "manic-depressive illness."

In England madness was spreading quickly throughout the sixteenth century, by the end of it being considered—as we learn from *Hamlet*—a special mark of English society. In the seventeenth century madness was observed in the rest of Great Britain and in the English colonies overseas, but was as yet completely unknown in Continental Europe. Visitors from foreign parts considered it an object of great curiosity and called it "the English malady." However, when nationalism developed in France by the end of the eighteenth century, madness arrived there too, and later—with nationalism—spread to the German principalities and to Russia. At first in all these countries it affected almost exclusively the elites—people who actually enjoyed the dignity, the liberty, and choice implied in the national consciousness. As the values of nationalism penetrated deeper into the masses of the population, insanity (the word is another early synonym for "madness"), too, became proportionately far-reaching. In the nineteenth century the rates of insanity increased as the national society became more inclusive, as new groups gained membership in the community of equals, and as more choices became available to more people.

Why do the secular focus of nationalism and the two principles embodied in the society constructed on its basis lead to madness—or schizophrenia and manic-depressive illness? All three of these features place the individual in control of his or her destiny, eliminating the expectation of putting things right in the afterlife, making one the ultimate authority in deciding on one's priorities, encouraging one to strive for a higher social status (since one is presumed to be equal to everyone, but one wants to be equal only to those who are superior), and giving one the right to choose one's social position (since the presumption of fundamental equality makes everyone interchangeable) and therefore identity. But this very liberty, implied in nationalism, both empowering and encouraging the individual to choose what to be—in contrast to all the religious pre-national societies in which no one was asked "what do you want to be when you grow up?" since one was whatever one was born—makes the formation of the individual identity problematic, and the more so the more choices for the definition of one's identity a society offers and the more insistent it is on equality. A clear sense of identity being a condition sine qua non for adequate mental functioning, malformation of identity leads to mental disease, but modern culture cannot help the individual to acquire such clear sense, it is inherently confusing. This cultural insufficiency—the inability of a culture to provide individuals within it with consistent guidance—was named *anomie* by Durkheim.

Though realized in vastly different ways (depending on the manner in which this form of consciousness developed in a particular society), the three principles of nationalism—secularism, egalitarianism, and popular sovereignty—affect the formation of the individual identity in nations necessarily. A member of a nation can no longer learn who or what she or he is from the environment, as would an individual growing up in an essentially religious and rigidly stratified, nonegalitarian order, where everyone's position and behavior are defined by birth and divine providence. Beyond the very general category of nationality, a modern individual must decide what s/he is and should do, and thus construct one's identity oneself. Schizophrenia and depressive (bipolar and unipolar) illnesses, I argue, are caused specifically by the values of equality and self-realization, which make every individual one's own maker—and the rates of such mental diseases increase in accordance with the extent to which a particular society is devoted to these values, inherent in the nationalist image of reality, i.e., in the national consciousness, and the scope allowed to the freedom of choice in it. This turns the prevailing view of the mental diseases in question upside down.

The argument implies, above all, that, while there may be biological predispositions, genetic or other, which influence who succumbs to this disease and who does not, the disease itself is not a disease of the body (the brain), but of thinking—it is truly a disease of the mind. The agent of the disease—the functional equivalent of AIDS's HIV, or malaria's mosquito—is not physical, but cultural, in other words. Though opposition to the prevailing biological view is not unheard of and the voices against it at times even combine in a small choir—the week I am writing this an extended comment on recent books by three reputable authors experienced in dealing with mental illness appears in the *New York Review of Books;* each of them, despite differences in emphasis, "subscribes to the popular theory that mental illness is caused by a chemical imbalance in the brain"—

nobody has yet offered an alternative explanation that could stand scientific scrutiny.[4] The undisputed authority of the biological paradigm in general may make the present argument appear quite controversial. Of course, the claims advanced by the two previous books on which it builds, too, appeared controversial at the times of their publication and came to be regarded as far less controversial since then. I therefore expect that the same will happen to this third, admittedly even more unusual, argument in the natural course of things. But I am getting older and feel that the natural course of things often takes too long, and I also think that it is incumbent on me—in this concluding articulation of the interpretation of nationalism and modernity, developed over two decades of research on modern experience—to locate the entire project amid existing traditions and areas of study with which the reader may be familiar and thereby save some unnecessary discomfort.

The subject of this book—culture—places it within general, theoretical anthropology and sociology, as well as within theory or philosophy of culture, if these can be separated. Its specific preoccupation with nationalism and modern culture makes it a book in historical sociology, which is but a form of history, while the focus on psychiatric illness necessarily connects it to the disciplines of psychology, psychiatry, and even neuroscience. It is relevant to all these areas of research and belongs within none of them exclusively, just as *The Spirit of Capitalism* was relevant to economics, intellectual history, economic history, political economy, and sociological theory, but belonged exclusively within none of these specializations; and *Nationalism* was relevant to comparative politics, history, sociological theory, and history and sociology of science, literature, and religion, among other fields of expertise, without falling exclusively within any of them. Like the previous two books, this book seeks to connect all these areas of human experience, contributing to the study of all of them and the construction of a unified science of humanity. My position on this matter is well summarized by a pioneering French psychiatrist, Jules Baillarger, who will figure in one of the chapters below: "Man is one, despite the distinct elements of which he is formed. In a marvelous manner combine in him the . . . forces, which can be conceived in isolation only outside him."[5] Thus it is, inevitably, also a book in philosophy.

Its methodology, which, in general, is guided by the rules of the scientific method of conjectures and refutations,[6] namely, of logical formulations of hypotheses then methodically tested against empirical evidence (i.e., tested against *all* the available relevant evidence), follows the lead of three giants of the human sciences, who were also philosophers among other things: Émile Durkheim, Max Weber, and Marc Bloch, alternately claimed by anthropology and sociology; sociology, cultural history and economic history; and history and sociology. Specifically, it adopts Durkheim's "rules" of treating every social fact as a thing and of careful, unprejudiced definitions as the first step in attempting any explanation, and combines these with Weber's "methodological individualism."[7] From Bloch it takes the distinction between "intentional" and "unintentional" evidence, and the preference for the latter (sources not intentionally related to the phenomenon one seeks to explain, and serving, as it were, as "witnesses in spite of themselves"); the tactic of cross-examining the evidence—or juxtaposing it at every point with evidence derived from elsewhere; and the reliance on language as both evidence and an instrument of analysis.[8] Durkheim, Weber, and Bloch (I list them chronologically) are unassailable authorities in the social sciences. But, quite apart from the fact that their major theories, all of which treated social—namely, cultural, economic, political— phenomena of great importance, though proposed a very long time ago if measured in life spans of theories in science, have not been superseded, but retain a canonical status for anyone wishing to work in the areas to which they pertain, I rely on them because all three also thought of a unified science of man (or human sciences), and defined it, whether they referred to it as "sociology," as did Durkheim, "history," as did Bloch, or sometimes "history" and sometimes "sociology," as did Weber, as the mental science. This may be lost in translation when Durkheim's use of the word "mental" in French is rendered "social" in English, or glossed over in the case of Weber's insistence on subjective meaning as the defining feature of social action. But in Bloch's explicit formulation it cannot be missed. "In the last analysis," he says, "it is human consciousness which is the subject-matter of history. The interrelations, confusions, and infections of human consciousness are, for history, reality itself."[9] I consider myself belonging to the same "mentalist" tradition in the human sciences.[10]

Of the three classics, Durkheim, it will be easily seen, is most prominently present in these pages. This is not only because, not wishing to discriminate between the two founding fathers of my official discipline and eager to pay filial homage to both, I had to privilege him, having done so for Weber in my previous book. It can even be argued that this project continues the project of Durkheim begun in *Suicide*. Durkheim chose to focus on suicide, of all acts the most personal, most individual, and seemingly independent from social influences, to demonstrate the empirical, and yet not material, reality of society (reality consisting mostly of mental "collective representations") and its priority over the psychology of the individual, embedded in human biological reality. Similarly, focusing on the admittedly biologically real diseases of schizophrenia and manic depression and offering a cultural, historical explanation of a significant health problem, I sought to demonstrate in a most dramatic manner the reality of the symbolic, nonmaterial factors and their profound, all-pervading effect on human life.

Of course, intellectual filiation is not as simple as that. One does not begin with selecting an authority to follow (at least, I don't) and then model one's project on the example of that authority. The project, rather, forms in one's mind, inspired by whatever else is going on there (for instance, one's other projects, or thinking about other, non- work-related events in one's life), and then spontaneously connects to the examples of similar projects stored in one's memory, which, from that moment on, become an important point of reference. But, in my case, Durkheim's presence, nevertheless, may be said to be over-determined, because it is from him that I have borrowed—some twenty-five years ago already—my central explanatory concept: anomie. A condition of structural inconsistency, that is, a systemic inconsistency among collective representations, anomie directly affects individual experience, creating profound psychological discomfort. This discomfort motivates participants in a given social situation to resolve the bothersome inconsistency. Therefore, the concept encompasses the most generally applicable theory of social change, a theory, moreover, which is the only one to lend itself easily to the probe by empirical evidence, because it points to the (psychological) mechanisms that connect the cause and effect in any particular case. Anomie was central in my explanation of the emergence of nationalism in *Nationalism*, and it was the pervasive anomie in American society in particular, which became starkly evident to me in the course of the examination of the American economy for *The Spirit of Capitalism,* which first made me think about its psychological implications.

The Empirical Focus

Clearly, even without Durkheim's *Suicide,* today in America there would be plenty of excellent reasons to focus on schizophrenia and manic-depressive illness. It was the ubiquity of depression among very young Americans (among whom I spent most of my time as a mother and a college teacher) that originally sensitized me to this kind of mental illness, making it a personal problem. As an adolescent in the Soviet Union and during my university studies in Israel (two countries obviously beset with most serious objective problems of individual and/or collective survival), I had never encountered such widespread hopelessness and unhappiness in this segment of the population, which, surely, of all others, could be expected to be most hopeful and happy. Young Americans' familiarity with depression was striking. Once, in class, comparing modern society to the feudal one, I tried to make my students—about forty bright undergraduates—imagine what it was like to live in near-constant physical pain. That was, in fact, the condition of vast numbers of people in medieval Europe.[11] There were no over-the-counter painkillers to treat a common headache or, worse, a toothache, no anesthesia during surgery or (which was plainly inconceivable) delivery. But broken bones were an everyday occurrence, limbs were routinely sawed off, kidney stones were not unknown, women hardly enjoyed any respite between pregnancies, and teeth would hurt before rotting completely and falling out when one approached the ripe old age of forty. For Americans of college age in the past ten or fifteen years, the idea of a toothache evidently has become as foreign as that of an amputation with nothing but a ball of cloth between the teeth for relief. I did not know that; and my students' reaction to the descriptions of their ancestors' experiences caught me by surprise. Instead of sympathizing with the unfortunate sufferers, they suggested that physical pain must have been much less painful in the Middle Ages than it is now (in the rare cases in which they were willing to admit it exists), because, they said, first, medieval humans must have become accustomed to it since it was so common, and, second, surely they would have invented something against it if it were really bad. Faced with the problem of making that optimistic crowd recognize the possibility of unbearable suffering, which does not kill fast enough and therefore must be born, and to alleviate which, short of killing oneself, one can do nothing, I asked them a question: "Who of you has ever gone through, or has seen someone close to you go through, a depression that required treatment?" Their bright faces darkened, eyes turned thoughtful and sad, and each one of them raised a hand. After that, they found it easy to imagine how it feels to have a toothache for days and maybe even what it is like to have one's leg sawed off without anesthesia.

The problem of depression, thus, was unquestionably an American problem—a problem of a particular society. My impressionistic conclusion that this was a colossal social problem affecting fearsomely large numbers of people was constantly confirmed by statistics, for mental disease, I discovered, was a favorite subject of calculation. Suffice it to adduce the two most recent examples that came to my attention. One is the already mentioned review, " The Epidemic of Mental Illness: Why?" in the *New York Review of Books* of June 23, 2011. It starts:

> It seems that Americans are in the midst of a raging epidemic of mental illness . . . The tally of those who are so disabled by mental disorders that they qualify for Supplemental Security Income (SSI) or Social Security Disability Insurance (SSDI) increased nearly two and a half times between 1987 and 2007—from one in 184 Americans to one in seventy-six. For children, the rise is even more startling—a thirty-five-fold increase in the same two decades. Mental illness is now the leading cause of disability in children, well ahead of physical disabilities like cerebral palsy or Down syndrome . . .

The review then asks some questions to which we will later return:

> What is going on here? Is the prevalence of mental illness really that high and still climbing? Particularly if these disorders are biologically determined and not a result of environmental influences, is it plausible to sup-

pose that such an increase is real? Or are we learning to recognize and diagnose mental disorders that were always there? On the other hand, are we simply expanding the criteria for mental illness so that nearly everyone has one? And what about the drugs that are now the mainstay of treatment? Do they work? If they do, shouldn't we expect the prevalence of mental illness to be declining, not rising?[12]

The second example of the recent confirmations of the extent of the problem is a three-part series of articles, "Students in Crisis," published in my campus newspaper, *BU Today,* that April. It also does not mince words, declaring: "Depression and anxiety on college campuses have risen to epidemic proportions. . . . the alarming trend . . . is supported by numerous studies, including a February 2010 Healthy Minds Study finding that 20 percent of BU students surveyed fit the criteria for anxiety or depression."[13]

Agreements and Disagreements on the Subject

There is no question for me that "the prevalence of mental illness [is] really that high and still climbing," and that it is high time to stop it. But then my argument is that some, the most severe, in fact, of these disorders are not "biologically determined" and are indeed "a result of environmental influences," specifically influences of a particular culture and image of reality implied in it. For those who believe that mental disease is essentially a reflection of physical, biological disorder, such declarations—and the consistent statistical findings on which they are based—remain questionable, because what they logically imply (an ongoing and environmentally unprovoked change of the physical human nature itself) is impossible and, therefore, cannot be true. What this means is that the persistence of the belief in the biological causation of all mental disease prevents serious (i.e., among other things, massively funded) consideration of alternative, nonbiological explanations of mental illnesses, and makes impossible both their cure and formation of policies that could arrest the rise in their rates. We could continue debating whether the increase in their prevalence, which the statistics report, is "real" or not until the end of time. I can disclose to my readers already at this point that this has certainly been debated—in the very same terms—since at least the beginning of the nineteenth century, and no conclusion has been arrived at thus far.[14]

The unquestioned (and, like all deeply held beliefs, unquestionable!) assumption of the biological nature of all mental diseases has been an obstacle to the understanding of the most disabling of them—schizophrenia and manic-depressive illness. Statements of leading experts (psychologists, psychiatrists, and neuroscientists) suggest that these particular diseases are no better understood today than they were two centuries ago, when psychiatry was born, despite the enormous accumulation of every kind of biological knowledge about them. To quote just one, but very weighty and representative authority, Norman Sartorius, the former president of the World Psychiatric Association, former director of the World Health Organization's Division of Mental Health, and retired professor of psychiatry at the University of Geneva, he said in 2007: "Despite advances in our knowledge about schizophrenia . . . nothing allows us to surmise that the causes of schizophrenia will soon become known."[15]

It may be argued that the biological bias in mental illness conceptualization and research cannot alone be held responsible for this unsatisfactory state of art, since the biological position was not the only position to enjoy a wide popularity for long periods of time. Indeed, since its earliest days the psychiatric establishment in the United States (as well as everywhere else) has been split between two approaches to insanity specifically, or, as an anthropologist put it in a 2000 monograph, has been "of two minds" in regard to its "big three"—schizophrenia, bipolar disorder, and major depression.[16] The specific contents of these approaches have changed many times in the course of the last two centuries, but in their general outlines and philosophy they remained the same—"biological" vs. psychodynamic. The "biological" approach could be summed up in the claim that psychiatric diseases are fundamentally diseases of the brain, while the psychodynamic approach, seemingly much less committed as to the ultimate cause of the complaint and focused on habit and behavior, has rather inclined to seek it in the constitution of the individual personality. The best-known example of the psychodynamic approach was Freudian psychoanalysis, extremely influential in American psychiatry in the half century between 1930 and 1980, and still important as therapy, in particular of milder forms of mental illness. But the actual difference between the two approaches has been that in the degree to which their assumption of the biological causality was explicit, and not in the presence of this assumption versus its absence: Freudian psychoanalysis, after all, also presumed that instincts and tendencies that were repressed and/or underdeveloped were "natural," i.e., reflected the universal, biological constitution of the human organism. For sociological reasons—that is, reasons pertaining to the social circumstances of the lives of psychiatrists—the explicitly biological approach in our scientific age (in which the psychiatric establishment was born) was assured overall dominance. With the body as its subject, medicine was a scientific profession to begin with. Subscription to the principles of science was the most direct road to prestige and authority for its first specialization even before Darwin's evolutionary theory divided the educated public into two camps: the majority (Bolsheviks, so to speak) who interpreted the theory to mean that only empirical demonstration justified belief, and the minority (Mensheviks), perceived by the majority as reactionary and obscurantist, who persisted in believing without the slightest empirical support that there was more to empirical reality than met the eye.[17] After the publication of Darwin's great book, the prestige of science (biology, in particular) skyrocketed: one could not question the biological paradigm and remain in a medical field.[18]

In Germany, a concerted effort began to improve the scientific credentials of psychiatry. Around the turn of the twentieth century, mental diseases remaining within the jurisdiction of the profession (after epilepsy, paresis, and, to a large extent, puerperal insanity were removed from it into the respective care of neurological, infectious diseases, and gynecological specializations) were minutely classified, named, and described in preparation for analysis. German-language psychiatry rose to a position of undisputed leadership in the international community of experts. The division of major psychoses of unknown etiology, or insanity, into the broad classes of schizophrenia and manic-depressive illness dates to that time and, though certain subcategories were added to it in the course of the twentieth century, still forms the framework for the understanding of these diseases.[19]

The contributions of German-language psychiatrists continued to be particularly prominent throughout the first four decades of the twentieth century. Since then the world center of psychiatric research has been in the

United States. The ready availability of government support with the foundation of NIMH significantly strengthened the explicitly biological position in this country. After the discovery—however accidental—of anti-depressant, mood-stabilizing, and antipsychotic drugs, effective in some cases of schizophrenia and/or manic-depressive illness, first in the 1950s and then in the 1980s, the powerful interests of large pharmaceutical companies also lined behind it. In the past thirty years or so, the explicitly biological approach has ruled virtually uncontested.[20]

Remarkably, though the literature on schizophrenia and manic-depressive illness, already voluminous, in the past quarter century has been increasing at an ever accelerating pace, now informed by new kinds of research that were inconceivable several decades ago, the psychiatric understanding has remained very close to the one achieved before World War II—a fact widely recognized by members of the research community. Virtually no new interpretations have been proposed in the period that elapsed since the 1940s, the neurobiological revolution that has been occurring during the recent decades being, in psychiatry, but a revolution in its traditional sense—i.e., it put an end to the prevalence of psycho-analysis and brought about a revival of the explicitly biological paradigm which had reigned in the beginning of the twentieth century. By World War II, however, early twentieth-century psychiatry, as is generally acknowledged, had reached an impasse: no existing interpretation was able to take into account all the aspects of schizophrenia and/or manic-depressive illness and the partial theories, beyond leaving much unaccounted for, as a rule contradicted the evidence they left out of its purview. As a result, no cure was found for either of the two diseases, patients languishing in ever-increasing numbers of hospitals ever growing larger and often dying there.[21]

With the introduction of lithium, especially, as well as of some effective antipsychotics, the containment of most immediately dangerous expressions of schizophrenia and manic-depression became feasible out of the hospitals. This pharmacological development combining with the reformist spirit of the 1960s led to a major reorganization of the services to mentally ill in this country. The inpatient population in the United States today is relatively small and nobody for a long time already would see in it a gauge of the total number of severely affected individuals. The reorganization of mental health services, however, reflected a change in the attitude towards, not an advance in the understanding of, the two mental diseases: there is still no cure for schizophrenia and manic-depressive illness. Some symptoms may be contained, but no one, once affected, can be declared schizophrenia- or manic-depression-free, the affliction is chronic and recurrent. A flare-up with its worst consequences is always possible, and families who are now responsible for the care of their mentally ill members must always be on the alert. Thus, the costs of this disease category, economic, social, and personal, would have probably grown with deinstitutionalization even if the rates of prevalence remained stable.

Today we know an awful lot about schizophrenia and manic-depressive illness. An enormous amount of information has been collected about the psychological and biological expressions of these diseases—about the personal experience and outward behaviors corresponding to them, the anatomical abnormalities which show themselves in certain groups of patients and neurochemical dynamics characteristic of others; about patterns of their transmission in families and certain genetic elements involved. But this information refuses to combine into a "case"—an explanatory argument based on the available evidence: there are gaping lacunae where pieces of the puzzle are supposed to dovetail; and none of the things we know can be said to constitute the smoking gun. We still do not know what causes these diseases and thus can neither understand their nature nor cure them. After two-hundred years neither of the two approaches—the biological and the psychodynamic—in which psychiatry put its hopes brought these understanding and cure any closer. Therefore, I feel justified to offer a new—radically different—approach that has never been tried.

The historical recency, the timing of the spread in different societies, and the increase in the rates, of mental disease of unknown etiology indicates that it cannot be understood in terms of any universal, biological or psychological, propensity of human nature, or explained by the characteristics of the individual human organism or personality as such. The observable trends (however incredible) pertain to and distinguish between specific societies and historical periods, and therefore must be accounted for historically. However, before proceeding any further, I must add a caveat. My intention is not to prove either the biological or the psychodynamic approach to mental disease wrong, but to complement them, adding to psychiatry a necessary element that has been heretofore missing. All the findings of the biological research, specifically, should be consistent with the approach I propose and, in cases they are not, the fault would lie with the approach rather than the findings. Culture, personality, and biology are different but not mutually exclusive realities, and for this reason cultural, psychological, and biological arguments should not be mutually exclusive. It is obvious that every human individual is affected by the surrounding culture at least to some extent, and every effect on the individual must be experienced through the body. To the extent that neurotransmitters or blood flow participate in any experience of any cultural effect, such effect must be reflected in neurotransmitters or blood flow. To the extent that neurotransmitters and blood flow are genetically regulated, genes allowing for such reflection must be present in order for the cultural effect to occur. The approach I propose should not be inconsistent with psychodynamic approaches as well, though because the latter are often purely speculative, it may be in disagreement with particular variants.

A position with which I do disagree, though deriving from the very same biologistic persuasion, combined with the same evidence, ironically, is the one prevailing among Western social scientists—anthropologists, sociologists, and historians studying psychiatry—who conclude that madness is a largely invented problem, a modern "discursive artifact" for the description of extravagant and deviant behaviors, strictly analogous to the equally false "social constructions" of witchcraft and possession of other cultures, but dressed in a scientific garb and unjustifiably enjoying the authority of science in ours. Underneath this view also lies the presupposition that human nature is the same everywhere, and that if mental disease does not exist (at all or at a certain rate of prevalence) in any one society, neither can it exist at the given rate in any other. Of course, the biological reality of madness has been proven by neuropsychiatry beyond any doubt. And whatever happens in other societies, severe, debilitating mental disease, which causes tremendous suffering to its victims and their families, is common in ours. In fact, one does not need statistics to know this. Any parent who pays attention to what happens in our high schools, in which depression is an epidemic, and any college professor who actually takes the time to get acquainted with one's students, is aware of and overwhelmed by it. When an eminent statistician declares "mental illness is the chronic disorder of young people in our nation," this does not come to such a parent or professor as a surprise, nor does the parallel drawn by a famous psychiatrist between insanity in the Western world and the plague appear much of an exaggeration.[22]

My particular point of contention with such social scientists is historical. The incontrovertible historical evidence of the recency of the diseases that came to be known as schizophrenia and manic-depressive illness in general and their being more recent in some societies than in others are just some of the facts in which these specialists, focusing specifically on the historical and cultural context of psychiatry and mental illness appear to be peculiarly uninterested. Mental diseases, obviously, have existed since time immemorial and have been recognized, and named, as such since ancient times and in all cultures. The brain is a part of the body and, insofar as they affect the brain, numerous physical conditions have been known to produce mental symptoms. In the Western world a rich vocabulary for mental disorders originated in the medical literature of ancient Greece and was used by physicians throughout the Middle Ages. Weak-mindedness, or idiocy, and geriatric dementia are also historically universal conditions. "Madness," however, was not a part of this vocabulary and did not refer to such conditions. It was a new word, coming into use in sixteenth-century England and indicating that something was abnormal in the old, familiar experience of mental abnormalities.

Many of the signs of madness were similar to the symptoms of familiar mental abnormalities. In particular, both madness and some previously known organic conditions would express themselves in behaviors with abnormal affect—extreme excitement and paralyzing sadness, respectively referred to (in original Hippocratic parlance) as mania and melancholia. But the difference was that in organic disorders these symptoms were temporary. They ended with the underlying organic ailment itself either in a return to normal mental functioning or in death. Madness, in distinction, appeared to be an existential, permanent condition, and its symptoms, once manifested, were chronic. It must have been this existential character of madness which distinguished it so sharply from the known, accidental, forms of mental affliction, in the eyes of the first generations that had experienced it, as to require a neologism. But there were other differences as well.

The first victims and/or observers of the new phenomenon were not necessarily medics, the new form of suffering being so different from the familiar forms of bodily suffering. The thinking of the age was not as decidedly monistic in regard to the perceived dual aspects of reality, as is ours, and treated the spirit with at least as much respect as the matter. Thus first attempts to interpret it were as often informed by astrology or theology as by medicine, another new word, which emerged as a synonym of "madness," indeed being "lunacy." It took close to two centuries for the scientific tenor to prevail over the other voices and for madness to be assimilated to earlier, organic, forms of mental disease and appropriated by medicine as a problem obviously belonging within its jurisdiction. Contrary to a common assumption in the history of psychiatry and related academic areas that the phenomenon of madness is as old as history, preceding by centuries the medicalization of mental dysfunction, which ostensibly took place with the emergence of modern psychiatry, in fact, mental disorder has been a legitimate (if not exclusive) province of medical expertise since time immemorial, and it is madness that is new.

A cursory analysis of the sixteenth- and seventeenth-century descriptions of madness reveals that what we today consider the two (or three) discrete diseases of major depression, bipolar disorder, and schizophrenia was experienced and perceived as forms or expressions of the same condition, which modern psychiatrists would call "psychosis." These forms were distinguished by the affect that accompanied it and by whether it was restricted to specific spheres of life or was all-pervading. In terms of affect, madness was clearly regarded as a bipolar disorder, though the manic state was much more rare than the depressive one. The psychosis of both mania and depression could be focused on a particular subject, or diffuse and attaching to everything in the patient's experience. The all-pervasive form of madness (which we would term "schizophrenia") was the worst form of all and indicated the point of no return. The focused psychotic attitude to the boundaries between the bodily self and the outside and, specifically, to food (today's anorexia) was frequently present with any of the other expressions of the condition.

The essence of the disorder, which the word "madness" referred to, was its delusionary quality. "Delusion" is usually defined as the inability to distinguish between fact and fiction, truth and untruth, or reason and unreason. I propose to define it instead as the inability to distinguish between information originating outside the mind and information generated by the mind (or inside the brain). For it must be remembered that human reality is a culturally constructed reality: what we experience, i.e., what is empirical for us, in the vast majority of cases, is symbolic, meaningful, even if material, and most of what we experience is not material to begin with. Social *facts* (as Durkheim pointed out a century ago) differ from one's fantasies only in that they face the individual from the outside. A widely held idea (say, that hell awaits those who eat flesh on Fridays, or that all men are created equal) is no less a reality for people in the community holding the idea, than the Atlantic Ocean, and only at a great peril can be crossed (out) as fiction. Therefore, however unreasonable or untrue certain statements may sound to the materialistic Western ear, they may be perfectly factual in the experiential actuality of another time or place. This approach to the diagnostically necessary concept of "delusion" extricates it from the logical difficulties it encounters when defined as the inability to distinguish "truth" from "untruth" or "reason" from "unreason," and from the irrelevant comparisons with experiences of bewitchment, possession, and religious ecstasy, which lead so many specialists (psychiatrists, and psychiatric anthropologists, historians, etc.) to diagnose entire cultures as psychotic, to retroactively pronounce medieval saints schizophrenics or, alternatively, to declare mental disease, as such, a myth.[23]

The delusion of the etiologically uncertain psychosis, whether focused or all-pervading, in particular disturbs the experience of self, confusing one regarding one's identity, making one dissatisfied with, and/or insecure in, it, splitting one's self in an inner conflict, and in most severe cases dissolving it altogether into the environment. Sixteenth-century English phrases such as "losing one's mind," "going out of one's mind," and "not being oneself" capture this disturbed experience at the same time as they construct a differentiated, dynamic concept of the self and the mind (who does the mind belong to, so that it can be lost? who is it going out of one's mind? what is one who is not oneself?). This experience expresses itself in out-of-control behaviors (namely, behaviors out of one's control, out of the control of the self), that is, in the impairment of the will in action and in speech and, as a result, in maladjustment and functional incapacitation.

The population of madmen and lunatics in sixteenth-century England was miniscule in comparison to the nation-within-a-nation existing today in these former English colonies, but it was visibly growing. This was also a new experience. The baseline rate of insanity was calculated at 1 person per 1,000 adults or 2,000 of the general population: this is, roughly, the number of people who would suffer from mental symptoms related to congenital defects, infectious disease or malnutrition, of women who would fall victim to puerperal insanity and of individuals who would go insane as a result of substance abuse—in short, all those affected by organic mental disease.[24] However reliable (or unreliable) this estimate is for Western societies before the age of madness, it still reflects rather accurately the mental health condition of many non-Western nations. It is a stable rate, one of those reminders of life's unfairness with which one learns to reconcile. In sixteenth-century England, very clearly, judging by the sources, insanity had already become far more common than one mentally ill person per 1,000 adults who were well and seemed to become increasingly noticeable every decade.

At any rate, it was noticed by Englishmen first, then—since the seventeenth century—also by foreigners. For at least two hundred and fifty years, madness appeared to affect only England and the British dominions, and was, judging by all accounts, entirely absent from the European Continent. By late seventeenth century, indeed, it acquired the reputation, and by mid-eighteenth century, the name of "the English malady."[25] It was a national characteristic. Since this was precisely the period of the country's spectacular rise to European (and then world) supremacy, England was closely watched and imitated by its neighbors, in particular by France, which saw its own position of influence threatened. From mid-seventeenth century on, following the Puritan Rebellion, English ways of thinking were imported into France and English institutions copied. The 1656 transformation of the Bicêtre prison in Paris into a mental hospital was one case of such importation. But it is almost certain (that is, as certain as anything may be in history) that this happened not because madness arrived, but because it was misunderstood, in France. A whole century later, as we know from the correspondence of the philosophes, even the most acute of the pre-Revolutionary French thinkers still could not fathom, much less identify with, the peculiar English experience of mental disease. By early nineteenth century, this had already become possible. Yet, when we remember that psychiatry as a medical specialty was born in France (its birthday symbolized by Pinel's famous liberation of Bicêtre's inmates from their chains) in 1793, the reasons why this long-since international profession has been so unsuccessful in penetrating its subject become much clearer.[26]

What becomes absolutely clear is that Michel Foucault's theory of the social construction of madness, the main source of inspiration behind the literature to which I am referring here, could not possibly have any explanatory value. "Madness," a new word invented to capture a new experience, which the existing vocabulary failed to capture, was translated into French as "folie," an old word, an equivalent of "folly" in English, which referred to forms of mental disturbance known from before. It was, in other words, mistranslated to begin with, separated from its meaning because the experience it connoted did not exist in France at the time. When Foucault, himself a sufferer from severe depression, thus a "madman" in sixteenth-century English terminology, wrote his *Folie et déraison*, which was translated into English as *Madness and Civilization,* he wrote both about the new, functional and existential, form of mental disease and about the old, organic and accidental, ones, but the word "folie," used for both, blinded him to the fact. He was writing about two different—and, in fact, unconnected—subjects, while believing that he was dealing with one. His theory of "the great confinement" in the Age of Reason, undertaken in order to stigmatize deviance and exclude extravagantly behaving "fools" from the orderly bourgeois society, is based entirely on the assumption of equivalence between madness and older forms of mental disorder, which was favored by the French language. Proving this assumption unwarranted renders this theory null and void.[27]

Epistemological Foundations of the Argument

Resolving the Mind-Body Problem

But even the best-supported causal argument will not be persuasive if the translation of the cause into the effect (in this case of modern, nationalist, culture into biologically real mental disease) is logically inconceivable and the mechanisms of the causation cannot be imagined. Such translation is, however, logically inconceivable, given the current philosophical assumptions underlying much of the popular attitudes to scientific research. These assumptions are very old, predating science capable of progressive development (i.e., modern science) by over 2,000 years. The most important of these assumptions is that reality, which is presumed consistent, expresses itself in two fundamentally heterogeneous, mutually inconsistent ways, the material and the spiritual, or the physical and the psychical. In the past century and a half, these expressions of reality are often referred to as the "real" and the "ideal" (which, obviously, suggests that only what is material is real, while the spiritual is but a product of ideation and does not really exist; this, in fact, is the position of the great majority of people engaged in science and is likely shared by most of the population of modern societies). In relation specifically to humanity, this dual conception of reality takes the form of the mind/body vision.

This psychophysical, or mind/body, assumption has been at the root of the central philosophical problem in the Western tradition since the time of Plato, because no satisfactory solution could be found to the connection between the two heterogeneous expressions: both are a part of every human's experience and clearly influence each other in it, but it is impossible to account for this coexistence and influence either logically without contradicting this experience or, for that reason, empirically by showing how precisely one translates into the other. Depending on the intellectual fashions of the time, one or another monistic position would be accepted without debate, which would pose that only one of these expressions of reality was real in the sense of being causally active, the other being merely apparent or epiphenomenal, a secondary expression of the first one. The causally active factor was for a very long time believed to be the spiritual one—creative divine intelligence. But for the last three centuries or so, matter has held the position of the causal factor, and the spiritual element— human consciousness, mind, culture—was gradually reduced to the status of only apparent reality, an epiphenomenon.

Within this philosophical framework, my argument that culture (an ideational, symbolic, nonmaterial phenomenon) causes a biologically real (material) disease appears quite incredible. This lack of credibility is, in the first place, a function of the credit given today to the materialist interpretation of the psychophysical relationship. But the real problem lies not in one or another interpretation, but in the assumption of this relationship itself. In most areas of life and of science this philosophical assumption is of no importance—it may exist in the back of our minds but is very rarely, if ever, brought to the surface, and does not in any way interfere with our daily activities. In psychiatry and human neuroscience, however, it forms an impassable obstacle to the understanding of the very phenomena those engaged in these fields aim to understand, for there is no more logical possibility, in the framework of the dual mind/body view of reality, of translating material events occurring in the brain into the symbolic events of human consciousness, than in translating a symbolic cause into a material effect. So long as there remains the unresolved philosophical mind-body problem, no significant advance in human neuroscience and, therefore, psychiatry, would be possible. Any claim on a subject involving human consciousness, whether from a materialistic or idealistic perspective, and whether appearing credible or incredible, will remain purely speculative and of little relevance to real-life empirical problems. The first order of the business is, therefore, to escape the mind-body quagmire.

A number of preliminary, logically consecutive steps will help the reader to approach my central argument prepared to consider it on its own terms, without the fear that one is committing scientific heresy. The first chapter, "The Premises," demonstrates that it is neither logically nor empirically necessary to imagine reality as expressed in two fundamentally heterogeneous, mutually inconsistent ways. The recognition that this long influential image was a product of a particular historical time and place, thus arbitrary from the point of view of science, makes it easier to give up. Instead, I propose we regard reality, for heuristic purposes, as consisting of three autonomous but logically consistent layers, the physical layer of matter, the organic layer of life superadded to it, and the symbolic layer of culture and the mind superadded to the organic layer. This view is implied in Darwin's evolutionary theory and is to no small extent responsible for the spectacular development of biology in the past century-and-a-half. Because the advancement of biology before then was only marginally impeded by the psychophysical assumption, the layer view was never considered as a solution (in fact, elimination) of the mind-body problem. But Darwin did, in fact, transcend the old ontological view and made possible the one suggested here. The presuppositions of logical consistency with the underlying layer(s) and of autonomy make both upper layers of reality in the layer view what philosophers would call "emergent phenomena," irreducible to, but by definition existing within, the boundary conditions of the elements of the underlying reality out of which they have emerged.[28]

Both the organic and the symbolic emergent phenomena are essentially processes that occur in time rather than substances taking place in space (though to different events in the process may correspond specific constructions in space); therefore, they cannot be simply defined as material. No one would judge unreasonable the claim that organic processes are empirical phenomena that are a proper subject of science. Thus, there is nothing unreasonable in treating similarly symbolic processes such as human consciousness, or the mind, and culture.

Mind and Culture as an Emergent Empirical Phenomenon

The decision to consider human consciousness as an emergent phenomenon, logically consistent with the biological and physical laws but autonomous, logically leads to certain conclusions that are the subject of Chapter 2, "The Mind as an Emergent Phenomenon." I argue that, like life, the symbolic process occurs simultaneously on the collective and the individual levels, that is, as mind and as culture. The mind, therefore, can be seen as "culture in the brain" or "individualized culture," while culture is

3. The emergent layer of symbolic reality: culture and the mind

boundary conditions created by the organic layer of life

2. The emergent layer of organic reality: life

boundary conditions created by the physical layer of matter

1. The fundamental physical layer of reality: matter

The layered view of reality replacing the dualist conventional ontology and resolving the mind-body problem quite accurately imagined as "collective consciousness."[29] This makes both stages in the causal chain from culture to mind to a biologically real disease easily conceivable and no more shocking or mysterious than the translation of a visual perception of an environmental sign, for instance, light, by an animal into the physicochemical events in the animal's brain, even though, obviously, more complex.

Just like a species' habitat and the species itself for an organism, the symbolic process on the collective level, culture, represents the environment in which the mind (and, therefore, the brain which supports it) functions. This cultural environment shapes both the contents with which human mental processes operate and the essential "structures" (necessary processual configurations or functional systems) of the mind. These "structures" or functional systems are also necessarily supported by the brain, but they are made necessary by the special character of, and exigencies of adaptation to, the human, cultural, environment, and on the psychological level represent the different aspects of the self or "I." They are identity (relationally constituted self); will (the acting self or agency); and the thinking self or the "I of self-consciousness". Identity and will are closely related and work, as it were, in tandem, the relationally constituted self providing the scale of priorities and the acting self deciding on the course of action under different circumstances. These two mental structures are functional requirements for the individual's adaptation to the cultural environment. The thinking self, which under normal conditions is perfectly integrated into the individual mental process, in distinction, is a functional requirement for the perpetuation of the cultural process in general; therefore, it is functionally independent from the other two structures. It can function on its own. Culture calls into being and shapes the structures of the mind, but it never determines them, for the necessary participation of the brain in every mental process precludes the possibility of such determination and instead makes every individual mind a (more or less) junior partner in the self-creative cultural process.

Interpreting Schizophrenia and Manic-Depressive Illness

Schizophrenia and manic-depressive illness provide the crucial test for this underlying approach. If we are able to explain mental disease as a function of the mind, consciousness, affected by the open modern culture, then we have the green light for the scientific study of the nonmaterial reality of the mind, in general (making it as proper a subject for such study as gravity or evolution), and, with it, finally, for a real, cumulative, science of humanity. Accordingly, the two opening chapters, which spell out the philosophical assumptions behind the argument, are followed by a part that may be characterized as psychological. It probes the current state of the art and science of psychiatry insofar as the understanding of schizophrenia (Chapter 3) and manic-depressive illness (Chapter 4) is concerned, analyzing contributions of the various sectors of the mental health research community—clinicians, neurobiologists, geneticists, epidemiologists, and experimental psychologists—working on the subject. The view that the mind is a cultural phenomenon and that madness (schizophrenia, mania, depression) is a disease of the mind rather than the brain, permits the advancement of a comprehensive interpretation of the underlying psychological structure of the disease(s) in question—at present lacking in the field—which leaves out and contradicts nothing of what is known about the phenomenon.

The argument of this part is that the psychotic disease of this kind is fundamentally a malfunction of the "acting self" (the functional system or "structure" of will). It is experienced as a loss of the familiar self and as a loss of control over one's physical and mental activity. The three varieties of madness, distinguished today (unipolar depression, bipolar depression—that is, depression with mania, and schizophrenia) may, to begin with, be placed on a continuum of the complexity of the will-impairment experienced, from the loss of positive (motivating) control in action and content of thought in depression, through the loss of positive and negative (restraining) control in action and content of thought in manic-depression, to the complete alienation of the acting self, i.e., complete loss of cultural individualization and loss of positive and negative control in action and both content and structure of thought in schizophrenia. More complex forms of the disorder should not be equated with more severe ones: clearly, in terms of danger to life that it poses, depression must be considered the most severe of the functional psychoses. What further contributes to the complexity of such disorders and, in particular, is responsible for rendering the most complex of them, schizophrenia, so bizarre is the involvement of the third, autonomous mental structure: the thinking self. As long as only the content of thought escapes the control of the will, the thinking self remains to a certain extent integrated with the rest of the individual's mental process, i.e., it does the mind's thinking. The liberation of the thought structure from the control of the will indicates complete disintegration of the individual's mind and, leaving the thinking self (which serves the function of the cultural process in general and not of the individual) on its own, changes its function. It becomes the observing self, the "I" of (unbidden) self-consciousness. In observing the dissolution of the self as agency, and observing itself observing it, it uses the resources of culture in general, of culture not individualized for the purposes of the individual's adaptation. This explains not only the nature of schizophrenic delusions, but the strange hyper-reflexivity of schizophrenics, their intellectual hyperactivity and cerebral, detached approach to reality, incongruously combined with what appears as a loss of "higher intellectual functions" and of "ego-boundaries," for which current interpretations cannot account. It also explains the extraordinary linguistic creativity of many patients, their sensitivity to the semantic multivalence of words and propensity to neologisms, as well as their tendency to switch between contextual logics, which may appear and is often interpreted as the loss of ability to think logically. Having vast cultural resources as if free ranging in their brains and no mechanisms to rein them in and channel them into personally relevant directions, schizophrenics, in a way, have culture, always multiperspectival, think for them and language, always multivalent, speak for them. Thus it is possible to have full-blown schizophrenia without displaying any of the neurobiological abnormalities expected and in many (though never all) cases present with the disease.

This, at last, puts us in the position to tie the mental diseases in question directly to the cultural and historical phenomenon of nationalism, to which I devote the last three chapters of the book. The reason for the dysfunction of the acting self lies in the malformation of identity. It is possible that the complexity of the original identity problem (the depth and number of inconsistencies in the relationally constituted self) contributes to the complexity of the disease; for instance, in a case of dissatisfaction with one's nevertheless clearly experienced identity causing depression, and in a case of no clearly experienced identity, combined with numerous competing

possibilities, producing schizophrenia.[30] It is modern culture—specifically
the presumed equality of all the members of the society, secularism, and
choice in self-definition, implied in the national consciousness—that makes
the formation of the individual identity difficult. A member of a nation can
no longer learn who or what s/he is from the environment. Instead of pre-
scribing to us our identities, as do religious and in principle nonegalitarian
cultures, modern culture leaves us free to decide what to be and to make
ourselves. It is this cultural laxity that is anomie—the inability of a culture
to provide the individuals within it with consistent guidance (already in the
beginning of the twentieth century, recognized by Durkheim as the most
dangerous problem of modernity).[31] Paradoxically, in effect placed in control over our destiny, we are far more likely to be dissatisfied with it, than
would be a person deprived of any such control: not having a choice, such a
person would try to do the best with what one has and enjoy it as far as
possible. A truly believing person would also feel s/he has no right to find
fault with the order of things created by God, much less to try and change
it to one's own liking—one's situation in life would be perceived as both
unchangeable and just. Conversely, the presence of choice, the very ability
to imagine oneself in a position different from one currently occupied or
that of one's parents, and the idea that social orders in general are created
by people and may be changed make one suspect that one's current situation is not the best one can have and to strive for a better one. The more
choices one has, the less secure one becomes in the choices already made
(by one or for one) and making up one's mind—literally, in the sense of
constructing one's identity—grows increasingly difficult.

It is for this reason that the malformation of the mind—quite independent of any disease of the brain—becomes a mark of nations. The sooner a
society defines itself as a nation, the sooner diseases of the mind appear in
it, and the more dedicated it is to the ideals of equality and liberty, the
more perfectly the twin principles of nationalism are realized in social,
political, and economic institutions, the more widespread they can be
expected to be. Since, in addition to values (which encourage one to take
advantage of opportunities), one's choices are also affected by the practical
exigencies of the situation and are likely to be more numerous when the
nation is prosperous and secure than when it is poor and embattled, the
rates of such diseases would be greater in affluent and generally secure

societies. This reasoning fits perfectly the history of schizophrenia and manic-depressive illness from its inception in sixteenth-century England, and explains why they spread through Europe and North America in the order they did, and why Britain, who led the way for so long, ceded the palm of this dubious priority to the freer, more egalitarian, and more prosperous United States.[32] And as the same logic applies to groups within societies as to societies in their entirety, it also explains why in all these nations these diseases first and most gravely affect the strata whose possibilities of self-realization are least limited and whose members face the largest number of choices.

The theory I offer for your consideration combines philosophical, psychological, historical, and sociological arguments. The problem before us does not belong to any particular discipline and the project is, therefore, necessarily transdisciplinary. There are no transdisciplinary specialists: this would be a contradiction in terms (though there are, clearly, as there should be, transdisciplinary thinkers). This book is not written by a specialist or for specialists. I hope, of course, that the experts on whose separate fields of expertise it touches will find it of interest and read it. But I entertain the same hope in regard to everyone who is interested in the problem I discuss, experts or no experts, and it should interest very many. No specialist knowledge is needed to follow the discussion or to form one's own judgment about it. Throughout the book I try to provide the reader with everything needed for this. I attempt to define all my terms clearly and to formulate my propositions in a manner that makes it easy to perceive their logical implications and to contradict them if need be. Wherever I rely on specialist literature (in neurobiology, psychiatry, and psychology), the reader can double-check the accuracy of my knowledge and understanding. Most of the book does not rely on interpretations of other scholars. The historical discussion is based mainly on primary materials, and the ideas are original.

If I were to suggest a guiding principle for the reader, it would be the motto of the Enlightenment, *Sapere aude*, "dare to know."[33] It is astonishing how much depends on this one act of will. And also: enjoy. This book is neither short nor simple: its tremendously important and somber subject would not allow that. And yet, it was so exciting to write that I firmly believe some of this excitement, at least, will be communicated to the broad audience for whom it is intended and that some of its readers, at least, will find it enjoyable.

It may be apposite to conclude this introduction by stressing what is added to the specialist perspectives with which the subject of this book may be associated. To reiterate, this is a book of history, philosophy, psychology, and sociology. Its empirical focus—the severe mental disease(s) of schizophrenia and manic-depression—is a subject of psychiatry and neurobiology, and its argument, therefore, has significant implications for these two professions as well. But:

1. Though it necessarily touches on it, this is not a book in the history of psychiatry (or of medicine more generally) because its focus is not the healing profession's development and approaches to mental disease, but the disease itself.
2. For the same reason, this is not a book in the sociology of mental health, though, again, it necessarily touches upon social attitudes toward mental disease, the institutions within which it is treated or contained, and its distribution among different social groups.
3. Its contribution to psychology, philosophy of the mind, psychiatry, and neurobiology is contained in its central argument, viz.: that the mind and diseases of the mind are cultural phenomena, that the mind cannot be understood in isolation from culture, that, because the two are one and the same process on different levels, the mind transcends the individual by whose brain it is supported, and that, therefore, the focus on the individual alone (as in traditional philosophy of the mind, psychology, and psychiatry) or on the brain alone (as in neurobiology and philosophy of the mind in recent years) narrows the attention to but a small and not the most important element of the mind.

It should be evident from the nature of the arguments exposed here that I do not believe that any individual can be considered the sole author of one's own ideas. The mind is individualized *culture*. It is always culture that is the true innovator and discoverer, the true author of anything worthy. The individual is privileged to be invited as a junior coauthor, when culture is ready for a breakthrough. Very often, an appearance of an idea that strikes everyone as obvious after it appears is delayed precisely because culture is not ready before. My arguments, therefore, necessarily build upon the contribution of generations of thinkers (in addition to the three great human scientists I mentioned in the beginning of this Introduction and Charles Darwin), and yet do not derive from the thought of any particular past (or present) authority.

Why some individuals are privileged to participate in culture's movement forward while others are not probably depends on the cultural resources that one appropriates in the course of one's experience: the mind, after all, is *individualized* culture. I am sure I would not have the opportunity to author this book had I not been brought up in Russia in the family of two hereditary physicians, one of whom was a frustrated historian and the other, a frustrated physicist, and encouraged to follow my parents' passions rather than their profession; had I not been brought up in admiration of Western Europe, particularly France and England, which made me, from very early on, feel at home in a number of worlds in which I never physically lived; had sociology not have had, in the Soviet Union, the taste of forbidden knowledge, which determined my decision to study it in Israel; had my Israeli teachers not been European immigrants and their sociology so informed by history, in its turn so philosophical and so psychological; and, finally, had I not then arrived in the United States to be struck by its extraordinary openness and pluralism, astonished by the multiplicity of possibilities it offered, and shocked by the normality of depression in it, so common that it was considered natural in teenagers.

Having been so privileged, the individual, as such, contributes little to the work culture does in him or her. The mind must reach the conclusions contained in the premises and give them expression, that is all. Of course, sometimes the individual comes uninvited, forcing oneself on culture that can never yield what is not in it, or fails to draw the conclusions from the premises, and contributes nothing. This is a frightening thought and I hope, naturally, that such is not my case.

I

PHILOSOPHICAL

1

Premises

Let us begin with a little experiment: consider your daily experiences from the moment you wake up to the time you are falling asleep at night.

Give yourself two minutes.

What are these experiences? What do they consist of and where do they happen?

Remember: you hear the alarm. The first thing you feel is, perhaps, irritation: "Oh, gosh, it's time to get up again," you say to yourself. Or, perhaps, your first experience of the day is joy: you say, "Aha, another day—so many wonderful things will happen!" and imagine these wonderful things. You get out of bed, your cat rubs against you, you say to the cat, "Hello, gorgeous," and think, "Oh, darling, darling kitty! Isn't it a privilege to share one's life with such creatures!" Or, perhaps, not; perhaps you feel that old pain in your back and think, "One day I'll have to get this thing checked." The whiff of coffee reminds you of that day, long ago, in your grandmother's kitchen, and its smells, the touch of your grandmother's hand, the feel of that kitchen flood you for a moment, but you switch on the radio and hear a favorite melody; its sounds bring with them different images and replace your grandmother. You brush your teeth, notice their perfect whiteness, congratulate yourself on choosing a great cosmetic dentist and spend a moment smiling at your own reflection in the mirror. Your mood changes when the morning news reports on another turn in the presidential campaign and you express your disgust in a manner that causes your cat to raise its tail and walk out of the room. Or something else. Your feelings prompt your thoughts, these thoughts provoke other feelings, and so it goes until, fourteen hours later (or eighteen hours later, if you are twenty) you close your eyes, and thoughts, feelings, and images become blurred and transform, and whirl wearily, and you lose consciousness of yourself.

All these experiences are mental. Even if they have a physical aspect to them, they are mental, and most of them lack physical aspects: sounds you hear are mostly noiseless, sights that present themselves clearly to your "inner eye" occur irrespectively of what you are looking at. An overwhelming majority of these experiences are also symbolic: they are thoughts and emotions that involve words and images. They happen in our heads; they are experiences of the mind.

The sum of these daily experiences is our Experience with the capital *E:* it is the only direct knowledge we have of reality; it is, in fact, what reality *is* for us, for whatever it is for subjects of other kinds—for gods or dogs or trees—for human beings reality is only that which we know of it directly, by experience, while everything else we believe we know we extrapolate from it and is a matter of interpretation. In other words, we have no empirical proof of anything else, because "empirical," from the Greek *empeiria* ("experience"), means "experience."[1]

You have just demonstrated that we have abundant empirical evidence for the existence of the mind.

Most languages do not have a word for "mind;" they refer to it as "soul" or "spirit" (*psyche* in Greek; *anima* and *spiritus* in Latin; *âme* and *esprit* in French, *Seele* and *Geist* in German, *dusha* and *dukh* in Russian, etc.). In English, these words ("mind," "soul," and "spirit") are synonyms; they emphasize different aspects of the phenomenon, but denote the same referent. For instance, the proper vernacular rendition in English of the famous "psycho-physical" problem is the "mind-body" problem.[2]

You have just demonstrated the empirical reality of the soul.

The goal of this project is to offer a scientific analysis of this empirical reality.

But everyone, scientists foremost, would tell you that this is impossible. Everyone knows that the problems of the soul are eternal and insoluble. Science, however, is the art of the soluble, ergo the soul (or call it the mind) is not a scientific subject. Scientific subjects, after all, must be objective and material. And the mind (the soul)—as you have just established—is neither. Let us examine these claims.

Science is the only epistemological system that has consistently led to humanity's greater understanding, and control, of certain aspects of empirical reality. It is the only known way to objective, universally valid, knowledge and has been generating it since the seventeenth century. In the sense that it systematically increases the amount and depth of such knowledge, it is progressive. It is the only intellectual endeavor that may be said to progress. Why has it not led to the increased understanding of, and never even attempted to analyze, the soul (or "mind" in English)? To answer this, we must first dispel several misconceptions about science.

Modern science (namely science since the seventeenth century) is based on the premise that empirical knowledge, experience, offers far more reliable access to the understanding, and ultimately control, of reality than belief, or dogma. Science is only interested in the understanding of empirical, i.e., experiential, reality (what may be experienced). As a social institution—which is one useful way of imagining it—it represents a patterned activity oriented to the understanding of empirical reality and achieving this understanding by the method of conjectures and refutations—specifically, logical formulation of hypotheses, followed by a methodical attempt to refute them with the help of empirical evidence.[3] Logic and direct knowledge, experience, are its twin pillars. As a matter of principle, science suspects the authority of secondary interpretations and eschews belief.

Yet, science (as an organized, collective enterprise) is not consistent in its self-understanding. This has led to remarkable contradictions in the assumptions and orientation of scientific research in the past two centuries. For example, the obvious reason for the lack of any attempt of an empirical, scientific study of the mind—what we are going to attempt here—is the attitude of scientific skepticism (the wariness of belief, characteristic of science). The belief in the reality of the soul has been for millennia one of the core and most powerful religious beliefs. The close association of the soul with religion naturally renders the soul suspicious for science. What is less obvious is that, despite the plentiful and, as you noticed in the course of our little experiment, easily available empirical evidence of the soul's (mind's) existence, science has transformed its suspicion by association into a belief (dogma) and, in the face of this plentiful empirical evidence to the contrary, assumed that the soul does not exist, that it is not an empirical reality.

This glaring contradiction in the attitude of science of the past two centuries towards the mind points to the overall importance of belief in the practice of science, which opposes reliance on belief in principle. In practice, science, taking its normative orientations (its principles) at face value, and leaving its reliance on beliefs concealed, often substitutes these beliefs for empirical evidence, assuming that what a scientist believes is actually what he or she experiences. Some of the beliefs of science are fundamental—that is, irreducible to evidence and unjustifiable logically, but essential for human survival; it is important to be aware of the purely dogmatic quality of fundamental beliefs. In addition, some beliefs are necessary in the sense that science would be impossible without them. It is important to remember this dependence. Other beliefs are unnecessary: they do not enable scientific activity and, in fact, hamper it in many cases. It is important to be able to distinguish between these types of belief and question the unnecessary ones.

Recollect our little experiment. Our reality, what we experience, is, by definition, empirical, but, as you have just empirically proven, it is also mental, that is, subjective. We are enclosed in the subjectivity of our mental experience; there is no possibility to transcend it. That such a possibility does not exist empirically is obvious, but it also does not exist logically, and only our ability to live perfectly contented with gross logical contradictions saves us (every single one of us) from being paralyzed by the reasonableness of solipsism—the proposition that reality is the product of my imagination, and that I am all there is.[4] There is no way of proving this claim wrong, and this puts us in a difficult position in regard to all other claims. If I cannot be certain—logically and empirically—that I am actually holding a computer on my lap, that there is such a thing as my lap, which is independent from my mental experience of it as such, or as a computer, independent from my imagination, and that I am typing these words on it, how can I be certain of the material—or, alternatively, God-given, essentially spiritual—nature of reality, of the evolution of *Homo sapiens* from other animal species—or of the creation of man on the sixth day of

Creation; of the neurons firing in my brain when my husband comes from work in exactly the same pattern they fire, apparently, in the brain of a romantically inclined male rat—or of that I rejoice at seeing my husband because I see relations between men and women in terms of Shakespeare's *Romeo and Juliet*?

Yet, science—together with all of us in the lay population—holds the irrefutable solipsistic proposition irrelevant and firmly believes in the objective world around us, in the construction of which our imagination plays no role. It is utterly dependent on this belief, as we all are. This fundamental belief in the objective world is necessary: if we did not believe in it, we would die.

In addition to the rest of humanity, science is also dependent on the belief that this objective world is consistently ordered; after all, it is this order that science seeks to uncover. But, while science is dependent on it, this belief in the consistent order in the universe (unlike the belief in the objective reality) is not fundamental. It is reducible to certain experiences and certain type of empirical—historical—evidence: meaning that there are societies in which people do not believe in it, but, rather, assume chaos as the condition of reality. Such, clearly, were the polytheistic societies, which, to boot, instead of imagining the objective world as a *universe,* that is, as one entity, saw it as a conflicted multitude regulated by warring egocentric gods. It was monotheism that united this chaotic multitude under one timeless order. The conception of the objective world as an ordered universe is a necessary belief for science. It is based on this religious conception.[5]

Science would be impossible without monotheism for more than one reason. Not only do we owe this grand, originally Jewish, religious philosophy the idea of the ordered universe, but we also owe it that pillar of science—(Aristotelian) logic based on the principle of non-contradiction. This principle is inconceivable in a polytheistic reality, which presupposes no unifying order, and this—and only this—explains why the famous transition from *mythos* to *logos* in ancient Greece, which, we are told, signaled the birth of philosophy as such,[6] began, was first conceived of, when exiled Jews in Babylon combined the texts of the Old Testament in the first redaction of the Hebrew Bible in the early sixth century BC. An alternative to the polytheistic chaos emerged, and a sixth-century Miletian, Thales, figured out that this alternative view implied the principle of no contradiction—an unchanging organizing principle, which, in turn, implied a standard applicable to all statements about this ordered universe. This provided a dimension along which arguments—if they were about the ordered universe—could be placed, related, and compared, and made them rationally arguable. No longer were means to decide arguments limited to the use of physical or emotional force, blackmail, and intimidation. Opponents could be brought over to one side of their own accord, by willing obedience to that remarkable rule.[7]

People who do not distinguish between Greek (ancient) and modern science consider Thales the first scientist. They do so with good reason. Only logic based on the principle of non-contradiction, formalized by Aristotle a century and a half later, makes it possible to formulate hypotheses so that they can be tested—contradicted—by evidence. Logic is a result of a historical accident, the rise to dominance of one, peculiar, system of beliefs among others, but science would be impossible had this accident not occurred.

INTERIM CONCLUSION 1: All scientific propositions, therefore, have a good share of belief in them; it is these beliefs, which they presuppose, that give them meaning in the first place, not direct, empirical, knowledge of reality. Science is, therefore, as dogmatic as any other system of beliefs: there are certain beliefs that it simply cannot give up. The difference between science and Judaism or Christianity, for example, lies mainly in that, while Judaism and Christianity proudly assert their dogmatism and say "Amen" ("Believe!" in Hebrew), science denies it.

The dependence of science on logic and the conception of reality that implies logic, paradoxically, make science more dogmatic than any monotheistic religion. Monotheistic religion, proud of its faith, seeks no justification of it. It is not bothered by the lack of correspondence between belief and reality, and therefore accepts reality as it is; it does not deny experience. Because faith is free and is a matter of individual responsibility, a true believer is aware that his or her faith is one among others and is not bothered by the existence of those whose faith is different: he or she knows that they are wrong. Not so in science. Many (if not all) scientists believe absolutely, though for the most part implicitly, that the ordered universe is what there is—that it *is* the empirical and objective reality. They do not consider it one conception—belief—among others or even raise the possibility that this might be so.[8] Thus, they believe absolutely that empirical reality, which, as all of us, they must consider objective, is actually based on the principle of non-contradiction, that it is actually a logical reality. They equate the logical, the objective, and the empirical—and deny the reality, the empirical character, of experiences that are not objective and not logical. Science, therefore, only accepts reality to the extent reality accords with its beliefs. It denies much of reality as it is.

All of human reality, as you have established, whatever else it may be, is the reality of the mind. We cannot transcend the mentality of what we experience. What is literally empirical for us is, therefore, necessarily subjective. Scientists are human. How can science deny the reality of the empirical and yet use empirical evidence for the testing of its propositions? The short answer is: it cannot. The claim that scientific evidence is empirical evidence is yet another misconception about science (that is, a belief about it, held by most scientists, which is unsupported by empirical evidence). As a rule, the evidence on which scientific propositions rely is not empirical.

None of the scientific propositions I mentioned before in connection with the solipsistic hypothesis have been proven empirically—neither the one regarding the material nature of the objective world, nor the one about the evolution of *Homo sapiens* from other species of animals, nor that pertaining to the firing pattern of neurons in my brain resembling that of a romantic male rat. They could not have been empirically proven, because I (and any of you) have never experienced, and could not have experienced these *interpretations:* causality, some sort of which all of them imply, does not belong to the sort of things that can be experienced, and, while it can be derived from experience, none of us has had the experience—that is, direct knowledge—of the pattern in which our neurons fire or the creation of the universe and humanity.[9] To many of you these interpretations, of course, make more sense than others that I mentioned as alternatives. But for something to make sense there must be someone to whom it would be made: interpreting my feelings for my husband as a product of the idea of love introduced by Shakespeare makes much more sense to me than interpreting them as a reflection of the similarity between me and a male rat, but, I am sure, my views on love would represent a minority position in any gathering of neuroscientists and even psychologists.

Additionally, these interpretations have the merit of logical consistency, the first two of them—though certainly not the third, as I hope to demonstrate shortly—perhaps, being more consistent than their alternatives: both the proposition that there is creative intelligence of a personal God behind the universe and that man was created on the last day of Creation have been known to give trouble to some very powerful logicians. Let us keep this in mind. But the evidence that supports them is not empirical. Science, which is secretive about this, in fact recognizes this lack of empirical proof. This is why even the most successful theories remain *theories*, possibilities, and are not considered by scientists certain knowledge.

The only thing for which we have truly empirical proof is the existence of the mind. Not coincidentally, this also is the only thing of which we can be certain beyond any doubt, this certainty, as you surely know, being recognized (by Descartes) in the proverbial "I think, therefore I am." Both by definition (for it is constituted by thinking), and also as we know by experience, as you have established in the course of the little experiment with which we began, this "I" consists of words, images, implicit understandings—symbols; and emotions, feelings, sensations, provoked by or associated with symbols.[10] Everything else we think we know about the world is a matter of belief, and the evidence for our beliefs, in cases it is adduced at all, is not empirical, but circumstantial.

Circumstantial evidence is itself an interpretation in which logical considerations are paramount. It is not direct knowledge, but a logical construct, an inference—based in small part on experience and in large part on beliefs we hold about the objective world—from circumstances which make sense to us only if interpreted in its terms. It is, in other words, not the smoking gun. To demonstrate the difference between empirical and circumstantial evidence, or between direct knowledge and knowledge mediated by beliefs, let us first consider the insufficiency of sensual perception as the direct way to knowledge about the objective world.

As we by now agree, there is no possibility to prove the objectivity of our empirical reality either empirically or logically, but we must assume it. We must assume that what we experience is objective, that each one of us is surrounded by beings with essentially identical experiences. Having assumed this, it is reasonable to assume further that our physical senses—sight, hearing, smell, taste, and touch—afford us direct access to knowledge about the physical world outside, which is what most scientists (and non-scientists) do. We believe, in other words, that we see something, hear something, touch something, and therefore know it. The actual process of the transformation of a physical perception by our bodily organs into the knowledge about the world may be complex, it may occur in several stages and involve several parts of the brain, but the content of knowledge is not affected by this complexity, nothing intervenes between perception and received/stored information: what we see is what we get (as knowledge). It is in this sense that we consider a formula such as $E=mc^2$ empirically based.

This, however, implies that the only difference between scientific knowledge, consisting of such propositions and formulas and the knowledge of a dog gained from smelling around a bush is the difference in the form in which the two instances of knowledge are expressed (since dogs, obviously, do not record their findings in letters of the Latin alphabet). This implication is patently wrong. The meaning inferred by a dog is fully contained in the information the dog has gained through the nose, the animal's brain may have to draw from this information some conclusions, but these conclusions are in the empirical premises and, as in the simplest Aristotelian syllogism, only one inference from them is possible. In contrast, people always have a choice as to the meaning with which they invest their sensual perceptions. Information that influences this choice necessarily intervenes between our sensual perceptions and our knowledge about the outside world. This information consists of beliefs we already hold, which are not supported by empirical evidence. (This, incidentally, explains why rats in neuroscience labs perform so much better on transitive inference tests than do humans when confronted with IQ questions.) Again, most of what we consider scientific knowledge consists of these beliefs.

Here is a very simple example. In a classroom at the Hebrew University, I once saw a three-letter word in my native tongue, Russian. Russian uses the Cyrillic alphabet, and so there was no mistaking the word's Russianness. I was brought up in Russia (and in Russian) until the age of seventeen, was eighteen at the moment, and my Russian was as good as it gets. The word had only three letters, I sat staring at it and could not make it out; not only could I not decipher its meaning, but I could not read it, that is, say it in my mind. Now there is a set of very common words in Russian that are considered (and referred to as) unprintable and which are not pronounced in polite society. These are obscenities as exist in many languages, but in Russian they have almost a magical status—speaking them places one outside of a certain circle. I sat staring at this word, intently trying to read it and quite aware of my curious difficulty, and, when I finally did say it in my head and simultaneously became aware of its meaning, it came to me as a shock, I was physically startled and became red in the face. A whole culture intervened between the very simple information my eyes perceived and my knowledge of what I saw. The reason I could not get the meaning of the information I perceived was that I believed the meaning it actually conveyed was impossible: no matter what the evidence of my senses was, this word could not be there, my knowledge about the objective world precluded my learning about it. In the end, the clash between what I saw and my belief that I could not see it became too much and evidence of my senses triumphed. But I was not at all invested in my belief of what Russian words could or could not be on the blackboard (of a Hebrew course on the logic of scientific discovery, as it happened, the perception-to-knowledge message of which I am now disputing); it was not made explicit until after the fact (as the explanation of my unusual difficulty), and I did not come to the experience with any preconceptions. The contradiction between sensual evidence and my belief in its impossibility could not have been stronger, and yet it would have to be stronger for the evidence to win, were this belief explicit and had I been invested in it when I first saw that writing on the blackboard (as scientists are in the knowledge with which they approach evidence). Usually we perceive only that which we are ready to perceive, only that, in other words, which we believe could be there.

That is why "normal" science, in the words of Thomas Kuhn, or science as it is practiced usually, most of the time, consists not in the advancement of knowledge, but in the application, or in establishing the consistency, of the dominant understanding of empirical reality (the dominant belief as to how things are) to more and more cases. What Kuhn calls "anomalies"— inconsistencies between examined cases and the dominant understanding or belief—are likely to be disregarded or attributed to problems with evidence (because we do not believe in them), much rather than (as Kuhn believed) cause us to question the belief.[11] Advances in understanding, however, happen only when the beliefs are reconsidered, when we conceive of (not perceive) possibilities that previously were inconceivable. This happens very rarely and only when our investment in the previously dominant belief has been for some reason emotionally (not logically, through inconsistencies with evidence) weakened.

Since, as a matter of fact, what you see is not what you get, but, rather, what you get (know already) is what you see, and our senses—unlike the senses of a dog or a rat—do not lead directly to the knowledge of what we perceive through them, the evidence science adduces for its theories is logical, rather than empirical. Have you ever seen, heard, touched gravity? No? Neither have I. However, this force, which nobody ever saw, heard, or touched, offered the only logical explanation of apples stubbornly falling down, rather than floating in every conceivable direction, besides the possibility that God personally interfered in the fate of every individual apple (and feather, and ball, and bomb) and carried it down at a certain velocity, when it was ripe enough to leave the parental branch. Isaac Newton, who came up with the theory of gravity, while a very religious man, did not believe in the personal intervention of God in such mundane affairs; he thought that God in his infinite wisdom had created the universe in such a way that it could take care of itself in a perfectly consistent, that is logically perfect, manner. The idea (not the sensual perception, not the experience) of gravity was the only way to account for the stubborn downward inclination of inanimate objects in the context of a perfectly consistent creation of the perfect divine mind. Thus Newton (and all of us after him) took the consistency between a new idea, an old system of beliefs, and the phenomenon to be explained (why objects fall) for empirical evidence. Such substitution of logical consistency for information of sensual perception is what circumstantial evidence is. It is constructed in science in precisely the same way as in law. (Incidentally, it is circumstantial evidence constructed in this very manner that supports the claim that logic based on the principle of non-contradiction was ushered into the human world thanks to the first redaction of the Hebrew Bible.)

INTERIM CONCLUSION 2: The twin pillars of science, it turns out, are in fact one pillar: science, ultimately, rests on logic. In distinction to all other epistemological systems that investigate empirical reality, science uses logic systematically. Only science insists on the logical formulation of conjectures, so that they may be contradicted by other elements within the (circumstantial) evidence it constructs to test them. This is particularly clear in physics, where logic, formalized to the highest degree, becomes mathematics and thus allows for the detection of the subtlest contradictions. The protection against contradiction mathematics offers physical theories enables post-Einstein physics to virtually abandon the pretense of relying on empirical evidence. In turn, the great extent, unparalleled in any other science, to which physics relies on mathematics is a function of the original definition of physical reality (by Newton, among others) as perfectly logical.

Because logic is the only way to make arguments about an ordered universe (which we assume) rationally arguable and because science prioritizes logic to a far greater extent than any other epistemological system that investigates empirical reality, science is the only approach we have, likely to result in objective, universally valid knowledge about empirical reality. This leads to two further conclusions: (1) Despite all the shortcomings of science we have discussed, despite the fact that science is, like any cultural activity, based on beliefs and would, as such, be impossible without some of them, that it is as dogmatic as religion, and sometimes more dogmatic than religion, and that the evidence it relies on is not strictly empirical, but circumstantial—despite all this, we have no other choice but to turn to science if we wish to attain objective knowledge about the subjective empirical reality of the mind. (2) *Given that what distinguishes science from every other epistemological system that investigates empirical reality is its normative attitude to logic (the fact that it is used systematically) and the far greater extent (which results from this normative attitude) that it relies on logic, and given that the evidence for scientific theories is not empirical, but circumstantial (i.e., logically constructed) which we take for empirical, there is no reason why the empirical reality of the mind—or the soul—cannot be a proper scientific subject and why there cannot be a proper, as logical as any other and as empirical as any other, science of the mind (or the soul).* In fact, such a science would be more in accordance with the declared principles of science, such as the preference for empirical evidence over belief, than any other science, because, in distinction to every other science, the science of the mind (or the soul) does, as you have demonstrated in the course of our little experiment, have actual empirical evidence to rely upon—in addition to the ability to construct logical circumstantial evidence, which it shares with all other sciences.

To conclude our discussion of science, it remains for us to cross the t's and dot the i's. We must understand what brought the normative structure (normative attitudes) of science about, allowing for its progress and the expansion of the scientific project as far as it has expanded. And we must account for the ascendancy in science of the philosophical materialism—the belief, quite exceptional historically, in the essentially material nature of reality—which has precluded the expansion of science into human reality, arresting its progress into the area most important for humanity.

Science as an organized continuous activity—i.e., as a social institution—emerged in seventeenth-century England.[12] It did not exist as such before. Of course, there had been great scientific achievements throughout the period between Thales's discovery of how to make arguments rationally arguable and the formation in 1660 of the first strictly scientific research center—the Royal Society of London. But they were few and far between; long periods of scientific inactivity separated them, during which past achievements could be obscured and forgotten, so that a scientist interested in the area in which they were made often had to begin anew, on one's own, as if nobody preceded him (it was always "him") in his investigations. Individual scientists—namely people interested in understanding, gaining reliable, objective, knowledge about, empirical reality and determined to do so logically—existed, but as a collective, continuous enterprise, spanning generations and allowing for the building on past achievements, science did not exist. Therefore, there was no scientific progress.

The emergence of science as a social institution (what we call "modern science") in the seventeenth century and not before had several reasons, the most important being the relative lack of interest in empirical reality, the experiential world, in earlier times. The image of reality that people had then, what they considered the objective world that they inhabited, was the image of a vast cosmos, most of which transcended experience. Their objective reality, in other words, unlike ours, was not empirical; most of it—a far, far greater part—was transcendental. Transcendental forces (in monotheistic cultures, God) ruled this reality and gave meaning to every element of it. The empirical world—the world of human experience—was one of these elements; meaningless and valueless in its own right, it derived all its meaning and value from the grand transcendental scheme of which it was a part. Thus, it was not a very interesting subject for investigation. The curiosity of the curious, their desire to know, was focused on the transcendental.

In monotheistic cultures, which conceived of the objective reality as the universe ordered by One Almighty God, and therefore, privileged logic as an epistemological instrument—though never above faith—it was possible to gain some knowledge of the transcendental sphere through the use of reason. But God and his designs could not be rationally known in principle: they were unfathomable. So the power of human reason was limited, and there was not much incentive to cultivate logical thinking as well.

All this changed with the radical transformation of belief, which occurred in England in the course of the sixteenth century. This transformation of belief was brought on by an equally dramatic change of experience, first among the most talented and educated members of the English people, and then among the English population, in general. A civil war, called the War of the Roses, between two branches of the Plantagenet royal family and their supporters in the later half of the fifteenth century decimated the English feudal aristocracy and extinguished the royal family. A very distant relation of the winning Lancaster branch, Henry Tudor, neither wealthy nor influential himself, ascended the throne as Henry VII. Willy-nilly, the new king had to turn to commoners for support, which could not fail to increase their self-respect and sense of authority. The top of the social hierarchy left empty, they began to move up. The king needed an aristocracy to help him rule; by the beginning of the sixteenth century a new aristocracy was created, recruited among petty nobility and people from below.

The consciousness of the time, the prevailing beliefs and the image of reality associated with them, could not make sense of this new experience. Social reality was imagined as based on the Providential Plan, the will of God, who for his higher reasons, unfathomable for mortal beings, shaped it in the form of three hierarchically arranged orders: the military nobility on top, the laboring common folk on the bottom, and the clergy—a kind of learned estate—in the middle. These orders (in particular, the upper layer and the rest) were, in principle, hermetically closed to each other: social mobility, a regular feature of social life for us, was both illegitimate and virtually incomprehensible. I.e., it was believed impossible, it could not be—and yet, here was the empirical evidence of it.

The experience of the upwardly mobile commoners was a positive one—they cherished it, they were vested in it. The emotional hold on them of the beliefs that denied this experience was, therefore, weakened. They groped for a new belief that would make good sense of their mobility, that is, both explain and approve of it. They found it in the idea of the nation.

Of course, this was not a conscious search. They were bewildered by their experience (just like I was by the sight of that naughty Russian word on the blackboard) yet unwilling to explain it away because it was positive. The idea of the nation saved them from this bewilderment, and they became deeply committed—converted—to this idea.

The word "nation" at that time referred to the groups of extremely high-placed individuals who represented different positions at the Church Councils. These elite individuals were the bearers of the political and cultural authority; the word "nation" thus meant "a political and cultural elite." Some time at the very beginning of the sixteenth century, someone among the members of the new English aristocracy equated "nation" with "people," making the two words synonyms. The word "people," however, at that time, referred mainly to the lower classes of society; it had been the synonym of "rabble" or "plebs." Making it, instead, the synonym of "nation" elevated Englishmen of all classes to the dignity of the elite and declared them the bearers of political and cultural authority. This semantic fiat legitimated social mobility and explained why any Englishman, no matter where born, socially speaking, could find oneself occupying any of the most influential positions in the land. But, in addition to this, it fundamentally changed the image of society (the beliefs as to what a society was) and, with it, the view of reality, in general.

The definition of the people, the entire population of the country, as a nation implied the fundamental equality of the members of the national community, which made them interchangeable and social mobility legitimate and sensible. The fact that the people were invested with political authority, in particular, implied the principle of popular sovereignty, which made the government representative (however that representation was arranged). This investment of the community of living individuals with political authority divested of it particular families and lineages, whose hereditary right to rule rested on tradition and Divine sanction. This, in turn, divested of authority God himself. In social life, God became irrelevant: people now organized their affairs on their own, and made their own laws. But social life—going about their business, whatever it was, in society, getting married, raising children, teaching them to say prayers, participating in religious rituals on certain days and going to market on others, etc.—occupied most of people's attention during their everyday existence, just as it does of yours today: making God irrelevant in social life focused the mind on the secular world to virtual exclusion of the others.

The new image of reality that resulted from the equation of the concepts of "people" and "nation" forms the core of modern consciousness. Societies constructed on its basis are very different from the European feudal "societies of orders" which they replaced and from other types of society. Their social structure is relatively open, mobility is its central feature; its chief political institution, the state, is impersonal and, therefore, in principle representative, it embodies the idea of popular sovereignty. Because these modern societies, beginning with England, are called "nations," the image of reality (the system of beliefs) that underlies and informs them is called "nationalism."

INTERIM CONCLUSION 3: Nationalism as a system of beliefs, or this, national, modern form of consciousness, which—examine yourselves—all of us share, whatever other beliefs it may contain in any particular case (such as American nationalism, Russian nationalism, etc.), always contains these three: (1) the belief in the fundamental equality of those considered members of the nation; (2) the belief that the national community is self-governing, the source of authority and law; and (3) the belief that this empirical world, the objective world accessible to our experience is inherently meaningful and autonomous, that, whether or not transcendental forces had anything to do with it at the time of creation, they have nothing to do with it at present. This last belief, as you have already concluded, I am sure, elevates empirical reality to the top of our intellectual priorities, the top of the list of things we want to understand. In other words, nationalism, because of its secular focus, prioritizes the exploration of empirical reality over other intellectual pursuits and reliable (objective and universally valid) knowledge of empirical reality over other types of knowledge. Logic already being the privileged epistemological tool for the development of such knowledge, this calls for, makes imperative or normative, the systematic use of logic and brings about science as a social institution.[13]

It is important to realize that, while the secular focus of nationalism is logically related to the beliefs in the fundamental equality of membership and popular sovereignty, themselves logical implications of imagining the people as a nation, the eventual secularization of our entire worldview—i.e., the replacement of the belief that the objective reality is mostly transcendental with an insignificant secular/empirical corner in it, with the belief that the objective reality is essentially secular—is not logically related to them. (Remember, Newton was a deeply religious man.) This replacement, rather, is the result of the purely emotional weakening of the religious faith, the fading of God from memory.

I often start my courses on nationalism or any aspect of modernity with asking students to draw a pictogram of their world—all that is significant for them. I have done so many times in the United States and twice at a Summer University in Switzerland, which brought together students from around the world. The pictograms are always essentially the same: Americans draw the globe or one's head, and on the globe or in the head symbols of human relationships (little people in various poses), symbols of nature (little trees), of one's individual interests (books, music, etc.); students from other countries, in addition, in a large minority of cases draw the globe with geographical contours of their country on it and the flag or some other national symbol. After they explain the meaning of their pictograms to the class, I ask how many of them believe in God—a majority of both American and international students usually raise their hands. Then I ask them where is God in their drawings; there is a minute or two of stunned looks in silence and then they realize that they had only believed that they believe in God, that, on self-examination, this turned out not to be so: God is absent from their world. (Try it on yourself; examine whether God is actually found in yours. If you do this honestly, in nine out of ten cases you will find that your world is entirely secular as well.) I like to compare these pictograms to the paintings, let's say, of El Greco, to take a later example: this—earthly—world is crowded at the very bottom of the canvas, the eyes of the diminutive mortals focused on the large scale fig- ures of saints and angels who occupy most of the painted surface above them; all the action, everything of significance is happening there, in the sphere of the transcendental.

This dramatic change in the image of reality and the nature of our beliefs about it is not a result of conscious, logical examination of our beliefs vis- à-vis the evidence (empirical and circumstantial), it is a result of the nat- ural, biological process of forgetting. God is not of much use to us anymore; the use of God's name, talking about God is no longer emotionally charged—even for people who truly believe themselves Christians, or Jews, or Muslims, it is far less charged than talking about politics and mentioning the name of a favorite (or most detested) presidential candi- date. And so the memory of this religious belief, which might never have been consciously discarded, becomes harder and harder to recall in the physical, neurobiological sense of the word "recall."

The premise on which the scientific project has been based in the last two centuries, the belief that empirically knowable reality is material, is a result of a similar emotional, rather than logical, process. The reality we know empirically is mental and symbolic. It belongs squarely within the "psycho-" compartment of the colossal psychophysical conundrum, the mind-body problem that humanity (at least in the monotheistic cultures) has not been able to resolve since Plato (through Socrates) first posed it 2500 years ago. Since Socrates, Western metaphysical philosophy, and therefore epistemology, has been based on the idea that objective reality is dual, that it consists of two disparate, heterogeneous elements or sub- stances: one material, the other spiritual.[14] Humanity contained both of these elements in equal parts: it was both material and spiritual, thus, dual, like objective reality; the rest of the natural world (organic and inorganic) was, for all intents and purposes, material, but the transcendental forces (gods and ancestral spirits of Greek and Roman antiquity, and, of course, the One Almighty God, the Creator of Judaism, Christianity, and Islam) were spiritual. For those who came to see the world as one ordered uni- verse and incorporated logic (in their thinking and in their physical being, i.e., in the neurobiological sense of conditioning), this duality became a problem, because it was a radical contradiction. Nobody doubted for a moment the reality of either spiritual or material element, because nobody doubted or questioned the objectivity of one's experience. Yet this experience undermined the essential consistency of one ordered universe, which could not be questioned either. The law of non-contradiction ruled that a thing could not *be* and *not be* at the same time, have and yet not have the same quality, but both the world and humanity did. The world was both material and not material, spiritual and not spiritual; men were, like all organic bodies, mortal, but, as spirits, they could not be subject to death. (Recall that what distinguished the gods for the Greeks was their immortality, that is, in every other respect they were like men; the Latin root for the word "man"—*homo*—is cognate with "burial," making man one who is buried, i.e., dies, unlike gods who do not die, yet, unlike mortal animals who have no spirit which requires burial. The duality of human nature must have been recognized very early, but before logic it was not seen as a problem.)

Since Socrates, philosophy has been vainly trying to resolve the psychophysical problem. The proposed solutions have been of two types that came to be called "idealist" and "materialist."[15] For most of the two and a half millennia after Socrates, philosophical idealism was dominant. Idealism gave causal priority to the spiritual element and, though it obviously did not deny the empirical reality to the material element, it denied the material element significance and causally reduced it to the spiritual element. In the last three centuries, however, philosophical materialism became dominant. Materialism gives causal priority to the material element, denies the significance of the spiritual element and causally reduces it to the material element. In addition, in contrast to the idealist philosophy, materialism (or, at least materialists) very often denies the empirical reality of the spiritual element.[16]

The mind, we are saying (I am saying this with you, for I hope you have considered your experiences and have arrived at the conclusion I am stating on your own), is not a material reality. The soul, the spirit (use whichever synonym you choose) exists, and it is the only fact of which we have direct knowledge. We have empirically overturned the premise on which the scientific project has been based in the last three centuries: the premise that empirically knowable reality is material. But materialism, like every position that is not based on direct, empirical, knowledge, is a matter of belief. It is the dominant epistemological belief in modern societies and, for this reason, it makes sense to the great majority of people, while opposing beliefs (such as, for example, the Old Testament belief that the mind is what God breathes into a new human life) appear to them devoid of any sense whatsoever. I am sure that until this very moment many of you have never felt a need to question it, even though your experience constantly contradicted it; it made perfect sense to you.

The dominance of the materialist belief, like that of any belief which is not necessary for human survival, is explained historically. After over two millennia of feeble opposition to the dominant spiritualist, or idealist, conception of reality and several more centuries of an uneasy truce with it when this, secular world emerged as the focus of human consciousness and the human community replaced God as the supreme lawgiver, materialism eclipsed idealism as the sensible option simply because, matter allowing manipulation and intentional experimentation, scientific exploration of the secular world began with the exploration of matter, and physics, for a long time, existed unrivalled as the model science. Newton and other natural scientists of his time were philosophical idealists. Scientific exploration of empirical reality, however deep, does not contradict a religious belief in its divine creation and does not in the least presuppose philosophical materialism and, specifically, the belief in the material nature of empirically knowable reality. This materialist belief is dominant today because of the weakened emotional hold of religious beliefs in modern society, not the other way around.

The materialist premise of contemporary scientific project overturned, where does this leave us? Are we to return to idealism? The dualist epistemological system in the framework of which all the pursuit of knowledge in monotheistic, logic-based cultures has taken place in the last 2,500 years—the philosophical tradition we call "Western"—after all does offer us only two options. If the reality is not essentially (that is, ultimately reducible to) a material one, it is essentially ideal, or spiritual. We cannot even opt for the dualistic tolerance of assuming that some aspects of reality are of one kind and others are of the other, because than we would have to accept that the world is not consistently ordered, in which case we deprive ourselves of the use of logic, without which science, and the acquisition of reliable knowledge, is impossible. Our study would, indeed, deteriorate into pure speculation. So idealism does seem to be the only solution.

But what if the image of reality we have held for two and a half millennia is wrong? Make an effort, try to imagine this possibility. Western philosophical tradition is venerable, but venerable traditions have been overturned, beliefs of even longer standing have been proven wrong. However agnostic we must remain in regard to some aspects of the Creation story, we know that it cannot be right as to the time it took, for instance. So, perhaps, reality does not, as we have for so long believed, consist of two heterogeneous elements or substances, the matter and the spirit. Yes, this is—so we are told—how we experience reality, and there is much historical and anthropological evidence that this experience of duality of the human nature is very widespread and not limited to our monotheistic, logical civilization. But, remember, what you get (what you believe) is what you see. And, obviously, before or without logic one could not even make arguable arguments about one's experience or reality. Outside of the framework of Aristotelian logic one cannot argue (and, therefore, rationally understand) that the belief in the objectivity of the world one can experience only subjectively is a purely dogmatic notion, unsupported by a shred of empirical or circumstantial evidence. Perhaps Socrates (or Plato), who was one of the very first thinkers to apply logic to human experience, did not examine the duality proposition and took it for granted, transmitting it, empirically and logically unwarranted as it was, on to future generations bolstered by his enormous authority? We—you and I—know that our experiences, as we actually experience them, are not material. They may be caused materially and may be reducible to something material, but we have no empirical evidence of that. The only thing we know by direct experience is that what we experience is not material. Matter, whatever is material, however, has certain qualities; it can be positively defined. Whatever is spiritual, in distinction, is chiefly defined by that it is not material. This means that, if we are not certain that there is a material side to our reality, it makes no sense at all to call the reality we are certain about "spiritual." There is something we experience—"I think, therefore I am"—but we do not know what this "I" (and, therefore, everything else) is. So, it stands to reason that the image of reality which has served as our epistemological foundation since time immemorial was a misrepresentation, or, to turn the metaphor, *when subjected to logical examination, the dualist image of reality, presumed to consist of the material and the spiritual elements or substances, falls apart.* We are fully justified with replacing this belief with something else.

The most important consideration here is that the dualist epistemological system is no longer useful. It ceased to be useful already in the nineteenth century, when it prevented the advancement of objective, universally valid, knowledge in biology. Darwin's theory of evolution, which made possible this advancement, presupposed different metaphysics and suggested a different epistemology. It is this metaphysics and epistemology that I propose we follow.

Up to the publication of Darwin's *On the Origin of Species* in 1859, biology did not advance because it was clear that life cannot be explained by the laws of physics. The science of life was stuck between philosophical materialists, who claimed that, when we know more about both life and physical laws, we would be able to so explain it; and philosophical idealists, called *vitalists,* who claimed that there was a sort of vital spirit—*élan vital*—behind or in every living thing and it was this spirit that created life. Neither philosophical materialism, nor philosophical idealism, however, allowed their proponents in biology to do any scientific work. Both were reduced to description, on the one hand, such as categorizing and creating typologies of various species and organs (that is why biology consisted of descriptive subdisciplines, such as botany, zoology, comparative anatomy), and philosophizing—speculating, on the other. (I wonder if any of you, interested in human neurobiology and humanity in general, perceive a parallel between the state of biology then and the condition of some other disciplines now.)

Already then, a solution to the psychophysical problem was needed that would reconcile the heterogeneity of the objective reality with the idea of one consistently ordered universe. (Remember: we cannot give the belief in one ordered universe up, because neither logic, nor, therefore, science and accumulation of objective, universally valid knowledge, would be possible without it.) Specifically, for biology to exist as a science, it was imperative to prove that the phenomenon of life, while consistent with the laws of physics, was autonomous, i.e., had its own laws, that its irreducibility to inanimate matter was rationally (logically) intelligible within one ordered universe.

This is precisely what Charles Darwin accomplished with his theory of natural selection. On the basis of meticulously constructed circumstantial evidence (that is, pieces of empirical evidence, gaps in empirical evidence, considerations of scholars in other fields, specifically geology, certain beliefs regarding the nature of reality, contradictions in other beliefs regarding it, etc., that were fitted perfectly together, creating a logically watertight argument) Darwin proved that there was a law pertaining to the development of life on earth that had nothing whatsoever to do with laws of physics, and yet was logically consistent with them, because it operated within the *boundary conditions* of the physical laws. That is, in distinction to philosophical materialists, Darwin proved that life indeed could be irreducible to inanimate matter, but, in distinction to philosophical idealists, or vitalists, who claimed that life was independent from the material reality studied by physics, he proved that laws of life could only operate within the conditions provided by physical laws. By proving that life was an *autonomous* reality, Darwin made biology *independent* from physics: biologists now could take physics for granted and explore the ways biological laws operated.

Millions of people today believe in the theory of evolution. However, while scientific understanding progresses, beliefs do not: recent beliefs are not more correct than those of times past, and sharing in a contemporary belief does not make one smarter than those who hold on to beliefs of long ago, only more conformist. Very few people among those who believe in evolution understand Darwin's theory. For example, some very important philosophers think that he established a unified framework in which everything can be understood, when, in fact, he established precisely the opposite.[17] Did his theory of natural selection signify the victory of materialists in the dispute between them and the idealist vitalists? No, it transcended this dispute and made both positions quite irrelevant. (If we define matter as it is defined in physics, clearly, the theory of natural selection implies that the phenomenon of life is only partly material, that there is more to it than matter. Matter is essentially a spatial phenomenon; it is defined by taking place in space. There is much that is spatial in every living organism, but the great biological law is historical, evolution by natural selection occurs in time. Time, as we know from Einstein, is not a physical phenomenon, it is not an element of material reality, but only of our knowledge of material reality, that is why it is relative to the observer—us again; it does not have any physical qualities. A phenomenon which is essentially a process happening in time, rather than a substance existing in space is material, strictly speaking, only to a certain extent.)

After Darwin, it became possible to envision the objective world not in terms of the materialist/idealist duality, but in terms of *emergent phenomena*.[18] An emergent phenomenon is a complex phenomenon that cannot be reduced to the sum of its elements, a case in which a specific combination of elements, which no one element, and no law in accordance with which the elements function, renders likely, produces a certain new quality (in most important instances, a certain law or tendency) which in a large measure determines the nature and the existence of the phenomenon, as well as of its elements. Life, as might be expected, is the original referent of this concept. Life is irreducible to the inanimate matter of which, and only of which, every living cell is composed; it is a quality—a tendency—beyond and apart from this matter, which exists in the boundary conditions provided by it, yet shapes it at the same time, insofar as this matter belongs to the living thing. The irreducibility of the emergent phenomenon implies that at the moment of emergence there occurs a break in continuity, a leap from one interconnected world or reality into another one, essentially disconnected from, yet fundamentally consistent with it, a transformation the mechanism of which, by definition, cannot be traced exclusively to the first reality, and is, at least in part, extraneous to it.

CONCLUSION: The important point to make here is that the recognition of the tremendous world of life as an emergent phenomenon proves that such improbable new autonomous worlds are possible. And this, in turn, suggests that experiential reality which is conceived of since the beginning of the Western philosophical tradition as having only two aspects, the real or material and the ideal or spiritual (both or only one of which may be considered essential and autonomous), may be approached from an altogether different perspective. *Reality may be imagined as consisting of three autonomous but related layers, with the two upper ones being emergent phenomena—the layer of matter, the layer of life, and the layer of the mind.* This opens the way to the scientific investigation of the mind.

2

The Mind as an Emergent Phenomenon

Now that we have cleared the major obstacle on the way to our investigation—the universal claim among scientists that the mind is not a scientific subject and any pronouncements about it must be considered pure speculation—and escaped the epistemological vice in which our thinking has been held for 2,500 years, let us analyze our empirical evidence and see what, in fact, the mind—or the soul—is.

Since we have agreed to regard the mind as an emergent phenomenon, it would make sense to begin with the elements out of which it is emergent and which serve as boundary conditions for its existence, and then proceed with the analysis of the quality—in this case, the tendency or law—which has been added on to these elements. We do not have to analyze the elements themselves, because, while they make the emergent phenomenon possible, they cannot explain it, but must only list them, after which they should be taken for granted.

The Elements

The elements out of which the mind emerges to become more than their sum are organic, that is, they are structures, processes, and functions of life, and, as such, are products of the biological evolution through natural selection. They are *three* in number. Two of these are specific bodily organs, one of which—the brain—common, in the specific evolutionary form apparently required to make the mind possible, to several biological species at the very least; while the other—the larynx—in that specific evolutionary form is unique to the human species. The third element that has made the mind possible is a certain evolutionary stage of the process or function of perception and communication of perception within a biological group— the perception and communication by signs.

It is humbling to realize that of these three elements only larynx is unique to the human species. This means that, had the larynx of the wolf, the chimpanzee, or the dolphin—to name only the best recognized competitors of the so-called *Homo sapiens* for the palm of superiority in brain power—been structured and positioned like ours is, they and not we might conceivably be the rulers of the earth today. Can we really know how *sapiens* the obviously wily *Canis lupus*, who does not talk to us, is? The larynx gives us the mechanical ability to speak, namely to articulate sound, which no other animal possesses to anywhere near the same degree. But it goes without saying that it is not this mechanical ability that has created *Hamlet,* the theory of evolution, or free markets. Such creativity is peculiar to man. Yet, on logical examination, there could possibly be no evidence that the brains of a wolf or a dolphin would not be able to support it, had they been given the chance— that is, no evidence for the frequent claim that art, science, or the economic organization of Western society emanate from the human brain.

The human larynx must be a result of the natural selection for procreation of certain genetic traits particularly well adapted to a very specific environmental niche, i.e., the environmental niche existing at the moment when the immediate ancestor of our species reached a certain evolutionary stage (the one which made the larynx particularly adaptive) and which, therefore, existed only for this our immediate ancestor. Not so with the brain and signification. These two obviously related features of the organic (life) process have developed in numerous species.

All living beings are in contact with the environment and for animals, at least, this environment is changeable from minute to minute. In the environment of a gazelle, one minute there may be a certain predator on the prowl, another minute may be free of danger, allowing the gazelle to concentrate on feeding, and then, suddenly a completely different predator may appear. In the course of evolution, animal species evolved mechanisms and techniques for adapting to a changeable environment, that is, for reacting properly to different environmental stimuli. Various organs of perception developed to alert individual organisms to these stimuli and various behavioral sequences were genetically encoded to follow the perception of stimuli that were frequently encountered. The nervous system functionally united these organs and issued commands to deploy behavioral sequences to the organism.

Both the organs of perception and genetically programmed reactions to many of the stimuli involved the use of *signs*—an aspect of a stimulus, or of the encoded reaction to it, signifying the stimulus, respectively, to the perceiving organism and to members of the organism's group. The appearance of *significance* is one of the many astonishing effects of the emergence of life on earth—the appearance, that is, of beings to whom the world signifies—and, with them, of what we vaguely and indiscriminately refer to as "consciousness." Consciousness, on the most elementary level, is indeed the reading and communication of signs. There are no signs and no consciousness in the world of stones; the environment of a stone, whatever cataclysms may be occurring in it and however dramatic effect they may have on the stone, does not signify, it has no one to signify to. Life, in distinction, is full of significance. Everything in it is a sign; signs are the very web of the organic world, what ties the different strands of it, the different links of the great chain of the organic being, together. Each link or species may be constituted genetically, but it is the signs that regulate how lions and antelopes and zebras and leopards and cheetahs and all the rest of them of the Serengeti, or wolves and bears and deer and caribou and hares and foxes and other living things of the European forests and steppes live together. A whiff of odor signifies the presence of a prowling lioness or a leopard to a gazelle; it utters a cry which signifies it to others in the herd, they spring into flight; a tiny fawn just born is abandoned by his mother, it had no chance to learn anything about the world yet, but the reading of the signs is encoded in its genes and so it lies motionless, pretending not to be alive, so long as it reads the signs of the predator's presence and intentions.

The more complex the environment, the more complex is the nervous system. The brain—its governing organ—corresponds to very complex environments. At the same time, the more complex the environment, the more of the genetic programming for the nervous system must be left open. The genetic program for the nervous system is a relatively open program even in simple organisms: though the repertory of responses may be very limited, the nature of every stimulus cannot be predicted, and, by definition, each "stimulus-response" sequence cannot be encoded genetically. In complex environments the great amount of unpredictable stimuli require that an organism be adept at recognizing them for what they are on one's own (without the help of the genetically built-in information): for the wildebeest a lion is a terrible danger to flee, but what is a Land Rover or a two-legged animal getting out of it? The organism then must integrate such previously unfamiliar stimuli into its internal system by means of a mental (synaptic) record. Neuroscientists refer to these two mental acts, respectively, as "learning" and "memory." What these "learning" and "memory" involve is interpretation and acquisition of an ability to read new signs. Unlike human society, the natural world has zero tolerance for stupidity: the ones who cannot learn die. The brain which evolved to such a prodigious extent in mammals and birds because of its adaptive capacity in very complex environments (that is, because the learning disabled were not selected for procreation) has a lot of work to do—it must be active and in good working order at every moment.

The Emergence of the Mind

Nothing in even the most highly developed brain can produce a mind. Nor can the most extensive and complex set of signs imaginable do so. And even the combination of the two has no such creative or causal power. The addition to this combination of the ability to articulate sound, inherent in the peculiar structure and position of the human larynx, however, has led to the mind's emergence. Not that it made the mind in any way likely. The biological species of *Homo sapiens* had completely evolved—brain, larynx, and all—more than 100,000 years before the mind made its first appearance among its members.[1] This means that it was not caused by the organic combination that made it possible, but was the result of a most improbable accident—the transformation (a complete change in character) of one of its elements. When this transformation occurred, the emergent phenomenon of the mind was in place, and, being autonomous—self-regulating, self-sustaining, self-generating, and self-transforming (like life)—*it caused itself.*

It is absolutely impossible to reconstruct *how* this happened. But it is possible to understand—i.e., deduce logically—*what* happened. A very large plurality of the signs used by *Homo sapiens,* because of the biological constitution of this species, were vocal signs. The ability to articulate sound allowed for playing with it. For hundreds of thousands of years, *Homo sapiens* cubs—children—probably had a lot of fun with making various meaningless noises, noises which could be intentionally produced, as if one was reading or communicating a sign, but did not signify anything. Then, 20,000, maybe 30,000 years ago, one particularly *sapiens homo* recognized that sound signs could be intentionally articulated, and *intentionally articulated signs are symbols.*[2]

The intention that stood between the environmental stimulus and its sign, and which separated one from the other, transformed signs into symbols. Unlike signs, symbols represented phenomena of which they were not a part—in this sense they were arbitrary, dependent on choice. The meaning (the significance) of a symbol was not given in the phenomenon it was signifying—its referent, or genetically; it was given to it by the context in which it was used, and increasingly this context became mostly the context of other symbols. Thus the significance of symbols constantly changed. Unlike signs, which could be very many, but whose number was essentially limited by their referents in the environment, symbols were endlessly proliferating. (The very introduction of a symbol would change the environment and initiate a symbolic chain reaction.) Unlike signs, which exist in sets, they, from the first formed *systems,* ever changing and becoming more complex and connected by constantly transforming ties of interdependence. Symbols, in other words, constituted a world of their own; an autonomous, self-creative world in which things were happening according to laws of causation that did not apply anywhere else.

Symbolic Reality

The new reality that emerged out of the combination of the three organic elements, the highly developed brain, the human larynx, and the use of signs, was, to begin with, a *symbolic reality.* Unlike the organic reality which provided the boundary conditions for it, and in which every stage and level of the organic process occurring in time corresponded to a specific, definite, and peculiar to that particular stage state of matter occurring in space, the symbolic reality was *essentially historical.* It was a process that occurred without any specific reflection in substance. This process, like every process, occurred in time; but in distinction to the organic process, its relation to space was tenuous. It created material by-products and left material side effects, but all this was only after the fact—there was no material aspect to its actual happening.

It happened, however, *by means* of the organic process and the corresponding material structure of the brain. It is by means of the brain that the introduction of the very first symbols initiated the endless and ever more involved symbolic chain reaction, transforming a singular event into an emergent reality: the use of every symbol, the perception of its significance, its maintenance and transformation was supported by the mechanisms of the individual brain and reflected in some, not necessarily specific, physicochemical neuronal activity. This was thus a *mental process*. And it is this *symbolic* (therefore, *historical*) and *mental* process, this reality emergent out of the combination of the developed brain, the human larynx, and the use of signs, that we experience as the *mind*.

Mind and Culture

Of course, the overwhelming majority of the symbols in the mind process, as you know from our little experiment in the beginning, most of the words and visual images, for instance, that sound and show themselves in our heads, have not been created by the particular mind that happens to experience them at any given moment. No, they have been created by other minds, in some cases, minds that are contemporary with the experiencing mind, but in an overwhelming majority of cases minds that had existed generations, often multiple generations before the experiencing mind. This *symbolic common wealth*, every single bit of which had been produced in some mind, that every experiencing mind makes use of, can be referred to as "collective mind" and was referred to by one great student of this symbolic and mental reality, Émile Durkheim, as "collective consciousness." But there is no need for such confusing metaphors (which stress and deemphasize individuality at the same time), because this is precisely what we mean by the word "culture" today.

While culture can be referred to as "collective mind," the mind can be conceptualized as "culture in the brain," or "individualized culture." These are not just two elements of the same—symbolic and mental—reality, they are one and the same process occurring on two different levels—the individual and the collective, similar to the life of an organism and of the species to which it belongs in the organic world. The fundamental laws governing this process on both levels are precisely the same laws and at every moment, at every stage in it, it moves back and forth between the levels; it cannot, even for a split second, occur on only one of them. The mind constantly borrows symbols from culture, but culture can only be processed—i.e., symbols can only have significance and be symbols—in the mind.

It follows that having the mind and culture does not simply distinguish humanity from the rest of the animal kingdom, but separates it drastically from other species of life. Dependent on the organic laws, but autonomous, humanity functions in accordance with symbolic and historical laws instead, to the extent of modifying organic laws on many occasions. Defined thus by the emergent phenomenon of culture and the mind, it must be regarded itself as this emergent phenomenon. It indeed becomes a reality *sui generis,* of its own kind.

Language

The original form the reality of the mind and culture took was, undoubtedly, that of spoken language. Language lies at the very core of the culture process, because it is the chief symbolic means of transmitting culture across generations (i.e., long periods of time) and large distances. Even today, preparing other elements of cultural reality for such transmission, we package them in language. Its impact on the life of our animal species at the dawn of our transformation into humanity must have been colossal. When knowledge about the environment had been transmitted by signs, only the organism to whom a particular stimulus had been communicated directly (for instance, the *Homo sapiens* animal smelling the presence of a predator, or a cheetah who learned from her mother how to hunt a particular prey) could communicate it to others (the frightened *Homo sapiens* to the rest of the group, or the well-informed cheetah to her cubs) and only to others within its immediate vicinity. Only *direct learning* was possible and the transmission of information about the environment, which was not genetically encoded and, therefore, had to be acquired through learning, was extremely limited. Language allowed *indirect learning* and the acquired information expanded to the extent of rendering genetically transmitted knowledge about the environment superfluous, in effect replacing it.

Spoken language was the original symbolic system. But no symbol and no symbolic system exist alone. In the presence of brains they produce symbolic chain reactions and endlessly proliferate. Undoubtedly, very quickly other languages, other symbolic systems, must have been added to the spoken language—the language of visual images and body language, above all. Our reality, the world we inhabit as human beings, represents a multidimensional fabric of symbolic systems, interwoven, crisscrossing, and diverging in most intricate ways. Because we are symbolic creatures, everything around us becomes a symbol. A bow, a glance, a smile, a hand-shake are symbols. It is on symbols of this silent kind that the nodal cul-tural structure of social stratification, for instance, rests to a far greater extent, than on language proper, whether written or spoken. In context, a casual bow may signify a relationship of equality, a passing glance, superi-ority and, perhaps, contempt, a forced smile, subservience. All these ges-tures may also signify something entirely different. The meaning of these symbols, making certain reactions adequate to and others inconsistent with an action that elicited them, changes with time, but also depending on the sphere of social life of which the gesture exchange in question forms a part. Today, a casual bow to a salesclerk in a store would be adequate enough, but highly inappropriate to one's academic advisor in a corridor.

The service of language as the chief medium of the transmission of sym-bolic information across generations accounts for the mistaken notion that language is first and foremost a system of communication. But, while not the least, this is certainly not the most important function language per-forms for us. For language also lies at the core of the process of the mind—that is, of the symbolic process on the individual level. There, it is responsible for the existence of *consciousness* in its most distinctive human meaning of self-consciousness, which we can never ascribe even to very complex animal organisms. Half an hour of careful introspection will reveal to you that *language is the medium of thinking. Thinking* may be defined as explicit mental processing of symbolic stimuli, the mental pro-cess which involves not only the consciousness of environmental stimuli (in our case overwhelmingly symbolic), but also the consciousness of this consciousness. Whichever symbolic system occupies our mind at any given moment, if we are processing it explicitly, namely, being conscious of processing it, we process it in words and may be said to engage in thinking. Results of some forms of symbolic processing may be recorded in symbols other than language—for instance, in mathematical formulae or musical notation. But only a few symbolic systems have their own media of expression; complex symbolic systems of gestures and interactions, such as the system of stratification, for instance, or systems such as cuisine, fashion, politics, and so on, lack such specialized media and so must be expressed through language. Thus language intervenes in systemic relations of other symbolic systems. It has the ability to modify the significance of every other symbol. Clearly, other symbols possess this ability to some extent too: the meaning of words may be affected by intonation or gestures (as when one croons, caressing a pet, "Oh, you most terrible, horrible, bad boy"), as it may be affected by a tune to which words are sung. But no other symbolic system has this ability to anywhere near the same extent as language. Moreover, only language can reconstruct the mental process even in those few cases when a specialized medium of recording its results are available. Only language actually turns consciousness upon itself, making it a distinctly human consciousness. It does not merely make thinking possible—it is the very source of thinking. It is through language that the "I" of "I think, therefore I am," the "I" of Descartes, comes into being. It is, therefore, an absolutely essential element of the fully realized symbolic process on the level of the individual mind.

Both culture and the mind occur by means of individual brains, but both come to the brain from outside of the biological reality altogether, thus it takes time for a young *Homo sapiens* animal to acquire culture and the mind. It takes time, in other words, for a member of the human species to become human. Humanity, when analyzed logically, is an acquired characteristic; as such, it is not genetically heritable. Having two human parents does not make one, by definition, human. A child acquires the mind, and therefore, becomes human, somewhere around the age of three. Our ability to store symbolic memory (the kind of memory that can be recollected and experienced the way you have recollected and experienced your daily experiences in our little experiment in the beginning) signifies the accomplishment of this acquisition. Indeed, our earliest memories (consider yours) never go farther than this point: we start to remember symbolically only when we start to remember ourselves—when we acquire that Descartes' "I," the "I" of consciousness turned on to itself, when we start thinking. The mind we acquire as young children, though not fully developed (it takes, I would say, at least another ten years of immersion in culture to fully develop it) has all its qualities of self-creative symbolic process that make it what it is. The moment we acquire it we are utterly transformed, and, from a biological, animal being emerges a cultural being, a human. This means that the acquisition of the mind is not gradual, it is a quantum leap—indeed an emergence in the sense in which we have been using the word in the concept of "an emergent phenomenon." It happens in each one of us as we figure out that signs can be created intentionally and so turn them into symbols, at the same time guessing what turns symbols of a kind into a system.

The manner of language acquisition demonstrates this most clearly. Language, obviously, is not the only symbolic system which is acquired at this early stage, in fact, because it is so very complex, it may in numerous individual cases, be acquired later than simpler symbolic systems (themselves, on the collective level, brought into being by language). But its tremendous intricacy and formality (in comparison with body language, for instance), makes its acquisition easy to observe. And what do we observe? No child, between the day it is born and the age of five, is systematically taught—or can be systematically taught—the English language as it exists today and (which is not exactly the same thing) as it is encoded in the new edition of the *Oxford English Dictionary*. And yet, somewhere between the ages of three and five, as any parent among us would know, the child may be said to have acquired the language and starts using it, by and large correctly by the standards of its environment, that is, according to numerous rules of grammar and syntax, of which he or she could not have heard, and often creatively, guessing at words outside of the actually learned vocabulary, understanding these words without ever hearing them before—both easily finding the proper medium for expressing what he or she wants to express and interpreting the meaning of others' expressions reasonably well. Of course, one does not have the capacity for introspection or explicit interest in it to watch this quite miraculous process closely, when one acquires one's mother tongue. But, as adults we sometimes have the possibility of observing ourselves as we learn a foreign language. There, admittedly on a lesser scale, the miracle repeats itself. We spend weeks, perhaps months, laboriously memorizing words which make very little sense at first and combining them in simple sentences, according to the rules explained in the exercise books, and then one day suddenly find ourselves swimming in the new language, feeling it, reading without a dictionary! We figure out the organizing principle of the system. As in childhood, most of our new proficiency comes from this ability to understand, implicitly, but surely, what connects the different symbols together. It is by this means—i.e., owing to our ability to figure out, to discover, the principles of consistency in accordance with which symbols of a kind constitute a system, and then complement, and greatly augment the little that we know—that a language goes on living, and the same applies to other symbolic systems, from the etiquette of drugstore shopping (and evidently there is such a thing) to high diplomacy, and from cuisine to philosophy.

Two Important Implications

These considerations have serious implications for the way we answer the tremendous question, when does human life begin? The conventional options—that it begins (1)at conception, (2) some time during pregnancy, (3) at birth—are all wrong. The life of an animal organism, obviously, begins at conception. But human life begins only at the moment that the animal has a mind—transforming into a self-generating, creative, symbolic and mental process in addition to representing a specific materialization of the organic process. In some, very fast developers, this can happen at the age of one year, maybe even before one; in a large majority of cases this happens between two and three years of age. Does the understanding that human life begins much later than previously thought give an adult the right to terminate the life which has begun at conception but is not yet human? Does it, in other words, resolve the question of the morality of abortion? No. It removes the arbitrage in the case from the jurisdiction of biology and makes the question one of purely moral choice and, therefore, more difficult to resolve. Rather than being the question about at which point an adult person may be said to commit child murder (only at birth, if life begins at birth, let us say), and thus become criminally liable, abortion becomes one about whether one has the right at any point to destroy the possibility of a human life—which begins at conception.

The understanding that humanity—the quality of being human—is not a *natural* quality of the animal species *Homo sapiens,* but is something acquired, quite by accident, by this species, and that human life begins significantly later than animal life, and only with the acquisition of the mind and culture, the internalization of the principle of the intentionality of signs and figuring out the organizing principle(s) of one or more symbolic systems, changes how one thinks of human life in yet another way. It strongly suggests that members of species other than *Homo sapiens* may be human as well. That remarkable bird, Alex, the African gray parrot, who did not know the word for cake, and therefore called it "yummy bread," could not pronounce the letter "p," and therefore referred to an apple as "banerry"—part banana part cherry, and who, parting from his featherless teacher and companion the night before he died, told her, "I love you," certainly was human. Literally, not metaphorically, human.[3]

This has been long acknowledged however tongue in cheek, by many, including some famous professional philosophers, in regard to dogs, as when Schopenhauer remarked, "I am often surprised by the cleverness, and now and again by the stupidity, of my dog; and I have similar experiences with mankind."[4] Now we can put the tongue back in its proper place, for, upon logical consideration, this is nothing to laugh at. Descendants of the wolf—the superbly intelligent wild animal, the only animal species besides *Homo sapiens* able to adapt to life everywhere on the planet—dogs have been living with us, in a "domesticated state," we say, almost since we ourselves have become human. As we, in return for many services, have thrown them scraps of our food (which they, more often than not, helped us to secure), we have thrown them scraps of culture and, therefore, have given them nascent minds. In their necessarily limited, unsophisticated and unthinking because speechless, way, they have been able to communicate and cooperate with us, often more efficiently than we communicate and cooperate amongst ourselves, and have adapted to our every society. In recent centuries they have become our pets, members of our families, assuming ever more complex and mentally involved roles in our lives. Like the overwhelming majority of hominid humans—a humbling fact we must always remember—they do not have the ability to write *War and Peace,* but they make excellent companions and, so I hear, very reliable nurses, general assistants for disabled, emotional healers, and police officers.[5] The fact that they lack the mechanical equipment for speaking severely limits their ability to use language internally. Apparently, congenitally deaf persons have a similar limitation: although sign language provides an adequate system of communication, no such person has ever been known to become a great—or even mediocre—creative writer. An early deployment of the mechanical ability to use language seems to be essential in its successful acquisition, even when one's larynx is in order. This is demonstrated by the virtual inability of feral children of seven or eight years of age to learn more than a couple of words. (A famous example is that of the Wild Boy of Aveyron, studied and treated in the early nineteenth century by the French physician at an institution for the deaf, Jean-Marc Gaspard Itard. The boy of about seven was found wandering, naked, dirty, and insensitive to heat and cold, in the woods of Aveyron. His only means of expression were inarticulate grunts. Itard took the child into his home, where, after about two years, the boy became affectionate and obedient, sensitive to comforts of a human home and to temperatures outside, very attached to Itard, and obviously capable of understanding human speech directed at him. In all these respects, he became like a dog. The only thing that distinguished the boy from a dog in terms of behavior was that he learned to articulate two words: "milk" and "God.") Clearly, as humans, dogs are severely handicapped by their physique. But should their physical disabilities, in our eyes, deny them humanity?[6]

The physical disability of the four-legged humans with tails and the absolute dependence of the human way of life on a purely physical organ of the larynx are most evident on the collective level. However intelligent and creative they may be (and a dog who can diagnose correctly the severity of his master's distress and, when it is unusually severe, dial 911 and whine into the phone, asking for help, is, clearly, very intelligent and creative), they could not transmit their acquired minds and, therefore, have never developed a culture of their own—all this because they do not have the larynx. The symbolic process on the collective level, culture, however, is essentially a process of transmission.

Culture and the Mind

One useful way to define culture is, in fact, as the process of transmission of human ways of life. This definition points to a crucial difference between humanity as a whole and all other species of life and underscores the break in continuity between the organic process and the human one. The comparison with animals inevitably leads to this definition. Humans are the only biological species, the continuation of whose existence is dependent on symbolic transmission, which is qualitatively different from genetic transmission. Thus culture is what distinguishes humans from the rest of the living world—it and none other is the distinguishing, defining, characteristic, which makes of humanity a reality *sui generis,* a reality of its own kind.

It has been long misleadingly assumed that this distinguishing characteristic is society—that is why "social sciences" is the preferred appellation for academic disciplines focusing on humanity, the most general of which, indeed, is called "sociology." However, society—structured cooperation and collective organization for the purpose of collective survival and transmission of a form of life—is a corollary of life in numerous species above, perhaps, the most primitive: it exists among birds and bees, ants and antelopes, fish and crocodiles, not to speak about such highly intelligent mammals as lions or, again, wolves. Social sciences focus on social controls over individual behavior, the ways it is shaped, if not determined, by social pressures. Social structures, they teach us, form "iron cages"—a favorite metaphor—around each of us, limiting the freedom we derive from our animal nature. But there is no freedom among animals; their lives are strictly regulated down to the smallest detail, and human society differs from theirs most saliently in the degree of its laxity, the weakness and malleability of its structures, the possibilities of escaping the so-called cages—which, on closer examination, turn to be made of something more like paper than iron.

The social orders of all other animal species are biologically, genetically, determined and transmitted. An individual ant or even wolf is an essentially social being, even if separated from the colony or pack from birth, because it carries the ant or wolf society—with all its controls and bonds—in its genes. A human being lacks such genetic determination and acquires a social nature only in the actual presence of the group; if separated from human society at birth or in early infancy (as we know from the few examples of feral children), this genetically pliable being, in fact, and as we concluded logically a moment ago, cannot even become human. In distinction to all other animals, humans transmit their social ways of life symbolically, rather than genetically. The word "culture," therefore, properly refers to all that is distinctively human in human society. Everything that is not culture in it is animal, and should be studied by biologists.

The products of cultural or symbolic processes are stored in the environment within which our biological life takes place, thereby dramatically altering the nature, including the physical nature, of this environment: they are stored in buildings, tilled fields, technological implements from hoes to computers, books, paved streets, unpaved streets, breeds of domesticated animals, articles of clothing, and so on. One can call such storage facilities for symbolic information—or such physical record of cultural processes—"cultural memory."

Culture, as we have stressed time and again—and which bears repeating until it is finally lodged in our brains as a physical record of neurobiological memory—is a symbolic process. Symbols, in turn, are vehicles of meaning. They are signs whose significance changes according to the context, or the other symbols among which they are used. This makes culture an historical process: it occurs in time, every unit (period) of which is unique and absolute, the preceding units serving as necessary conditions for—though never determining—the succeeding ones.[7] The contents of culture, the meanings and information that symbols convey, are never exactly the same, they are constantly changing, which helps to understand the relative flexibility of social arrangements based on culture, in distinction to organizations embodying genetic information. It is never precisely the same society that one generation—be it in the family, the church, the economy or politics—transmits to another. Culture never stands still; for this reason, "structure" is a poor metaphor for it, it fails to capture this pervasive fluidity.

In its constant change it constantly creates enduring material structures, transforming (permanently for beings with our lifespan) its environment. We humans, who live in changeable, lax, fundamentally unstable societies, developing autonomously from our biological constitution (which only provides the boundary conditions for them), have thoroughly adapted the environment to our ways of life, humanized it, appropriated it in the sense of making it a part of our ways of life, constructing a sort of *cultural capsule* around us, a world within a world. The outer world intrudes on us from time to time in the form of snowstorms that stop traffic, hurricanes that flood cities, earthquakes that destroy highways, and that other kind of natural disaster—organic disease (that also comes from the outer world, although it uses our bodies as a way in). Yet, we rarely take that outer world into consideration as we go about our daily business. Even our physical environment has become cultural, man-made, obedient to our wishes: beyond the obvious buildings, cars, shirts on our backs, or square watermelons, there are fields because we cleared them, forests because we planted them, miniature dachshunds and blue Abyssinian cats because we bred them, and Canadian wolves in Yellowstone because, after destroying the native population, we have brought them there from across the border. And still, as you have demonstrated, most of our environment is not physical, it is symbolic to begin with: our human world is a world of meanings, not of things, and even things we experience through the meanings suggested to us by culture.

To say that symbols are vehicles of meaning, however, implies that meanings no more inhere in them than passengers inhere in buses in which they ride. The ever-changing cultural process leaves permanent traces everywhere around us, but all such traces—products of cultural activity— whether we are talking of steel and concrete constructions, Granny Smith apples and Jaffa oranges, or of words printed on paper or written on vellum—are fossils of culture, its dead remains stopped in time. Disciplines in the humanities, literature, history of art, archeology, classics, history of material culture, etc., focus on such fossils. It is important to focus on them. It is also important to remember that culture is alive only as it actually happens, and it happens—that is meanings attach to symbols, exist, transform, etc.—only in us, by means of our brains. The perception of symbolic stimuli (i.e., of culture) by the brain creates the emergent phenomenon of the mind—the one active element in culture.

And thus by another route we arrive at the same conclusion that culture and the mind are not simply intimately related, but that the two are, in fact, one: the same process occurring on different levels. Note: our original argument to this effect was deduced from the proposition that the mind is an emergent phenomenon—we followed the logical implications of this proposition and in the course of doing so discovered culture. Our second argument was prompted by the comparison—the single most important tool for the construction of circumstantial (taken for empirical) evidence—between humanity and all other animal species, this comparison demonstrated that cultural transmission is the distinguishing characteristic of humanity, and a most cursory examination of culture (where we see the traces of the process and where it occurs) brought us back to the mind.

The mind—the emergent process that happens in the boundary conditions of our organic being and, specifically, by means of our brain—is a cultural process. Culture—the process of symbolic transmission of human ways of life that happens in the mind—is a mental process. We can never talk just about the one or the other, we must remember that it is always *mind-in-culture* or *culture-through-mind* that we are discussing. For this reason, psychology, whether of the psychodynamic or neurobiological variety, which focuses on the mind alone, can never tell us much about it. This, obviously, also applies to neuroscience itself.

Capacities of the Animal Brain

Let us now see what the comparison with animals can teach us about the mind.

Cognitive Capacities

We have already briefly discussed the necessity for the biological mechanisms enabling the individual animal to recognize (i.e., interpret) new signs, that is signs that are not genetically encoded, and quickly acquire the ability to read them in an environment of any complexity. The more complex the environment the more important are these skills, which neuroscientists call "learning" and "memory," for the survival of the animal, the more adaptive are, in other words, the mechanisms that enable them, and the fewer are the chances of those animals who lack these mechanisms to be selected for procreation.[8] Thus, it is reasonable to assume that the highly developed animal brain, adapted to the very complex environments in which most birds and mammals live, is highly capable of learning and memory, and this assumption is supported by a wealth of observations and experimentally obtained data. These are, therefore, evolutionarily produced capacities of the animal brain and we humans share them, as animals, with other animals.

The cognitive processes involved in learning and memory are far more complicated than they appear at first sight and than the words "learning" and "memory," as used in neuroscience, suggest. "Learning," connoting a process common to a primitive organism such as the sea slug Aplysia (which has been the focus of some very important research in the neuroscience of learning) *and* humanity, is used in neuroscience in the sense of experience of contact with the environment. But, clearly, the ability to recognize new signs involves much more than such an experience. To begin with, it involves a comparison—usually, a series of comparisons—with the already known signs. For instance, a lion cub knows that the sight of an approaching buffalo means danger that requires that the cub run away or hide. The smell of an approaching buffalo also means that. Then the cub experiences an approaching Land Rover. Its sight is quite similar to the buffalo: it is big, dark, it is moving swiftly, trampling everything on its path. The smell of the Land Rover, however, is very different from that of a buffalo or of any living thing the lion cub knows genetically. Does it signify danger too? Should the cub run and hide? The vehicle moves quickly, making strange noises: the conclusion also must be reached quickly. The lion cub hides, but his companion, another cub, does not. The Land Rover stops and appears completely uninterested in pursuing and harming the cub, who did not hide. An unusual- looking living thing (judging by the smell) emerges out of its belly, looks at the cub and, moving its paws unthreateningly, lifts and holds at its face an object. The cub concludes that a buffalo-resembling thing that is not alive with a living thing looking like no other living thing in it, while certainly a sign of curiosity, is not necessarily a sign of danger. But he is a very intelligent cub, who is suspicious of generalizing from one instance. Next time he and his less suspicious companion encounter a moving Land Rover our cub still hides. The big dark thing stops, a strange living creature appears, lifts an object that makes loud noise, and the trusting friend of the cub falls dead. It did not take time to *consider* the new sign. The intelligent lion cub makes a further comparison: the object in the paws of the living thing, which killed its hapless playmate, looked and smelled different from the object the living thing held to its face on the previous occasion. It concludes: guns kill, cameras do not; a moving Land Rover signifies danger unless proven harmless by the absence of a gun in the living thing's paws. "Learning" thus consists not simply in perceiving the unfamiliar environmental stimulus, but in *analyzing it in comparison* with what the animal knows already (from previous learning experiences or from the genetically encoded information). And it is the lesson learned through this analysis that the organism then records in its memory.

Neuroscientists use the term "memory" in the sense of a record of the organism's contacts with the environment. This record can be declarative or non declarative and can represent numerous aspects of the contact that is recorded: visual, spatial, temporal, emotional, olfactory, audial, tactile, etc.—i.e., it can preserve whichever aspect of the contact was perceived, that is sensed, captured by the nervous system. What is recorded, however, is the *learning experience,* which, in addition to perception, involves its analysis and interpretation, a cognitive, intellectual procedure performed by the brain with the information available to it, some of it newly acquired, some genetically encoded, and some already stored in memory. And it is this experience, part experience of a contact with the environment, part that of reprocessing and manipulation of already known information that is recorded in memory.

In a well-known experiment Dusek and Eichenbaum have taught a sample of healthy rats a number of associations with odors presented in different sequences and established that rats are capable of nothing less than transitive inference—namely, drawing valid logical conclusions from a set of premises, a mental procedure represented in the form of categorical syllogism. The animals are first trained to recognize patterns of sequential pairing of odors, which can be called A-B and X-Y. Trials after this training present the rats with an initial odor A and the option of choosing between odors B or Y. The correct choice, based on the cue of odor A would be to choose its pair of odor B and thus garner a reward for the animal (a Froot Loop)—if the initial cue is odor X, then the correct choice out of options B or Y would be Y. The pair associations are then expanded by the introduction of odor pairs B-C and Y-Z and then tested in the same way. In a third testing trial, all the rats responded correctly to a novel pair sequence where the cue and the choices were only indirectly associated (i.e., A and

C or X and Z) thus exhibiting the capacity for transitive inference, or for the interleaving of stimuli based on associative relationships.[9]

This intellectual performance is not different from a person "figuring out" the principle uniting a series of perceptually dissimilar objects into a category, as one frequently has to do in IQ tests or, in a far more complex and already mentioned case, of a child figuring out the principles of the mother tongue. The cue for the rats' astonishing behavior is not a part of the sensorially perceived features of the environment with which the organism was in contact. The inference that "if A leads to B, and if B leads to C, then A leads to C" is not information supplied by the environment—the clever rodents *create* it inside their brains; they guess, or *imagine* that this is so. When we say, in the human context, of simple syllogisms such as the one above, that the conclusion is "contained" in the premises, we use the word "contained" metaphorically, meaning that anyone with enough intelligence to recognize that the two propositions have the same middle term, will envision the conclusion in the premises. But, as is obvious from the fact that, unlike the rats in the present case, who perform uniformly well, some people do better than others in IQ tests that offer to them the same sorts of logical puzzles to complete; not everybody sees the conclusion in the premises: they need to perform some mental work to put it there first.

The ability of an animal to adapt to a complex environment and react appropriately to new stimuli within it, therefore, in addition to perception and committing to memory of information offered by the environment, depends on the mental process of creating supplementary information inside the organism. Such creativity, the ability to complete within the brain the information received from outside by adding to it the unknown information necessary for adaptation is not recognized among animals and therefore goes without a name. In humans, we call the ability to do so "imagination." Clearly, animals are capable of it at least to the extent required by the complexity and indeterminacy of their environment.

The fact that animals are able to *imagine* suggests that the new information can be generated inside the brain unconsciously—in the sense that the imaginer is not aware of the steps that lead from the perceived and stored to new information, but, so to speak, "jumps to conclusions" over these steps. Imagination, therefore, like learning and memory as defined by neuroscientists, is a capacity of the animal brain and should not be confused with *thinking.* Humans, obviously, too, very often imagine (supplement the information from outside and that already stored in memory) unconsciously, the imaginer being unaware of the intellectual steps he or she takes and only in rare cases and retrospectively being able to reconstruct them or think them through. (An example of such rare retrospective reconstruction is Einstein's musing on the question "What, precisely, is thinking?" in the context of an attempt to account for the manner in which he arrived at the theory of relativity in *Autobiographical Notes.*[10] It requires an exceptional mind to do this.) Logically, there is no reason why animals should be able to think, while there are weighty reasons why they should have the capacity for imagination. The empirical (circumstantial) evidence, constructed in accordance with the rules of logic but independently of these logical reasons, therefore is perfectly consistent with them: there is plenty of evidence of animals' imaginative capacity, but—unless we take into account some unusual behavior of our humanized pets—none of their ability to think.

Emotions

In addition to considering the cognitive, intellectual capacities of the animal brain, we must also consider its emotional capacities. This, among other things, will allow us to distinguish among several kinds of emotional experiences, which will be of service when we move on to the analysis of the mind.

It is obvious that animals are capable of *sensations*—that is, physical experiences—very similar to ours: they as well as we have the same physical senses, though not all of them equally developed. Thus, like us, they experience pain and pleasure, fear, positive and negative excitement (joy and anxiety), hunger and satiation, and likely deploy the very same neurobiological mechanisms, while having these experiences, as we do. These sensations may be called *primary emotions* because very often they represent the direct reaction of the organism to the stimuli of its physical environment. But, probably, in various combinations, they can also accompany and physically express more complex emotions that lack a physical expression specific to them. For example, it is clear that animals are capable of affection. Quite beyond the exceptional cases of the wolf who comes to give himself up to be killed by men whom he successfully evaded for ten years, because they captured his mate, or the lioness who adopts an infant antelope and stops hunting because she has no one to keep an eye on her hoofed baby—cases of affection so intense, self-denying, and doomed, that they can only be characterized as love tragedies, we see it plainly in the species of birds (penguins, swans) and mammals (wolves) who mate for life and in the relations between mothers and their young among numerous species of mammals.[11] Physically, affection is, most probably, expressed through sensations of pleasure and joyful excitement. Animals that are capable of affection are also capable of sorrow—which must express itself as a kind of, and through similar neurobiological mechanisms as, pain— the emotion they experience when they lose the object of their affection. Mothers losing their babies, babies losing their mothers, a frequent occurrence in the animal kingdom, provide us with ample evidence of that. Species in which affection extends beyond the nursery are also capable of sympathy and pity. Great apes, as well as wolves, furnish numerous examples. Finally, anger—an outraged authority—is also not unknown in the rigidly structured societies of the wild: this is what moves a dominant baboon to inflict a beating on an adulterous female in his harem or the male of the pride to discipline an upstart adolescent.

These emotions, which are once removed from their physical expression, may be called *secondary emotions*. Unlike primary emotions, their function (or the reason for them) is not to increase the chances of the individual organism's survival within the social order of its species, but, rather, to strengthen this social order and, therefore, ensure the survival of the species. The capacity for secondary emotions is genetic; it is built into the organism just like the mechanisms for sensations. Wolves are relatively small predators, preying on relatively large, often very large, prey; their chances of survival outside the pack are slim. Thus they mate for life, generate extended families, and share responsibilities in caring for their young. Their superior capacity for affection towards other individuals in their group reflects and cements their social order. Bears, who share the wolves' habitat, are large and omnivorous, both males and females survive perfectly on their own, thus they mate and part from their mates without a second thought, and the only affectionate relationship among them is the one between the female and her cubs, which must be taken care of for a relatively long period of time.

Primary and secondary emotions form important categories of our emotional experience as well. But most of human emotions are more complex, *tertiary emotions,* twice removed from their physical expression. These, though not unusual among our pets, do not exist in the wild. Tertiary emotions are emotions such as love, ambition, pride, self-respect, shame, guilt, inspiration, enthusiasm, sadness, awe, admiration, humility and humiliation, sense of justice and injustice, envy, malice, resentment, cruelty, hatred; one can go on almost indefinitely. They are not capacities of the brain and are not built into the organism, but are products of culture; their explanation is not, therefore, functional or teleological, but historical. The brain supports, but does not provide for, them. And, as they necessarily express themselves in the brain through the limited repertoire of physical sensations, neuroscience has no means whatsoever to access them empirically.

Animals also, to some extent, have moods. Moods are not specific emotions, but are, rather, general predispositions for emotions of certain kinds. There are, in fact, only two moods: good mood and bad mood; the other attitudes that are referred to as moods (such as "fighting mood" or "tearful mood") are, in fact, too specific to be so called—they imply a specific behavior and, therefore, a specific emotion. Moods may be, partly in humans and wholly in animals, a reflection of natural temperament; that is, the chemistry of the brain, but in the wild nature does not allow for temperamental variation beyond very narrow limits. Good mood is a general predisposition to react to things as if they were likely to be pleasant: one often observes it among young animals. The young animals that abandon themselves to this mood, however, are unlikely to survive for very long. The bad mood, a general predisposition to see the world as a source of pain, is not observed in the wild, probably because morose attitude spells almost instantaneous death. Humans are not hampered by moods: neither of them endangers their survival, though cheerful disposition, by definition, makes life more pleasant. It is a mistake to equate *happiness* with good mood, as is often done lately.[12] Happiness is not a predisposition to view the world in a rosy light; it is one of the most complex tertiary emotions known to humanity and to humanity only.[13] As a tertiary emotion, it must be experienced through physical sensations of which animals are as capable as we are. But the animal brain lacks the capacity to produce it and cannot be regarded as its source.

Emotions express themselves physically: we feel them; this is the central characteristic of this mental process that distinguishes it, in the human context, from the cognitive processes of thinking and symbolic imagination. Because in the organic world signification is essentially physical as well (that is the world signifies to the animal through physical sensations), cognitive processes in animals, such as learning and imagination, which lead a rat to a fruit loop through a transitive inference, must be at once cognitive and emotional. This suggests that human cognitive process, especially when un(self)conscious, also has an important emotional component, that our symbolic imagination and even explicit thought are emotionally colored, as it were, and it is impossible in fact and unwise in theory to separate sharply between cognitive and emotional functioning.

Adapting to the Symbolic Environment

Darwin's theory of evolution through natural selection makes it clear that the environment of any life process forms an essential part of, and represents the crucial creative or causal factor in, it. It is the environment, after all, that is the agency of natural selection, the environment that kills the weak, the less adapted, and selects the fittest for procreation. Life, therefore, can be properly understood only in its environment (most of it itself living); thus ecology is an extremely important field in biology. In the study of inanimate matter, the environment matters at least as much. It is the environment that gives rocks a certain shape, the environment that causes colossal pieces of them to fall into the ocean and raise enormous waves that, having rolled over vast distances, crush as tsunamis on the shores of far away continents, the environment that creates magnetic fields and holds planets in their orbits. Both matter and life are imbedded in their, physical in one case, organic in the other, environments, because, with these environments, they belong to the same interconnected universes, no single piece of which exists or can be understood in isolation. This seems rather unproblematic. The logic behind the principle advanced here, that the mind cannot be understood in isolation from culture, is not different. Why, then, has it taken us so long to arrive at it and why is it still so controversial?

There is no mind without culture, for it is culture that creates the mind, but it is the mind that makes culture a creative process. The two cannot be understood in isolation, and yet, this is the only way they have been studied. The humanities have focused on the fossils of culture—culture separated from the mind and therefore dead. Psychology and neuroscience have concentrated, allegedly, on the mind alone, cut from the environment that every nanosecond of its existence makes it what it is. (And social "sciences" have been preoccupied with other subjects.)

Neuroscience is the science of the day and its voice sounds loudest. Prisoners to the dualist philosophical tradition that has shaped all our thinking, neuroscientists, obviously, subscribe to its materialist variety. That is to say, they believe that the material aspect of reality alone is essential and autonomous, and that the spiritual aspect (e.g., human thinking) is somehow determined by or reducible to the material one. Thus they consider the mind as an emanation of the brain.[14] Based on the assumption that humanity is just a very highly evolved animal species—namely, that all the differences between us and amoeba are strictly quantitative—they mercilessly prick sea slugs on their sides and ply innocent rodents with electrodes, learning very interesting things regarding their captive subjects, and then extrapolate from these experiments with animals to the ways we think, feel, reach policy decisions, write books, and come up with scientific theories. So far, regarding humanity, one would be able to conclude on the basis of this work that humans are a very sophisticated but confused kind of rat: four-legged rats easily surpass us in simple Aristotelian logic. This leads one to suspect that a rat might be capable of a more reasonable extrapolation from the experiments with rats than the people who design these experiments. What a pity that rats do not publish scholarly papers and we, therefore, cannot put this hypothesis to a test.

Logically, it is not difficult to understand why experiments with animals cannot teach us much that is useful about the mind. To use a simple analogy, it appears obvious to anyone that lungs would be affected by the kind of air that one breathes or stomach by the kind of food one eats.[15] Why would the input of the environment into the brain have no effect? Clearly, the brain too must be affected by the kind of stimulant that is put into it. Similarly to the stomach that would process differently fatty foods and carbohydrates, or lungs that would react differently to oxygen and carbon monoxide, events in the brain should reflect whether the information it receives is sensory or symbolic. Studying the brain without taking into account the nature of the environment to which it reacts (not being aware of this environment, in fact) is similar to studying the stomach while giving no thought to its possible contents. Yet this is what is done when we extrapolate from experiments with animals to our experience.

Neither can this procedure be justified by the claim that our brains are more complex than those of the animals on which we experiment and, for this reason, produce reactions to the environment that are more complex: where aplysia contracts in reaction to a prick, we may, simply as a result of our complexity, react with a poem on spleen, for instance. We do not say, after all, that the food we eat is a product of our stomach (however complex it may be in comparison with that of aplysia), we are aware that it comes from outside and we only process it. Why should poetry—or language, to take a more common example of brain-specialists' discussion—be a product of our complicated nervous system? The mind is no more a product of our brain than this chapter is a product of the highly sophisticated word processor that is supporting my writing. It is produced *in* the brain *by* culture.

The Self-Sufficiency of Human Consciousness

Culture is the environment in which the process of the mind occurs and only in which it can occur. The qualitative differences between humans and animals have to do, first of all, with the fact that the complexity of the human environment is not simply greater than that of animals in the wild, but that it is of an altogether different order of magnitude. Animals carry their immediate and most important environment—their social environment, the organization of interaction with other organisms in their species—in their genes; it is a part of their biological constitution. Therefore, while members of other animal species have to adapt only to their physical environment and the organic environment of the species, human individuals have to adapt, above all, to their immediate, most pertinent, intraspecies environment— human society. They do not, like other animals, carry the constitution of society in their genes: it is genetically undetermined; they chart it symbolically (by symbolic means) and thus construct culture. We know this because of the almost infinite variability of human societies.

With the addition of symbolic stimuli and experience (with the emergence of the new reality of culture and the mind), the complexity of the environment increases exponentially and proportionally increases (as, we are told, it does even in rats brought up with stimulating toys) the mass of the brain.[16] This jump—between the natural animal and human-cultured brain—is so great, that all additional increments in the human brain mass (owing to the relatively greater complexity of the already cultural environment) may be considered negligible. This means, of course, that humans normally learn by an order of magnitude more than the most intelligent wild animals and store much more and much more varied information from the outside (the overwhelming part of which is qualitatively different—symbolic) in their memory. Much of this learning and memory takes place and is formed in infancy (probably, as was suggested earlier, while the child acquires language). And then, we manipulate this vast amount of information acquired from the outside—complete it, construct or create new information through imagination, and store products of our imagination, or records of our inner experiences, in our memory, to manipulate it again and again. A snowball effect is created. Most of the stimuli of the symbolic—primary for humans—environment are in fact products of the mental process itself. With the emergence of culture and the symbolic environment, in other words, *human consciousness* or *mental life* (though not the mental life of every human) becomes self-sustaining, i.e., independent.

Specifically, it becomes independent of learning above a certain minimum. Above a certain minimum, which may be received in childhood, the mind needs very little stimulus from the outside; instead it manipulates and remanipulates—namely, augments through imagination—information already stored in memory, much of which, to start with, it has created at an earlier point. Memory becomes the major reservoir of stimuli for the continued activity of the nervous system/the brain. In a way it competes with the environment; for some it becomes more important than the environment in the individual's efforts to construct the state of equilibrium/comfort. Or, perhaps, we can say that the cultural environment enters the brain in a major way to start operations there (thus returning to our definition of *the mind as culture in the brain*), thereby allowing the brain—or, at least, some brains—to contribute in major ways to the creation of this environment—something that does not happen in animals.

Symbolic Imagination

In addition to placing most of the resources of our symbolic environment
at our individual disposal in the mind and thus transforming the process
of consciousness from one consisting mainly in the reading of the environment to the one almost exclusively self-stimulated and creative, culture
also changes the nature of imagination. *Symbolic imagination,* that is,
imagination that operates with symbolic stimuli, differs significantly from
imagination that manipulates only sensual stimuli. The laws guiding symbolic processes (which one can observe in the development of Elizabethan
vocabulary out of fifteenth-century English or of higher mathematics, as
well as in the dynamics of American presidential elections or the New
York Stock Exchange) are irreducible to the laws of brain operations, if
only for the reason that symbolic processes, as was already mentioned, are
essentially historical, with the possibilities of any given moment or stage
being inevitably dependent on (though not fully determined by) what went
on in relevant symbolic processes in the past.[17] While brain processes, like
all the processes of extended matter, occur in a certain space, with the time
during which they occur having little significance (i.e., it may be extremely
important that a certain process takes place in a frontal lobe or the hippocampus, but it is of no importance whether it happens in the spring or
fall of 1917; on a November night in 1928 or 1938; on the ninth or the
eleventh of September in 2001), symbolic processes are nonextended and
happen in time, rather than in space. Thus the exact date on which a process occurs in the mind of a person will be of tremendous importance for
its nature and outcome: the symbolic imagination of a Russian would flow
in altogether different directions during the February and October
Revolutions, as would that of a German Jew before and after Kristallnacht,
or of an American previous to and on the day of the momentous terrorist
attack. The emergent regularities of culture and the mind are not reducible
to the potentialities of the animal brain. And, while the latter serve only as
boundary conditions, outside of which the cultural process cannot occur,
powerless to shape the nature and direction of cultural processes, culture
itself consistently orients the human brain, forcing its mechanisms into
patterns of organization and operation, which (though, obviously, not

impossible) are most improbable given all that we may know of the biological functioning of the brain.

There are very good reasons, for instance, why rats are, in general, better than humans at solving logical puzzles. An animal exists in a world naturally limited by the place its species occupies in the evolutionary process, its own evolutionary niche to which it is, by definition, well adapted, and which it, therefore, perceives as consistently ordered. It does not and, unless caught by us, cannot know any other reality. The physical environment presents itself to an animal in terms of signs, which, unlike symbols, are not open to interpretation. A piece of food is a piece of food, and cannot under any circumstances turn into a representation of a divine power or be experienced as "impure" and, as a result, become inedible; a predator feeding on one's kind is a danger to be escaped and will not be interpreted as a possible partner in peaceful coexistence. This, and the biological intolerance of physical contradiction (stimuli, whether genetic or environmental, which simultaneously instruct the organism to do A and to do −A) necessitate that any relationship between quanta of environmental information present itself to the animal in accordance with the strictest rules of logic. A rat, of course, does not know that it makes a "transitive inference": in this sense, its mental—imaginative—process literally represents "jumping to conclusions," i.e., traveling unconsciously some distance over individual links of a logical chain. But its conclusions, which supplement and modify information received from the outside, nevertheless remain fully consistent with this information; its imagination, in other words, is allowed no flight, it is dependent on and restricted by logic.

It is not so with humans. Humans, clearly, retain the biological intolerance of physical contradiction, which could translate into the Aristotelian principle of non-contradiction. However, our—largely cultural—environment presents itself to us in complex systems of symbols, rather than signs, and to most symbolic systems this fundamental logical principle which states that a thing may not *be* and *not be* at the same time, does not apply. (This makes it very unlikely that a culture not based on logic—as ours is—would ever even issue stimuli that could be experienced as a physical contradiction.) In the human world, a thing may very well be and not be (or have and not have some quality) at the same time, and usually is. There is no contradiction in Jesus Christ's being a man and not a man, God and not God at the same time. The idea of the Trinity denies the fundamental principle of logic twice. A piece of food may be perfectly appetizing, a man fully prepared to consume it, but, if a man is an Orthodox Jew and it is revealed to him that the appetizing morsel is pork, it would immediately become revolting and inedible on the account of its ritual impurity, and, if the man was hasty enough to taste of it, may even cause symptoms of poisoning, such as nausea, vomiting, and abdominal pain.

In fact, any and every symbol denies the principle of non-contradiction, for it is what it is, and yet so much more than what it is at the same time, that what it is (as a matter of actual fact) becomes totally insignificant and irrelevant to understanding what it is. A word, "mama" let us say, is just a combination of four letters, two of each kind, but for most people "mama" is an emotional, sensual, and cognitive reality which can make them jump for joy under some circumstances, become terribly sad under others, suddenly feel pangs of hunger and a craving for an apple pie, or experience a feeling of satiation and emotional fulfillment. Symbols, as already mentioned, necessarily exist in systems. This means that the relationships among them are organized and the principles of their organization have a degree of binding power. Some symbols go together, some do not, i.e., some are *consistent* and some are *inconsistent,* but not in the Aristotelian sense. Any set of principles of consistency (let us call it "operative logic") in accordance with which elements within a system combine and develop, that is based on the denial of the fundamental Aristotelian principle on which the deductive logic of propositions and quantification (which guides reasoning in rats, as we have seen, among others, and for which the name "logic" is usually reserved) will be essentially different from this logic proper. Only when symbols are reduced to signs, i.e., when all further possibility of their interpretations is precluded by an elaborate system of definitions, as in mathematics (and with a lesser success in other forms of disciplined, methodical discourse, oriented towards eliminating inconsistencies and uncovering hidden systematic relations between phenomena— i.e., science and philosophy), or by a system of rules, as in traffic lights, may principles of deductive logic apply to them. A red light signifies "stop" and is not allowed to be interpreted as "go" or even as "let's see, maybe if I drive through the intersection very slowly, it will be OK." It is a subject to the principle of non-contradiction in all its life-threatening severity. Neither can two plus two signify anything but four, not even a tiny bit more or a tiny bit less. And even when symbols are reduced to signs and are completely and inseparably identified with certain physical things, as in music (where a C-sharp under all conditions signifies C-sharp and cannot, do what you will, be interpreted as a B-flat or anything but a C-sharp) the "operative logic" of the system—namely, principles of its consistency—may not be deducible from the principle of non-contradiction. In music, clearly, the propositions "if A leads to B, and B leads to C" does not render the conclusion that "therefore, A leads to C" valid. That is why, among other things, implications of a musical proposition are referred to as "variations." Logic, obviously allows no such variability. The relationship between principles of musical validity and deductive logic is a complex issue.

In all other symbolic systems—that is, systems in which symbols remain symbols and are not rigidified into signs—operative logics are different from the deductive Aristotelian logic. Therefore, new information created within the human mind (by means of brain mechanisms) in the process of symbolic imagination not only supplements and modifies information learned, or received from the outside, but may also, and is quite likely, to contradict it (in terms of deductive logic) or be inconsistent with it (in terms of the specific operative logic of the symbolic system under consideration).

Only we human beings, and only human beings with a most powerful imagination—i.e., an imagination capable to traverse great distances over the links of a specific logical chain—can articulate a logic. Formal logical systems are, therefore, a creation of our imagination. But the fundamental principles which underlie logical systems are not our creation in the same sense: we do not create but *discover* them, that is, *become aware of their existence,* in the same manner as we discover, or become aware of, certain empirical regularities. Such discovery may be a result of introspection as well as of observing reality around us. The principle of non-contradiction, which is the fundamental law of logic proper, for instance, was discovered by Thales, the forefather of philosophy and science, in the image of one ordered universe made available to him by the first comprehensive formulation of Jewish monotheism. Rats do not have to discover logic: their world *is* inherently and unchangeably logical, so they know that a thing cannot be and not be at the same time (which, we are bound to conclude,

makes rats very much like scientists). Unlike rats, we, in our human experience, constantly encounter evidence to the contrary. The valid conclusion
from the premises "All swans are mortal" and "Zeus is a swan" is "Zeus is
immortal," which denies the principle of non-contradiction, and not "Zeus
is mortal," which affirms it. And there is no purely experiential (i.e.,
empirical) evidence to the statement that two plus two equals four, for this
is only so predicated on the abstract notion of a number and the definition
of experiential reality in terms of this notion. Two apples and another two
apples make four apples, only if a natural fruit is taken to be the unit of
apple matter. But what if this matter is experienced (i.e., empirically perceived through the sense of satiation) in ounces? In this case, two and two
units may equal half an apple, or three natural apples, making, empirically,
four equal three, or four equal one-half, namely, be and not be four at the
same time. (This can be also demonstrated using an example from the
Chinese philosophy of language—regarded in the West as an alternative
logical tradition. A self-evident presupposition that all linguistic distinctions, such as "large" or "small" are relative and imply no constant standard
of comparison, leads one to deduce that "reality has no distinctions in
itself," i.e., that "everything is one." In this case, our statement refers to
everything. This, however, renders everything, which equals one, and the
reference to it, making two. These two would be "everything," which is
two, but is one, and referring to this in language would make three, that is
"everything is one, is two, is three," and so *ad infinitum.*) Einstein only
generalized this inconsistency between human experience and the fundamental principle of logical thinking, when he declared, "As far as the laws
of mathematics refer to reality, they are not certain; and as far as they are
certain, they do not refer to reality." And yet, he also said, "One reason
why mathematics enjoys special esteem, above all other sciences, is that its
laws are absolutely certain and indisputable," which, in logical terms, contradicted the previous sentence.[18]

Though logic proper is the only logic with invariable first principles,
while in other "logics" such principles are context-dependent, historical,
and constantly changing, these principles are also "discovered," rather
than intentionally created. In fact, *symbolic imagination* in essence consists
precisely in the ability to discover and rediscover them in different situations and, on the basis of such discoveries, construct one's behavior. Of

course, "discovered," in the case of other symbolic "logics," means only that their organizing principles are metaphorically "contained" in the "premises," or pieces of evidence that one is given—just as the conclusion is "contained" in the premises of a syllogism; for a mind to actually perceive what is so contained, it has first to create new information within. The nature of the process of imagination—i.e., internal mental generation of new information—thus remains basically the same, whether we are concerned with essentially historical (and changeable) symbolic systems such as language or class structure, or with logic proper and mathematics which involve invariable first principles, and thus, on the level of mechanisms, the process of limitless, uniquely human *symbolic imagination* may remain basically the same as the limited imagination of rats. But because, the principles of other symbolic "logics," unlike those of logic proper, are context-dependent, evolving, and historical, and therefore binding only to a degree, there is more than one set of principles that may be "contained" in the same set of evidence, what one "discovers" may be different from that which is "discovered" by another, and mistakes—i.e., "discoveries" obviously inconsistent with a specific "logic" in retrospect—become institutionalized as a result of historical accident. In consequence, the imaginative process is far more difficult to reconstruct; and because it is so difficult to reconstruct, it appears so far more mysterious.

The subject is further complicated by the fact that we must always navigate between numerous interdependent and yet autonomous symbolic systems, each with an operative logic of its own. We are given very little information, i.e., we can learn very little from the environment, on the correct path of action in most situations we find ourselves in. But on the basis of the few pieces of data our imagination provides us with the clue to the puzzle—the logic operative in any particular case—and so supplies the missing information. Our—correct and incorrect—behavior then becomes a lesson, an additional piece of information to others and to ourselves, and so it goes, a symbolic system is maintained, the cultural process continues.

Take, for instance, a simple and limited symbolic system such as fashion. The Middle Ages did not recognize it. Everyone knew precisely what fabrics, cut, and color one was supposed to wear, depending on one's station; to transgress against this knowledge was a social offense, and mixing clothing appropriate to different positions represented a contradiction. But what about today? On the face of it, anyone can—and does—wear whatever one wants. And yet, we immediately recognize people who, as we say "have "taste" and those who do not. What we recognize in fact by saying so is precisely consistency in one case and an inconsistency in the other. What makes a combination of certain articles of clothing consistent and others inconsistent—after all, fashion changes all the time? Nothing but context. Once wearing an expensive fur with tattered jeans would be literally inconceivable; today they mix perfectly; once a flowing garment in silk charmeuse would be appropriate only in the bedroom; today it is equally fitting as formal evening wear at a most anonymous and crowded public gathering. And yet, despite these swings of fashion logic, we know when one is doing the right thing and when one gets it all wrong, and, what is perhaps even more curious, people are quite consistent in either having or not having taste: they either have a fashion-imagination or don't, either are sensitive to inconsistencies within this symbolic system or are not.[19]

Symbolic imagination, probably, is the central faculty of the human mind, on which every one of its functions and its very formation and perpetuation (thus the cultural process itself—the transmission of culture) depends in the sense that all of these other functions and processes occur by means of symbolic imagination. Our mental life, that is, the process of human consciousness, consists mostly of the "discoveries" of organizing principles and flights over links of various "logical" chains, very rarely made explicit and analyzed retrospectively, making imagination far, far more common than thinking. One is not human without the capacity for symbolic imagination, but certainly not all humans have the ability to think. This means that human consciousness in the great majority of cases operates most of the time unconsciously in the sense of not being conscious of itself, and that emotions play a much greater role in it than thought.

The Mind's Anatomy

Symbolic imagination is analogous to the tendencies or faculties of a living entity, such as the tendency towards homeostasis or breathing (rather than to organs or organisms) and to physical forces such as gravity (rather than to structures such as crystals), which can be perceived only in their effects. Such faculties and forces may be operative throughout the particular reality—physical, organic, symbolic—across various levels of complexity or hierarchy of structures. So, breathing is involved in every function and affects every organ of a living organism within a species, and were the individual organisms to stop breathing, the species itself would immediately cease to exist. Nor does gravity, apparently, discriminate among more or less complex physical structures, distributing itself equitably throughout the physical world on Earth. Other crucially important phenomena or processes of the mind, which are patterned or systematic (and must, for this reason, be supported by analogous, patterned and systematic, processes in the brain), can be envisioned differently. For heuristic purposes, it is useful to see them as structures, by analogy to organs and organisms. The mind itself, as suggested earlier, though a process, can be likened to an individual organism, which exists in a larger structure/process, analogous to a species—a culture. Within the mind, culture, supported by the imaginative capacities of the animal brain, transformed by the symbolic environment into the specifically human, symbolic imagination, necessarily creates three such "structures," which further distinguish the human mind from the mental life of animals. These structures are compartments of the self or of I and include (1) identity—the relationally constituted self; (2) agency, will, or acting self, the acting I; and (3) the thinking self, "I of self-consciousness" or the "I of Descartes."

Identity

The term "identity," in the sense pertaining to this discussion, refers to symbolic self-definition. It is the image of one's position in the sociocultural "space" *within* the image of the relevant sociocultural terrain itself. It contains and provides information regarding one's social status and one's standing vis-à-vis nonhuman symbolic presences, such as angels, ancestors, or the nation; one's relevant others, mortal and immortal, individual and collective, and the types of relations one is supposed to have with them, one's significant symbolic environment, including one's immediate and more remote social and cosmic worlds, expectations one may have of one's environment and vice versa, conduct proper to one under various, likely to arise circumstances (i.e., foods one should like or dislike, clothes one is supposed to wear, questions one is supposed to ask and issues one is supposed to be interested in, emotions one may legitimately experience and ones of which one should be ashamed, people one may befriend, marry, respect, despise and hate, and so on). In short, one's identity represents an individualized microcosm of the particular culture in which one is immersed, with the image of one's particularly significant sector in it (which may include God and his angels, paradise and hell, or one's immediate neighbors, colleagues, and fellow Red Sox fans) magnified and highlighted.

Identity is a logical implication of the nature of the human environment. Since the primary environment for humans is cultural and since, above all, individuals have to adapt to the intraspecies environment of the human society in which they happen to live, a cognitive map of this cultural social environment must be created in the brain. This cognitive map, which is the representation of the surrounding culture, and the social order (always in relation to the cosmic one), constructed on its basis, in the individual's mind (thus, individualized culture), may be accomplished by something like place cells which are responsible, as neurobiologists tell us, for the spatial representations—maps of the changing spatial environment—in the brain of a rat.[20] The individual's identity is his/her place on this multidimensional symbolic map. Like the indication of the rat's place on the spatial mental map, it defines the individual's possibilities of adaptation to the environment—or to refer to specifically human reality, "powers," "liberties," and "rights." Because the cultural environment is so complex, the human individual, unlike the rat, is presented by the cognitive map with various possibilities of adaptation, which cannot be objectively and clearly ranked. They must be ranked subjectively, i.e., the individual must choose or decide which of them to pursue. This subjective ranking of options is, in the first place, a function of one's identity.

Neuroscience fundamentally misunderstands identity. In the beginning of an authoritative popularization of the latest findings in that authoritative discipline, *Memory: From Mind to Molecules* (the title indicating the direction of scientific progress in the field), by two eminent neurobiologists, one of them a Nobel laureate, the authors, Eric Kandel and Larry Squire, propose to rephrase Descartes' statement "I think, therefore I am." It should instead say, "I am, therefore I think," they argue, because "all the activities of the mind arise from . . . our brain." They further state that there is "a second and larger sense in which Descartes' original statement is wrong.

We are not who we are simply because we think. We are who we are because we can remember what we have thought about. . . . every thought we have, every word we speak, every action we engage in—indeed, our very sense of self and our sense of connectedness to others—we owe to our memory, to the ability of our brains to record and store our experiences."[21]

We have already addressed in passing the logical fallacy of these authors' first criticism of Descartes.[22] Their second one concerns the nature of identity. Descartes' statement, however, does not touch upon this issue at all. It certainly does not mean that one's identity (as, say, the subject of the French king, or as a Catholic) is exhaustively defined by one's ability to think. In fact, the ability to think, in most cases should have nothing at all to do with the construction of one's identity. Identity (which is experienced, in part, as "our sense of connectedness to others," for instance to other Catholics or other subjects of the French king) is constructed by symbolic imagination out of the symbolic materials and perceived relations of a particular historical context. The cognitive map that represents this context is configured (i.e., figured out) by the symbolic imagination. Symbolic imagination, as was suggested earlier, is, probably, a largely unconscious process; it is not explicit and does not involve either thinking or the I constituted by thinking.

As the cognitive map is configured out of the information derived from the cultural environment, it is subject to change with some, but not all, of the changes in that environment. Only a most dramatic change of the map, as a whole, as a result of the virtual transformation of the environment is likely to affect one's own place on it, that is, change one's identity. This should be so because, at first, cultural stimuli enter the new human's brain as a jumbled mess: their organizing principles must be figured out. As the child figures out the organizing principles of various symbolic systems and begins to deploy the symbolic imagination, he or she also figures out where precisely he or she belongs in and vis-à-vis the symbolic environment, which is still in the process of being constructed itself. The significance of other objects on the map is then assessed in relation to that place. One's identity organizes the mess and the cultural environment is observed from its perspective. This means, among other things, that, rather than being determined by our experiences, as the neurobiologists above suggest, the nascent identity ranks these experiences, storing those it *selects* for memory in accordance with their subjective significance and forgetting most of them altogether.

How this happens is an important question that we are unprepared to answer at present. But both the little we know and ever-helpful logic suggest that the process of identity formation, like the process of symbolic imagination by means of which identity is formed, is a largely emotional process. Most of mental life, human and not human, is emotional to the extent that it is physically felt. Thus perceptions, in addition to information about the outside world (which contribute to the organism's or person's *knowledge* of the environment or what neuroscientists, speaking about animals on which they experiment, call "semantic memory"), that is, in addition to its cognitive content, have an emotional content. Environmental stimuli are delivered with an emotional charge, in other words. (In the example we have already had an opportunity to consider of the Wild Boy of Aveyron, the two words the feral child was able ultimately to learn— "milk" and "God"—could only be chosen because of the enormous emotional charge that they carried. "Milk" was emotionally charged because it signified the liquid apparently associated with a great physical pleasure; "God" must have been actually *delivered* very emotionally by people around the boy, who worshipped God and wished to impress his tremendous power and benevolence on this temporarily abandoned creature.) This emotional charge may be positive or negative and may vary in intensity. It is reasonable to suppose that identity is created out of the stimuli with the strongest emotional charge and, where there is a choice, those charged positively.

Because of its essential ranking function, identity must start forming early. As we know from experience, however, the process of its formation may be long and is not always successful. Identity formation is likely to be faster and more successful the simpler the (always very complex) cultural environment in which it is formed is—i.e., the fewer and the more clearly defined the relations that must be taken into account in the relationally constituted self are. For instance, in an isolated village community, in which all the denizens are practicing the same religion, obey the same authorities, speak the same language, wear habits of the same kind, enjoy (or suffer from) the same level of prosperity, it may be expected to form easily and quickly. But in a large cosmopolitan metropolis, in which people of different religions, political persuasions, levels of wealth, styles of life, and linguistic backgrounds mix, it would take more time and for many people would never be complete, especially if the metropolis is also pluralistic and egalitarian, and therefore the cultural environment does not rank its different populations itself, but leaves all the ranking to the individual. An implicit ranking often emerges naturally, or survives from the times of lesser pluralism and egalitarianism; in this case, one can expect that the characteristics ranked highest, i.e., assigned the most significance by context, would form the core of most individual identities, but this effect is likely to be mediated by details of individual biographies.

The relationally constituted self is the core element of the self. Identity is the central "structure" of the mind. Because it is formed by symbolic imagination, that is largely unconsciously, it is rarely made explicit. In general, people tend to *think about it* or to *think it through* (analyze it) only when it is problematic. History, however, especially comparative history, offers us numerous opportunities to observe it from outside. The last fifteen years of the twentieth century, for example, revealed that ethnic nationality, *believed* to be genetically ingrained and carried in blood, uniformly trumped citizenship, religion, language, political sympathy, and *personal experience* as the source/basis of one's identity in societies, often multinational, which have developed the ethnic-collectivistic variety of nationalism.[23] The powerful resurgence of national hostilities in Eastern Europe and Eurasia, which surprised observers in the individualistic nations of the West and which resulted in what these observers called "ethnic violence" on the scale unseen since World War II, was the reflection of this mental structure, of people seeing themselves, in the first place, as members of ethnic communities. This character of Eastern European/ Eurasian identity explained how an evocative retelling of a story of a centuries-old defeat, of which one could have no memory in the neurobiological sense, inspired thousands of Serbs to forget their political unity with other Yugoslavs (i.e., Southern Slavs) and, despite their neural memory, stored in the brain and easily recoverable, of consistent personal experience of good relations with those of them whose ancestors once converted to Islam, take arms against these people. In an individualistic nation, such as the United States, which offers its members an enormous variety of choice in regard to self-definition, the power of identity (of relationally constituted self) over personal experience is demonstrated in less dramatic circumstances. While native-born Americans find it difficult to understand the raging passions in Eastern Europe (or the Middle East), to naturalized Americans from these regions the intensity of Americans' party affiliations, i.e., their commitment to either the Democratic or Republican Party, is nothing less than astonishing. To the nonnative eye, there are no significant differences between the platforms of these parties, and whatever subtle differences between them may exist are assiduously obfuscated during presidential campaigns which seek to appeal to the everyman in the center. Yet, generations upon generations of *hereditary* Democrats and Republicans would vote for their party's candidate, even though, as their conduct during primaries shows, they may, in fact, detest and mistrust him, and even though the specific policies he (yes, we still must use the male pronoun) advocates happen to go against their interests.[24] To claim that our identity—"our sense of self and connectedness to others"—is a reflection of our personal experiences stored in the neural memory, against this background, is to treat evidence rather cavalierly.

Similarly to the mind in general, of which it is the central structure, but to a greater extent and in a more specific sense than other mental structures and processes, identity, while necessarily a physicochemical representation in the brain, is a reflection and a representation of the particular cultural configuration of the time. Thus it is a part of the environment of the mind and the brain, as well as a part of the culturally modified structure of the brain itself. It is at once internal and external to the brain. As a representation of the (particular cultural) environment, identity should force itself upon the brain as any external stimulus. It, as it were, issues commands to the brain. Identity is a *symbolic* self-definition, a *relationally constituted* self, an image a human individual has of oneself as a cultural being and a participant in a particular cultural universe. At the same time, it is clearly an essential element of human mental—cognitive, emotional, and pertaining to social adjustment—functioning and health. Changes in certain peripheral aspects of identity are possible, but any change in its core (i.e., crises of identity, doubts about one's identity, multiple identities) translate into mental problems, affecting one's ability to learn and commit information to memory, the adequacy (in other words, cultural propriety) of one's emotional reactions, and the degree of one's social adjustment.

How problematic any change in identity is depends on which of its many aspects lies at its core in any specific case (e.g., being a Christian or being an American) and which undergoes the change (the core or one of peripheral aspects). Identity mediates between one's natural or animal capacities to learn, memorize, adapt to the environment—the capacities of one's animal brain—and one's functioning as, in fact being, a person, one's humanity. Obviously, an individual endowed with different natural mental powers from those of somebody else would learn, memorize, and adapt differently, but so most certainly would an individual with equal natural powers but a different identity: somebody who defines oneself as essentially an independent actor would have much greater difficulty to learn, memorize, and adapt to an environment in which independent action is frowned upon than a person of equal natural abilities defining oneself as a cog in a machine. Similarly, a damage to one's natural capacities (as a result of physical trauma or impaired growth) will undoubtedly be reflected in one's mental performance, but a damage to one's cultural identity (as a result of a traumatic experience, such as immigration or "loss of face," or in consequence of impaired formation) will alter mental performance as dramatically.

Like all mental processes, identity must be supported by brain mechanisms, thereby representing a process that can be studied experimentally with methods of neuroscience. But this mental process is unique to human beings, it is a constituent process of the human mind—an essentially symbolic, cultural phenomenon—and therefore it cannot be studied and understood by neuroscience unless in designing their experiments neuroscientists factor in the constant, pervasive and transforming, influence of culture on the animal nature in humans. So far, unfortunately, neuroscience has added nothing to our understanding of the mind. Fortunately, logic, comparative history, comparative zoology, and introspection contain a vast wealth of evidence and can bring us a long way towards such understanding.

The Will (Agency, Acting Self, "the Acting I")

Identity, which is the agent of a particular culture, does not issue commands to the brain directly; it does so through the "structure" of human *agency, will,* or acting *self,* the creation of culture in general. Human beings are carriers of will and discretion; they are—each one of them, if normal—independent actors in the sense of being capable of action and not just reaction, whose actions (except involuntary reflexes) are products of decision and choice. This *will* is a function of symbols—to operate with these intentional, thus arbitrary, signs, we internalize the principle of their intentionality; the will, therefore, like identity, is logically implied in the symbolic reality of the mind. When reacting to a cue, whether externally or internally generated (for instance, the election of a new president or a spontaneously firing nerve that triggers a memory-recall of an unpleasant incident at a doctor's office), we are capable of voluntarily interrupting the ensuing mental process, saying to ourselves, for example, "I don't want to think about this now," "I do not want to react to this in such-and-such a way," and thereby of shaping our response. It is to this intermediate stage between stimulus and reaction/action, in which, for humans, the nature of response is still indeterminate and must be decided that the word "consciousness" is frequently applied.

Conscious recall, in this specific, peculiar to human experience, sense of intentional, actively—though not necessarily or even often self-consciously and explicitly—*willed recall,* is something of which animals seem to be incapable. Indeed, there is no evidence to the contrary, and, logically speaking, there is no reason for them to be capable of it. Rats, even rats brought up with stimulating toys, seem to be making very few decisions, such as "even though I know that the Froot Loop is in cup D, I don't want to dig for it." If a—hungry—rat knows, it digs; and it is precisely the fact that rats lack an independent will and may be assumed always to want what they are genetically programmed to want, that makes possible learning experiments with them. In this they are dramatically different from my dog who, when offered perfectly edible and nutritious meal at the time he may be safely supposed to be hungry, usually takes his time *deciding* whether or not what is in his bowl corresponds to the nutrients he craves at this particular moment, and, if his decision turns to be negative, expresses his lack of excitement by an obviously disappointed vocalization and plainly tells me, "Forget it. I don't really know what I want, but if you won't give me what I want, I am going on a hunger strike." A human subject, indeed, unlike a rat, may decide to dance on the sand concealing the

Froot Loop, and this decision is independent of the subject's intelligence or capacity for transitive inference.

Moreover, humans are capable of independently, i.e., *at will,* generating cues and starting mental processes. For instance, a person may say to oneself, "I want to remember such-and-such episode" or "I want to begin thinking about such-and-such subject," and thereby start the process of memory recall or manipulation. One can study transitive inference in rats among other things because rats do not have a will: there is no doubt that they will want the Froot Loop—they are forced to want it. Humans are not genetically forced to want almost anything—perhaps to evacuate and to sleep—every other genetic imposition, including hunger, sexual desire, and pain, can be resisted by the will. How do we acquire binding volitions, i.e., desires that compel us to act?

The mind must include "structures"—mechanisms capable of blocking the biological information the brain generates, when this information interferes with the processing or creating of symbolic information. More generally, it must contain mechanisms that, for every event, select the "operative logic" (or logics) appropriate to the context, while suppressing other "logics." The will, or agency, or acting self—that part of our mind that makes decisions, is such a structure or set of mechanisms. What does the *will* do, specifically? It arbitrates in cases of contradictory stimuli. Most often, such arbitrage is unconscious and involves no effort (of will) on our part: we simply receive, and obey, an instruction of the sort: "In the case of the Christian doctrine (or the Jewish law, or ancient Greek mythology, or a grammatical structure, such as the affirmation that "nobody understands me") you will forget rules of Aristotelian logic." It is this ability to block one logic to attend to another that explains how people can live quite ordered and contented lives in a contradictory environment. (In the Soviet Union and Soviet-dominated Eastern Europe—to use an example from ancient history—such ability, evident from the fact that everybody knew that the social system was based on a pack of lies and yet staked one's entire life on the validity of its presuppositions, was attributed to the development of a "double consciousness."[25] In actuality, if a consciousness can be equated with a particular symbolic logic, we all necessarily develop multiple consciousnesses and, depending on the occasion, skillfully select among them the appropriate one.)

But the will's arbitrage may involve a conscious effort, and it is for the cases when it does that the language—at least, in the West—reserves the concept of the "will." For instance, one may be tired and wish to lie down, but have unfinished work (such as formulating the present thesis), in which case the *will*, will instruct the organism: "You will pay no attention to your fatigue, but will be guided by the logic demanding you to finish the work you have started." Late in the evening, however, it will issue a different instruction: "You will now lay down your work, though unfinished, and take care of your fatigue, (because otherwise you won't be able to continue your work tomorrow)." Or, in the case of a soldier fearing for his life, the *will* may declare, "The logic you will obey at present is that of a collective military enterprise. Therefore, you will expose your life to danger and disregard the survival instinct which instructs you to run away and hide." Or, in the case of a scholar building a career, the *will* may prompt the person to prefer the logic of scientific inquiry ("Go and raise questions about the dominant theory, on the acceptance of which your promotion depends, because you know this theory to be erroneous") to the "logic" of collegial harmony and career building ("Keep your mouth shut and pretend to accept the dominant theory, though you know it to be erroneous, because your promotion depends on such acceptance"). It is in regard to such choices that we talk of the "free will." By definition, the *will* is free: it is always up to the human *agency,* to the (acting) *self* (though not always to the human being) to decide which symbolic tack to take. Everything else in a person may cry against a certain action, and yet the person's will, the agency, will impose itself and the person will do its bidding. (I am referring here to cases such as a person *submitting* to an arrest or a painful or dangerous operation. Clearly, he or she would not like to submit, but the will, deciding the situation, concludes that the other courses of action are inappropriate—because unrealistic, for instance—and makes the person submit.)

We refer to that will as a "strong" one, which systematically imposes on the person the "logic" considered to be more difficult to follow. Of course, what is so considered changes with the context, and so do the "logics" of symbolic systems themselves; these "logics," let us repeat, are context-dependent and, for this reason, essentially historical: they evolve with the system, and with the system in which the particular system evolves, and thus do not have first, fundamental, principles. All culture-based "logics," but one, are variable. The only invariable logic is the logic based on the principle of non-contradiction. Therefore, this logic, from which all the other "logics" are different, this logic proper, remains the only standard, the only universal medium of translation, and the only way to formally and explicitly resolve and eliminate inconsistencies between other logical systems. But the will follows this logic rarely.

Symbolic imagination is travel over the links of various "logical" chains. Will, agency or acting self is the mechanism for making choices or decisions. We are able to deploy our imaginative capacities correctly, namely, in accordance with the appropriate symbolic "logic" thanks to the arbitrage of the will, while the will's arbitrage, much as our capacity to learn and memorize, is mediated by identity (the relationally constituted self). Clearly, it would be much easier for a person unambiguously self-defined as a soldier to risk his life in the face of mortal danger, rather than try to save himself; his identity will, in effect, screen the logic of self-preservation from him, making him, so to speak, "single-minded" in his sharp awareness of the dictates of proper soldierly conduct. A person unsure of whether being a soldier is really "him," in contrast, will be much more likely to hesitate and run for cover. Similarly, a person lacking intellectual confidence (i.e., suffering from self-doubt and uncertain of the validity of one's ideas) would be more sensitive to fatigue and ready to procrastinate and be distracted from unfinished work, than one who has a clear identity as a thinker and so does not question one's ability to produce scholarship of fundamental value. Problems with identity impair the will, making the person indecisive and unmotivated, while an impaired will interferes with routine functioning of symbolic imagination. (This, as will be seen later, is, schematically, my view of functional mental disease.)

The will/agency/acting self is the function of the *autonomy of human consciousness*—i.e., the mind's independence from the natural environment and from learning and memory related to the natural environment, the mind's being self-sustained, which makes possible a multitude of desires—and of identity (or relationally constituted self), which represents to the individual his/her options. Thus, it is the expression of *subjectivity*. There is no subjectivity in rats or even monkeys, unless these are pets, even though, given the nature of learning and memory, every rat's and certainly every monkey's brain is unique, and there is individuality in monkeys and rats. But because monkeys and rats do not have choices, the uniqueness of every animal's brain does not give rise to subjectivity, and there is no need in agency, will, and self. However unique, the knowledge and action/reaction of a rat or a monkey are objective (shared by others within the species), making every rat or monkey a representative of all rats or all monkeys.

One can speculate about the system in the brain that supports the will. Perhaps, it is neurons similar to those that make possible in rats the perception of the stimuli which require an adaptive reaction, transmitting to other neurons the command "do this or that," neurons whose function it is to sense desires imposed on animals by their genes, but in us culturally constructed and mediated by consciousness and structures of the self (even though not necessarily consciously mediated: a person is not always fully aware of what he or she wants). Whatever that brain system, culture determines the individual's likes and dislikes, programming the brain to will certain things—programming the will, like the rat's "will"(i.e., the rat)—is programmed genetically. Identity presents to the individual the possibilities for the given historical time, helping to establish their subjective ranking: because you are what you are (a Catholic or a Muslim, a wife or a soldier, a member of the aristocracy or a registered Democrat) you must will this and not this. It commands the will what to choose and to decide. In every specific case the will and the identity are determined by culture. The vast majority of the records or representations in memory are also determined by culture—the contents of memory, thus, the raw material of the imagination, are culture-given. What is done to these records in the brain (i.e., how they are manipulated) depends both on the brain and the organization principles of the particular symbolic system(s). But cultural selection—i.e., the social success of some imaginings and the failure of others depends exclusively on the historical context, that is, again, on culture. It is important to keep in mind that, unlike natural selection, cultural selection does not weed out imaginings not selected for success at a certain historical moment: they are not killed, but only left latent. In changed historical circumstances or in the presence of a genius there is always the possibility that these temporarily unselected imaginings will have their day.

The "I of Descartes"

Finally, there is the tremendously important structure, the structure of consciousness turned upon itself, to which Descartes referred in his great statement "I think, therefore I am" and which I, therefore, called the "I of Descartes" or the "I of self-consciousness." It is the thinking part of us. In distinction to all other processes and "structures" of the mind, which I have postulated in this chapter, the existence of the "I of Descartes" is not a hypothesis. It is, rather, the only certain knowledge available to us. We are all aware of it. We all know directly by experience, that is, we all know empirically, that it exists. This knowledge is absolute; it is impossible to doubt it.

It is very good that this is so, because the logical reasons for the existence of this mental structure are less obvious than those that help us to account for identity and will. Given the character of human environment, both these structures are necessary for the adaptation to this environment and, therefore, for the survival of every individual one of us. But one does not need the "I of Descartes" to adapt to life within culture. Dogs, for example, seem to adapt to the symbolic environment without necessarily developing the ability to think, as we have defined it. And, if they can do it, we, presumably, can do it too. One can argue, of course, that a fully human existence would be impossible without it, but such quantitative judgment is quite likely to lead us eventually to the unacceptable conclusion that only a genius (a very rare, thus abnormal, human condition that indeed depends on the "I of Descartes") can be fully human.

The logical necessity for the "I of Descartes" is of a different kind. While human beings can well do without it, human existence without it would be impossible. It is a necessary condition for the culture process on the collective level: what makes possible self-consciousness for any one of us is precisely that which makes possible indirect learning and thus the transmission of human ways of life across generations and distances. A functional (logical) explanation is not the only explanation and (with the exception of the mathematically based physics) rarely the best one. Lots of cultural and organic phenomena exist "just so," because they have happened to evolve, for reasons that are purely historical. Still, functional explanations are heuristically helpful and, besides allowing us to deduce the existence of the phenomenon from its context, aid us in analyzing it, that is deducing its special features.

In history, where functional explanations rarely, if ever, apply, we must rely heavily on circumstantial evidence. Most of the circumstantial evidence regarding the mind comes from comparative history and comparative zoology—comparisons between different cultural environments (the simple fact of their variety suggests the structure of identity, for instance) and between humans and wild animals (all our hypotheses in regard to the self-sufficiency of human consciousness and its largely inexplicit and emotional character, to symbolic imagination, and to will or agency are deduced from comparisons between our environment and its demands, on the one hand, and the environment of organic life and the animals' responses to it, on the other). Similarly, it is from comparative zoology we deduce that to transmit human ways of life we need the "I of Descartes." In the sense that it exists in all cultures it is a universal human characteristic, but it is not certain that it exists in every human being. I have already mentioned such an obviously humanized species as dogs, wonderfully adapted to our symbolic environment. It is not even clear that every ordinary human of the titular *Homo sapiens* variety thinks; all jokes aside, it is quite possible that, unless specially prompted to do so, many do not, i.e., they lack an impulse, a necessity to think.

Based both on the circumstantial and on the empirical (direct, therefore, introspective) evidence, there are a few things we can say about the "I of Descartes." Among all the symbolic mental processes, it is the one which is *explicitly symbolic;* it is not just a process informed and directed by our symbolic environment, but it is as essentially symbolic process as is the development of language, or of a musical tradition, or an elaboration of a theorem—or as is the transmitted culture, in general—in the sense that it actually operates with formal symbols, the formal media of symbolic expression. This is the reason for the dependence of thought on language, which has been so frequently noted. Thinking is only possible if such formal media are available, as they are in music, mathematics, visual art, and in language, above all. Our thought extends only as far as the possibilities of the formal symbolic medium in which it operates.

This presents an enormous problem for neuroscience: how to account conceptually for the perception, storage in memory, and recall of purely symbolic stimuli which may only acquire sensual components in use, after they are conceived in the mind, and these components are necessarily minimal (e.g., these words I am typing and you are reading acquire a visual component only after I have thought them and you perceive them at once visually and in their meaning, which touches only your mind, but none of your bodily senses). What *is* a perception of an idea? What is perceived and which organ perceives it? The translation of such stimuli into the organic processes of the brain, which must occur, because everything that happens in the mind happens by means of the brain, is beyond the current ability of neuroscience to imagine. Perhaps neuroscientists are blissfully unaware of this problem, because, even though they often talk, they rarely think of the specifically human mental functioning.

In the framework of the layered view of reality, however, this problem of translation is easily resolved. We, therefore, have all the reasons to hope for a development in the science of the mind similar to that which happened in the biological subdiscipline of genetics, which, called into being by Darwin's evolutionary theory, started to reveal the specific mechanisms of evolution through natural selection some forty years after Darwin had postulated it. Similarly to the process of breaking organic processes into its physicochemical elements that happens in the translation of organic stimuli, including the process of perception itself, into physical and chemical reactions in the brain, a process of breaking (from top down) of symbolic stimuli into its organic elements (reconstructing symbols as signs that are sensorially perceived, for instance) must be responsible for such translation, which would differ from the biophysical translation only in degree of its complexity, i.e., quantitatively. We are capable of perceiving, storing in memory, and recalling at will various aspects of our environment. It makes sense that we would intuit—but intuition would break into perception—and thus perceive and recall a string of information couched in formal symbols in the formal symbols in which it was couched; that is, perceive and recall a word not sensually, but by its imaginary sound, a geometric shape by its imaginary sight, and a melody by the imaginary sound and/or the sight of the corresponding notation. Do we actually *hear* the words and melodies in our heads? They are there, but the great majority of words in our vocabulary we have never actually heard, for we know them from reading only, some of them we have, like Alex, the remarkable human bird, invented, and a composer hears the music before putting it on paper or trying it on an instrument, and can do so, as the astounding example of Beethoven proves, even while being physically deaf. The actual confusion of these inner sounds with sensual hearing is called, as we soon will be discussing, "auditory hallucination" and is commonly considered a sign of a severe mental dysfunction, specifically of schizophrenia. This suggests that mentally dysfunctional individuals do not distinguish between symbolic and sensory stimuli and, specifically, do not distinguish between culture within (symbolic stimuli without a sensory component) and outside (symbolic stimuli with a sensory component) their brain. This also means, in regard to mentally functional humans, that we are actually processing—and experiencing—unembodied sounds, sounds that do not have any material and, therefore, sensual reality (though they can acquire both these realities, when outwardly expressed or objectified in the course of the cultural process). The experience is possible because the symbolic (meanings) naturally breaks into the sensory (signs).

Our conscious recall of such non-sensual information would necessarily be an explicit recall. The act of will, under different circumstances implicit and, as a result, unobserved, in cases of recalling explicit symbolic information (human semantic memory) will be self-observed (by the "I of Descartes") and become a subject of self-consciousness. The opportunities for observing one's consciousness are numerous: we might recall stored explicit information for comparison with any new learning experience with explicit symbolic systems in the environment, that is, with music, mathematics, visual art, but, above all, anything at all in language, and then we might wish to recall and manipulate and remanipulate it again and again. Then not only the process of consciousness and symbolic imagination, in general, which is largely unconscious (in the sense of unselfconscious and inexplicit), but also the process of thinking—of talking to oneself in language, mathematics, music, and explicit visual images—becomes self-sustaining and self-sufficient. I suppose this is what we mean when we talk about the "life of the mind." The "I of Descartes," which does not have to be involved in regular mental processes on the individual level (such as symbolic imagination which is for the most part unselfconscious) in such cases, is perfectly integrated with and involved in them. It performs the function of the *thinking self* and becomes an integral part of the mind as individualized culture and of the person. But it is important to remember that this is not the essential function of this mental structure, its essential function is to assure the symbolic process on the collective level. It is enough that some humans develop an active "I of Descartes" for this process to continue and for culture to be maintained. And because it is unnecessary, it is unlikely that the thinking self and the life of the mind in its specific meaning of the life of thought would be all that common.

It is, however, precisely the process that must occur in the uncommon cases of *genius*. A genius is a mind coordinated with culture to an unusually high degree. This close coordination between the symbolic process on the individual level and the symbolic process on the collective level is expressed in the complete individualization of the "I of Descartes," its appropriation as the *thinking self* and full integration with other, necessarily individualized, mental processes. As a result, it is characterized by an unusually powerful symbolic imagination, capable of leaping huge distances over particular "logical" chains. This also means that an imagination which is not symbolic, is not enough, and not even a wolf intelligent to the point of uniqueness, i.e., an exceptionally intelligent member of an exceptionally intelligent species, can be a genius. The same, I am sorry to conclude, is true for dogs. Dogs can equal people in intelligence and they have symbolic imagination, but there can be no geniuses among them, because the unusually powerful symbolic imagination in genius is powered by formal symbolic systems. There are not many geniuses in the whole of human history, and they are recognized, indisputably, only in a number of areas: in literature, in mathematics, in science, in music, and in visual art. Too often even in these areas we use the word imprecisely, as an intentional exaggeration; whenever we use it in other fields we, consciously or unconsciously, use it as a metaphor. Like so many other concepts that capture an important reality, the word "genius" is rarely defined and is used mostly without a precise meaning behind it. And yet, there is a close to universal consensus in regard to a very small number of people throughout the Western tradition, that these are geniuses. What they share may be said to constitute genius. These people, whose right to be so called is very, very rarely disputed, include in visual art Rembrandt and the High Renaissance trio of Leonardo da Vinci, Michelangelo, and Raphael; in literature, Shakespeare; in music, Mozart and, perhaps, Bach; and in mathematics and science, Newton, Darwin, and Einstein. There are some others whose claim to the status of genius is rarely disputed, but they are not as universally known; there are, clearly, also a number of geniuses rarely, if ever, so called (the word acquired its present meaning only in the eighteenth century and was not, except in visual art, in which special right to it was asserted, applied too far in retrospect), but who must be so called, if we are to define genius as what unites these nine or ten universally acknowledged geniuses. But this is beside the point.[26]

What unites these undisputed geniuses in art, literature, music, and mathematics/science is their ability to establish the organizing principles of a particular "logic" of great complexity on the basis of relatively limited learning experience and then make it explicit, i.e., think it through, or reconstruct it in an explicit symbolic medium. The complex "logic" in question may be that of biological evolution (perceived and explicitly reconstructed/formulated in language by Darwin); it may be the organizing principles of a new form of social experience and organization, which came to be called "modernity" (perceived and captured in words by Shakespeare—a subject to which much attention will be devoted in subsequent chapters); it may be the "logic" of musical resources inherited and perfectly realized in the inimitable oeuvre of Mozart or of the visual aspects of the human form at the height of physical perfection, fully imagined and explicitly reconstructed by Michelangelo, Leonardo, and Raphael, and of the actual, ever and, with age increasingly, imperfect human form, made glorious by Rembrandt, or the iron, mathematical logic of Newtonian physics, presented in the formulas of *Principia Mathematica*.

The outcome in all these cases of ultimate creativity on the individual level of the symbolic process is a new page in cultural development on the collective level, a dramatic cultural change. Genius either brings to a full realization and so exhausts the symbolic resources of the time (in the respective symbolic system) or, uncovering new resources, it outlines the framework in which activity in the area continues until the system exhausts itself. Only new directions were possible after Mozart and after Rembrandt, they could be imitated only intentionally and thus were truly creatively inimitable, and it is not coincidental that the style of Mannerism (i.e., intentional and exaggerated imitation, working in the manner of) followed

High Renaissance art. In science, Newton defined physics from his day to the end of the nineteenth century; Einstein did the same for the later period, and Darwin provided the foundation for contemporary biology with all its ramifications. As to Shakespeare, we still live in the world he did more to construct than any other single individual and perhaps many a social force combined of numerous individuals. (Postpone judgment of this statement for now; we shall have many opportunities to discuss it.) The phenomenon of genius allows us to articulate the mechanisms that make the mind and culture interdependent. The relationship obtaining between the symbolic process on the individual level and that on the collective level in the cases of the mental structures of identity and will (or of the relationally constituted self and acting self) is reversed in the case of the "I of Descartes" appropriated as the *thinking self.* While it is evidently culture that creates identity and will in the mind, it is the thinking self of the individual mind that generates culture.

Evidently, certain characteristics of the individual brain contribute to the making of a genius, as they do to other, less unusual cases of artistic (broadly defined) and scientific creativity. It is not clear what these characteristics are. Surely, they are not the ones measured however accurately by IQ tests. Superior intelligence (capacity for logical thinking) is, probably, involved in genius in science and mathematics, but does not seem of particular importance for one in music or literature. The definitive characteristic of genius, undoubtedly, is a characteristic of the mind not of the brain. It is having the vast resources of a certain sphere of culture at the mind's command, at one's *willed* recall—that is, the complete individualization of the mental structure of "I of Descartes," its perfect integration with the structures of identity and will, and becoming a component of the self. It is not the degree of development or activity of this structure that matters, but its integration with the other two processual systems that reflects the unusually close coordination between the mind and culture. A very developed and active "I of Descartes," often combined with acute intelligence, may lead to madness as well as to genius, and, if we remember how much more abnormal (that is rare) the condition of genius is from that of madness, is rather more likely to lead to the latter. In this case it must change its function too. Instead of being the "I of self-consciousness," which the "I of Descartes" is by definition, it must become the *eye of unwilled self-consciousness,* culture not individualized observing the mind and experienced as an alien presence within the self.

We are now in a position to attempt a new culturalist interpretation of schizophrenia and manic-depressive illness. Let us see whether the clinical descriptions and the findings of neurobiological, psychological, and epidemiological research justify the thinking that leads to it.

II

PSYCHOLOGICAL

3

Madness in Its Pure Form

Schizophrenia

Despite advances in our knowledge about schizophrenia in the past few decades, nothing allows us to surmise that the causes of schizophrenia will soon become known.

—Norman Sartorius, "Twenty-Five Years of WHO-Coordinated Activities Concerning Schizophrenia," *Recovery from Schizophrenia: An International Perspective; A Report from the WHO Collaborative Project, the International Study of Schizophrenia* (Oxford: Oxford University Press, 2007)

State of the Art 1: Current Definition and Classification

Schizophrenia is widely considered the most severe and least susceptible to treatment of severe mental diseases, "the cancer of the mind," "madness in its pure form," "the quintessential form of madness in our time." Its causes are unknown and there is no cure for it. A world's leading expert on this condition, Irving I. Gottesman, wrote in 1999:

> Many scientists from various fields have studied this most puzzling illness closely for nearly 200 years. . . . Dozens of therapies for severely disordered minds have been tried, from spinning chairs to bloodletting to psychoanalysis, to no lasting avail. It was not until the early 1950s that specifically antipsychotic drugs successfully came into use, not as a cure, but as an aid in alleviating some of schizophrenia's most troubling symptoms—the delusions, hallucinations, and disordered thinking. Neuroscience and social science have explored blind alleys, as well as many avenues that have yielded new understanding of how the brain and nervous system function and how drugs affect them. *Still, we have no clear consensus among experts on the cause or causes of schizophrenia, and it does not yet have a cure.*[1]

The defining feature of schizophrenia is psychosis. In this it differs from the other two of psychiatry's "big three"—the bipolar, or manic-depressive, disease and the major unipolar depression—which may also present with psychotic symptoms, but not as defining features.[2] According to the latest so far, fourth, edition of the *Diagnostic and Statistical Manual of Mental Disorders* (*DSM-IV*), the definition of psychosis itself is problematic:

> The term psychotic has historically received a number of different definitions, none of which has achieved universal acceptance. The narrowest definition of psychotic is restricted to delusions or prominent hallucinations, with the hallucinations occurring in the absence of insight into their pathological nature. A slightly less restrictive definition would also include prominent hallucinations that the individual realizes are hallucinatory experiences. Broader still is the definition that also includes other positive symptoms of Schizophrenia (i.e., disorganized speech, grossly disorganized or catatonic behavior).[3] Unlike these definitions based on symptoms, the definition used in earlier classifications (e.g., *DSM-II* and *ICD-9*) was probably far too inclusive and focused on the severity of functional impairment, so that a mental disorder was termed 'psychotic' if it resulted in 'impairment that grossly interferes with the capacity to meet ordinary demands of life.' Finally, the term has been defined conceptually as a loss of ego boundaries or a gross impairment in reality testing.

Specifically in schizophrenia, *DSM-IV* continues, "the term psychotic refers to delusions, any prominent hallucinations, disorganized speech, or disorganized or catatonic behavior." But in some other psychotic disorders, "psychotic is equivalent to delusional."[4] "Schizophrenia" itself is defined as "a disturbance that lasts for at least 6 months and includes at least one month of active-phase symptoms (i.e., two or more of the following: delusions, hallucinations, disorganized speech, grossly disorganized or catatonic behavior, negative symptoms)." To qualify for the diagnosis these signs of the disorder must be associated with marked social or occupational dysfunction and cannot be attributed to "the direct physiological effects of a substance or a general medical condition," that is, the disorder cannot be considered organic. Schizophrenia is a mental disorder "without a demonstrable brain disease."[5] It is this that distinguishes it most sharply from organic psychotic disorders, which are numerous.

As was mentioned in the Introduction, the diagnosis of schizophrenia is a product of the late nineteenth-century classification revolution in psychiatry, which not unexpectedly began in Germany. The revolution was led by Emil Kraepelin (1856–1926), a psychiatrist and then professor at Heidelberg, who believed that schizophrenia was a brain disease and devoted his life to finding what kind of a brain disease it was. As in many other fields, of which economics, perhaps, represents the most striking example, in Germany psychiatry emerged some three hundred years later than in England and at least half a century later than in France, and it emerged as first and foremost an area of research and theoretical discussion.[6] Where their British and French counterparts tried to devise means to treat and take care of those who suffered from mental disorder that they observed as physicians, lawyers, and policy makers, the first German psychiatrists focused on the concepts with which to analyze it. Thus both the name of the field—"psychiatry"—and most of its lexicon came from Germany.

As concerns specifically schizophrenia, "the definitive categorizer" Kraepelin at first used the French term *demence precoce* (early loss of mind, *dementia praecox* in Latin), which was coined in 1860 by Benedict Morel, to distinguish a form of dementia with an early onset and rapid development from the common geriatric dementia.[7] Kraepelin then separated *dementia praecox* from manic-depressive insanity (called by the French *folie circulaire* or *folie à double forme*), with which until his classification revolution it was believed to constitute the general category of insanity (*madness* or *lunacy* in the original English), and distinguished within it a number of varieties, such as catatonia, hebephrenia, and paranoia—an old term newly used for delusions of grandeur and persecution. Central to Kraepelin's diagnosis of *dementia praecox* were delusions (of the paranoid kind, among others) and hallucinations, which imply imaginative hyperactivity. But the term he kept suggested something different: a progressive mental lethargy—the loss of mind, similar to the geriatric dementia. The influence of Morel's original conception and term proved so profound that, throughout the twentieth century and despite the replacement of the initial name by "schizophrenia," the psychiatric community in general continued to interpret the disease as implying mental degeneration (explicitly argued by

Morel), and specifically as the degeneration of cognitive or ratiocinative capacity.[8] Kraepelin himself lent considerable support to this view, for the basis for his distinction between *dementia praecox* and manic-depressive illness was precisely the course and outcome of the two forms of psychosis, *dementia praecox* being supposed to steadily progress towards and almost invariably terminate in a complete loss of mind; it is likely that he adopted not just Morel's term but his concept as well.

The evidence has consistently contradicted this classic interpretation, the signal mark of schizophrenia being not the weakening of the intellect or inability to think, but its bizarre character, the inability to think normally, i.e., in the commonly accepted way. Indeed, a compatriot and near contemporary of Kraepelin, Karl Jaspers, known more as a philosopher than a psychiatrist, characterized the thought of a schizophrenic as "ununderstandable" to others, but itself exhibiting a "fine and subtle understanding" and revealing the grasp of "the profoundest of meanings."[9] A century after Jaspers, an experimental psychologist Louis A. Sass dedicated a hefty volume to the demonstration of the intellectual acuity of schizophrenia, assembling very large quantity of data collected by researchers and clinicians throughout the twentieth century on the subject, which allowed him to argue that schizophrenic thought and expression display "the sensibility and structures of consciousness found in the most advanced art and literature" of our day. Schizophrenia, he insisted, is associated with "a heightening rather than a dimming of conscious awareness," and can well be interpreted not as an escape from but as too much consciousness.[10] At the end of the twentieth century, despite all the evidence for it, this view was still very unusual in the schizophrenia research community.

The other part of Kraepelin's original definition—the postulate that schizophrenia almost always ended badly—was also contradicted by evidence. "Since the early 1980s, a body of epidemiological evidence has taken shape . . . challenging the early Kraepelinian view that the long-term prognosis for schizophrenia was almost uniformly poor." The series of the relatively recent (1973–1996) WHO-sponsored cross-cultural epidemiological studies of schizophrenia, which is the main source of current knowledge about this disease around the world, found, in fact, that in the "developing" countries both short- and long-term outcomes varied mostly between "good" to "excellent" and could hardly be more "at odds with the more pessimistic view."[11] Yet, schizophrenia is still considered a sort of dementia, i.e., a disease primarily expressed in the weakening of the mind, and it is still distinguished from manic-depressive illness on the basis of its course of steady deterioration towards the outcome of increasing cognitive deficit.

To avoid the misinterpretation of schizophrenia as a progressive deterioration of the intellect, obvious to an unprejudiced clinician (that is a clinician not educated to see the disease as such), and focus attention on its symptoms, which accompanied delusions and hallucinations, a Swiss psychiatrist Eugen Bleuler in 1908 proposed the term "schizophrenia," meaning, "splitting of the mind."[12] Bleuler wished to stress the dissociation of various mental processes, the cognitive and emotional ones, in particular. The disease, according to him, consisted primarily of "the four A's": abnormal thought associations, autism (self-centeredness), affective abnormality, and ambivalence (inability to make decisions). The two first of these features could be characterized as cognitive impairments, the third pertained to emotional functioning, and the forth was a problem of the will. Delusions, hallucinations, and catatonia, emphasized by Kraepelin, were, in Bleuler's view, secondary to these.[13] Bleuler, however, was influenced by Freud, and therefore tended to see mental dysfunction as mental retardation, the inability to develop higher intellectual functions as a result of unresolved childhood conflicts, for instance dismissing the "very common preoccupation of young hebephrenics with the 'deepest questions'" as "nothing but an autistic manifestation."[14] Thus psychoanalytically inclined followers of Bleuler also failed to see the significance of the hyperactive intellect in schizophrenia.

The diagnosis of schizophrenia continued to evolve into the 1930s. An eminent German psychiatrist of the time, a student of Jaspers, Kurt Schneider, postulated the so-called "first-rank symptoms," the possession of which allowed to classify a patient as a "nuclear schizophrenic." These included:

1. Voices speak one's thoughts aloud.
2. Two or more voices (hallucinated) discuss one in the third person.
3. Voices describe one's actions as they happen.
4. Bodily sensations are imposed by an external force.
5. Thoughts stop and one feels they are extracted by an external force.

6. Thoughts, not "really" one's own, are inserted among one's own.

7. Thoughts are broadcast into the outside world and heard by all.

8. Alien feelings are imposed by an external force.

9. Alien impulses are imposed by an external force.

10. "Volitional" actions are imposed by an external force.

11. Perceptions are delusional and ununderstandable.[15]

The current classification of schizophrenia in *DSM-IV* (and its World Health Organization's counterpart *ICD-10*) still reflects the thought of these four German-language psychiatrists. Until quite late in the twentieth century, American and Western European psychiatric research and respective practices differed in emphasis, Americans preferring Bleuler's approach associated with psychoanalysis, which was dominant in the United States, while their colleagues in Europe favored the "more scientific" understanding of Kraepelin. Since Bleuler's diagnostic criteria were wider, many more cases of mental disorder in the United States were diagnosed as schizophrenia than in Europe. When the American and the British practices were compared in the famous 1972 US-UK Diagnostic Study, it became clear that conditions classified on this side of the Atlantic as schizophrenia would, in the old world, be treated in 75 percent of the cases as bipolar or manic-depressive illness.[16] In the last thirty years, owing mostly to the accidental discovery of anti-depressant and antipsychotic drugs, which were, in some cases, effective,[17] psychoanalysis lost its caché in the United States, the stock of neurobiology rose, and American psychiatry converted to the Kraepelinian (called now neo-Kraepelinian) paradigm of our European brethren.

The symptoms of schizophrenia today are divided into positive ones, referring to distortions or exaggerations of normal functions, such as delusions (distorting inferential—logical—thinking), hallucinations (distorting perception), disorganized speech (affecting the normal organization of thought and language), and bizarre behavior monitoring (distorting the behavioral function), on the one hand, and, on the other, negative symptoms, lessening or diminishing normal functions. These include alogia—lack of fluent speech, affective blunting—lack of facial expression, avolition—lack of motivation and drive, anhedonia—lack of capacity to enjoy, and asociality—inability to interact with others or social maladjustment. These negative, non-psychotic (and only quantitatively different from the normal) symptoms would, obviously, impair the patient's everyday functioning at least as much as positive and specifically psychotic ones (qualitatively different from the normal). Negative symptoms are also more often resistant to drug treatment. Two types of schizophrenia are recognized, Type I, which mostly presents with positive symptoms, and Type II, presenting predominantly with negative symptoms. The outcome is generally better for Type I, as is its responsiveness to drugs and, remarkably, premorbid adjustment. All around it seems to be better to be delusional than to suffer from disorders of will and affect.[18]

In addition, *DSM-IV* distinguishes five subtypes of schizophrenia: paranoid, disorganized, and catatonic; and in addition residual and undifferentiated. Paranoid schizophrenia is characterized by preoccupation with delusions and hallucinations and shows no disorganized speech, catatonia, or flat affect; disorganized schizophrenia is especially marked by disorganized speech and behavior, and often inappropriate affect, but does not meet criteria for catatonic schizophrenia, while this latter is diagnosed when the patient shows at least two of the following: (1) motoric immobility, catalepsy, stupor; (2) excessive motor activity that is apparently purposeless; (3) extreme negativism or mutism; (4) peculiarities of movement, stereotypies, odd mannerisms, or grimacing; (5) echolalia or echopraxia. All these three subtypes, it is important to stress, present with positive symptoms, all of which, specifically in schizophrenia, as already indicated, are equated with psychosis (though only delusions would qualify as psychosis in other forms of psychotic illness). This leaves one somewhat uncertain as to the nature of Type II schizophrenia, schizophrenia being defined as a psychotic illness to begin with.

According to the *DSM-IV,* the onset of schizophrenia usually occurs in the late teens to early thirties, with modal age of onset being eighteen to twenty-five for men and twenty-five to thirty-five for women. Men are believed to be more susceptible to the disease and face a worse prognosis. The disease is usually chronic, only 22 percent of patients having only one episode and no residual impairment. 35 percent have recurrent episodes, 8 percent have recurrent episodes and develop significant impairment, and 35 percent have recurrent episodes, develop a significant impairment, and the impairment is becoming worse with time. Seventy-eight percent, therefore, do not recover. The great majority never marry or have children, and most are unable to support themselves. Thirteen percent of diagnosed schizophrenics commit suicide.[19]

Separate schizophrenic episodes proceed through three characteristic phases: the prodromal phase with little if any functional impairment, manifesting itself in certain behavioral, emotional, and cognitive abnormalities (some of which correspond to negative symptoms) which usually go unnoticed before the disease is diagnosed, though being quite striking in retrospect, that precedes the presentation of obvious psychotic symptoms, sometimes by many months; the active phase of psychosis; and the residual phase which is similar to the prodromal phase, though functional impairment is more noticeable (whether because it is greater or because it is expected) and psychotic symptoms may continue. Remarkably, schizophrenia presented with an acute onset, obviously psychotic from the beginning, has a better prognosis than the one with a prolonged prodromal phase (insidious onset). Since good prognosis in schizophrenia is atypical, this suggests that acute-onset schizophrenia corresponds to the atypical one-episode/no residual impairment schizophrenia. If this is indeed so, this renders suspect findings regarding schizophrenia in "developing" countries, where, it appears, at least the plurality, and sometimes the majority, of cases identified are those with acute onset and, as already noted, good outcome.[20] Could it be that many of these cases, then, are not cases of schizophrenia at all or a type of schizophrenia very different from the one observed in Europe and North America? Most descriptions naturally focus on the active phase of the syndrome and pay certain attention to the residual one. An extensive discussion of the prodromal phase is rare.[21]

State of the Art 2: Current Views on Etiology

Despite prodigious developments in biology and in neuroscience, in particular, schizophrenia is still diagnosed on the basis of its psychopathology (observed abnormalities of language and behavior), just as it was in the days of Kraepelin and Bleuler. The breakthrough is imminent, insists Gottesman, but "there is not yet a blood test; urine or cerebrospinal fluid analysis; or CT (computerized tomography), rCBF (regional cerebral blood flow), PET (positron emission tomography), or MRI (magnetic resonance imaging) brain-imaging scan that can establish an unchallenged diagnosis of schizophrenia." This is because no biological abnormality has been found that is specific to schizophrenia and exists in all cases. Indeed, *DSM-IV* stresses: "no laboratory findings have been identified that are diagnostic of Schizophrenia [though] a variety of laboratory findings have been noted to be abnormal in groups of individuals with Schizophrenia relative to control subjects."[22] This "scientific" uncertainty as regards the diagnosis makes the search for an organic cause, however relentless, futile. As in any other field, in biology, one cannot explain a problem when one does not know what the problem is.

As in much biological research, statistics plays the role of the searchlight. Several correlations have been considered suggestive and several causal avenues explored. For instance, it has been "shown convincingly" that being born in winter-spring correlates with an increased risk of developing schizophrenia.[23] The common explanation for such seasonality is epigenetic. However, it is difficult to explain epigenetically why, of all possible birth dates, the risk is highest for those whose life begins on Halloween, the thirty-first of October.[24] Thus the significance of seasonal variations remains a mystery. The same may be said of a correlation established between high heels and mental disease, and between the population of pets in a society and specifically schizophrenia in it.[25] The latter is considered by one of the most eminent schizophrenia experts of our day, E. F. Torrey, as the proof for his theory that schizophrenia is an infectious disease, spread by pets.[26] The theory is reasonable, and a certain parasite, responsible for several, mostly neurological, diseases, *Toxoplasma gondii*, whose *definitive carrier* is the cat, has been found. But the parasite is carried by almost half the human population, less in those areas where pets are common, and indoor, pet, cats have been entirely cleared of the awful suspicion cast upon them: they and *Toxoplasma* do not keep company. It is important to keep in mind that believing in the significance (not just statistical) of a possible statistical finding is the main reason for undertaking a statistical study. A correlation, when established, reinforces this belief, and we forget that statistics is a descriptive, not an explanatory, tool. It is absolutely certain that, were we to try, we would find statistically significant relations between schizophrenia and color of one's eyes (as in, "having green eyes increases your risk by so-and-so much"), one's height and weight, or one's predilection for Assam as opposed to Ceylon tea. We do not check for these possibilities because the hypotheses, to begin with, appear to us absurd. Unexpected statistical findings may often be very suggestive, but alone, statistical findings never explain anything.

The most "scientifically" promising area in the search for the organic causes of schizophrenia in the past one hundred plus years has been genetics. Darwin suggested in *The Descent of Man* that certain mental capacities and personality traits among humans may be hereditary, as in animals, and it was Darwin's cousin and the father of human genetics, or eugenics as he called the new discipline soon to become so important, Francis Galton, who in his 1869 book *Hereditary Genius* devised a statistical method for calculating traits' heritability, still used in macrogenetic research, and pioneered the study of such capacities. But the first to undertake a genetic investigation in psychopathology was Emil Kraepelin. In 1915, having completed much of his classificatory work, he founded a research institute which was to focus on the genealogy of psychiatric patients, choosing a certain Ernst Rüdin as director. Rüdin was to become mainly known for his contribution to the purification of the German genotype by means of the Nazi Law to Prevent Hereditarily Sick Offspring (responsible, among other things, for the execution by experimental methods, such as gassing, of about 100,000 mental patients). But before turning his attention to the improvement of the racial stock, he published in 1916 the first systematic study of heredity in schizophrenia, done with "proper statistical methods," which concluded that having a schizophrenic parent or sibling significantly increased one's risk of developing the disease and that, therefore (here followed a very important non sequitur) schizophrenia was genetically transmitted.[27]

Today, extensive research in psychiatric genetics of the type undertaken by Rüdin (i.e., nonmolecular and based on Galton's calculation of genetic overlap between relatives) and consisting of family studies, adoption studies, and twin studies, leads to the congruent conclusion. The risk of schizophrenia among relatives of schizophrenics appears to be significantly greater than among general population and roughly proportional to the degree of genetic overlap. This is still regularly interpreted as suggesting that "there is a big genetic component" in the etiology, or causality, of schizophrenia, but such interpretation remains unwarranted. It should be remembered that an overwhelming majority of schizophrenics do not procreate (which, somehow, does not result in the selection of alleged schizophrenigenic genes out of the genetic pool), that 89 percent percent of schizophrenics do not have schizophrenic parents and 81 percent do not have first degree relatives who are schizophrenics, as a result of which the numbers with which we are dealing are remarkably small.[28] The optimal research design, controlling for the environmental input, is the study of identical twins, separated at birth and brought up apart, at least one of whom is a schizophrenic. But life does not cooperate with the statisticians: by 2001, only fourteen such cases were described in the literature—"a dangerously small sample for any generalization." (So says the author who then proceeds to generalize: "the shared genotype seems to matter much more than the shared experience.")[29]

The small numbers would not matter in two cases. If (1) all the relevant environmental socio-cultural factors were identified, attention equal to the one paid to the possible effect of genetics were paid to these factors, and the findings of equally careful studies in regard to their effects were fully consistent with the findings of macro psychiatric genetics; or if (2) a specific gene were identified in molecular genetic research either actually causing schizophrenia (as in Huntington disease or phenylketuronia) or without which it could not possibly happen (a necessary condition though not a cause). But neither of these cases obtains. Whatever attention was paid to the sociocultural environment focused only on a few factors consistent with the prevailing psychiatric approach, extremely limited in its understanding of the environment at all times. Significant cross-cultural variations in the course and outcome of schizophrenia (such as the relative immunity of the "developing" countries to severe form of the disease with insidious onset, chronic course, and poor outcome, affecting prosperous Western nations with depressing regularity), observed time and again by participants in the WHO-sponsored epidemiological studies, by 2000 convinced these researchers in that the affliction they "observe, measure, contend with, and treat is not nature's mischief alone, but the work of culture too." But, declared the editors of the report of these path-breaking studies, the International Study of Schizophrenia, urging the exploration of "an 'upstream' (or primary causal) role for psychosocial factors in the development of schizophrenia.":

The sustained inquiry and customized tools needed to take the measure of "local moral worlds" were conspicuous by their absence in [the earlier of] these studies. . . . Fifteen years later [2006], we still lack even the limited cultural data collected early on by the [earlier] substudies that would make for modest comparative analysis. Nor have we made substantial analytic headway in resolving the "dilemma of context" . . . [30]

Thus the environment—and most factors in it that could be relevant—was never analyzed. And there is now a consensus that no specific, causal "schizophrenia gene" exists. All that the existing macro psychiatric research allows us to conclude in the absence of "the schizophrenia gene" in fact is that "genetic factors may be responsible for a certain portion of the vulnerability to schizophrenia," that is for a person's individual (inborn or acquired before the onset of the disease) predisposition to it.

There is a consensus that 70 percent to 80 percent of such vulnerability is accounted for genetically.[31] The figure is impressive, but let us examine the logic. Individual predisposition is at most a condition for, not a cause of, developing schizophrenia; and we do not know whether this condition is necessary. One may have no predisposition for developing the mental habits of a scientist, or an MD, or a lawyer, or a violin player, but, pressed by one's environment (the prestige of science, medicine, law, art; the desires of one's parents, etc.) go through an appropriate schooling and develop them nevertheless. Granted, one is not likely to become a brilliant scientist or concert soloist in such a case, but one certainly can become a member of a team at a research institute, a music teacher, and even a very successful cosmetic surgeon or lawyer. Why should this be different with the mental patterns (otherwise: habits) of schizophrenia?

It has been established that the vulnerability to schizophrenia, like most human genetic traits, is polygenic. Gottesman explains:

The numerous polygenes associated with a particular disease coact with each other and other factors to produce pathology, . . . each has only a small effect on trait variation [in our case on the predisposition to schizophrenia] as compared to the total variation for that trait. Therefore, the expression of the trait depends much less on which polygenes in the specific system a person has . . . than on the total number pulling him or her toward an extreme. A feature of special interest in the study of schizophrenia and other major mental disorders is the ability of such polygenic systems to store and conceal genetic contributors to the liability to developing the disorder.[32]

In other words, given that the trait in question is only a condition for, rather than a cause of schizophrenia, it cannot be expressed unless the disease is actually caused by something else. Even presuming that vulnerability is a necessary condition for schizophrenia, its causality may be analogous to infectious diseases such as tuberculosis or AIDS. It is quite possible that a certain genetic makeup is necessary to succumb to either of these dangerous illnesses, carried by specific agents (the *Mycobacterium tuberculosis* or the HIV), but such genetic makeup becomes a vulnerability only in the presence of the agent; no agent—no vulnerability, in other words.

Perhaps, we tend to assign such great importance to "vulnerability" in the case of schizophrenia because we interpret it as a latent part of the disease itself and assume that, as such, it represents an abnormality, in the sense of being a feature of a small minority of the population. But we do not have a good reason for such an interpretation. By 2007, "research has begun to identify some of" these vulnerability or susceptibility genes.[33] A particular gene, related to the serotonin system, has been isolated, whose main function is to regulate another gene, producing the protein (disabled by Prozac in cases of depression) that transports serotonin away from the synapse. All of us have two copies of this regulating gene, which exists in a long form and in a short form. The large majority of the human population (68 percent) have at least one copy of the short form, while slightly less than one-third minority have two copies of the long variant. Having two copies of the long form of the gene is abnormal—it is a characteristic of a minority of human population. But it is the short form of the gene in question—the normal variant—that has been found to contribute to the "liability of mental illness"![34] There is a definite possibility, therefore, that it is human nature that predisposes us to schizophrenia. To the extent that human nature is genetically shaped, there is indeed a big genetic component to this predisposition. However, this also means that such ubiquitous vulnerability is not a latent element of a disease and that its explanatory value is nil.

No amount of genetic research can possibly lead us to the discovery of the "bacterium schizophrenicus" or a mosquito that may serve as its vector. In 2007, Norman Sartorius, the President of the World Psychiatric Association, the former Director of the WHO Division of Mental Health, and a Professor of Psychiatry at the University of Geneva, published the following statement: "Despite advances in our knowledge about schizophrenia in the past few decades, nothing allows us to surmise that the causes of schizophrenia will soon become known."[35] All this does not mean that the knowledge we have accumulated—anatomical, neurochemical, and genetic—is worthless. In a completed solution of the schizophrenia puzzle it will undoubtedly have its place, most probably answering the many questions as to how the cause leads to the various aspects of the disease. Only that the many pieces of this useful knowledge do not combine into an account of schizophrenia and leave the question of its etiology open. We still know nothing about what causes the disease and nothing we know points to where we should look for it. For this reason, preeminent experts warn, we have no reason to hope that "the prevention of the disorder will become possible in the immediate future" or "that it will become easier to help people with schizophrenia."[36] We must look for circumstantial evidence— the circumstances in which people who develop schizophrenia are placed, not in, but around them. Since statistics—in this case epidemiology—has been the tool used within the schizophrenia research community, we should start with the consideration of epidemiological findings.

State of the Art 3: Epidemiological Findings

"*The* definitive source book" on the disease, *Schizophrenia Genesis*, opens with the following declaration: "If madness is as old as humankind, we might be tempted to assume that schizophrenia, one of today's best known and most common forms of madness, has been present since the dawn of civilization. No conclusive proof of that assumption exists."[37] E. Fuller Torrey, called "the most famous psychiatrist" in this country today,[38] is one of the very few people who consider the absence of evidence for the historical ubiquity of schizophrenia important. As mentioned earlier, he argues that schizophrenia, together with manic-depressive illness, is indeed a new, previously unknown disease, transmitted by an infectious agent, carried by pets, common (i.e., affecting more than an occasional individual here and there) only since the eighteenth century, and spreading with their popularity. As noted above, the argument has some serious weaknesses and is generally dismissed by Torrey's colleagues and the wider public, but it is encouraging that the fact that there is no evidence of schizophrenia at least before what can be called "the early modern period" is nevertheless taken seriously, as, of course, it should be, by some schizophrenia researchers. The historical recency of schizophrenia (which must be assumed unless evidence to the contrary is found) in turn suggests that the disease may affect only select populations at present as well. This would be consistent with what we know of physical diseases. Changes in the repertoire of our bodily afflictions are not unknown (think, for example of AIDS). And the repertoires themselves vary across populations, depending on alimentary, chemical, or physical conditions, among others. Yet, though most epidemiologists believe schizophrenia to be a disease of the brain with a strong genetic component (i.e., a physical disease), the epidemiology of schizophrenia is based on the assumption that the risk of developing schizophrenia must be spread uniformly across human populations in time and in space.

It is a point of consensus among experts that the lifetime morbid risk of schizophrenia in the general population is 1 percent, specifically meaning that one in one hundred people will develop schizophrenia by age fifty-five. This is the "normal" rate across the world. If the rate actually found in any particular population is higher, it "must be due," says Gottesman, "to some increase in risk factors." The question what may account for a lower rate is not addressed. I had the opportunity to ask Michael Lyons, a distinguished epidemiologist of schizophrenia, why exactly 1 percent is considered to be the normal lifetime risk. His answer was: "One has to begin somewhere."

The actual basis for this presumed statistic seems hardly less arbitrary. Indeed, comments Gottesman: "the currently accepted value is not, after all, so far from the 'lucky' guess."[39] The value was calculated using census method and biographical method. The earliest census study of 1928, not unexpectedly coming from Germany and using "a very small sample," arrived at the figure 0.85 percent—not so far from 1 percent one may say—and, although the epidemiological community remained for quite some time satisfied with it, some doubts apparently persisted in Scandinavia, where two classic studies were carried out in the late 1940s, one census, one biographical, which established the standard of 1 percent as indisputable or, at any rate, undisputed.

In 1947, a team headed by Eric Essen-Moeller conducted a census of the 2,550 men, women, and children in rural southern Sweden—all the living inhabitants of two parishes. "Virtually everyone was interviewed," describes Gottesman, "and information gathered from them was complemented by data from official sources—schools, tax authorities, alcoholism registers, mental and penal institutions, and so on—and from family physicians. The data are a gold mine of information." The study found lifetime morbid risk of 1.12 percent and 1.39 percent, if four probable schizophrenics were included.

In a study published in 1951, Kurt Fremming, a Danish psychiatrist, conducted one of only three mental health studies that use the biographical or cohort method. It "differs from Essen-Moeller's census method chiefly in that Fremming counted the schizophrenics who died over the course of the follow-up period as well as those still living at the end of it: None of its subjects were older than fifty-nine. He began with 5,529 persons born between 1883 and 1887 on the island of Bornholm in the Baltic Sea between Denmark and Sweden and then traced them up through 1940. . . . The lifetime morbid risk for schizophrenia that emerged from this biographical method was close to 1.0 percent." "It is obvious," concludes Gottesman, "that allowing for schizophrenics who have died and dropped out of sight leads to a more accurate estimate of risk and to a more accurate benchmark value. By comparing the general population risk of 1.0 percent from the biographical method with the risk of 1.12 percent or 1.39 percent from the census method, we can conclude that they converge upon a more or less equivalent value; henceforth, we can depend upon the more practicable census method."[40]

Accepting that the two studies acquired their classical status owing to the stellar quality of their research design and analysis—that is, that they are as valid and reliable as epidemiological studies can be—what is the reason for taking the value of 1 percent at which they estimated lifetime morbid risk of schizophrenia in two rural Scandinavian communities as the "normal" rate of schizophrenia around the world? Nothing but the assumption that mental disease is spread uniformly across human population can justify the adoption of this benchmark. Yet, not only is this assumption unwarranted by empirical evidence, it contradicts what we know about physical diseases. Nobody assumes, for instance, that the life-time risk of tuberculosis is the same everywhere on earth—we recognize the tremendous contribution of the environment to the risk of this infectious disease. Neither do we assume that genetically transmitted diseases occur at a uniform rate in all societies—there is no "normal" rate for Tay-Sachs disease. In regard to "multifactor diseases such as diabetes, ischemic heart disease or cancer . . . 10- to 30-fold differences in prevalence across populations are not uncommon." "It seems," says epidemiologist John McGrath, "that some opinion leaders believe that schizophrenia stands out from all other human disorders."[41] Could it be that, while it is all right to admit that susceptibility to physical diseases varies across societies (whether because of genetic or environmental factors), the possibility that schizophrenia—"madness in its pure form"—strikes different human populations at a different rate is ideologically unacceptable and we insist on the uniform spread of this mental disorder because to concede that it could be otherwise would make us morally suspect?

Epidemiological studies have been carried out only in a few societies, an overwhelming majority of them based on the monotheistic tradition (a circumstance never paid any attention) and most of those relatively affluent industrial democracies. The number reported in "A Systematic Review of the Prevalence of Schizophrenia," published in 2005 by a team of Australian epidemiologists and based on all the studies with original data (188 in all) on the prevalence of schizophrenia, appearing between 1965 and 2002, is forty-six societies.[42] Twenty-two of these societies (and 127, i.e., 62 percent of, studies) are "Western" societies par excellence, that is countries of Western Europe, Anglo-America, Australia, New Zealand, and Israel; seven additional countries are the poorer relations of this rich and free world—thirteen studies have been done in Eastern European and Post-Soviet societies and one in Argentina, bringing the number of countries to twenty-nine. Six studies were carried out in four African countries, two in two Middle Eastern countries, two in two Caribbean countries, and one in Papua New Guinea. Finally, forty-three studies (many of them comparative and most conducted by Western teams) explored the problem in the tremendous population and landmass of East Asia—nineteen of them in India, seven in China, and six in Japan. Thus, most of our knowledge on the spread of schizophrenia is based on what happens in relatively affluent and free societies of the "developed" world; we have little knowledge on the problem in poor "developing" societies. Neither do we know much about societies based on religious traditions other than monotheism (for instance, China, India, and Japan).

In 2004, the WHO World Mental Health Survey Consortium in a publication regarding mental diseases in general stressed the "consistent finding" that prevalence is low in Asian countries (irrespective of level of development) and that, while serious cases, implying disability (which would, among others, include all cases of psychosis) are a minority every- where, they constitute 29 percent of the total counted in the United States and only 8 percent in the poorest and least developed of the countries compared, Nigeria.[43]

Considerable differences in frequency of schizophrenia specifically, as well as in its course and outcome, have been observed constantly. Jablensky, in 1997, stressed that the existence of unusual populations has been docu- mented for a long time. In a 1953 study, carried in the north of Sweden, the lifetime morbid risk of schizophrenia was found to be 2.66 percent (i.e., twice as high as the value of Essen-Moeller's study in the south, which, at 1.39, we take as proof of the "normal" rate of 1 percent). The replication of this study in 1978, also found an unusually high rate of prev- alence of 17 per 1,000 persons. This rate was attributed to a founder effect in an isolated population, but the study of pedigrees failed to support this interpretation. In addition, unusually high rates were found in several other sites in Sweden, as well as in Croatia, Ireland, and, not the least, in the United States—clearly, before the 1972 U.S.-UK Diagnostic Study, which established, among other things, that four times as many schizo- phrenics were diagnosed in this country as in the United Kingdom, and in the more recent study of 1994.[44] Populations virtually immune to schizo- phrenia were also observed, but these observations were not based on accepted epidemiological methods and, therefore, elicited the reaction of "rude skepticism" on the part of the "educated public." In 2005, Saha and team drew attention to notable international differences. The 1,721 preva- lence estimates from the 188 studies they reviewed (based on an estimated 154,140 potentially overlapping prevalent cases) rendered the following numbers per 1,000 persons for the distributions for point, period, lifetime, and lifetime morbid risk: for point prevalence, 1.9–10.0, with the median value of 4.6; for period prevalence, 1.3–8.2 (median—3.3); for lifetime prevalence, 1.6–12.1 (median—4.0), and for lifetime morbid risk, 3.1–27.1 (median—7.2). They also reported: "The prevalence of schizophrenia in migrants was higher compared to native-born individuals: the migrant-to-native-born ratio median (10%—90% quantile) was 1.8 (0.9—6.4). When sites were grouped by economic status, prevalence estimates from 'least developed' countries were significantly lower than those from both 'emerging' and 'developed' sites."[45]

The most comprehensive research on schizophrenia in different countries, examining its incidence, characteristics, course, and outcome, is that of the already mentioned quarter-of-a-century-long series of studies began by the World Health Organization in 1967 with short-term follow-ups after two, five, and, for some sites, ten years, and a follow-up for the long-term course in the International Study of Schizophrenia (ISoS) in the last decade of the twentieth century. This research has consistently found that poor "developing" countries were doing considerably better than affluent "developed" ones across all dimensions: schizophrenia in them was not only probably less common (though this was not stressed), but, when found, was far more likely to be limited to a single episode with no residual deficits and, in general, less severe and characterized by a more positive outcome, caused significantly less functional disability and contributed less to mortality.[46] These findings supported the early anthropological accounts, "indifferent" to the principles of epidemiology and based on suspect methods, and their "claims of psychosis-free societies" outside the West, and strongly suggested the importance of culture, "ubiquitous, intuitively pertinent, if imprecise." But, as pointed out, cultural factors were not analyzed, and, on the whole, the influence of culture was assumed to be limited to the explanation of course and outcome of the disease, and not pertinent to the etiology of schizophrenia itself. Within the schizophrenia research community at large the consistent differences between "developed" societies and the "developing" ones were bracketed as "persistent puzzles," "the counter-intuitive, but persistent anomaly," leading to the question "what might be compromising recovery in the West?" but leaving unquestioned the assumption that schizophrenia is a genetically transmitted brain disease with the 1 percent "normal" rate of lifetime morbid risk across all populations.[47]

A common explanation for the rates above the assumed "normal" rate, which in all cases were found by careful epidemiological studies and thus in societies easily lending themselves to careful epidemiological studies, was that they must have reflected overdiagnosis. The team of the latest replication of the NIHM National Comorbidity Survey (NCS-R), however, is of the opinion that previous studies had systematically *under*estimated the prevalence of major mental illness. Statistics regarding the costs of schizophrenia to United States, Canada, and United Kingdom also suggest morbid risk far above 1 percent.[48]

The opposition to reports on extremely low incidence and prevalence of schizophrenia is more obstinate. These, coming from poor traditional societies, are invariably explained away as "only slightly better than anecdotal" and/or attributed to the low detection rate.[49] Where there is the will there is a way. Accurate epidemiological conclusions, apart from and before statistical methods, depend on the clarity and reliability of diagnostic criteria, but such clarity and reliability in the case of schizophrenia still evade us. This means, paradoxically, that, one can easily interpret the lack of any evidence for schizophrenia as evidence for the "normal" rate. Not unexpectedly, unlike early anthropological reports of psychosis-free societies, which are "rudely" dismissed, the anecdotes of psychiatric anthropologists, presented as such evidence, are usually considered reliable and few experts doubt these wonderful storytellers' ability to detect schizophrenia even where no apparent signs of it are known to exist. Of course, the symptoms may be indistinguishable from a psychosis due to medical causes, such as an infectious disease, or to substance abuse, or the patient may display conventional symptoms of bewitchment. When all one has to observe is an acute episode, which can be ascribed to any of these circumstances, there is no way to decide among them. But, tolerant as we are, we, Western scholars, know that illness may be experienced and expressed differently in different cultures and have no problem with such local details. Deploying our advanced knowledge and "praecox feeling" we clearly see behind them schizophrenia with its bizarre delusions. In the absence of a clear definition, anything remotely resembling schizophrenia may be defined as schizophrenia and the absence of evidence may be attributed to the unreliability of non-Western health agencies. But, given that schizophrenia is diagnosed solely on the basis of the specific manner in which it is experienced and expressed, selectively relying on anthropological evidence of schizophrenia around the world brings us very close to denying that this disease exists altogether.[50]

Some of the findings regarding differences in the frequency of schizophrenia are not disputed—they are simply not commented on. For instance, the evidence that urban birth and residence increases the risk of developing the disease, as does migration and, in particular, immigration, is now considered "robust."[51] This would seem to suggest that populations in societies with high degree of urbanization would be at a greater risk than largely agrarian ones, that is, that there would be different "normal" rates for the two groups of societies. The idea, however, is hardly popular. Neither does the robust evidence regarding migration, troubling as it might seem for genetic explanations, seem to bother anyone. Jablensky, for example, only notes—relative to the exceptionally high rates of schizophrenia among Afro-Caribbeans born in the United Kingdom (especially striking when compared to lack of evidence that schizophrenia is found in their home islands at any rate)—that this finding is not new, as it was already described in 1967, leading one to the conclusion that replication deprives it of importance.[52]

"Today we find human beings afflicted with schizophrenia in all societies and in all socioeconomic strata within societies," summarizes Gottesman these contradictory findings. "Overall, about one in one hundred persons will develop this condition by age fifty-five or so. Differences in frequency over time and space (cultures, subcultures) have sometimes been observed, but they are difficult to interpret. . . . Many of the reported variations must be artifacts of inaccurate reporting (untrained observers, small samples, idiosyncratic conventions about diagnoses), and perhaps simpler explanations relating to changes in life expectancy and to social mobility will suffice."[53]

The increasing life expectancy, indeed, is a cause of worry to those on the cutting edge of the schizophrenia epidemiological research. Given that neither understanding nor, therefore, the cure is forthcoming, writes Sartorius, "the increased life expectancy at all ages in most countries and the consequent increase in the numbers of young adults—the population group at highest risk for schizophrenia—allows the prediction that the prevalence of schizophrenia will grow significantly over the next few decades."[54] But life expectancy—and the population of young adults—is increasing most rapidly in "developing" societies where the prevalence of schizophrenia is low, and in most of the "developing" world life expectancy has not yet reached the one characteristic of the "developed" societies with the consistently higher rates of prevalence of schizophrenia, on the basis of which the "normal" rate was established. Cross-cultural evidence, in other words, contradicts the "increasing life expectancy" argument. As to social mobility, this brings us back to the problematic influence of the socio-cultural environment.

The reasoning in this "simple explanation" of differences in the frequency of schizophrenia among cultures and subcultures seems to be that social mobility increases morbid risk of developing the disease, perhaps because it implies an experience of social instability and instability is believed to be a measure of environmental stress. Such, at least, is the very tentative conclusion of the team of participants in the WHO international studies, attempting to account for the statistically confirmed and therefore undeniable, but still mysterious effect of "the black box of culture" on course (defined in terms of the quality of remissions between episodes) and outcome of schizophrenia. They write:

> For some, including those with a less favorable clinical picture, living in certain areas [countries] improves chances of recovery. The characteristics of an area were only crudely measured in this study, but stability of the area appears to be related to disability outcomes. We continue to question the predictive value of the developing-developed dichotomy based on the CART (Classification and Regression Trees) model: Given good short-term outcome, subjects in Chandigarh [India] urban had poorer long-term course than their rural counterparts. The challenge remains to open up further the black box of culture . . . [55]

The hedging and the discouraged tone of this quotation make it quite clear that to epidemiologists actually facing the evident for them influence of the socio-cultural environment, no explanation involving characteristics of this environment looks simple. In their view, there is no logic behind such explanations, even if it is themselves who are called upon formulating them. How can there be, if they lack concepts to capture the nature of the phenomena whose influence is so strongly suggested by their data?[56] A black box—that is what culture is for them: how are they supposed to discern the principles at work in its pitch darkness? Thus "stability": black boxes that are shaken can be differentiated from those that are not.

Apparently, initially, just as "developing" and "developed" were code words for "non-Western" and "Western," stability/instability were taken to stand for "developing" and "developed" countries: India is defined as a developing country, that is why researchers are puzzled by the difference between rural Chandigarh and urban Chandigarh, both equally Indian and thus equally "developing" thus stable, by definition, and yet, not equally stable as rated, rural Chandigarh receiving a significantly higher rating on the "variable" (1 as opposed to 1.9—on the scale of 1–3—for urban Chandigarh). Here again is an example of how language adopted for the interpretation of certain data obscures the reality of what is observed. In the early twentieth century, Western observers divided the world into "civilized" (active, industrious, changing the world around) and "primitive" (childlike, sleepy, unchanging) peoples. Within the "civilized" world they included members of their own societies, and within the "primitive" one all the rest. This general perspective did not necessarily change when the attitude to name-calling did, and, since the term "primitive" came to be seen as condescending, the dichotomy was rechristened: the "civilized" (we) became "developed" and the "primitive" (they) "developing." The logical connotations of "developed" and "developing" are, respectively, "that, which no longer is in the process of development," thus "stable," and "that which is in the process of development," i.e., constantly changing, thus "unstable." Obviously, a developing system, whatever it is, is less stable than a fully formed, developed, one. But because "developed" is a euphemism for "Western" and "developing" is a euphemism for "primitive," the obvious explanation for lower rates of chronicity and disability due to schizophrenia in "developing" countries becomes their presumed stability. Indeed, it is hard otherwise to account for characterizing as "stable" the site of Agra in India, which consistently showed the best results on all scores in the course of the WHO cross-cultural studies.[57] Here is the description of the site:

Agra is the third largest city (1.2 million population) in the northern province of Uttar Pradesh (UP), the largest Indian state with over 160 million
population. . . . In the 25 years since IPSS [the International Pilot Study of
Schizophrenia, 1973], the city and other parts of the catchment area have
had the phenomenal growth and have developed industrially; the decennial
growth rate between 1981 and 1991 was 25%. Consequently, Agra is very
densely populated, and its narrow roads are choked with traffic of all
sorts—automotive vehicles, rickshaws, scooters, cycles, bullock carts,
horse-drawn carriages, and stray cattle. . . . The nearby town of Mathura
has one of the biggest petroleum refineries in India, and the agricultural
sector of the area is undergoing a green revolution with farmers converting
to modern methods. Agra has two universities and scores of colleges and
has become a tourist center.

Among major historical events occurring in this region during those 25
years were the murders of two former Prime Ministers, Indira Gandhi and
her son Rajiv, and the destruction of Babri Masjid (Mosque) by Hindus,
resulting in nationwide tension between Hindus and Muslims. Political
awareness has reached the village level where women hold 30% of the positions as heads of village councils.[58]

Clearly, stability of the sociocultural environment is not what accounts for
the comparatively excellent chances of recovery of Agra area residents
diagnosed with schizophrenia. Neither does the explanation work for
other study sites or centers defined as "developing" (Chandigarh, rural and
urban, and Madras in India; Cali in Colombia, Ibadan in Nigeria, Hong
Kong, and Beijing), all of which showed "a more favorable picture" than
their "developed" counterparts (Dublin, Honolulu, Moscow, Nagasaki,
Nottingham, Prague, Rochester, NY, Groningen, Mannheim, Sofia, and
Washington, DC), repeatedly confirming what the very first of the WHO
cross-cultural studies found: the considerable "course and outcome advantage enjoyed by developing centers."[59]

How, in the late 1990s, it was possible to characterize Sofia as more
developed than Beijing is difficult to understand, but Sofia and the other
center in Eastern Europe, Prague, did contribute to the redefining instability as, specifically, a change in political regime. The reasoning behind
this was the following:

In the two-year follow-up, studies on the DOSMeD subjects report that those from Prague had outcomes as favorable as those in developing centers. . . . Thirteen years later, the Prague cohort had consistently poor disability outcomes. As is well known, Prague (as well as other eastern European countries) has undergone significant political and social upheaval. In their report on the Bulgarian ISoS cohort [the researchers] document that the sample has poorer outcomes on social disability and on symptoms than do samples from Chennai, Groningen, and Nottingham. Since Bulgaria underwent greater social upheaval than did these other areas, further credibility is lent to a hypothesis that the social stability of an area can impact levels of functioning.

Unfortunately, even this attempt to make the meaning of "instability" more precise did not help to make the stability argument more persuasive, because "persons in the Moscow center—whose area had been ranked high on social instability—[were] among those with better symptom and disability outcomes."[60] Moscow's "good" results might have been explained by the sad fact that so many of the patients either died or had no means to stay in Moscow and were lost to the follow-up study, but the collapse of communism in Eastern Europe still would not be able to account for the very low rates of recovery in Dublin or Rochester, NY, indeed consistent with the mostly insidious onset of schizophrenia among patients there and its continuously psychotic course in so many cases.

As of 2007, the most influential study of the incidence of schizophrenia internationally was the concluding study in the ISoS series—the so-called WHO *10 Nation Study,* somewhat puzzling in its title, since only eight sites in seven nations were examined.[61] For the fans of the "normal" rate the results were not entirely encouraging. Though the methodology was uniform across all eight sites, it was found that, whether the definition was narrow or broad, at least a twofold difference existed between the highest and lowest sites, which in the case of the broad definition was statistically significant. The incidence of schizophrenia (i.e., new cases over a period) was 7 per 100,000 in Aarhus in Denmark and 14 in Nottingham, England, when the narrow criteria (CATEGO S+) were used; when the broad criteria (IDC 9 schizophrenia) were employed, incidence was 16 per 100,000 in Honolulu and 42 in the urban Chandigarh in India. Perhaps, this was less important than the fact that higher incidence corresponded to the better course and outcome (raising the question whether one observed the incidence of the same disease). But, whatever the actual significance of the findings, J. J. McGrath commented in his probing 2004 NAPE lecture, "Myths and Plain Truths about Schizophrenia Epidemiology": "The study is frequently quoted as showing that there was no significant variation between countries in the incidence of nuclear schizophrenia as defined by the PSE/CATEGO system. However, it is more correct to say that the study had insufficient power to detect significant differences. . . . when a broad concept of schizophrenia was examined, the incidence varied fourfold. The Ten Country study is often cited, perhaps mistakenly, as providing the evidence for worldwide uniform incidence and symptom expression of schizophrenia."[62] The preliminary report of the study itself concluded: "The results provide strong support for the notion that schizophrenic illnesses occur with comparable frequency in different populations."[63] This statement, says McGrath continues to resonate within the schizophrenia research community nearly two decades later.

Where does all this leave us? While there is no evidence that schizophrenia in its chronic, incurable, continuously or repeatedly psychotic form, which justifies naming it "the cancer of the mind," exists "in all societies and in all socioeconomic strata" and affects all human populations at the "normal" rate of lifetime morbid risk of one in one hundred persons, there is plenty of evidence that it does not, but, instead, affects almost exclusively societies that are called "modern" in the specific sense of the word, that is, societies which are well-developed from the economic standpoint, being in most cases oriented to sustained growth and affluent as a result, or at least not subject to the traditional (Malthusian) cycles of growth and decline; professedly egalitarian and democratic, however the principles of equality and popular sovereignty are implemented; and, though fundamentally secular in outlook, rooted in the monotheistic religious traditions. To a far lesser extent it affects certain groups in societies of other types, influenced by modern societies. There is also evidence that modern societies are affected at a rate significantly exceeding the presumed "normal" rate of morbid risk. Some of this evidence is historical, which "the schizophrenia research community" considers irrelevant for science by definition and therefore blithely disregards; this evidence is to be discussed in later chapters. Some of it, as we have seen, comes from recent epidemiological research of the best repute and concerns the prevalence, the type, the severity, and the outcome of schizophrenia found in different societies. In addition, some suggestive evidence comes from studies of schizophrenia distribution by social class.

It has been found from epidemiological research on physical disease that of all the commonly examined social categories, such as ethnicity, occupation, marital status, religion, and emigration, social class shows a consistently stronger correlation with morbid risk. Epidemiologists of schizophrenia, therefore, have paid particular attention to social class in its classical sociological definition of socio-economic status (i.e., income/education/occupation). Already the first such study, carried out in 1939 by Chicago sociologists Robert Faris and H. Warren Dunham, found that incidence of schizophrenia (as reflected in first-admission rates) was more than four times greater among residents of central city slums than among those who lived in the affluent Chicago suburbs.[64] Since then it has been generally believed that lower class increased the risk of developing schizophrenia and many subsequent studies supported this theory. Variations similar to Chicago (that is incidence in poor central city vs. incidence in suburbs) were found in other cities, and in 1966 William Eaton, also a sociologist, has demonstrated that occupation could be used instead of the socioeconomic profile of the neighborhood as an equally powerful predictor, incidence among blue-collar male workers being five times higher than among the professional and technical groups.[65] The most obvious explanation for such regularities (because the standing Western explanation for all "social problems") was poverty. Poverty made people unhappy and was responsible for crime, broken families, and child abuse. Together, these stressful conditions increased the vulnerability of the lower class population to schizophrenia—the so-called "breeder" hypothesis. That poverty in the United States after the Great Depression was never of the absolute kind, suggesting starvation and homeless children wandering the streets, which is characteristic of the countries in which, given the evidence, chronic schizophrenia is found, if at all, at lower than "normal" rates, but, instead, has been only relative, namely "poverty" measured solely by comparison to a certain standard of riches, was not sufficient to reject this interpretation. Neither were the assumption that blue-collar workers (plumbers, electricians, builders, auto-mechanics, etc.) must be destitute and unhappy, and the association of such work with broken families (as if divorce among lawyers, college professors, and psychiatrists were not at least as common) considered unwarranted.

The "breeder" hypothesis, however, was supported only when social class was defined as that of the patient at the time of diagnosis. When the more usual for stratification/social mobility studies "class of origin" (or that of the schizophrenic's family of origin) was the variable examined, the opposite of the "breeder" theory held true, giving rise to the currently accepted "downward drift" interpretation. The 1963 Social Medicine Research Unit study in London compared the social mobility patterns of schizophrenic men with those of their male relatives—brothers, fathers, uncles, and grandfathers. It found that, while only 4 percent of patients belonged to the upper socioeconomic class comprising 16 percent of the general population, 21 percent of patients' brothers and 29 percent of their fathers belonged to this class, which meant that the upper class supplied many more schizophrenics than its share in the population warranted (over 20 percent of the schizophrenic population). Both the middle and the lower classes supplied fewer schizophrenics than was the share of these classes in the general population. While 58 percent of the general population and 56 percent of schizophrenics' brothers belonged to the middle class, only 48 percent of their fathers belonged to it (which means that at most 48 percent of the schizophrenics in the study were raised in middle-class families). The lower socioeconomic class at the time of the study comprised 27 percent of the general population; but, while 48 percent of the patients belonged to it at the time of the diagnosis, only 23 percent of their brothers and their fathers were in the lower class as well, meaning that at most this percentage of schizophrenics were raised in lower-class homes. When social class is defined as position among income groups, elderly population may well be subject to downward drift: therefore more fathers of schizophrenics could find themselves in both the middle and the lower classes at the time their twenty-five- to thirty-four-year-old sons were diagnosed with schizophrenia, than were there at the time when these children grew up, as a result of drifting from the upper and the middle class downward. At the same time, it is obviously possible, but only in a minority of cases, for one's income to reach its highest point after the usual retirement age. As to patients themselves, undoubtedly, their near absence from the upper class (4 percent), considerable presence in the middle class (48 percent), which is, however, considerably lower than expected if schizophrenia is spread uniformly across social classes (48 percent instead of 58 percent), and disproportionate concentration in the lower class (48 percent) in which only a minority of them could be born are a result of the massive downward drift associated with their disabling disease. The findings of the London study were replicated in several studies in the United States and the psychiatric community (in practice as well as in research) is currently in agreement regarding the reliability of the "drift" interpretation.[66]

Support for the downward drift hypothesis may not disprove the role for stressors, as some believe, but it certainly disproves the role of absolute poverty as a stressor, in increasing the risk of schizophrenia. It is also inconsistent with the claims that there is a "normal" risk for schizophrenia, that it affects people in all societies and in all classes of these societies, and, perhaps most important, that there is a significant genetic component to this disease. Clearly, if, in a mobile, open society, such as United Kingdom or the United States, the risk of developing schizophrenia is several times greater precisely in the stratum of the most successful people, by definition, in which there are fewest material contributors to this risk (such as poor nutrition, poor living conditions, lack of medical services, etc.), than in any other, the genetic element of it, if it exists at all, cannot be great. At the same time, the "downward drift" hypothesis, which implies that schizophrenia is a particular problem for the affluent strata with numerous choices in regard to consumption and occupation, is fully consistent with the evidence, however disputed, that it is a particular problem of certain types of societies—societies which offer its denizens the greatest number of such choices, "modern," prosperous, Western societies.

State of the Art 4: Current Views of Underlying Psychological Structure

There appears to be no reason to disagree with the statement of the clinical and experimental psychologist Louis Sass that, despite schizophrenia's being "psychiatry's central preoccupation . . . the attention lavished on this condition seems not . . . to have fathomed its many mysteries." Indeed, as we have seen, "to this day we remain largely ignorant of the causes . . . and even the precise diagnostic boundaries of this most strange and important of mental illnesses." To these unfathomed mysteries, Sass adds "the underlying psychological structure" of the disease.[67]

The interpretation of schizophrenia—the task of integrating all of its features into an understandable whole, to make sense of, if not to explain it causally, has proven as difficult and thankless as any other aspect of the solution of this puzzle. Unlike AIDS, heart disease, epilepsy, or certain developmental mental disorders, schizophrenia, as currently conceptualized, does not make sense. No way has been found so far to relate its positive symptoms to the negative ones, to understand how self-disturbances captured in Schneider's first rank symptoms are connected to the multiple peculiarities of the schizophrenic language, or what do hearing voices and the disregard for the principle of non-contradiction have in common. One never knows what to expect: the invariable feature of schizophrenia, it is claimed, is the extreme variability of its expressions. "Schizophrenics are idiosyncratic, unique, inappropriate or bizarre in their responses," write coauthors of a research paper in *Psychological Medicine*, "any further elaboration is impossible."[68]

And yet, this is so not for the lack of trying. Attempts to interpret schizophrenia are at least as old as the term. Interpretation is an intellectual exercise different from causal explanation and forms a necessary condition for the latter. It is a kind of extended description of a complex phenomenon, in terms that make clear why it constitutes a separate entity and points to the organizing principle that connects its parts. In this sense, it is analogous to definitions of simpler phenomena and similarly important for explanations of specific instances and expressions, and for causal explanation, in general. It is necessary to know what one is trying to explain before attempting an explanation. In the case of complex phenomena, one, presumably, seeks to explain their organizing principles.[69] Students of schizophrenia, even if not explicit as to the place of interpretation in their overall quest, undoubtedly have sensed the logical priority of the *what* question over that of *why,* and did their best to pinpoint the central dynamic that has woven the various symptoms into the classical syndrome and this syndrome and less common combinations into one disease, thereby figuring out its underlying psychological structure.

Definitions, as Durkheim has taught us in the human sciences, are best approached without prejudice. One is not supposed to know the explanation before one has defined the phenomenon, neither is one supposed to know the organizing principle of a complex phenomenon before one has studied it without preconceptions. Definition, or extended description—interpretation—is the first step in the explanatory process. The organizing principles are discovered, not given. This has been the Achilles' heel of the schizophrenia studies. The nature of schizophrenia's etiology has been presumed before establishing what schizophrenia, in fact, is. The prejudices on which interpretations of schizophrenia are based have been of two kinds and reflected the "two minds" of contemporary psychiatry: biological and psychoanalytical. They derived from the ideas, respectively, of Kraepelin and Freud.

Kraepelinian interpretations postulated that schizophrenia is a disorder of the brain, resulting in the disabling of an essential brain function, usually perceptual or cognitive. For example, Kurt Goldstein, a famous neurologist of the first half of the twentieth century, in particular interested in brain injuries, argued that schizophrenics lack the capacity for abstraction. He was led to this conclusion by the similarity he perceived between the behavior of brain-damaged patients whom he treated and performance of schizophrenics to whom other psychiatrists in Russia (where psychiatry from the start was strongly biologistic) and Germany administered sorting tasks. "There is no question that a very great concreteness is characteristic for the behavior of schizophrenics," he declared on this basis, and this "clinical picture," in his opinion, supported the idea of a brain defect.[70] "Abstract attitude," the loss of which Goldstein believed to be the "core disturbance" in schizophrenia, was essential for all higher mental functions, which was consistent with the definition of schizophrenia as a form of dementia or weak-mindedness. Unfortunately, though Goldstein's "concreteness thesis" remains (or, at least, remained in the 1990s) "the most famous interpretation of schizophrenic thinking," it left out of account much of the clinical picture, including the tendency towards what may be characterized as abnormally abstract attitude, at least as pronounced as the one towards "very great concreteness" (only the latter of which schizophrenics share with organic, including brain-damaged, patients). In fact, "the propensity to give responses at both extremes" of the concreteness-abstractness continuum appears to some researchers as deserving of attention as either tendency taken on its own.[71]

Other interpretations of the cognitive/perceptual defect variety include attributing schizophrenia to a breakdown in the Gestalt perception—that is the inability to see the forest behind the trees, which, again, while stressing the importance of one characteristic tendency, contradicts the evidence of an equally pronounced tendency to disregard details perceptible to everyone else for generalities which nobody else perceives; to the deficiency of "selective attention," which forces the schizophrenic to perceive every detail of every aspect of the environment and internal mental process, whether or not it has any practical relevance; and to a failure of logic (presumably hardwired into human brain), specifically, lack of sensitivity to contradiction in thought, resulting in what von Domarus calls "paralogical" reasoning.

The interpretations of psychoanalysts differ from those of psychiatrists with a more biological orientation only in that the deficiency or defect which they see as the source of all other problems in schizophrenia is attributed to arrested psychological development or regression to levels of consciousness as early as "fetal," where the "ego" does not yet distinguish between oneself and the world, or, in some interpretations, to the levels of "higher animals, children, the brain-damaged, and preliterate humans." For this reason, Silvano Arieti, for instance, refers to the schizophrenics' disregard for principles of Aristotelian logic as "paleological" thinking. From where one derives the knowledge about the consciousness of a fetus or of preliterate humans, for that matter, one can only guess; like all Freudian theories, psychoanalytical interpretations of schizophrenia are plagued by problems of empirical access. But, in general, they are neither better nor worse than neurological ones. To quote Sass regarding all of them, "though useful in many ways (particularly in highlighting the sheer variety of characteristic deviances), it seems fair to say that the overall attempt to discover some central deficit or tendency must be deemed a failure. The characteristic anomalies of schizophrenic thinking appear to be too diverse to be ascribed to any single factor, and too bizarre to be accounted for as simple errors or consequences of regression."[72]

Schizophrenia as Observed and Experienced

In this part I propose to undertake an interpretation of schizophrenia in the terms of the theory of the mind as a cultural phenomenon, the individualized culture in the brain. I shall do so, relying on detailed descriptions of schizophrenic experience by patients and clinicians. Characteristic expressions of schizophrenic disorder, from the fullest to barely suggestive, according to most descriptions, arrange themselves in the following sequence:

Full-blown psychosis:	1. Delusions
	2. Acute psychosis: acute experience of the loss of self; hallucinations
Middle Stages/Bleuler's "fundamental features":	3. Formal thought disorders; language abnormalities
Prodrome:	4. Confusion; self-reevaluation; changes in the sense of reality

The negative symptoms of schizophrenia are present during all of these stages.

A Typical Delusion

Schizophrenic delusions are the best-known feature of the disease—at least, among the laymen. Very often they take the form of the belief in the "influencing machine." In fact, the very first clinical record of schizophrenic delusion, that of James Tilly Matthews, recorded by Dr. John Haslam in his famous *Illustrations of Madness* of 1810, and as recently as 2001 still cited as the typical case, belonged precisely to this variety.[73] James Matthews was a patient of Bethlem (or Bedlam) Hospital since January 1797, admitted there on the petition of his parish officers. In January 1798, he was placed in the incurable ward and was there for over a dozen years when, in 1809, his case was reviewed by Haslam, then apothecary to the hospital, or its medical attendant. All these years Matthews and his family demanded his release, claiming that he was sane from the beginning or perfectly recovered, experts were called on their side and the side of the hospital, and the matter was decided in court. The necessity to pronounce yet again on the patient's sanity was the reason for Haslam's publication of Matthews' case.[74]

Matthews was a tea broker in London who spent some time in Paris, spoke good French, an obviously educated man, and, as will become evident in a moment, very intelligent and articulate. His delusion was that there existed in London gangs or bands of French agents, very knowledgeable in advanced science and skillful in technology, whose goal was to weaken Britain by all means possible, in particular, by disclosing to the enemy its military and diplomatic secrets and republicanizing its people. These bands operated by means of Air Looms—elaborate machines, constructed in accordance with the principles of the science of Pneumatic Chemistry—which, if positioned at a distance of less than 1,000 feet from their human target (whether or not separated by a wall), could, by emitting warps of magnetic fluid, exert virtually irresistible mental influence on the targeted person, determining the person's thoughts, emotions, and actions. The many ways in which this pneumatic influence was exerted were called "assailments." To become a subject for assailment, the person first had to be saturated with a magnetic fluid, which was effected by "hand-impregnation": an inferior member of the gang was "furnished with a bottle containing the magnetic fluid which issues from a valve on pressure. If the object to be assailed be sitting in a coffee-house, the pneumatic practitioner hovers about him, perhaps enters into conversation, and during such discourse, by opening the valve, sets at liberty the volatile magnetic fluid which is respired by the person intended to be assailed. So great is the attraction between the human body and this fluid, that the party becomes certainly impregnated, and is equally bound by the spell as . . . the harmless fly is enveloped in the shroud of the spider."[75] Being so "impregnated," the person becomes a helpless tool in the hands of the French agents and the unwitting means to the ruin of Great Britain. A detailed drawing of the air-loom used in the assailment of Matthews himself attested to his fine draftsmanship (as well as to his minute familiarity with contemporary machinery) and explained in the accompanying notes how "the assailed object is affected at pleasure: as by opening a vitriolic gas valve he becomes tortured by the fluid within him; becoming agitated with the corrosion through all his frame, and so on in all their various modes of attacking the human body and mind, whether to actuate or render inactive; to make ideas or to steal others; to bewilder or to deceive; thence to the driving with rage to acts of desperation, or to the dropping dead with stagnation, &c. &c. &c."[76]

The magnetic fluid was a combination of various mineral and organic effluvia and compressed vapors, most of them, apparently extremely malodorous, and different formulas were utilized in different assailments. The assailments themselves were as numerous as forms of torture in the repertoires of most accomplished henchmen, causing the victim terrible mental and physical suffering. Two of the most important—because these were the main ways in which the French agents communicated to the magnetically enslaved Britons their wicked assignments—were *brain-sayings* and *voice-sayings*. Brain-sayings were defined as "a sympathetic communication of thought, in consequence of both parties being impregnated with the magnetic fluid, which must be rarified by frequent changing and rendered more powerful by the action of the electrical machine. It is not hearing; but appears to be a silent conveyance of intelligence to the intellectual atmosphere of the brain, as subtle as electricity to a delicate electrometer: but the person assailed (if he be sufficiently strong in intellect) is conscious that the perception is not in the regular succession of his own thoughts." Voice-sayings, in distinction, were "an immediate conveyance of articulate sound to the auditory nerves, without producing the ordinary vibrations of air; so that the communication is intelligibly lodged in the cavity of the ear, whilst the bystander is not sensible of any impression."[77] Other assailments included *fluid-locking:* "a locking or constriction of the fibres of the root of the tongue . . . by which the readiness of speech is impeded"; *cutting soul from sense*—"a spreading of the magnetic warp, chilled in its expansion, from the root of the nose, diffused under the basis of the brain, as if a veil was interposed; so that the sentiments of the heart can have no communication with the operations of the intellect"; *thigh-talking*—the direction of the gang's voice-sayings "on the external part of the thigh, that the person assailed is conscious that his organ of hearing, with all its sensibility, is lodged in that situation. The sensation is distinctly felt in the thigh, and the subject understood in the brain"; *kiteing*—lifting into the brain some particular idea, "as boys raise a kite in the air . . . by means of the air-loom and magnetic impregnation, [which idea then] floats and undulates in the intellect for hours together; and how much soever the person assailed may wish to direct his mind to other objects, and banish the idea forced on him, he finds himself unable; as the idea which they have kited keeps weaving in his mind, and fixes his attention to the exclusion of other thoughts. He is, during the whole time, conscious that the idea is extraneous, and does not belong to the train of his own cogitations"; *sudden death-squeezing,* also called *lobster-cracking*—"an external pressure of the magnetic atmosphere surrounding the person assailed, so as to stagnate his circulation, impede his vital motions, and produce instant death." There was also *lengthening the brain,* analogous to the lengthening of one's countenance in the cylindrical mirror reflection. "The effect produced by this process [was] a distortion of any idea in the mind, whereby that which had been considered as most serious becomes an object of ridicule. All thoughts are made to assume a grotesque interpretation; and the person assailed is surprised that his fixed and solemn opinions should take a form which compels him to distrust their identity, and forces him to laugh at most important subjects. It can cause good sense appear as insanity, and convert truth into a libel; distort the wisest institutions of civilized society into practices of barbarians, and strain the Bible into a jest book." *Thought-making* was a result of one member of the pneumatic gang "sucking at the brain of the person assailed, to extract his existing sentiments," while another member of the gang, "in order to lead astray the sucker (for deception is practiced among themselves as a part of their system; and there exists no honor, as amongst thieves, in the community of these rascals) will force into his mind a train of ideas very different from the real subject of his thoughts, and which is seized upon as the desired information by the person sucking." *Laugh-making* contorted the face muscles of the assailed into a frozen grin;[78] *poking,* or *pushing up the quicksilver,* by a manipulation of magnetic fluid disarmed the particularly intelligent victim of assailments, ready to revolt and resist them, and cowed him into absolute submission; *bladder-filling* partially dislocated the brain with the goal of eventually making the victim weak-minded; *tying-down* relaxed the victim's control of his own thoughts; *bomb-bursting* caused an electrical shock—"a powerful charge of the electrical battery (which they employ for this purpose)"—to the whole physical and nervous system of the victim. And there was more.[79]

Most of the victims of the pneumatic gangs' assailments were British ministers of state and members of high command. James Matthews, however, was targeted in particular because of his remarkable intelligence (which allowed him to discover the machinations of the French agents and penetrate the mysteries of their pneumatic chemistry), his untiring solicitude for the good of the British nation (by which he was compelled on numerous occasions to issue warnings, by letter and in person, to all the high-placed personages of the kingdom, who were in danger of falling into the snares of magnetic impregnation and air-looms), and his unbreakable spirit (which, despite all that he had endured, would not let him be totally subjugated to the pneumatic French cabal). According to Matthews' own testimony, "the assassins opened themselves" to him "by their voices" in 1798, more than a year after he was admitted to Bethlem Hospital. But, he wrote, he had already in 1793, while in France, "sufficient information" about French plans to spy upon and republicanize Great Britain and Ireland, and particularly to disorganize the British navy. After he alerted "each of the 1796 administration," the gang, "having found my senses proof against their fluid and hand-working, as it is termed, were employed to actuate the proper persons to pretend I was insane, for the purpose of plunging me into a madhouse, to invalidate all I said, and for the purpose of confining me within the measure of the Bedlam-attaining-airloom-warp, making sure that by means thereof, and the poisonous effluvia they used, they would by such means keep me fully impregnated, and which impregnation could be renewable and aggravated at their pleasure, so as to overpower my reason and speech, and destroy me in their own way, while all should suppose it was insanity which produced my death." His efforts, he was satisfied, were not in vain: his "incessant and loud clamours, almost daily writing to, or calling at the houses of one or other of all the ministers in their turn, conjuring them to exert themselves to prevent wretches from disorganizing the British navy [resulted in] that in truth [the gang] could not make any way therein while I was at large: and to this solely was owing their not having been able to fulfill their engagements with the French, to have the British fleet in confusion by the time stipulated." Unfortunately, having him "safely immured, the experts went to work again boldly, and then, in less than three months blew up that flame in the British navy, which threw the three great fleets into open mutiny, about Easter 1797 . . ."[80]

With Matthews rendered powerless against them, the villains became quite open with him regarding their planned activities, and, calling him their "Property and Talisman," confided in him which of the British ministers they intended to make their puppets, assassinate, etc. In addition to direct communications with Matthews through brain-sayings and voice-sayings, transmitted by the air-loom adjacent to Bedlam, the gang, especially appointed to assail him, communicated with him by signs, only partially explaining the significance of the message by brain-sayings. For example, seeing daily in the papers advertisements of Philanthropic Insurance, signed by William Ludlam, Matthews would understand that the reference was, in fact, to his Lordship (Ludship), Erskine, Grenville, or William Lord (Lud) Grenville, and the brain-voices would cry in their native tongue, "Voilà la Victime." Later, when Ludlam was caught, pistol in hand, jumping through the window of the London Tavern and ordered by Lord Erskine under the care of the psychiatrist Dr. Monro, Matthews writes,

I mentioned their pretexts and sent out a memorandum thereupon, stating that, though they were active to prevent my perceiving all their drift, I feared they intended to make Lord Erskine mad; for they often asserted, that with but half stress on the fluid with which he was impregnated, he would become weak in intellect; and as it was to my wife, I could not help saying, "Notwithstanding the readiness to act as Counsel for me in 1797, which Mr. Erskine professed, yet, when you called upon him to ask him from me to mention my case and imprisonment in Bedlam in the House of Commons, he would not do so; and for which the assassins boasted once they stagnated him in the House of Commons, by an air-loom warp, attaining him from no great distance; and would have killed him afterwards there as an example in their pretexts but for my exposing their infamous threats; he now cares no more for me than he does for the dogs in the street." "Enough (they cried) we'll shew you." At a subsequent time when it was said that the Lord Chancellor, passing along Holborn, saw several persons pursuing and beating a dog in order to kill him, pretending he was mad; "Aye, (they cried) that's as you say we pursue you pelting you with our murderous efforts;" but he not thinking any madness appeared about him, ran into the midst of them, and taking the dog up in his arms, rescued him from their fury, and ordered him to be conveyed to his stables and taken care of: "Yes, (said they) that part is the derision of the event; we have commemorated your words; he does care about the dog, but you may lie in the stable (a term used by them for being placed on the incurable establishment in Bedlam) and be damned."[81]

Matthews knew his assailants by sight as well, although the warp of magnetic fluid that allowed him to see them rarely offered more than a brief glance. Thus he was able to describe in some detail their apartment, the location of the air-loom and other furniture, the personages themselves (there were seven—four men and three women), the functions they fulfilled in the gang (the duty of one was to summarize the group's deliberations in shorthand—just invented, it reflected the network's technological sophistication), their habits, clothes, and characters, and the relations among them. There were some he liked more than the others, some (the woman Charlotte, for instance, who was mistreated by the rest), for whom he even felt sympathy.

Altogether, his delusion is a remarkably engaging story, which is no more implausible than many an example of the better kind of spy fiction. Even simplified and foreshortened in this necessarily brief summary, it reveals a knowledgeable, politically engaged person, a true patriot, willing to risk his life for the common good and national interest. Clearly, Matthews' is not a problem of lethargic and degenerating intellect; his mind would be more accurately characterized as gifted, rather than weak. His delusion testifies to an exceptional fertility of imagination, unusual powers of observation, and evidently above average intelligence (specifically, the ability to make sense of the observed). His fantasy world is an alternative reality, marvelously organized. What gives it its realistic feel is that he is so attuned to his contemporary society. His world is, unmistakably, the world of England in the first decades of the Industrial Revolution: the world of newly omnipotent science, rapidly developing technology, and shorthand. There is no such science as pneumatic chemistry, but it could well exist, and one does not have to stretch the imagination too far to conceive of an air-loom, given the general excitement over power-looms, and the centrality in contemporary life of valves-and-tubes contraptions that turn vapor into a powerful force capable of producing material effects at a distance.[82]

Matthews' politics and political concerns are those of British patriots in

the Britain engaged in a great war with France. Napoleonic Wars are as
defining a conflict for the Britons of the late eighteenth and early nineteenth centuries, as the cold war was for the Americans of the 1950s
through the 1980s. There is nothing strange in his sentiment or those he
attributes to the villains of his treacherous gang. If his ideas of psychological influence smack of Mesmerism, which appears foolish to us in the
twenty-first century, surely the prominence of psychoanalysts in the service of evil in our popular cold war spy novels would appear equally absurd
to readers of the next, if not the present, generation. Matthews' villains are
as multidimensional as any villain wishing to sell the secrets of Great
Britain to the French may be expected to be (as any villain of Dickens, for
that matter), as are the dynamics of relations between them; given the
believable wickedness of their motives, they are believable individuals,
down to the styles of clothes they favor and the accents they affect.

The phenomenological description of Matthews' own condition is precise and detailed: obviously, he is to an unusual degree capable of introspection and self-analysis. He is also a tolerably good writer with a talent
for vivid, original, metaphoric descriptions (think, for instance, of *kiteing*).
His explanation of his psychological state as a result of air-loom assailments is somewhat unorthodox, but not more bizarre to a person of different education (and less inconsistent with the experience and observation)
than neurobiological interpretations equating schizophrenia with defects
in perceptual or cognitive brain mechanisms, or the psychoanalytical ones,
seeing in it regression of the ego to the fetal level. In fact, the only thing
that renders Matthews' fantasy bizarre and makes it a delusion is his being
unaware of his own authorship, his sincere belief that he is caught in the
snares of the pneumatic practitioners and their infernal scientific machine,
his inability to place himself outside his own creation, convinced as he is
that this *is* the outside.

This confusion of the subjective mental process with the objective reality
alone transforms what could be otherwise just an engaging piece of fiction
into a characteristic expression of schizophrenic disorder. Delusion is the
inability to distinguish between the mind as culture in the brain and culture outside, i.e., between the cultural process on the individual and collective levels. Only in this sense, one can see in schizophrenia the "loss of
ego-boundaries," the phrase indeed introduced—in 1919 by a member of

Freud's original circle, Victor Tausk—in relation to a delusion very similar to Matthews' and also involving an "influencing machine."[83] The problematization, for the schizophrenic, of the sense of self (the so-called "self-disturbances" or "I-disorders") is obvious: it is the perception of this problematization from the outside that is the source of the "praecox feeling," which, in the pre-*DSM* era, had been so often the only basis for the diagnosis of schizophrenia. It is also this problematization in the experience of self that is captured by Schneider's First Rank Symptoms: "all these symptoms," comments Sass, for instance, "are quite specific, and all involve passivization or other fundamental distortions of the normal sense of volition, inwardness, or privacy." However, the equation of this experience with insufficiency of mental faculties ("little capacity to reflect on the self," or the lack of "observing ego") and its attribution to regression to, in Anna Freud's words, "those primitive levels of mental life where the distinction between the self and the environment is lacking" serves to obscure the nature of the problem, instead of revealing it.[84] In general, an undifferentiated concept of self and of the mind does not allow for the understanding what precisely the problem is. At the same time, inattention to the mind as an empirical reality of its own kind—namely, symbolic reality—as a result, for example, of the exclusive focus on the brain, makes the definition of delusion itself, and therefore, psychosis, impossible. Without a clear understanding that this central symptom of schizophrenia is a sign of a fundamental problem of the mind as symbolic reality, one is unlikely to explore what the mind consists of and arrive at a differentiated concept. Thus schizophrenia cannot be either interpreted as an entity or causally explained.

Matthews exemplifies every single one of Schneider's First Rank Symptoms. His thoughts are "sucked" out of him and pronounced aloud, discussed by members of the gang, while he himself hears the discussion (physically), whether in his actual ear or with this hearing organ relocated into the thigh—these are the voice-sayings, which Schneider calls "hallucinations." Brain-sayings and the techniques of kiteing and thought-making insert thoughts into his mind and he is aware that they are not his own. His brain is "lengthened" and his opinions are perverted. Feelings that he does not want to experience (such as doubt of the meaningfulness of what he always thought meaningful, contempt for the Bible or British institutions) are imposed on him, so are painful bodily sensations. His reason is overpowered and his speech impeded; he is turned into a helpless plaything of wicked machinists, who at their pleasure actuate him or render him inactive; make ideas or steal others; bewilder or deceive; and eventually drive him with rage to acts of desperation, or to the dropping dead with stagnation. In his concluding comments on Matthews' fantasy, John Haslam writes: "Although the fable may be amusing, the moral is pernicious. The system of assailment and working events deprives man of that volition which constitutes him a being responsible for his actions, and persons not so responsible, in the humble opinion of the writer ought not to be at large."[85] Matthews could not be released from Bethlem Hospital, in other words, because he was a danger to himself and others; his delusion clearly demonstrated to Dr. Haslam that the patient was not a free agent.[86]

In terms of the present theory, Mathews' experience was that of the loss of the acting self, or will. His powers of perception, observation, and reasoning were intact, and he was clearly aware that he no longer was in control of his actions and thoughts. This was, obviously, a very painful, disorienting, and all-embracing experience; Matthews' thinking self was focused on it. Evidently, while he took his fantasy world for objective reality, to which others could find proof, he insisted, on the streets of London and in the *Chambers' Dictionary* of 1783, he knew that he was the author of his notes on this world, and therefore, conscious of his thinking self. He also, as he jotted down these notes and conversed about the delusional world in which he believed himself living, was aware of his relationally-constituted self: he knew himself to be a British subject, a tea broker, the husband of his wife, and he remembered his sojourn in France in the years past and was well informed about the national and international situation before and during his isolation at Bedlam. It is obvious that, while writing about or discussing the assailments of the pneumatic chemists, he was not assailed: rather, he recounted the events and experiences of the past. He was calm and collected and could well appear reasonable to a number of reputable physicians called upon to pronounce judgment on the state of his mind. He was, as Dr. Haslam pointed out, delusional, and therefore, psychotic, but he was not acutely psychotic. He described, however, experiences of acute psychosis—that stage in his disease (which at the moment of calm recollection he did not consider a disease) when the loss of the acting self was experienced as great suffering. His delusion was, in Freudian terms, a rationalization of that experience. His will was still impaired, but, subjectively, it was no longer problematic for him, no longer a source of suffering. His elaborate delusion (temporarily) resolved the subjective problem.

The Acute State

When we move (backwards) to the stage of acute psychosis, it is the experiences Matthews described and accounted for as the effects of French agents' air-loom and magnetic fluids, which become central. In Matthews own case, of which little is known besides the information contained in Haslam's little volume, it is clear that during the stage of acute psychosis his relationally-constituted self was lost as well: he was not aware of his identity and claimed, rather, to be, in Haslam's words, "the Emperor of the whole world, issuing proclamations to his disobedient subjects, and hurling from their thrones the usurpers of his dominions."[87] The full title he assumed on such occasions was "James, Absolute, Sole, & Supreme Sacred Omni Imperious Arch Grand Arch Sovereign Omni Imperious Arch Grand Arch Proprietor Omni Imperious Arch-Grand-Arch-Emperor-Supreme etc." This is how one such proclamation is signed. He ruled over OmniEmpire Territories, which, though perhaps not coextensive with the whole world, included, by name, most of the countries known at that time in Britain.[88] It is also clear that during acute psychotic episodes Mathews, while self-observing, experienced his thoughts as inserted by someone else, had the consciousness of "an automaton moved by the agency" of the air-loom gang, which (the consciousness and the gang) he would later, in the period made lucid by his delusion, describe. It is the torment of the acute period which his elaborate vocabulary of assailments—lengthening the brain, kiteing, separating soul from sense, bomb bursting, and fluid-locking, among others—attempts to capture. Thus, he had no self altogether, experiencing neither his acting self, nor his thinking self, in addition to being completely confused as to his identity.

The experience of acute psychosis is often described in clinicians' interviews with schizophrenic patients, but it is important to realize that these interviews rarely take place at the time when acute psychosis is experienced, but usually after that, though not necessarily during the moments of relative self-possession (the return of the relationally constituted and thinking self), accomplished by delusional imagination. During acute psychosis, schizophrenic patients (in this instance, I use the word in its original sense of "sufferers") cannot be talked to—they are not there to be talked to—but, rather, have to be restrained and medicated. As is often noted, coming to grips with their experience of acute psychosis, the patients "manifest the so-called 'I am' sign—the habit of repeating over and over to themselves some desperate litany such as 'I am'; 'I am me, I am me'."[89] They are attempting to put together the dispersed aspects of their selves. The "thinking self," which is the last to be alienated, is also the first to return. Remarkably, schizophrenics' sensitive analysis of acute psychosis experiences makes it evident that "thinking self" is never lost; present throughout, constantly self-observing and meticulously recording its observations in memory, it simply changes its function: from the "thinking I" or "I of self-consciousness" the structure turns into the "eye of an external observer." In terms of the theory presented in Chapter 2, the mind loses its individualization and reverts into the general cultural process. In acute psychosis it is no longer individualized culture (which is the mind), which exists by means of the individual brain, but culture as such. The brain by the means of which the process of observation and memorization happens may be completely healthy. The disturbance is not in the brain. It is in the cultural, symbolic, structures of the mind. When the acute stage is past and the "thinking self" is reappropriated as such, the patient may recall the memory (at will) and speak of oneself experiencing the loss of self, as in "I get all mixed up so that I don't know myself. I feel like more than one person when this happens. I'm falling apart into bits. . . . I'm frightened to say a word in case everything goes fleeing from me so that there's nothing in my mind. It puts me into a trance that's worse than death." (People who put their trust in Foucault or Szasz should consider such testimonies before they claim that mental illness is a social construction.)

Moreover, the experience of observation by the alienated "thinking self" is also stored in memory. Often, the state of acute psychosis is remembered as a state of being watched. As a result, patients recall, as does the person quoted, "a critical self who gave me no peace," an "outside agency" communicating to her "the feeling of being an observer of myself: of seeing everything I did, as though I were someone else." The recollection continues: "I lie down and try to think, but the voices interrupt, pass comment and criticize." It is the voices (for culture in general speaks with many voices) of the alienated "thinking I," which takes on the function of the "eye of an external observer," that patients hear in their characteristic auditory hallucinations in acute psychosis. Sass writes: "By far the most frequent kind of hallucination in schizophrenia is, in fact, of highly intelligible voices; and these voices (unlike the auditory hallucinations of patients with alcoholic hallucinosis, the other group that very commonly hears voices) generally have more of a conceptual or cognitive than a sensory or perceptual taint, as if heard with the mind rather than the ear. [These voices] seldom occur early in the course of the illness; and they tend to escalate during circumstances of passivity and social isolation, and to diminish when patients interact with other people."[90] Almost by definition, at the state of acute psychosis the patient is incommunicative. The fact that communication diminishes auditory hallucinations in schizophrenics, points to the importance of directed culture for the function of the mental structure of "thinking I"/"eye of an external observer." Culture is usually directed in the fact of its individualization: the mind is the mechanism with the help of which the individual adapts to his/her symbolic environment and it (specifically, the structure of the will, the acting self) directs cultural resources, including the thinking self, to the solution of specific adaptive problems. In the mind as individualized culture, all the mental structures are integrated and serve (make functional) the individual. Willed thinking or willed self-consciousness, in other words, is always functional—it enables the individual to function and to adapt to the symbolic environment. For this reason, it is wrong to suspect self-consciousness as such in contributing to mental disorder. The cause of mental disorder (dysfunctional mental processes) is disintegration of the mind and, in particular, the impairment of the will, which prevents it from regulating the other mental processes. Unwilled thinking, i.e., thinking out of one's control, independent of one's acting self, becomes undirected process by definition (there is no agency to direct it) and is experienced as an alien consciousness. The "thinking I" turns into the "eye of an external observer." But culture can also be directed actually from outside—i.e., by an agency which is clearly and unproblematically recognized by the thinker as someone else, another person, and this actually outside direction can turn the "eye of an external observer" back into the "thinking I," reattach it to the mind, as it were.

Schizophrenic patients themselves are remarkably sensitive to what I envision as "free-ranging" or undirected, general culture in their brain; to the complex, composite nature of their minds; and to the connection between the acting and the thinking aspects of their self, or between the structures of the will and that of the "I of Descartes" (though, obviously, they do not call the latter by this name). One very articulate patient "describes himself as largely withdrawn from 'sensor motor activity,' and as dominated, during all his waking hours, by 'ideological activity—that is, central-symbolic, particularly verbal' forms of thought . . . tends to experience himself as passive, a mere observer of a process in which, as he puts it, 'concepts sometimes shift from one stratum to another'. . . . [He] states that his 'hallucinoid ideological stratum has its origin in the foreign content of the thoughts-out-loud experienced by the writer. That is, it is that part of ideas expressed by the hallucinatory allied phenomenon of minimal, involuntary, subvocal speech which the writer's self classifies as being foreign." Another one talks of "the splitting 'dialectic' and the splitting 'egos which inspect each other.'" These inner processes which she experiences and is able to describe and analyze, but is unable to stop, cause her suffering: "then I, through this combination of myself projecting into the other person, and the other person in itself, am monitored to react as expected, and that happens so rapidly that I, even if I had wanted to, am unable to stop myself. And after that, I am left by myself and very lonely." The disappearance of the "acting I" and, with it, of intention, makes simplest actions troublesome and forces the "thinking I" to take the place of the will, as if the person tried consciously to will oneself to will. One patient describes: "I am not sure of my movements anymore. It's very hard to describe this. . . . It's not so much thinking out what to do, it's the doing of it that sticks me. . . . I found recently that I was thinking of myself doing things before I would do them. If I am going to sit down, for example, I've got to think of myself and almost see myself sitting down before I do it. . . ." He adds, wistfully: "If I could just stop noticing what I am doing, I would get things done a lot faster"; the problem is he is not noticing what he is already doing, he must consciously create a blueprint for doing before he can do anything. In some

patients, this atrophy of the will and confusion between functional structures of the mind go so far that, according to Sass, they are no longer
capable of experiencing instinctual desires and, specifically, "gradually
cease to have any sexual feelings at all."[91]

Bleuler's Fundamental Features

While the sense of the loss of self, or loss of one's mind, reaches its terrifying peak during the phase of acute psychosis, when it is experienced
most directly, neither observed by the yet functioning "thinking self," nor
represented by elaborate delusions, as something else, the process begins
much earlier in the episode and can be seen in what Bleuler considered the
fundamental features of schizophrenia, to which delusions and hallucinations were secondary: formal thought disorder and abnormalities of schizophrenic language. The formal thought disorder—in distinction to the
disorder in the thought content (elaborate delusions and "monomanias" or
"overvalued ideas") is captured in the term "disassociative thinking": the
inability to privilege normal (i.e., conventional, common, socially accepted)
associations in thought. Another suggestive term for what, in the theoretical scheme of this book, clearly represents an abnormality of the structure of symbolic imagination, is Paul Meehl's "cognitive slippage," which
"brings out the unanchored and vacillating quality of schizophrenics'
thinking."[92] Bleuler, like many others after him, specifically emphasized
that disordered thought seemed not to serve any purpose for the thinker, it
was not goal-directed—therefore, again pointing, as noted above, to its
source in the impairment of the will, willed thought being directed by
definition. Characterizing schizophrenic thinking as "unanchored" and
"vacillating" also draws attention to this impairment.

Normal associations, i.e., associations of the vast majority of people, in
our—logical—civilization, first of all, mean associations following the
implicit rules of Aristotelian logic.[93] Schizophrenic thinking, as we saw, is
often considered logically deficient, "paralogical" or "paleological," and,
depending on whether the observer is a neurobiologist or a psychoanalyst,
respectively attributed to a brain defect or psychological immaturity.
Logic, however, is an historical, thus cultural, phenomenon, not a universal, inherent human ability. We assume absolute need for Aristotelian

logic in formal thought. There in no such absolute need. In a civilization that does not privilege logic as we do, normal associations won't follow its rules. It is, however, likely that they would follow some rules. But where the switchman of the will is absent, different sets of rules will intermix, and no particular set will be privileged. Schizophrenic impairment of will precludes the choice of logic as the framework of thought—thus we perceive in their thinking a dizzying multiplicity of points of view. With their will impaired, their symbolic imagination is, in fact, unanchored in any one of them, and naturally vacillates, and the more mentally developed and educated they are (i.e., the more symbolic material they have in their perfectly working memory), the more unanchored and vacillating, the more bizarre, it would seem to us.

Another way of putting this is to say that schizophrenic thinking is unconstrained (by logic, first and foremost, but by the conventions of the culture that is relevant to their social adjustment, in general). Instead, it is really free, and we necessarily regard its freedom as "pathological."[94] It is free because culture in general contains numbers of possibilities by many orders of magnitude greater than the culture of any specific group or any individualized culture, the mind. Culture is personalized, rendered practical, for each individual through the mental structures of identity and will (which works in tandem with identity). But in the "I of Descartes" it exists in its impersonal—and, for this reason, impractical—form. The "I of Descartes" can observe the rest of the mind, because it is, in a way, always outside it; it has an outsider's perspective. When, in the course of the disintegration of the mind, this one's "thinking I" attempts to take on the functions of the disabled will, it necessarily performs these functions differently, in an unfocused, unintentional, not goal-oriented way. "When one expresses a thought," already one of Bleuler's patients tried to explain, "one always sees the counterthought. This intensifies itself and becomes so rapid that one doesn't really know which was the first."[95] This must be a dizzyingly confusing experience. The "pathological freedom" of schizophrenic thinking, its not being anchored—through the mechanisms of identity and will—in reality relevant to the individual, is very likely to present them at some point in their disintegrated mental process with the possibility of solipsism, which was considered in the first chapter. Since, unlike the rest of us, they lack the ability to will themselves away from this possibility (which is what we all do), they are forced to let it, so to speak, "get to them" and become virtually paralyzed. In the Rorschach test, patients with a diagnosis of schizophrenia sometimes demonstrate "contamination percept"—a response almost never observed among other patients with psychosis, in which several possibilities present themselves to the mind at once, and the patient interprets the blot as a "dog rug," "bloody island," or "a butterfly holding the world together."

Changing its function from the original one of the "thinking I" to that of the "eye of an external observer" the mental structure of the "I of Descartes" acquires quite eerie analytical powers. Recalling experiences from this phase of self-alienation, patients characterize them as explicitly felt paralysis of will. One of Sass's patients explained his incommunicative (actually, mute and nearly motionless for days) behavior, saying that "he had felt unable to 'exert his will-power' because, he told [Sass], he had to deal with too many 'echelons of reality'—there were 'so many innuendos to take into account.'" Patients are also often acutely aware of not being the source of the possibilities they suggest and go as far in their explanations as to point to a general creative force that prompts these suggestions. One patient, asked why he sees "embryonic warthogs" in a Rorschach card, says: "Anthropomorphized. I take snapshots. Mind is a camera. On one of the takes they were anthropomorphized. Half human, half warthog." The mind with which this patient takes snapshots is not himself. His wording is mechanistic and reminds one of a common neurobiological position: the brain is a camera, a machine for taking pictures of reality. In the formulation of this patient, however, the camera is not a machine, but an artist: it creates reality. Another patient says in an interview: "Yes, we all have perspectives, everyone does, and then you ask the perspective spirit to help you find a home you can live in, if you don't have one, and so . . ." At this crucial point, the patient is interrupted by the interviewer! A "perspective spirit"— spirit with numerous perspectives—who suggests to the patient possibilities as unexpected by the patient as by the patient's interlocutors, speaks out of the patient; it, and not the patient's self is at home in the patient; the patient is homeless, evicted, and asks the perspective spirit for help to find a home where the self can live. "Perspective spirit," so *chez soi* where the self is supposed to be, is culture. In the disordered schizophrenic mind culture processes itself. A home for self is individualized culture. If only the interviewer were a bit more patient, perhaps the patient would be able to finish this tremendously suggestive thought and receive some help.[96]

Besides "cognitive slippage" or "pathological freedom," which, obviously, takes numerous forms, there is one specific abnormality common to schizophrenic thinking. Their thought lacks the temporal dimension—they seem to inhabit a timeless, spatial only, world. The reality they experience is in fact timeless. In moments of psychosis, not yet contained through elaborate delusions, their mind (mental process) takes the form of free-ranging culture in their brain, completely out of their control. They, therefore, exist as culture; experience their minds as impersonal, not individualized, culture. The integrated self, the ordered mind, of course, exists only in time, which necessarily colors the cultural space, constrains, limits, individualizes it. Each one of us—the mentally healthy—inhabits a certain absolute cultural time, which our minds represent. But few of us are truly conscious of the historical nature of culture; on the collective level, culture appears to most of us as timeless, with accumulated cultures of successive times overlaying each other, and layers melting into a timeless mass analogous to Oriental lacquer. Culture in general necessarily extends far beyond the time/space any of us occupies and represents. The fact that schizophrenics lose the temporal (cultural) dimension of their experience, but retain the spatial (material) one more or less intact (they orient themselves in space quite well) points to the cultural nature of their disorder, which does not necessarily affect their (animal) brain. It is the symbolic process (the change of meanings in accordance with the changing symbolic contexts) that introduces time into our experience, necessarily making us aware of the irreversible past-present-future relationship. Conversely, it is the mind that constitutes time into the relationship of past, present, and future. The cultural process outside—history—reflects it, so one can learn this from history; still, it is the mind that discerns, supplies the organizing principle to the perceived phenomenon—therefore supplies time—not the free-ranging culture. When we lose the sense of our specific location (it is remarkable that we all must use the language of space to capture the experience of time) in the symbolic process, which is inherent in the sense of self, time disappears or completely changes its feel.

This change is prominent in schizophrenics' recalled experiences. A patient of Jaspers remembers his psychosis: "The play with time was so uncanny . . . an alien time seemed to dawn." Almost a century later another patient complains: "I feel as if I lost the continuity linking the events of my past. Instead of a series of events linked by continuity, my past just seems like disconnected fragments. I feel like I'm in the infinite present."[97] Yet another sufferer describes watching the hands of a clock: "The hand is constantly different: now it is here, then it jumps so to speak and turns. Isn't this a new hand every time? Maybe somebody is behind the wall and keeps replacing the hand with another one at a different place each time. You get absorbed in the observation of the clock and lose the thread that leads you to yourself."[98]

Sass brings an example from "a major textbook on diagnostic testing" of a patient's responses to the Thematic Apperception Test, in which subjects look at pictures and must tell (1) what activity is going on in the scene depicted; (2) what led up to this activity; (3) what the outcome will be; and (4) the thoughts and feelings of the characters. In the example a young hospitalized man must respond to a card showing two people facing each other and in close physical contact. He says: "Before this picture, these two people, ah, hated each other. . . . And then they were accidentally thrown together in some situation and just before this picture, a miraculous change took place which I can't describe. In the picture they—they feel as if they are a picture—a complete thing. And they are aware of their limits and they accept them and after the picture they leave each other um—and the picture. [What are the limits? asks the testing psychologist. The patient responds:] The boundaries of the picture." It is evident that the patient not only substitutes the (physical) dimension of space for the (symbolic) time, but altogether loses the distinction between symbols and their referents, the understanding that symbols are arbitrary vehicles for meanings, which is the foundation of cultural experience. For the schizophrenic the symbol becomes the referent. Sass stresses the disturbed sense of semiotic relationships and comments: "Among patients without demonstrable brain disease . . . it is only schizophrenics who deviate from [the normal narrative spread with a past, present, and future] in a way that indicates a profound difference in the very structure of their experience,"[99] i.e., in the very way their mind operates. Patients themselves notice that the change in their perception of time is associated with increased cerebration (the hyperactivity of the "I of Descartes" oscillating between the functions of the thinking self and the "eye of an external observer") and the general feeling of profound insecurity, having no ground under one's feet. As experiences understood to be mental and symbolic are replaced by ones that are perceived to be coming from outside of oneself as the undoubted and only reality, and the continuity supplied by the mind disappears, a person indeed must feel as if he or she is at every single moment encountering a different world. Says one patient:

> I look for immobility. I tend toward repose and immobilization. I also have in me a tendency to immobilize life around me. . . . Stone is immobile. The earth, on the contrary, moves; it doesn't inspire any confidence in me. I attach importance only to solidity. A train passes by the embankment; the train does not exist for me; I wish only to construct the embankment. The past is the precipice. The future is the mountain. Thus I conceived of the idea of putting a buffer day between the past and the future. Throughout this day I will try to do nothing at all, I will go for forty-eight hours without urinating. I will try to revive my impressions of fifteen years ago, to make time flow backward, to die with the same impression with which I was born, to make circular movements so as not to move too far away from the base in order not to be uprooted. This is what I wish.[100]

As we saw, the one invariable characteristic of schizophrenic thinking is the extreme variability of its abnormalities. It is as likely to be abnormally concrete as abnormally abstract, for example. However comfortable within (one or the other interpretation of) the dual mind-body ontology, experts on schizophrenia through their unguarded formulations testify to the impossibility to even describe this otherwise than by reference to culture. Sass writes,

> The salient feature seems to be simply the sheer peculiarity of their generalizations and sortings—the use of principles that are highly personal, private, or bizarre, *less likely to be shared, or readily understood, by other members of the culture.* . . . In fact, responses [such as those of schizophrenic patients on various psychological tests] would seem to have sprung from an enhanced ability to perceive nonobvious similarities. . . . What is striking and undeniable about [them] is their *sheer unconventionality* . . . not so much an

incapacity for selective attention [which is often attributed to schizo-phrenics] as an unusual manner of allocating attention—a quality likely to derive from . . . their eccentric and often impractical or goalless orientation to the world.[101]

The circular nature of this statement helps to underline the predicament in which even the most sensitive members of the schizophrenia research community find themselves: there is no exit from this labyrinth so long as we let the mind-body view stand; nothing but understanding that mind is an emergent, and essentially cultural, phenomenon can solve the tragic puzzle of schizophrenia.

As any thought, disordered thought is most commonly expressed in language; language abnormalities characteristic of schizophrenia therefore, correspond to abnormalities of schizophrenic thinking. Again, Sass notes:

> The oddities of schizophrenic language . . . salient though they are, . . . have always been exceptionally difficult to characterize, let alone to explain. This is due partly to their daunting variety [and] the inconsistency and vari-ability of the characteristic peculiarities. . . . it is not surprising that schizo-phrenic language should so often have been described in purely negative terms—as incomprehensible, unconventional, or idiosyncratic, for example; these, of course, are but ways of asserting the absence of something normal or expected without saying anything positive about the nature and sources of what is observed.[102]

I shall try to do just that, interpreting the nature and sources of schizo-phrenic language, as was done on the previous pages regarding schizo-phrenic thought, in the terms of the proposed theory of the mind as individualized culture.

Sass postulates that all the linguistic abnormalities of schizophrenia can be interpreted as instances of three general trends: desocialization, autono-mization, and impoverishment. He defines "desocialization" as "the failure to monitor one's speech in accordance with social requirements of conver-sation" [note once more the uncommented upon dependence of the symptom on the cultural context], such as the loss of the deictic, or pointing, aspect of speech (relating it to any context). Schizophrenic speech, in other—our—words, tends not to have a specific (always time-dependent) context and to be impersonal. This also can be attributed to the loss of self, and specifically, of the acting self and relationally consti-tuted self—the will and identity that individualize culture and create con-text. Sass believes that the use of neologisms, one of the more prominent though relatively rare characteristic schizophrenic abnormalities, and new, unusual, and strikingly vivid metaphoric word combinations, in which common words are employed in unfamiliar and, Sass says, "personalized" ways (such as we saw in Matthews' vocabulary of "assailments") should be regarded as examples of desocialization, because they, too, like deictic failure, obscure the meaning the patient attempts to communicate to his or her interlocutors. But schizophrenics do not try to communicate meanings to others: they, as so many experts agree, lack intention to begin with, feel that they do not control the meanings (thoughts) they produce, and in their terrible plight are most concerned in making sense of their inner experiences to themselves. The new words and word combinations they utter are better conceptualized under the second rubric Sass suggests: autonomization of language.

Autonomization refers to "tendencies for language to lose its transparent and subordinate status, to shed its function as a communication tool and to emerge instead as an independent focus of attention or autonomous source of control over speech and understanding." As was pointed out earlier, it is a mistake to see language primarily as a communication tool and as a tool, to begin with. Language is the central element of the culture process; therefore, it is, under all circumstances, autonomous. It is also the medium of thinking, which, to some extent at least, makes thinking a function of language for individuals whose minds are in no way disturbed. The differ-ence between such mentally healthy individuals and persons suffering from schizophrenia is not that language is autonomous in the case of the latter and not autonomous in the case of the former, but that the *mind* loses its autonomy in the case of the latter, while being autonomous in the case of the former. Thus mentally healthy individuals experience their own speech as controlled by themselves and speech (or writing) addressed to them as having a specific and understandable to them meaning; in fact, this is only partially true, in the sense that language is integrated as an element in an individualized process and channeled into directions relevant to and useful for the user. In distinction, schizophrenics, caught in the loss of self and disintegration of the mind, experience language as out of their control (which it is indeed), external to them. In schizophrenic thought disorder which gives the observer "the praecox feeling" and associations appear "pathologically free," multi-perspectival, bizarre, it is no longer the individual, but culture, which does the thinking; similarly, in the abnormalities of schizophrenic language, it is no longer the individual, but the language, which speaks. It is this that explains the remarkable linguistic creativity and sensitivity of schizophrenics: their "verbal keenness" and "magnificent" ability to find the right terms for describing and analyzing unusual experiences (recognized by many and incorrectly conceptualized as "control" over meaning), expressed in neologisms, striking word combinations, and propensity for punning. Because of the disappearance of the self, the schizophrenic in fact becomes a mouthpiece and sensor for the creative multidimensional powers of language itself. The general attitude to the utterances of schizophrenics, says Sass, at least in psychiatry and cognitive psychology, has been that, as a product of malfunction, they do not need to be understood and that interpreting them would be a waste of time. But, if indeed it is language itself that speaks through them, the value of schizophrenic linguistic usage for the study of language should be enormous, and these utterances, more than any other linguistic material, would deserve being carefully analyzed and interpreted.

According to Sass, autonomization of language expresses itself in glossomania, a suggestive term, which he defines as "the flow of speech, channeled largely by acoustic qualities, or by irrelevant semantic connotations of one's words," but which I would translate, rather, as "undirected rush of speech." Here is an example: a patient is asked to identify the hue of a color chip; he answers: "Looks like clay. Sounds like gray. Take you on a roll in the hay. Hay day. May day. Help." "Such discourse is led at least as much by rhyme and alliteration," says Sass, "as by any overarching theme or meaning." Indeed, and in this sense this is precisely what happens in creative literature—in the prose of such authors as Dickens, who so obviously like to play with language, and especially in poetry.[103] The word "discourse," probably, should not be applied to such activities, in which the author, quite literally, lets himself go, leaving the direction of the process to language itself. In the terms of the conceptual system presented here, what happens is that the author at will switches his will off to enable the mind's symbolic warehouse guide the imagination. The radical difference between the artist and the schizophrenic is that in the case of the latter the autonomization of language is not willed. Rather than letting oneself go to offer free play to language, the schizophrenic experiences language as an oppressive external force and feels forced to give utterance to words and sentences willed by someone else. "I often repeat the same words," says a patient, "but they don't mean the same thing. . . . I understand absolutely nothing of what I say. . . . When I stop it is because the sentence has just finished." Sass, who quotes this patient is puzzled:

> In these glossomanic ways of speaking, a certain disengagement or abdica-
> tion of responsibility seems to occur. Instead of being guided by an overall
> sense of intended meaning, the flow and sense of the message is determined
> largely by intrinsic and normally irrelevant features of the linguistic system.
> One consequence is that, when reflecting upon their own writing or speech,
> such individuals may come to find their words as opaque and ambiguous as
> their listeners do. . . . there may be a loss of feeling of initiating or intending
> one's utterances. . . . [Patients may] experience their own speech or writing
> as some kind of alien substance rather than as the medium they inhabit and
> imbue with meaning.

It is as if, he muses, "the patient were in no better position than the listener to interpret the meaning of the words he himself has uttered."[104] But, of course, he is not in a better position. He lacks intention. Intention is the work of the will, and his will is impaired, lost; the schizophrenic does not exist as the acting self.

Finally, there is the "impoverishment" of schizophrenic language, which Sass characterizes as "the most heterogeneous of the three features." It includes restriction in the amount of spontaneous speech—conceptualized by Matthews as "fluid-locking." It also includes poverty of the content of speech, i.e., "utterances that are adequate in amount, in sheer number of words emitted, yet that seem to convey little information because the language is 'vague, often over-abstract or over-concrete, repetitive, and ste-reotyped.'" Two additional expressions of "impoverishment" are the use of "the most lofty, affected phrases" to convey trivial ideas, noticed already by Bleuler, and blocking—sudden interruption of speech due to the inability to continue a train of thought. These may be connected to the character-istic of schizophrenics' sense of the inadequacy of language, its inability to explain—to themselves, in the first place—what is happening to them and to capture the alternating or even simultaneous feelings that the world has lost all meaning and that it has become palpably meaningful in every detail, which often signal the onset of the schizophrenic episode. The ideas a patient attempts to convey in lofty phrases may not appear trivial to him or her, for indeed schizophrenics are unusually preoccupied with subjects of very general significance. Like the loss of the deictic dimension of speech (pointing to a specific context) in what Sass names "desocializa-tion," this is consistent with the characterization of the schizophrenic mental process as impersonal, as culture processing itself, resulting from the disintegration of individualized culture and loss of self. The more accurate term in this case may be "deindividualization," rather than "deso-cialization"; and what Sass and others perceive as "impoverishment" of language may in fact reflect the embarrassment of riches, the individual brain being overwhelmed and inundated by the enormous wealth of cul-ture and language, no longer selectively allowed in at the sluicegates of identity and will and channeled by these functional structures of the mind, but descending on it all at once as if in an avalanche.

Prodrome to Schizophrenia

One can characterize the two stages of full-blown psychosis—the acute psychosis phase and elaborate delusional phase—as the stages in which the loss of self is clearly perceived by the patient (acute psychosis) and in which it is perceived by others (elaborate delusions). Psychotic episodes in schizo-phrenia, however, usually announce themselves in the perception of a change in the nature of reality. In this prodromal phase, the patient seems to focus on the world outside himself or herself, rather than on the self and the inner world, and the observer is likely to interpret whatever abnormal behavior that results from the patient's changed attitude, if such abnor-malities are noticed at all, as signs of eccentricity, often attributed to supe-rior intellectual abilities. The changed attitude to the world outside is captured in such phrases (all of German origin) as the "truth-taking stare"—riveted attention to certain aspects of surrounding reality, as if never seen before; *Trema*—a theater slang term for stage fright before performance, in which anxiety intermixes with exhilaration; and *Stimmung*, which Sass describes thus:

> The patient will be suspicious and restless, often filled with anticipation or dread. Normal emotions like joy and sadness will be absent, the mood veering instead between anxiety and a kind of electric exaltation. Generally the person has a sense of having lost contact with things, or of everything having undergone some subtle, all-encompassing change. Reality seems to be unveiled as never before, and the visual world looks peculiar and eerie— weirdly beautiful, tantalizingly significant, or perhaps horrifying in some insidious but ineffable way. Fascinated by this vision, the patient often stares intently at the world . . . (He may also stare at himself in a glass, as if transfixed by the strangeness of his own reflection—the so called *signe du miroir*.) Usually the person becomes quiet and withdrawn, though an abrupt and seemingly senseless breach of decorum or discipline may also occur. This mood is sometimes followed by the development of delusions, espe-cially the symptom called "delusional percept"—where a relatively normal perception is experienced as having a special kind of meaning, a meaning not obviously contained in the percept itself and with a special relevance to the perceiver. . . .
>
> This is a strange and enigmatic atmosphere, a mood that infuses every-thing yet eludes description almost completely. To judge from what the patients say, the world appears to be, in some sense, quite normal. At least at first, they experience neither hallucinations nor delusions, nor does their thinking or behavior seem disorganized to any significant extent. Still, everything is totally and uncannily transformed: the fabric of space seems subtly changed; the feeling of reality is either heightened, pulsing with a mysterious, untamable force, or else oddly diminished or undermined— or, paradoxically, things may seem . . . both "unreal and extra-real at the same time."
>
> Patients in these moments may have a feeling "of crystal-clear sight, of profound penetration into the essence of things," yet, typically, "there is no real, clear content to communicate." The experience can involve a kind of conjoint and rather contradictory sense of meaningfulness and meaning-lessness, of significance and insignificance, which could be described as an "antiepiphany"—an experience in which the familiar has turned strange

and the unfamiliar familiar, often giving the person the sense of *déjà vu* and *jamais vu,* either in quick succession or even simultaneously.[105]

While these experiences are characteristic of the prodrome phase of the schizophrenic attack, they happen throughout the course of the disease and are observed in milder schizophreniform and schizoaffective cases. Sass believes that they represent a fundamental feature of schizophrenia, responsible for "the famous 'praecox feeling,'" and serving as "the source for other, better-known symptoms, such as delusions or ideas of reference (the latter involves the belief or sense that one is somehow the center of attention, the object of all gazes and messages)." In accordance with his general, if implicit, interpretation of schizophrenia as alienation from the objective, natural and social, reality, he sees in the *Stimmung* the beginning of the "move away from the social, consensual world."[106] The recollections of patients he quotes, however, seem to fit the interpretation proposed here—schizophrenia as the deindividualization of cultural resources of the mind and loss of self (only barely perceived in this early phase of the episode) better. Here is how the *Stimmung* stage is remembered by a patient, "Renee":

> For me, madness was definitely not a condition of illness; I did not believe that I was ill. It was rather a country, opposed to Reality, where reigned an implacable light, blinding, leaving no place for shadow; an immense space without boundary, limitless, flat; a mineral, lunar country, cold as the wastes of North Pole. In this stretching emptiness, all is unchangeable, immobile, congealed, crystallized. People turn weirdly about, they make gestures, movements without sense; they are phantoms whirling on an infinite plane, crushed by the pitiless electric light. And I—I am lost in it, isolated, cold, stripped, purposeless under the light. . . . This was it; this was madness, the Enlightenment was the perception of unreality. Madness was finding oneself permanently in an all-embracing Unreality. I called it the "Land of Light" because of the brilliant illumination, dazzling, astral, cold, and the state of extreme tension in which everything was, including myself.[107]

This frozen picture already demonstrates the change in the feel of time: Unreality is timeless, in fact, it is a collection of discontinuous spatial perceptions, each one dazzlingly clear, but lacking context, and therefore senseless. It is Unreality, because there is only the brain, doing its work of perception faithfully. But the self that supplies the context and the sense is absent, lost and purposeless, says Renee, in the infinite, deindividualized, space. The "Land of Light" is lifeless, nothing is going on in it, because the life of Renee's mind has stopped: no connections are made between perceived things, no logical leaps—jumping to conclusions—occur. There is no agency. Unlike at the stage of acute psychosis, during the prodrome the disappearance of the acting self is perceived indirectly, through what happens to the outside world when it disappears. And the thinking self is already compensating for the impaired will. When visited by a friend, Renee recalls, she "tried to establish contact . . . to feel that she was actually there, alive and sensitive. But it was futile. Though I certainly recognized her, she became part of the unreal world. I knew her name and everything about her, yet she appeared strange, unreal, like a statue."

Renee is oppressed by the "mere being" of things—the fact that they are there, and yet entirely meaningless, which fills her with horror. She writes:

> When, for example, I looked at a chair or a jug, I thought not of their use or function—a jug not as something to hold water and milk, a chair not as something to sit in—but as having lost their names, their functions and meanings; they became 'things' and began to take on life, to exist.
>
> This existence accounted for my great fear. In the unreal scene, in the murky quiet of my perception, suddenly 'the thing' sprang up. The stone jar, decorated with blue flowers, was there facing me, defying me with its presence, with its existence. To conquer my fear I looked away. My eyes met a chair, then a table; they were alive, too, asserting their presence. I attempted to escape their hold by calling out their names. I said, "chair, jug, table, it is a chair." But the word echoed hollowly, deprived of all meaning; it had left the object, was divorced from it, so much so that on the one hand it was a living, mocking thing, on the other, a name, robbed of sense, an envelope emptied of content. Nor was I able to bring the two together, but stood rooted there before them, filled with fear and impotence.[108]

Under the conditions of a normal mental process, things that exist independently of the person perceiving them, nevertheless also exist in the mind of that person: our attention is selective, and we only perceive things that are meaningful to us. For Renee, things take on life—they force themselves on her perception without selection. (In a way this means that perception and memory become perfected: they take in all; there is no attention deficit.) Renee's conscious understanding (arrived at through explicit thinking) is also strikingly sharp: it was a profound insight on the part of the great Émile Durkheim to define a "thing," in opposition to a "mere idea," as a coercive power, forcing itself on us, and to advise that cultural facts, which are necessarily also ideas, that is, meanings which exist only in the mind, be treated by a sociologist as things. The remarkably intelligent schizophrenic girl Renee (described by her psychoanalyst as mentally functioning on the fetal level!) draws the same distinction; she understands that, having lost meaning for her, a jug and a chair become things precisely because they acquire a coercive power over her. They confront her "in the murky quiet" of her perception—where the mind is dead, but the brain still works perfectly. She attempts to escape the hold of things by asserting her control (the control of her self, her agency) through naming. But words escape her control and acquire a life of their own as well and she stands "rooted . . . filled with fear and impotence" (as my dog Billy stands when an unfamiliar model of a lawn mower springs to life in front of him, and he perceives but cannot make any sense of it). All she has now is the objective reality; the important, subjective world is gone.

Renee is aware that the life of things consists only "in the fact that they were there, in their existence itself." As yet, she is neither delusional nor hallucinating. Her disease is not caused by disabled perception, and she does not believe that items of furniture or crockery transform their inanimate nature into organic. Her experience is simply no longer that of constant give-and-take between the world that surrounds her and her own self, between culture and the mind. Her self can no longer take part in this give-and-take, it is lost, and therefore culture now forces itself on her. Also, because, unless the self connects things and invests them with meaning, they remain separate and meaningless, she experiences the world as fragmented.

Yet another one of the patients in Sass's description feels the need "to put things together in" his head. One always does it, of course—but unconsciously; schizophrenics, in distinction, have to do this consciously and

deliberately. They have lost the structure of the mind responsible for inexplicit, un(self)conscious, spontaneous consciousness, their acting self, will,
agency, and with it the I that is known through spontaneous consciousness. The structure of the mind that remains to them, their explicitly
thinking, verbal I, the "I of Descartes," now consciously takes on itself the
functions of other structures. It also observes the absence of the acting self.
Self-consciousness turns into the consciousness of no self. One knows
oneself dead; one actually sees oneself dead. Sass quotes a patient saying:
"I feel nameless, impersonal. My gaze is fixed like a corpse; my mind has
become vague and general; like a nothing or the absolute; I am floating; I
am as if I were not." And he comments: "The patient, it seems, is plagued
not so much by diminished awareness or ability to concentrate as by hyper-
awareness, a constant, compulsive need to exercise his own consciousness. . . . it introduces a potentially disturbing self-consciousness and
awareness of choice, a conscious, controlled mode of functioning that disrupts more automatic or spontaneous processes."[109]

Sass refers to the last aspect of the schizophrenic *Stimmung* as "the apophanous mood" (from the Greek for "to become manifest"). It is, in effect, a
psychological resolution of the problem of meaninglessness—the terrifying
sense of the inability to see the perceived as meaningful, which dramatically
changes the familiar experience of perception. Apophany returns meaning
to the world. Suddenly, everything becomes profoundly significant, and the
sense of meaninglessness is replaced with "a certain abnormal awareness of
meaningfulness." The meaning is new and at first cannot be specified or put
in words. In his *General Psychopathology*, Jaspers wrote of patients in this
phase: "'I noticed particularly' is the constant remark these patients make,
though they cannot say why they take such particular note of things nor
what it is they suspect. First they want to get it clear to themselves." The
relief brought by the return of meaning is not to be equated with relaxation:
the experience of the deep meaningfulness of reality, combined with the
inability to interpret it, of the certainty of significance the nature of which
is uncertain, is oppressive and creates a particular kind of stress—"delusional
tension." "The experience of apophany," writes Sass, "is shot through with a
profound and almost unbearable tension (in some cases combined with exaltation). In this state of pulsing significance, the very ineffability, uncanni-
ness, and precision of everything seem nearly intolerable, as if the human

need for meaning and coherence were being titillated only to be frustrated on the brink of its fulfillment." A patient describes: "Every single thing 'means' something. . . . This kind of symbolic thinking is exhausting. . . . I have a sense that everything is more vivid and important. . . . There is a connection to everything that happens—no coincidences."[110] Thus it is not surprising that schizophrenics often complain of the insufficiency of language: first words lose all their meaning and become "things" that express nothing and then they are inadequate to capture the meanings one senses. It is also not surprising that apophanous mood seamlessly transforms into full-blown delusions: creative interpretations of the sensed meanings; and that "delusional tension" dissolves itself in overt psychosis.

The root of the schizophrenic experience, from the earliest stages and throughout the episode, is the problem with the self, specifically the acting self: the dissolution of the will. The difference between the early, middle, acutely psychotic, and elaborate delusional stages for the patient consists in that, during the prodrome, the loss of the acting self is experienced indirectly, through changed experience of the outside world, becoming more and more direct through the middle stages, culminating in the sense of the loss of the mind (and both relationally constituted self and the thinking self) in the stage of acute psychosis, and continuing in a partial restitution of identity and the thinking self, or the reconstruction of the *self-in-the-world* in the elaborate delusion. The structure of self-consciousness or the "I of Descartes" is involved at every stage in the disease process, but it changes its function from that of the thinking self to the one of the "eye of an external observer" and back, or, in other words, transforms from the part of the mind (individualized culture) to culture in general and back, confusing the levels of the mental and symbolic process. The different phases or stages of the illness, obviously, cannot be strictly separated but seamlessly flow and transmogrify one into another.

I would like to draw the reader's attention to two points. (1) Seen in this light, as a mental, rather than a brain, disease, as the disorder of the mind, and therefore, a cultural phenomenon, schizophrenia appears to be of a piece. All of its symptoms (however contradictory they may seem when seen in other frameworks) can be accounted for by the loss of the acting self and related to each other through this overarching relationship to the impairment of the will. One is no longer forced to consider the extreme variability of abnormalities to be the single invariable characteristic of schizophrenia. There is, after all, an organizing principle that makes it possible to integrate all of its features into an understandable whole. (2) To arrive at this interpretation of schizophrenia and depict its underlying psychological structure, there was no need to step outside the theory of the healthy mind as outlined in Chapter 2. No abnormality was interpreted *ad hoc*, proving the sufficiency of this theory. The analysis of schizophrenia, it is possible to claim, provides a strong support for its hypotheses regarding the structure of the mind.

It still remains to us, of course, to explain schizophrenia causally. As was stated in the Introduction, the explanation I propose is that modern society, based on the principles of nationalism, is profoundly anomic and, as such, makes the formation of identity (the relationally constituted self) problematic. Malformed identity, in turn, necessarily impairs the will. This hypothesis will be tested in two stages: first, through an examination of a well-documented contemporary case (the case of John Nash) and then, much more thoroughly, on the basis of comparative-historical analysis of the development of relevant aspects of the modern culture.

Anomie—Identity—Madness: The Case of John Nash

The mathematician John Nash won the 1994 Nobel Prize in Economics and later became the subject of Sylvia Nasar's award-winning biography *The Beautiful Mind* and a popular motion picture of the same name. The Nobel Prize is a very great honor, but few of the winners have ever attracted such general attention. The reason that John Nash became its focus was that his fame was preceded by thirty-four years of paranoid schizophrenia.

He experienced his first psychotic episode at the age of thirty and the first half of Nasar's meticulously researched biography deals with his life before he became the victim of "severe delusions, hallucinations, disordered thought and feeling, and a broken will."[111] Thus, in the case of John Nash, exceptionally, we are in possession of a wealth of premorbid information, sadly lacking in most cases of schizophrenia.

The symptoms of Nash's malady were classic, as were the signs of the predisposition to it, which he exhibited since early adolescence. His personality was clearly schizoid. He was "obsessed with originality," "disdainful of authority," "jealous of his independence." "Eager to astound, he was always on the lookout for the really big problems." His "faith in rationality and the power of pure thought was extreme. . . . he wished to turn life's decisions—whether to take the first elevator or wait for the next one, where to bank his money, what job to accept, whether to marry—into calculations of advantage and disadvantage, algorithms or mathematical rules divorced from emotion, convention, and tradition. His contemporaries, on the whole, found him immensely strange. They described him as "aloof," "haughty," "without affect," "detached," "spooky," "isolated," and "queer." . . . Preoccupied with his own private reality, he seemed not to share their mundane concerns. His manner . . . suggested something 'mysterious and unnatural.' His remoteness was punctuated by flights of garrulousness about outer space and geopolitical trends, childish pranks, and unpredictable eruptions of anger."

After the onset of the actual illness, Nash believed himself to be a "messianic figure of great but secret importance," "a prince of peace," and a victim of political and cosmic persecution (by war-mongering United States and the Jews as the incarnation of evil, respectively). His thoughts raced, he heard voices, and wrote "torrents of letters" to people he knew and did not know. All this—delusions of grandeur and persecution, enveloped in elaborate theories, auditory hallucinations, strangeness, flat affect, private reality—reads like a page from *DSM* description of schizophrenia; flights of garrulousness, mood changes and unpredictable irritability, racing thoughts and incessant writing also bring to mind mania. In our terms, what is remarkable is the obvious dominance of the "I of Descartes"— the explicitly symbolic thinking—over the unconscious and emotional mental processes, and specifically over the will; and the unusual preoccupation with the definition of self or identity.

In two respects, Nash's schizophrenia may seem atypical. Based on the way his mind worked before the descent into madness and the contributions he made to pure mathematics, Nasar concludes that he was in fact a genius, and, though there are more exceptionally creative individuals (thus, presumably, geniuses) among the insane than in the general population, very few schizophrenics are geniuses. In addition, Nash, apparently, made full recovery in his late 60s, and only about 8 percent of schizophrenics make such recovery.[112] Paradoxically, this may be less uncharacteristic than it seems because of the extraordinary nature of the event that preceded this recovery—the Nobel Prize in Economics, awarded to Nash at the age of sixty-six, for the twenty-seven page long PhD dissertation, written when he was twenty-one. That the Nobel prize in a discipline ostensibly dealing with human motivations was awarded to a person who, by the very definition of his pathology, could have had no experience of and no sympathy whatsoever with what makes most people act, a man "so out of touch with other people's emotions, not to mention his own," raises serious questions in regard to the status of economics as a form of rational thought, not to say an empirical science, but does not detract from Nash's genius as a mathematician and an abstract thinker. In any case, Nasar takes the Nobel Prize at its face value, writing:

> he did contribute, in a big way. . . . Nash's insight into the dynamics of human rivalry—his theory of rational conflict and cooperation—was to become one of the most influential ideas of the twentieth century, transforming the young science of economics the way that Mendel's ideas of genetic transmission, Darwin's model of natural selection, and Newton's celestial mechanics reshaped biology and physics in their day.[113]

Background

The parents of John Nash were not people comfortable with their situation in life: it was not what they wished it to be, and they strove incessantly to make it look like it was. His father, John Sr. came from a family of teachers, déclassé owing to his own father's philandering, instability, and, finally, abandonment of his wife and children. He grew up in relative poverty, which he considered shameful for a family of education, and in a fatherless home, which was considered shameful by others. As a result, he had "a deep and ever-present hunger for respectability" and, as his daughter, Nash's sister Martha, remembered, "was very concerned with appearances, . . . wanted everything to be very proper." Interested from early on in science and technology, Nash Sr. earned a degree in electrical engineering from Texas Agricultural and Mechanical and for a short time worked for General Electric, leaving this job to enlist in the army when the United States entered World War I. Rather than resume it after the war, he joined his *alma mater* as a member of the faculty, perhaps, as Nasar surmises, in hopes of pursuing an academic career. After one year of that, however, he took a position with a utility company in Bluefield, West Virginia, and remained with it for the rest of his life.

In Bluefield, Nash Sr. married "one of the most charming and cultured ladies of the community," from a "well-to-do, prominent local family." One of four sisters with a university education, Virginia Nash was also a daughter of a university-educated mother, and, before her marriage at the age of twenty-eight, she attended additional courses at such prestigious universities as Columbia and Berkeley, and taught school for six years. The young couple first lived in the imposing house of the bride's parents with her mother and sisters, but by the time their first child, John, was born, four years into the marriage, in 1928, they moved to a rental house owned by Virginia's mother. Writes Nasar:

> More than anything, the newly married Nashes were strivers. Solid mem-
> bers of America's new, upwardly mobile professional middle class, they . . .
> devoted themselves to achieving financial security and a respectable place
> for themselves in the town's social pyramid.

Details adduced by the biographer to support her interpretation throw some doubt on it. It seems that Nashes' experience was not one of upward mobility, but rather that of being stuck on a lower social grade than the one from which John Sr.'s family and Virginia herself descended, and that the chief purpose of their striving was not financial security but getting back their lost status—that is, not a "respectable" place in Bluefield's strat-ification but a place at its top. To claim, and show that they had, this status, they pinched pennies, and the desire to live beyond their means made them worry about the means they had and constantly dissatisfied with them.

Despite becoming "Episcopalians, like many of Bluefield's more pros-perous citizens, rather than continuing in the fundamental churches of their youth," despite joining "Bluefield's new country club, which was displacing the Protestant churches as the center of Bluefield's social life," despite Virginia's diligent participation in "various women's book, bridge, and gardening clubs," and despite remaining, unlike so many, financially secure throughout the Depression of the 1930s, the Nashes were not successful in their quest. They managed to acquire a house in one of the best neighborhoods. Yet, their three-bedroom home was "modest" by comparison "to the imposing homes of the coal families scattered around" and the necessity to mingle with the neighbors (which, after all, was the reason for the choice of the location) likely underscored, rather than concealed, that they did not really belong to it. Nevertheless, writes Nasar, "however much they were forced to economize, the Nashes were able to keep up appearances."[114]

It was into this atmosphere of pervasive status-inconsistency and strident striving that John Nash was born and in which he grew up. He must have learned in infancy the discrepancy between what one was in fact and what one wished to be. The necessity to keep up appearances—that is, to pretend to be what one was not—must have been instilled in him by the time he learned to walk, and the frustrations of his parents were surely communicated to him in many subtle ways with his mother's milk. Much of the boy's early childhood was spent in his mother's parental home, the easy opulence of which, if not the actual comforts, must have contrasted jarringly with the publicly concealed but privately insisted upon asceticism of her own household, because John was painfully aware and ashamed of his family's (in effect self-imposed) impecunity and had developed an irrational regard for money—not the power of wealth, but the medium of exchange, which, throughout his life, he would treat as almost magical, respecting it for itself, down to the smallest denominations. Virginia, who, according to her daughter Martha, "wasn't just a housewife," made the education of her first-born "a principal focus of her considerable energy." She "became actively involved in the PTA, taught Johnny to read by age four, sent him to a private kindergarten, saw to it that he skipped half a grade early in elementary school, tutored him at home and, later on, in high school, had him enroll at Bluefield College to take courses in English, science, and math." In a way, like many a parent frustrated in her own life, she sought to achieve status vicariously through Johnny, and therefore, while obviously a caring mother, easily became anxious when he deviated from her image of what he should be like. John Sr. also, consciously or not, projected his interests and frustrations onto the boy. A neighbor remembered: "He never gave Johnny a coloring book. He gave him science books."

Johnny was, very clearly, uncomfortable in these incongruous surroundings, he felt acutely that he was not what he should have appeared to be, did not mix well and was socially awkward. His behavior in elementary school, no doubt, would today be characterized as attention deficit disorder: "he daydreamed or talked incessantly and had trouble following directions, a source of some conflict between him and his mother." Thus his teachers considered him an underachiever and failed to discover much promise behind his "immaturity and social awkwardness." The boy naturally preferred solitude. Instead of playing with other children, he read his science books. However, "the Nashes pushed Johnny as hard socially as they did academically." His lack of interest in children's games (which, otherwise, they in no manner encouraged) became "major sources of worry for his parents. An ongoing effort to make him more 'well rounded' became a family obsession." When the children grew older, the younger Martha who was much better adjusted (because, first and foremost, less of a focus for and so less consistently disoriented by her parents), was asked to involve John in her social life. Though embarrassed by her brother's social inaptitude, she did her best—without much success.

While John did not like the society, whether of children his age or of adults, he did appreciate an audience and "enjoyed performing in front of other children." The performances were shows of his superiority. He made good use of the science books his father gave him and by the age of twelve acquired a rather extensive knowledge of the natural reality. It was not his superior knowledge that he exhibited, though. "At one point, he would hold on to a big magnet that was wired with electricity to show how much current he could endure without flinching. Another time, he'd read about an old Indian method for making oneself immune to poison ivy. He wrapped poison ivy leaves in some other leaves and swallowed them whole in front of a couple of other boys."[115] His need to feel superior, to affirm his uncertain self, was also expressed in more troubling ways. A neighbor remembered:

> I was a couple of years younger than Johnny. One day, I was walking by his house . . . and he was sitting on the front steps. He called for me to come over and touch his hands. I walked over to him, and when I touched his hands, I got the biggest shock I'd ever gotten in my life. He had somehow

rigged up batteries and wires behind him, so that he wouldn't get shocked but when I touched his hands, I got the living fire shocked out of me. After that he just smiled and I went on my way.

Nash, we are told by his biographer, "rarely passed up a chance to prove that he was smarter, stronger," even if it was just smarter and stronger than a smaller child. Besides, we learn that he "enjoyed torturing animals." It is disturbing to think how prodigious must have been his need for self-affirmation, how deep the doubt of his own worth if proving himself superior to smaller children would gratify him. Or how much anger and resentment against the world he must have accumulated in his twelve years to find pleasure in the pain of others. While Nasar makes no allusions to nineteenth-century fiction—so focused on the experience of status-insecurity in a mobile, anomic society—no one familiar with this literature can miss the striking similarity between the pattern emerging from the story she is telling about the future Nobel Laureate and that one finds in the fictional narratives of Dickens or Flaubert. In fact, already the very first of these "psychological novels"—in this case a fictionalized autobiography—*Anton Reiser* by K. P. Moritz, draws the link between uncertain identity and self-doubt, on the one hand, and cruelty, on the other. Anton, caught between social strata and securely belonging to none in the eighteenth-century German society, also becomes a "bad boy" and soothes his frustrations by torturing a dog.[116]

At the age of fifteen, Nash with two other boys from his elite neighborhood began experimenting with homemade explosives. Apparently a remarkably enthusiastic experimenter, he at one time threw a beaker of nitroglycerin of his own making over the cliff at Crystal Rock which, as his surviving co-experimenter commented decades later, "would have blown off the whole side of the mountain," but "luckily, didn't work." The other coexperimenter did not survive, an amateur bomb exploding in his lap. There is no doubt that had this happened today, we would regard the ingenuity of the teenage John Nash in the same light we consider Eric Harris and Dylan Klebold of the Columbine disaster fame. Indeed, the experiences of these three unhappy adolescents were in numerous ways comparable. Following the accident the other boy who remained alive was dispatched to a boarding school, but it is not known what the reaction of Nash's parents was.

Though Johnny's experimentation with bomb making took place in 1943–44, it was not patriotically motivated. "The war," writes Nasar, "made a lot of Bluefield boys want to hurry and grow up lest the war be over before they were eligible to join. But Johnny did not feel that way." If anything in connection with that titanic struggle preoccupied him, it was the economic boom produced by the war effort in Bluefield and the new rich whose fortunes it made and for whom Nash had little sympathy. The secret codes he was inventing of "weird little animal and people hieroglyphics" were "sometimes adorned with biblical phrases: 'Though the wealthy be great/Roll in splendor and State/I envy them not, /I declare it,'" which made it quite evident that envy was not the least of the motives behind his preoccupations.[117] The great conflict in which his country was involved was not much on his mind. Already then the boy could be accurately characterized as alienated.

When the society in which one lives fails to assign one's identity, which was emphatically the case with our protagonist, one must choose an identity for oneself. An attractive choice emerged for John Nash when, at the age of thirteen or fourteen, he read the 1937 *Men of Mathematics* by E. T. Bell. The book which, according to Nasar, provided Nash with "the first bite of the mathematical apple" and offered him the first glimpse of "the heady realm of symbols and mysteries entirely unconnected to the seemingly arbitrary and dull rules of arithmetic and geometry taught in school or even to the entertaining but ultimately trivial calculations that Nash carried in the course of chemistry and electrical experiments," consisted of brief and "lively [but] not entirely accurate" biographies of famous mathematicians. Bell presented them as very attractive personalities in general, but above all as men of genius—that is, men capable of intellectual achievement, which was quite beyond the capacities of most of humanity. He also offered his young readers the opportunity to test themselves, including some problems previously solved by these men of genius. Bell's essay on Fermat (whose main interest was number theory) "caught Nash's eye . . . For Nash, proving a theorem known as Fermat's Theorem about prime numbers . . . produced an epiphany of sorts." Nasar considers this experience to be comparable to "similarly revelatory experiences" of "other mathematical geniuses," and adduces as an example a passage from Einstein's "Autobiographical Notes" in which that scientific genius described the impression made on him, as a twelve-year-old, by Euclid: "Here were assertions, as for example the intersection of three altitudes of a triangle at one point which—though by no means evident—could nevertheless be proved with such certainty that any doubt appeared to be out of the question. This lucidity and certainty made an indescribable impression on me."[118] But the two adolescents' experiences are completely different. While Einstein, very clearly, was delighted by an unexpected quality of geometry—its lucidity and certainty, Nash (who found Euclidian geometry dull), as Nasar herself writes, was rather "thrill[ed by] discovering and exercising his own intellectual powers." In other words, he delighted in the possibility that he might be a genius.

From then on mathematics replaced science and engineering as Nash's main interest. Fearful that mathematics was unlikely to lead to a secure job, such as his father's, which kept the family well fed and clothed through the worst economic times, he still intended to become an electrical engineer, though, probably, as his father, hoping for a career in academia, rather than in a utility company. With the war "making heroes out of scientists," electrical engineering offered one plenty of opportunities to prove one's intellectual superiority, and it is evident that, by the time he entered the high school, proving his intellectual superiority became a priority for Nash. His chosen identity was that of a genius. Though he failed to make the honor roll without cracking a book, as he promised himself and a couple of sons of Bluefield College professors, whom he selected among his classmates as his audience, "Johnny entered the George Westinghouse competition and won a full scholarship, one of ten that were awarded nationally. The fact that Lloyd Shapely, a son of the famous Harvard astronomer Harlow Shapely, also won a Westinghouse that year made the achievement all the sweeter in the eyes of the Nash family."[119] Then he left Bluefield for the Carnegie Institute of Technology.

Having chosen an ideal identity for himself—what he wished to be—Nash had necessarily zeroed in on a particular social circle in which this identity—that of a genius—had its utmost value. Unfortunately for him, Carnegie turned not to be it. It still "resembled the trade school for sons and daughters of electricians and bricklayers" and was "shunned by the local ruling elite, which sent its children east to Harvard and Princeton." Harvard, in particular, the magical name for those seeking status in the American academic world, became the object of Nash's aspirations. These aspirations were encouraged by his math professors. His experiences at Carnegie soon proved beyond reasonable doubt that he was not a genius either in engineering or, after he changed his major to chemistry, in this branch of science either, but it also made it obvious that his future lay in mathematics. Nobody was less certain of it than Nash himself, which testifies to how insecure he was in his chosen identity—he was trying it on, as a new cut of clothes which one admires on a perfectly proportioned model, while in the depths of one's soul suspecting, if not knowing, that on oneself it would look ridiculous; indeed, above all, he needed to prove his genius to himself. He doubted even that he could make it at all—that is, make a living—as a mathematician. It was his mathematics professors who persuaded him that he could; thus he changed his major again.

In his new department, for the first time Nash found himself surrounded by Jews. It was his fate to be always surrounded by Jews, at least until he lost his mind (when it became his fate to be pitied and supported by Jews). During his studies and later, at RAND, at MIT, at the Institute for Advanced Study, and at the Courant Institute of Mathematical Sciences in New York, his Jewish colleagues and former classmates were among his most steadfast friends. It was they who attempted most persistently to bring him back from the dark world of madness, to arrange for some part-time position, to secure some funding, to make possible treatment that was less degrading than hospitals for which his mother and sister believed themselves able to pay. In the end it was Ariel Rubinstein who insisted on his integration into the Olympian circle of mathematical economics and worked tirelessly to ensure that he would get the Nobel Prize, all because he believed it unfair that a brilliant thinker such as Nash would become a victim of schizophrenia and utterly unacceptable that, just because of thirty years of madness and absence from the profession, he would be deprived of the recognition that a mind such as his deserved: it went against the Israeli professor's sense of justice.

At the time of Nash's studies at Carnegie, Jewish refugees from Europe flooded with talent the rather sleepy hollow of American mathematics, raising many a math department to earlier undreamt of intellectual stature and rousing the field itself to a heretofore-unknown level of activity. This attracted students, and while Jewish professors from Europe were as—or, perhaps, more—likely to end up in Princeton as at Carnegie, American born Jewish students were perforce limited to second-rate technical schools. Nash's Jewish classmates who included him in their group, despite all the discrimination they inevitably faced while growing up, were more cultured and socially sophisticated than Nash who grew up in the no man's land between the confident upper stratum of the Bluefield society and the "strivers" just below it, and raised on a diet of scientific magazines and science and science fiction books. "'He was a country boy, unsophisticated even by our standards,' recalled Robert Siegel . . ."

One of the Jewish boys with whom Nash passed his time was a fifteen-year-old *wunderkind* Paul Zweifel. Nash suddenly "discovered," writes Nasar, "that he was attracted to other boys [and] during Thanksgiving break, in the deserted dormitory, Nash climbed into Zweifel's bed when the latter was asleep and made a pass at him." This behavior made Nash a butt of jokes. "While his professors singled him as a potential star, his new peers found him weird and socially inept. . . . 'Here was a guy who was socially underdeveloped and acting much younger. You do what you can to make his life miserable,' Zweifel admitted. ' . . . We were obnoxious. We sensed he had a mental problem.'" His classmates' teasing likely reinforced the sense of inferiority that must have plagued Nash in any event as a result of his status-insecurity and the vagueness of his identity. And this made him ever more insistent on his intellectual superiority. "Nash defended himself the only way he knew how. . . . He went for childish displays of contempt. 'You stupid fool,' he'd say,' Siegel recalled. 'He was openly contemptuous of people who he didn't think were up to his level intellectually. He showed this contempt for all of us.'"

But, of course, Nash didn't know that he was smarter: any of them, and not he, might as well have been a genius, and this was the worst of all. In fact, his classmate George Hinman made it into the top ten of the prestigious William Lowell Putnam Mathematical Competition for undergraduates in 1946, in which Nash too participated, but without any success. The first five were practically assured acceptance to the Harvard department of mathematics. Nash tried again the next year and now found himself among the top ten, like Hinman a year earlier. This was a crashing disappointment: he was, after all, not superior to Hinman. "Decades later," writes Nasar, "after he had acquired a worldwide reputation in pure mathematics and had won a Nobel Prize in Economics, Nash hinted in his Nobel autobiography that the Putnam still rankled and implied that the failure played a pivotal role in his graduate career. Today [in 2001] Nash still tends to identify mathematicians by saying, 'Oh, So and So, he won the Putnam three times.'" Nobody, however, had ever connected his disease to this event.

Despite his self-doubt, Nash was accepted to the four top graduate departments in the country, Harvard and Princeton among them. Princeton was at the time "the mathematical center of the universe," while Harvard, which refused to "take advantage of the emigration of the brilliant Jewish mathematicians from Nazi Germany," in contrast, had entered "a state of eclipse." Still, Nash wanted to go to Harvard. His biographer comments:

> Harvard's cachet and social status appealed to him. As a university, Harvard had a national reputation, while . . . Princeton with its largely European [read, Jewish refugee] faculty, did not. Harvard was, to his mind, simply number one, and the prospect of becoming a Harvard man seemed terribly attractive. The trouble was that Harvard was offering slightly less money than Princeton. Certain that Harvard's comparative stinginess was the consequence of his less-than-stellar performance in the Putnam competition, Nash decided that Harvard didn't really want him. He responded . . . by refusing to go there. Fifty years later, in his Nobel autobiography Harvard's lukewarm attitude toward him seems still to have stung . . .

Thus, his fear that he was not, in fact, what he wished to be—a genius— led Nash to opt for a milieu from which he felt alienated even before he arrived there. He chose a society to which he did not want to belong. Princeton was at that time unquestionably the most exciting place for a mathematician to be, but "the only thing Nash really knew about Princeton was that Albert Einstein and John von Neumann were there, along with a bunch of other European émigrés . . . the polyglot Princeton mathematical milieu—foreign, Jewish, left-leaning—still seemed to him a distinctly inferior alternative."

As he was not a patriotic American of a nativist (or any other) variety, the foreignness of the Princeton faculty could not have bothered him much and, being totally uninterested in ideological politics, he could not have known that it was left leaning. There was, it appears, only one reason why Princeton would be inferior to Harvard in the eyes of an aspiring star on the mathematical firmament: while the department at Princeton was far more selective in its admissions, "admitting ten handpicked candidates each year, as opposed to Harvard's twenty-five or so," Harvard remained a bastion of a different sort of exclusivity, and the thickly Jewish community of Princeton, despite the astonishing concentration of talent—genius—in it, did not confer the same social status as the racially more refined (and openly anti-Semitic) high society of the older university on the Charles. Genius was Nash's chosen ticket to status—Harvard, he feared, did not recognize his genius, but Princeton, which recognized it, could not offer him status. "Sensing Nash's hesitation," but clearly unaware of its nature, Solomon Lefschetz, the chairman of the Princeton department, added to the initial offer the most prestigious fellowship the department had to offer. "For Nash, that clinched the decision." The fetishist attitude to money, which made Nash attach great importance to trivial sums, was already clouding his perception of reality; and he "calculated Princeton's more generous fellowship as a measure of how Princeton valued him."

Another symptom of his still unsuspected disease presented at the same time:

> he became more and more worried about being drafted. He thought that the United States might go to war again and was afraid that he might wind up in the infantry. That the army was still shrinking three years after the end of World War II and that the draft had, for all intents and purposes, ground to a standstill, did not make Nash feel safe. . . . He . . . was obsessed with ways to defend himself against any possible threats to his own autonomy and plans.

It must have been exceedingly unpleasant to be around the twenty-year-old John Nash when he arrived at Princeton in the fall of 1948. "The first-year students were an extremely cocky bunch, but Nash immediately struck everyone as a good deal cockier." Handsome, he cultivated the look of an English aristocrat. His hair flopped over his forehead; he was constantly brushing it away. He wore his fingernails very long, which drew attention to his rather limp and beautiful hands. . . . Moreover, his expression was rather haughty and he smiled to himself in a superior way. . . . He seemed eager to be noticed and seemed to want to establish that he was smarter than anyone else in the place. . . . He seized opportunities to boast about his accomplishments. He was a self-declared free-thinker. On his Princeton application, in answer to the question "What is your religion?" he wrote "Shinto." He implied that his lineage was superior to that of his fellow students, especially Jewish students. . . . a fellow student who grew up in a poor family in the Bronx, recalled catching up with Nash when he was ruminating about blood lines and natural aristocracies . . . "He was opposed to racial mixing. He said that miscegenation would result in the deterioration of the racial line. Nash implied that his own blood lines [as opposed to those of the student from Bronx] were pretty good."

Such talk, addressed to a Jewish classmate three years after the Holocaust, was a different kind of cruelty from the one Johnny Nash practiced as a young teenager, but it was motivated by a similar desire to cause pain to another and thus assert one's superiority; it makes one consider seriously where would this brilliant mathematician end up had he been born ten years earlier and in Germany, rather than in the United States—would we find him seeking relief from his status-anxiety in the ranks of the SS? It also makes one think, more generally, about the connection between the problematic sense of self and evil. Perhaps, the source of the latter is not such a mystery after all? And, perhaps, what in the end leads to self-destruction and hospitalization in the United States may in a different time and place find release in the participation in a genocidal movement?

The very stridency of his efforts to have his superiority acknowledged by all around him makes it clear that Nash was very anxious—that is uncertain—about it. And it was especially difficult to prove oneself intellectually superior to those who surrounded him at Princeton. He was brilliant, of course, but every one of the handpicked rising stars was at least equally brilliant, many of them were to achieve mathematical celebrity greater and certainly sooner than Nash, and what they remembered of him at this stage in particular was "a tremendous amount of ambition."

Remarkably, unlike most great scientists and mathematicians of known biography, while obviously driven, Nash was driven not by an internal desire to understand or to resolve a particular problem, but by a desire to prove that he could resolve the most important problems, whatever they might be. Mathematics was not his passion, but the arena in which he knew that his passion could be satisfied. Thus he "really cross-examined people on what were the important problems": there was no point in wasting time on being brilliant where it could be overlooked. Nash displayed a similar attitude in his relations with his would-be teachers: all he wanted from them was to recognize him as a superior intellect, he was not in Princeton to learn. Nothing diverted him from his one goal—to become secure in his chosen identity. Nash "read astonishingly little . . . taking the attitude that learning too much secondhand would stifle creativity and originality." For the same reason, he did not become anyone's disciple and never chose an advisor in the literal sense of the word among his professors. A conventional path to recognition—passing general exams, writing a dissertation—against the urgency that he experienced must have appeared too long.

The presence of Einstein—the genius of geniuses—seemed to offer a shortcut. Were Einstein to declare that Nash was a genius, surely the entire world would immediately accede to this opinion. The twenty-year-old dreamt "how he might strike up a conversation, stopping Einstein in his tracks with some startling observation" and, for him, the daydreams were already acquiring the undeniable character of reality. "It was a measure of Nash's bravura and the power of his fantasy," writes Nasar, "that . . . just a few weeks into his first term at Princeton, [he] made an appointment to see Einstein. . . . He told Einstein's assistant that he had an idea that he wished to discuss with Professor Einstein." The idea was a hunch he had in physics, and "Nash had given [this] hunch enough thought to spend much of the meeting at the blackboard scribbling equations." Einstein gave him an hour of his time and listened with interest, but all he said in the end was "You had better study some more physics, young man."

Nash then tried approaching the second-ranking genius in Princeton—also a Jewish émigré—John von Neumann, whose attempt in the 1920s "to construct a systematic theory of rational human behavior by focusing on games as simple settings for the exercise of human rationality" by the late

1940s resulted in the emergence of a new branch of mathematics—game theory. The book von Neumann published in 1944 with Oscar Morgenstern, *The Theory of Games and Economic Behavior,* in which it was claimed that, in the framework of the theory "the typical problems of economic behavior become strictly identical with the mathematical notions of suitable games of strategy," was a hit among the economists. A reviewer jubilated: "Ten more such books and the future of economics is assured." (The fact that it was "'a blistering attack' on the prevailing paradigm in economics and the Olympian Keynesian perspective [with its] attempt to ground the theory in individual psychology" today, when this perspective is back in force and the Nobel committee distributes prizes to the so-called "behavioral economists," throws a melancholic light on this reception.) Though the Navy made use of game theory during the war and generously funded game theorists in Princeton, the pure mathematicians considered it as an applied branch of no great importance, even "trivial." "But to many of the students at Princeton at the time it was glamorous, heady stuff, like everything associated with von Neumann."[120]

Von Neumann's game theory was incomplete. The best-developed part of it concerned zero-sum two-person games of total conflict, which were believed to be less applicable to economics than games of more than two players. Von Neumann "couldn't prove that a solution existed for all such games." Proving this, Nash decided, would be worthy of his effort. In his second semester in Princeton, he wrote "his first paper, one of the great classics of modern economics," says Nasar.

> "The Bargaining Problem" is a remarkably down-to-earth work for a mathematician, especially a young mathematician. Yet no one but a brilliant mathematician could have conceived the idea. In the paper, Nash, whose economics training consisted of a single undergraduate course . . . at Carnegie, adopted 'an altogether different angle' on one of the oldest problems in economics. . . . By so doing, he showed that behavior that economists had long considered part of human psychology, and therefore beyond the reach of economic reasoning, was, in fact, amenable to systematic analysis.[121]

When the paper was published (in 1950 in *Econometrica*), Nash thanked Von Neumann and Morgenstern for reading and commenting on the first draft, but claimed later that he had been interested in the problem before attending the game theory seminar in Princeton. Von Neumann, a senior fellow at the Institute for Advanced Study, did not advise graduate students and, probably, did not read drafts of their papers; the game theory seminar was led by Albert Tucker, von Neumann's book was its "bible," and von Neumann at most gave a lecture or two in it. Nasar surmises that "very likely Nash sketched his ideas for a bargaining solution in Tucker's seminar and was urged by Oscar Morgenstern . . . to write a paper."

During the summer of 1949, Nash suddenly asked Tucker to be his thesis supervisor. Having had little out-of-class contact with the student, Tucker asked why. Nash's answer was that he had "some good results related to game theory." Tucker agreed that he was the appropriate academic advisor for the subject. Nash continued to mull his ideas over and by the beginning of his second year had "his brilliant insight into human behavior, the Nash equilibrium," for which forty-five years later he would receive the Nobel Prize in Economics. In the fall of 1949, however, Nash went to see von Neumann. "He wanted, he had told the secretary cockily, to discuss an idea that might be of interest to Professor von Neumann." It was not. Von Neumann, preoccupied with the development of the H-bomb, listened to Nash politely as the young man began "to describe the proof he had in mind for an equilibrium in games of more than two players. But before he had gotten out more than a few disjointed sentences, von Neumann interrupted, jumped ahead to the yet unstated conclusion of Nash's argument, and said abruptly, 'That's trivial, you know. That's just a fixed point theorem." "Trivial" was the word Nash used to characterize the ideas of his classmates whom he considered less brilliant than he was. "Von Neumann's rejection of Nash's bid for attention and approval must have hurt," writes Nasar, "and one guesses that it was even more painful than Einstein's earlier but kindlier dismissal. He never approached von Neumann again."

It was this work, however, which was several months later approved as Nash's PhD dissertation. Albert Tucker, Nash's nominal advisor, though surprised that Nash had completed a draft within such a short time, remembered later that he was not particularly impressed by the work: after all "whether or not this was of any interest to economists wasn't known." Thus Nash was leaving graduate school as only a very promising young mathematician, his identity as a genius still had to be proven and he remained uncertain of it. The stubborn refusal of the world to acknowledge that he was in fact what he wanted to be must have already weighed very heavily on him, and though he was only twenty-one, for him it was probably becoming too late.

And yet nobody around him suspected that he was in distress, that he was ill. His strangeness, which cried "schizoid" to anyone with even minimal knowledge of psychiatry, was attributed, basically, to mathematics: brilliant mathematicians, apparently, are supposed to be eccentric. The fact that Princeton was teeming with brilliant mathematicians, some of them of acknowledged and undoubted genius, who nevertheless were nowhere as bizarre as Nash, did not arouse any suspicions. He was respected for his obvious talent but unloved and considered simply a nasty character. "He was quite popular with his professors, but utterly out of touch with his peers. His interactions with most of the men his own age seemed motivated by an aggressive competitiveness and the most cold considerations of self-interest. His fellow students believed that Nash felt nothing remotely resembling love, friendship, or real sympathy, but as far as they were able to judge, Nash was perfectly at home in this arid state of emotional isolation."

At the same time, they were aware that Nash was prone to have "crushes"—fervent childish infatuations—for "other men, mostly brilliant mathematical rivals." His idea of wooing was as eccentric as anything he did and consisted—in addition to talking mathematics—of pestering and practical jokes, often cruel and sometimes very dangerous. It would be too time-consuming to offer examples. Attracted to Nash at first by the surprising and beautiful way in which his mind worked in mathematics (his imagination seemed to be free-ranging, not at all controlled by the established rules, it seemed to skip all the steps considered necessary, and yet, more often than not it led to the correct result) the men would befriend him in turn. But these friendships never lasted.

It is likely that Nash was truly unaware of his homosexual tendencies. Homosexuality certainly was not a part of his chosen identity—the way he had decided to see himself and wished to be seen by others. This chosen identity required that he get married and have children, and he was to do this within less than a decade of graduating. Before affiancing himself to a woman who corresponded to his image of the wife of a patrician and a genius, he had a mistress who clearly did not correspond to this image—an affair he kept secret from his colleagues—and had a child by her. In his relationships with both women he was unfeeling and often treated them with intentional cruelty. He had no interest in either of them as persons or in their circumstances, expressed no sympathy for their difficulties, took no responsibility for problems he caused them, and used them openly and unabashedly. Clearly, he did not think that there was anything wrong with this behavior.

The most astonishing—and most hurtful as far as the two women were concerned—was his attitude to money. He was glad to learn that his mistress was pregnant, but throughout her pregnancy offered no financial help to her or, after the birth, to his child; suggested that she give the boy up for adoption; and, when she refused, watched calmly as she, unable to support herself and the baby on her meager salary or even to earn it in a social climate in which single unwed motherhood was looked down upon as immoral and undeserving of consideration, moved his son from one foster home to another. It was Nash's parents, in the end, when the poor woman learned that he was going to marry another and demanded child support, who provided it, unwilling to force him to marry below his station. Still, John Stier, Nash's elder son, had a miserable, insecure childhood, in which real, not imaginary, poverty was the most stable element. But even with his wife, Alicia, Nash kept separate accounts and demanded that all the bills, down to the restaurant checks, be equally divided and that she pay for her expenses with her own money. Throughout all this period he was employed by prestigious and generous institutions, MIT and RAND, and more than comfortable financially.

Nash's crushes on men, and the attitude to money that had more in common with that of Moliere's Miser, pathetic and ridiculous already in the seventeenth century, than with the thinking expected of a late twentieth century Nobel Laureate in Economics, and that in particular characterized his relationships with women, were the only exceptions in a life that was experienced and lived as purely and unfailingly rational. In fact, it appears that Nash was quite incapable of symbolically inexplicit mental processes: his consciousness worked only as explicit thinking. This meant that, unless things were explicitly stated—in writing, in conversation, or in his mind—he was not aware of them. Most of the things in our lives are not stated explicitly. Apart from a few books on etiquette, there are no written rules for social conduct; our own reactions, our understanding of other people's emotions are based on no formal principles. Social and/or emotional idiocy combined with an acute ratiocinative intelligence is, in fact, a common feature of schizophrenic disorders. Nash's astonishing lack of tact, his coldness represented the other side of his all-pervading rationality. He was absolutely clueless as to what makes people tick: he could not read the inexplicit texts.

Nasar offers a telling example from Nash's Princeton days. With a couple of friends, among whom was Nash's "crush" of the moment, who wished to channel the "absurd behavior" of his besotted admirer in "a more intellectually constructive way," Nash invented a game, which he, characteristically, called "Fuck Your Buddy":

> Nash and the others crafted a complicated set of rules designed to force players to join forces with one another to advance, but ultimately to double-cross one another in order to win. The point of the game was to produce psychological mayhem, and, apparently it often did. [One of the group] remembers losing his temper after Nash cold-bloodedly dumped him on the second to last round, and Nash was absolutely astonished that [the other] could get so emotional. "But I didn't need you anymore," Nash kept saying, over and over.

Even more remarkable was Nash's reaction several years later to an experiment with Prisoner's Dilemma, "the most famous game of strategy in all of social science," run by two mathematicians at RAND the day they learned of Nash's equilibrium idea, to test whether his predictions would hold true in actuality:

> the results hardly resembled a Nash equilibrium. . . . Players tended not to choose Nash equilibrium strategies and instead were likely to "split the difference." . . . [They] chose to cooperate more often than they chose to cheat. Comments recorded after each player decided on strategy but before he learned the other player's strategy show that [one of them] realized that players ought to cooperate to maximize their winnings. When [the other player] didn't cooperate, [the first one] punished him, then went back to

cooperating next round. Nash, who learned of the experiment from Tucker, sent [the experimenters] a note . . . disagreeing with their interpretation: "The flaw in the experiment as a test of equilibrium point theory is that the experiment really amounts to having the players play one large multi-move game. . . . There is too much interaction. . . . It is really striking however how inefficient [players] were in obtaining the rewards. *One would have thought them more rational.*"[122]

Nash was a mathematician, not a scientist: empirical evidence was no evidence for him, and he was quite unconscious that rationality could as well obscure as reveal the real springs of human action.

Still, the most striking example of the opacity of Nash's mind one finds in his biography concerns neither games, nor game theory, but the serious business of sex. In the summer of 1954 Nash was arrested by the vice squad of the Santa Monica police. Picked up in a men's bathroom in a park, he was charged with indecent exposure and released. It happened early in the morning. The arrest, apparently, did not strike Nash as deserving a minute of his consideration; he actually went straight to his office at RAND and back to his mathematical problems. But at RAND mathematicians had access to top-secret information, Nash had a top-secret security clearance, and at the time security guidelines "specifically forbade anyone suspected of homosexual activity to hold a security clearance." The organization was informed of the arrest a couple of hours after it happened and had no choice but to cancel his consulting contract on the spot. The security manager Richard Best and his boss, Steve Jeffries, writes Nasar:

> went around to Nash's office and confronted him with the bad news themselves . . . Nash did not appear shaken or embarrassed. . . . Indeed, he seemed to be having trouble believing that Best and Jeffries were serious. "Nash didn't take it all that hard," said Best. He denied that he had been trying to pick up the cop and tended to scoff at the notion that he could be a homosexual. "I'm not a homosexual," Best quotes Nash as saying, "I like women." He then did something that puzzled Best and shocked him a little. "He pulled a picture out of his wallet and showed us a picture of a woman and a little boy." "Here's the woman I'm going to marry and our son."

In a postcard to his parents he blamed the withdrawal of his RAND security clearance on the Communist past of his mentor at MIT, Nathan Levinson.[123] It is obvious that he really believed that and was really unaware that his interest in men could be interpreted as homosexuality: after all, here was the picture—an explicit image of his heterosexual credentials. Apparently, homosexuality was not discussed among mathematicians in those days, therefore, for Nash it did not exist.

With his RAND contract lost, Nash spent the next few years working on problems in pure mathematics: there was no other way to the apex of the mathematical hierarchy, with its highest accolade—the Fields Medal—and a tenured position at Harvard or, at the very least, Princeton. During his sojourn at the Courant Institute of Mathematical Sciences, the "national capital of applied mathematical analysis," he solved a major problem in the field of nonlinear theory. As usual, the manner in which he did this was completely unconventional. This convinced many people around him that he was a genius and the solution got a lot of attention. Briefly, Nash became a celebrity; the Courant Institute made him "a handsome job offer" (which he refused, preferring to remain at MIT "because of the tax advantage of living in Massachusetts as opposed to New York"). But then he learned that a completely unknown young Italian mathematician, Ennio De Giorgi, had proven the same theorem a few months before him. He was terribly upset. He was twenty-nine years old. Writes Nasar:

Nash's thirtieth year was . . . looking very bright. He had scored a major success. He was adulated and lionized as never before. *Fortune* magazine was about to feature him as one of the brightest young stars of mathematics in an upcoming series on the 'New Math.' And he had returned to Cambridge as a married man with a beautiful and adoring young wife. Yet his good fortune seemed at times only to highlight the gap between his ambitions and what he had achieved. If anything, he felt more frustrated and dissatisfied than ever. He had hoped for an appointment at Harvard or Princeton. As it was, he was not yet a full professor at MIT, nor did he have tenure. . . . Getting these things after only five years would be unusual, but Nash felt that he deserved nothing less. But Martin [the chairman] had already made it clear to Nash that he was unwilling to put him up for promotion so soon. Nash's candidacy was controversial . . . just as his initial appointment had been. A number of people in the department felt he was a poor teacher and an even worse colleague. . . . Nash . . . was furious.

This was added to his despair "over the De Giorgi fiasco. The real blow of discovering that De Giorgi had beaten him to the punch was to him not just having to share the credit for his monumental discovery, but his strong belief that the sudden appearance of a coinventor would rob him of the thing he most coveted: a Fields Medal." The 1958 Fields Medal was awarded in August—not to Nash. A couple of months later he went mad.

The Course of Illness

Nash had presented the classical negative symptoms of schizophrenia since early adolescence, but they were at first considered as signs of somewhat unpleasant eccentricity natural to a particularly brainy youngster and later specifically attributed to his brilliance as a mathematician. As it happened, the central positive symptoms—the bizarre way of thinking that seemed not to follow accepted rules of logic and the particular delusions—were also long present and were also written down to either nastiness of character or genius, or—in the case of his paranoid obsession with Jews—to the idea that patrician boys will be patrician boys, which was just a fact of life. (After all, millions of Nash's near-contemporaries had a similar obsession without being ever suspected of schizophrenia; one may well wonder why.) It must be said that insanity was not entirely foreign to the mathematical community of which Nash was a part. Among a hundred or so mathematicians in his immediate circle at different stages of life Nasar mentions at least fifteen who are known to have suffered from a significant, though in all cases apparently affective, mental disorder, or whose first-degree relatives were hospitalized for mental illness, several of them with schizophrenia. Yet, not before Nash became obviously psychotic, and it was no longer possible not to recognize this, had anyone thought that he was mentally ill.

It took a number of months for the psychosis to become obvious. It was, as psychiatrists say, "kindling." During the summer of 1958 Nash became increasingly anxious about growing old and decided that he would prove the Riemann Hypothesis—"the holy grail of pure mathematics," which for a hundred years had resisted all attempts at proving it—promising explicitly to resolve the most challenging problem in the field. At the same time "Nash's somewhat compulsive attitude toward money blossomed into an obsession with the stock and bond market. An MIT economist, Solow, recalled:

> It seemed he had a notion that there might be a secret to the market, not a conspiracy, but a theorem—something that if you could figure it out, would let you beat the market. He would look at the financial pages and ask, "Why is this happening? Why is that happening?" as if there had to be a reason for a stock to go up or down." . . . Solow was aghast to learn that Nash was investing his mother's savings . . . "That's something else," said Samuelson [also friendly with Nash at the time]. "It's vanity. It's like claiming you can control the tides. It's a feeling you can outwit nature. It's not uncommon among mathematicians. . . . It's me against the world. . . . It's about proving yourself."

Nash's delusion of grandeur, which Samuelson so perceptively compared to claiming the ability to control the tides—one of the best known literary examples of madness (from Samuel Johnson's *Rasselas*), though he still believed it quite normal for a mathematician, was expressed in other ways as well. With the stellar Jewish economists such as Solow and Samuelson; with D. J. Newman (on whom Nash had a crush, despite saying that he looked "too Jewish"), Paul Cohen (a future Fields medalist, on whom Nash possibly also had a crush while fiercely competing with him for the title of the biggest genius), all the other brilliant young Jewish mathematicians with whom he was mostly hanging around, and the two Jewish Normans, Wiener and Levinson, as his mentors among his senior colleagues, Nash, while anxious to get tenure, was ever "more convinced that he didn't belong at MIT." For years open to the Jewish talent unlike many other institutions, MIT was a vibrant center of mathematical creativity, but Nash by the fall of 1958 did not see it that way. " 'I do not feel this is a good long-term position for me,' he wrote to Tucker. . . . 'I would rather be one of a smaller number of more nearly equal colleagues.' His sister Martha recalled that 'he had no intention of staying at MIT. He wanted to go to Harvard because of the prestige.' "

By December that year "Nash had already crossed some invisible threshold." And then in the course of the two following months underwent "a strange and horrible metamorphosis." He began telling people that abstract powers from the outer space and foreign governments were communicating with him through encoded messages in the *New York Times*. This was at first taken for a joke. He wrote a letter in four colors of ink to a French mathematician, saying "his career was being ruined by aliens from outer space." He handed one of his graduate students what he called "an intergalactic driver's license," which was in actuality his own expired driver's license, and, with this document, put him "in charge of Asia." He left in the departmental mail letters to all the foreign embassies in Washington, declaring that he was forming a world government. Levinson (whose daughter was hospitalized for manic-depressive illness and who himself had experienced severe depression) concluded that Nash "was having a nervous breakdown." On the basis of what he told her about this time in his life, Nasar writes that "Nash's recollections of those weeks focus on a feeling of mental exhaustion and depletion, recurring and increasingly pervasive images, and a growing sense of revelation regarding a secret world that others around him were not privy to." In the meantime, not only had the MIT department voted to promote and tenure Nash, but the University of Chicago made him an offer of a chair professorship. Nash thanked politely and declined, saying "he was scheduled to become Emperor of Antarctica." He also added that the chairman of MIT department, Ted Martin, was stealing his ideas.

And yet after all this the mathematical community still considered Nash only an exceedingly eccentric, because brilliant, individual and was with great anticipation expecting his proof of the Riemann hypothesis, which he was scheduled to present at a lecture, sponsored by the American Mathematical Society, at Columbia University in the end of February.

At first, it seemed like just another one of Nash's cryptic, disorganized performances, more free association than exposition. But halfway through, something happened. Donald Newman recalled in 1996: "One word didn't fit with the other. . . . It was Nash's first downfall. Everybody knew something was wrong. He didn't get stuck. It was his chatter. The math was just lunacy. . . . Some people didn't catch it. People go to these meetings and sit through lectures. Then they go out in the hall, buttonhole other people, and try to figure out what they just heard. Nash's talk wasn't good or bad. It was horrible."[124]

It took a horrible talk in mathematics to disclose to those mathematicians who were familiar with the subject discussed that in front of them stood a sick man in the state of acute psychosis. Mathematicians less familiar with the subject of the talk still did not understand this.

What followed was thirty years of nightmare. In an early moment of manic excitement Nash resigned his job at MIT. He believed himself in danger in the United States, several times left the country, wished to give up his American citizenship, and persistently but unsuccessfully petitioned various governments for political asylum. He imagined himself the Prince of Peace, "the left foot of God on earth," and a "religious figure of great, but secret, importance." From abroad he wrote countless letters, fantastically ornamented, "filled with numerology," sometimes containing poems and some written in a very beautiful unexpected language. In the United States he continued in the same vein. He was restless, unable to stay in the same place for long, constantly moving between Boston, Princeton, West Virginia, and visiting acquaintances elsewhere. He would stay in other people's homes. He lost all interest in his appearance, walking around with long hair and a full beard, wearing worn unmatched clothes. By his mid-thirties "he had decayed in a very spectacular way." His former colleagues time and again attempted to find him temporary positions that he might hold during brief periods of lucidity, but would obviously lose with ever-renewed psychotic episodes. He was poor. In the late 1960s he lived with his mother in Roanoke. Alicia divorced him in 1963, but continued to take care of him, and soon after his mother died in 1969, he would live with her and their son in Princeton.

Even with his body in one place his mind wandered:

in his own mind, he traveled to the remotest reaches of the globe: Cairo, Zebak, Kabul, Bangui, Thebes, Guyana, Mongolia. In these faraway places, he lived in refugee camps, foreign embassies, prisons, bomb shelters. At other times, he felt he was inhabiting an Inferno, a purgatory, or a polluted heaven ("a decayed rotting house infested by rats and termites and other vermin".) His identities, like the return addresses on his letters, were like the skins of an onion. Underneath each one lurked another: He was C.O.R.P.S.E. (a Palestinian Arab refugee), a great Japanese shogun, C1423, Esau, L'homme d'Or, Chin Hsiang, Job, Jorap Castro, Janos Norses, even, at times, a mouse. His companions were samurai, devils, prophets, Nazis, priests, and judges. Baleful deities—Napoleon, Iblis, Mora, Satan, Platinum Man, Titan, Nahipotleeron, Napoleon Shickelgruber—threatened him. He lived in constant fear of annihilation, both of the world (genocide, Armageddon, the Apocalypse, Final Day of Judgment, Day of resolution of singularities) and of himself (death and bankruptcy). Certain dates struck him as ominous, among them May 29.[125]

There was a method behind this madness. A certain theme remained permanent and, like a red thread, connected the seemingly disjointed elements of Nash's diseased imagination into a systemic worldview. This theme was the Jews as the incarnation of evil. Nasar writes:

> Before the 1967 Arab-Israeli war, he explained, he was a left-wing Palestinian refugee, a member of the PLO, and a refugee making a "g-indent" in Israel's border, petitioning Arab nations to protect him from "falling under the power of the Israeli state." Soon afterward, he imagined that he was a go board whose four sides were labeled Los Angeles, Boston, Seattle, and Bluefield. He was covered with white stones representing Confucians and black stones representing Muhammadans. The "first-order" game was being played by his sons, John David and John Charles. The "second-order," derivative game was "an ideological conflict between me, personally, and the Jews collectively." . . . It seemed to him also that certain truths were "visible in the stars." He realized that Saturn is associated with Esau and Adam, with whom he identified, and that Titan, Saturn's second moon, was Jacob as well as an enemy of Buddha, Iblis. "I've discovered a B theory of Saturn. . . . The B theory is simply that Jack Bricker [one of the young Jewish mathematicians on whom Nash had a "crush" during his early days at MIT] is Satan. 'Iblisianism' is a frightening problem connected to the Final day of Judgement." . . . the theme became predominantly perse-cutory. He discerned that "the root of all evil, as far as my personal life is concerned (life history) are Jews, in particular Jack Bricker who is Hitler, a

trinity of evil comprised of Mora, Iblis and Napoleon." These were, he said, simply "Jack Bricker in relation to me." At another point, he said, referring to Bricker, "Imagine if there would be a person who pats a guy on the back . . . with compliments and praises, while at the same time stabbing him in the abdomen with a deadly rabbit punch." Seeing the picture so clearly, he concluded that he must petition the Jews and also mathematicians and Arabs "so that they have the opportunity for redress of wrongs, which must, however, 'not be too openly revealed.'" He also had the idea that he must turn to churches, foreign governments, and civil-rights organizations for help.

Nash found great personal significance in the Biblical parable of Jacob and Esau and identified with Esau, tricked by his younger and smarter brother Jacob (for Nash representing the Jews) into selling his birthright of the elder son and so deprived of his inheritance. "I've been in a situation of loss of favor," he said. "If accounts are held for a trustee, in effect, who is as good as defunct, through lack of 'rational consistency.' . . . It's as if accounts are held for persons suffering in an Inferno. They can never benefit from them because it's as if they were supposed to come from the Inferno—to the bank offices—and collect, but they need, as it were, a revolutionary ending of the Inferno before having any sort of possibility of benefiting from their accounts."[126]

It requires no particular perspicacity to discern behind the idiosyncratic mixture of metaphors in this mad argument the all-too-familiar trope—familiarly phrased in terms of the Jewish patriarchal history—of the diabolical Jewry insouciantly triumphing over those who have every right to triumph, while pretending to be a persecuted and discriminated against tiny minority. A revolution against these illegitimate rulers of the world is fully justified, and the least one can do is to appeal to churches and civil rights organizations to put an end to the improbable, and therefore clearly supported by the forces of Evil, behavior (the resistance to being destroyed) of the Israeli State. The paranoid schizophrenic delusions of John Nash were not so bizarre, after all, and at least the psycho-logic behind them was as clear and conventional, as that behind Rosenberg's racial theory or the sympathy for the Palestinian cause on the campuses of the Ivy League universities. It was, in fact, a classic case of "transvaluation of values" resulting from *ressentiment* and, as in all such cases, reflecting above all the deep sense of inferiority. His Jewish friends and colleagues might have admired and encouraged him, they might have shrugged their shoulders when he would suddenly kiss the current Jewish object of his crushes on the mouth, voted to promote him or supported his applications for prestigious fellowships, but they got the medals he craved and the choicest positions, and they were not—he was certain—that impressed; they were always ready to deliver a deadly rabbit punch in the abdomen.

He was hospitalized on numerous occasions and the trajectory of his hospitalizations reflected the same "downward drift" that is generally characteristic of the life of a schizophrenic. Every step in his descent down the prestige scale of psychiatric facilities therefore aggravated the catastrophic disorder that made necessary his first commitment. This was at McLean Hospital in April and May of 1959. Nash was picked up on MIT campus by police and, after a scuffle, driven to Belmont "for observation." McLean is, perhaps, the most prestigious psychiatric hospital in the United States, so much so that, to be considered a *bona fide* Boston Brahmin, one could not until recently forgo having at least one relative among the inmates (just as at least one other had to be interred at Mt. Auburn Cemetery). One of the oldest "lunatic asylums" in the country, it was expressly built for the mad of the very best families, and continued to service "the wealthy, intellectual, and famous" long after it became impolite to refer to it as such. Built on the model of "a well-manicured New England College campus of late-nineteenth-century vintage," it consisted of small attractive buildings, some with suites with space for personal servants; one of them "Upham House, a former medical resident recalled, had four corner suites per floor and on one of its floors all four patients turned out to be members of the Harvard Club." Nash spent most of his time at McLean at Bowditch Hall, a locked facility for men, where he was joined by the poet Robert Lowell, "a manic depressive who was now enduring his fifth hospitalization in less than ten years"—as "thoroughbred mental case" as could be. The two men "spent a good deal of time together." The other patients "were polite, full of concern, eager to make his acquaintance, lend him their books, and clue him in to 'the routine.' They were young Harvard 'Cock[s] of the walk' slowed down by massive injections of Thorazine, yet 'so much more intelligent and interesting than the doctors,' as Nash confided. . . .

There were also old Harvard types 'dripping crumbs in front of the TV screen, idly pushing the buttons.'" Some "strutted around Bowditch late at night" in their "birthday suits." Thus, mere weeks after his status inconsistency became truly unbearable, Nash found himself precisely among the people with whom he believed he belonged—Harvard men, his kind: a patrician among patricians. Though affiliated with Harvard Medical School, McLean employed Boston University nurses respectful of their betters among the patients. They "brought him chocolate milk at bedtime, inquired about his interests, hobbies, and friends, and called him Professor." It was a madhouse nevertheless.

It was debated whether Nash was suffering from schizophrenia or from manic-depressive illness. The patient's class figured prominently in the diagnosis, and McLean was the upper-class establishment. Its patients were presumed bipolar until proven otherwise. Nasar writes:

> From the start, there was a consensus among the psychiatrists that Nash was obviously psychotic when he came to McLean. The diagnosis of paranoid schizophrenia was arrived at very quickly. . . . Reports of Nash's earlier eccentricity would have made such a conclusion even more likely. There was some discussion, of course, about the aptness of the diagnosis. Nash's age, his accomplishments, his genius would have made the doctors question whether he might not be suffering from Lowell's disease, manic depression. "One always fudged it. One could not be sure," said Joseph Brenner, who became junior administrator on the admissions ward shortly after Nash's hospitalization. But the bizarre and elaborate character of Nash's beliefs, which were simultaneously grandiose and persecutory, his tense, suspicious, guarded behavior, the relative coherence of his speech, the blankness of his facial expressions, and the extreme detachment of his voice, the reserve which bordered at times on muteness—all pointed toward schizophrenia.

In the course of his illness Nash would often display the classical symptoms of manic depression. With florid psychosis subdued by treatment, conscious of the bleak reality of his situation, he might become deeply depressed; this might be followed by a period of hypomania, when he would return to work, perhaps even write a paper, become very optimistic and expect "something wonderful" to happen, only to be grievously disappointed and descend into depression again or become acutely manic, with thoughts racing and speech (or, in his case, letters) becoming incoherent, quickly reaching the state of acute psychosis again. These phases of mania, hypomania, and depression followed each other in different sequences, but they were always there, if he was not on drugs (and sometimes he would stop taking medication because he wanted to hear his voices): the periods of lucidity, therefore, were periods of only relative lucidity; his delusions would be temporarily submerged, but he remained very ill. Nevertheless, after McLean the diagnosis of paranoid schizophrenia was no longer questioned. Nash was not as lucky as Robert Lowell: he was hospitalized at McLean only once. A facility for the elite, McLean was expensive. Nash's mother, sister, and Alicia, who would be responsible for his hospitalizations from then on, could not afford it. Other hospitals in which Nash would stay, such as Trenton State Hospital or even Carrier Clinic, catered at best to the middle class clientele and were used to see their patients as schizophrenics.

At Trenton State the nurses called Nash "Johnny": it was impossible to fall any lower. And yet, whenever his illness was contained by medication, and during periods of hypomania that was the closest he would come to his prepsychotic self he would be assailed by the frustrations of the world that he had left, resenting bitterly the recognition received by his former colleagues and fretting about his status. In 1966, after a hospitalization in Carrier, he was working at Brandeis, supported by Norman Levinson's NSF and Navy grants. A possibility was raised of his teaching at Northeastern University. He wrote to his sister Martha: "I'd rather be at a more famous place." "He thought," writes Nasar, "he would apply for a position at MIT instead. He wrote Martha that he felt MIT ought to reinstate him, adding, 'Of course, MIT isn't the most distinguished . . . Harvard ranks much higher.' Throughout the spring he would fret about being forced to take a position at a second-rate institution: 'I hope to avoid stepping down in social status because it may be difficult to come up again.'"[127] By the summer he was once more acutely disturbed.

According to Sylvia Nasar, in 1994, when John Nash received the Nobel Prize, he was in remission. He was still in remission in 2001, when Nasar wrote the epilogue to her book.[128] Was it a coincidence, a misinterpretation of calmly delusional state, as in Matthews' case, or was the Nobel

Prize—the supreme recognition of genius, which eliminated every trace of doubt in Nash's intellectual superiority and made him member of the most exclusive club on earth—actually the medicine capable of curing the otherwise incurable disease of paranoid schizophrenia? Nobel Laureates represent an infinitesimal proportion of human population, almost as uncommon as identical twins brought up apart from each other whose health history offers material for research on mental illness. The connection between Nobel Prizes and recovery from schizophrenia must be statistically insignificant.

This does not make the story of John Nash any less suggestive. It is mostly suggestive, of course, not because of what might or might not have cured him: even were the therapeutic powers of the Nobel Prize proven, the remedy would be so far beyond the reach of most patients as to render this irrelevant. The story of John Nash is suggestive because of what almost certainly caused his disease in the first place—anomie and resulting problems with identity, so patently evident at every stage in his tortured life, even though Nasar does not recognize it as the central element of the plot—and were we to prove that the Nobel Prize in Economics helped to cure him of it, this would only provide additional support for this causal explanation, not change it in any way. It is obvious that Nash was placed in the condition of acute anomie at birth, that all the personally pertinent symbolic information communicated to him in the course of his childhood was delivered to him in an emotionally ambivalent manner, that every experience of his early life carried a sign of distress: he could not delight in his mother's love, because this love was tinged with anxiety that he might fail to be what she wished him to be and could not fully delight in him herself; he could not enjoy the comforts of his parents' home because his parents found them wanting, or those, closer to ideal, of his mother's parents because of his parents' regret that they were not theirs. He was never allowed to understand who he was in relation to the people who surrounded him: the source of joy to his parents or the source of worry, an equal to his cousins and his neighbors' children or their inferior. For this reason, he did not know how to behave around these people and, naturally, could not enjoy their company. His emotional repertoire was necessarily limited, he was emotionally crippled, and as an emotional cripple he could not develop the relationally constituted self. His sense of identity was

problematic from the outset. From infancy, therefore, he was more recep-
tive to the impersonal information, delivered without an emotional charge.
His thinking self was overdeveloped and early on began to assume the
functions of the deficient and largely emotional mechanisms of identity
and will. Already as a child he became extremely dependent on explicit
mental processes, extremely cerebral and self-reflexive. The assault of the
agent of the disease (the symbolic "virus" or "bacillum schizophrenicus")
on him was so relentless and began at such a defenseless stage in the development of his mind, that it seems he was fated to become a schizophrenic.
Indeed, this is how the infection must happen. To be able to argue that it
does happen this way, we must prove that the connection between acute
anomie and acute psychosis, so clearly observable in the case of John Nash,
is systematic. This will be the task of historical chapters later.

4

Madness Muddled

Manic–Depressive Illness

Current Expert Position

The following discussion is based on the recent (2007) second edition of the authoritative *Manic–Depressive Illness* (hereafter referred to as *MDI*) treatise by Frederick K. Goodwin and Kay Redfield Jamison.[1] Over 1,000 pages long, this treatise summarizes all that is known about the subject to date and is the text used as reference both by clinicians and by psychiatrists in training. Before its appearance this role—of the last word in its area in psychiatry—was played by the first edition of the book, which came out in 1990. The second edition not only included the discussion of the new research that had accumulated in the intervening seventeen years, but added a subtitle: *Bipolar Disorders and Recurrent Depression,* to emphasize the unity of all the recurrent major mood disorders recognized today and stress the disagreement of the authors with post-*DSM-III* nosology, distinguishing between bipolar disorder and unipolar depression as separate diseases. Thus the treatise reasserted its adherence to the original classification of Emil Kraepelin.[2] The second edition, however, followed the *DSM-IV,* published in 1994, in its increased attention to the milder forms of the bipolar disorder, or the spectrum diagnoses, and, in particular, to the bipolar-II form of the manic-depressive illness, combining depressive episodes with hypomanic, rather than manic, ones.

The importance of this work in contemporary psychiatry cannot be overemphasized. Its authors, both professors of psychiatry, are recognized as leading experts in the profession and combine clinical and academic experience, Frederick Goodwin being trained as an MD, and Kay Jamison as a PhD. During the period between the publication of the first and the second editions of *MDI*, Dr. Jamison, a MacArthur Fellow, wrote two best-selling books on its topic, one—*An Unquiet Mind*—a memoir of her own battle with the disease. Excerpts from this autobiographic book are included among descriptions of patients' experiences in *MDI*. The precise degree to which current psychiatric thinking and practice reflects this text may be questioned, but it is certain that whatever is not discussed in it is not a part of the profession's concerns and understanding. One is, therefore, fully justified in confining the representation of this understanding to the contents of this one magisterial treatise.

Like schizophrenia, manic-depressive illness is a disabling, often terminal disease, and it represents a far greater public health problem: its rates are at least ten times higher than those of schizophrenia; these rates appear to be increasing, and we still lack the understanding of its nature, necessary to arrest this increase and to cure and prevent the illness, although there are certain pharmacological means to contain or manage the severity of its expression in some individuals.[3] It becomes obvious immediately that the general helplessness of the psychiatric medical establishment vis-à-vis this illness, like in the case of schizophrenia, is attributable to conceptual difficulties with its definition, both the vagueness of the notion of manic-depressive illness, and the assumption, not supported by any evidence, that it is a medical (which is to say biologically caused) condition. On the first page of their "Introduction" the authors write:

> Manic-depressive illness afflicts a large number of people—the exact number depending on how the illness is defined and how accurately it is ascertained. . . . To those afflicted, it can be so painful that suicide seems the only means of escape; indeed, manic-depressive illness is the most common cause of suicide. We view manic-depressive illness as a medical condition, an illness to be diagnosed, treated, studied, and understood within a medical context. This position is the prevailing one now, as it has been throughout history.[4]

The very fact that this view is explicitly stated—on the first page and following the admission of multiple possibilities of defining this condition—

raises questions about the statement. A statement of the kind in an authoritative text on heart disease, for instance, would be clearly out of place—it would be self-evident, true beyond doubt. It is not beyond doubt here, however. The authoritative text on manic-depressive illness starts with the statement of doubt about the position on which all the other statements in it are based.

Kraepelin bears the responsibility for the vagueness of the notion of manic-depressive illness. It was he who decided that what his French predecessors since the mid-1850s called *folie circulaire* or *folie à double forme* should be considered as a separate psychotic disease, specifically, separate from *dementia praecox* which was later named "schizophrenia." Both were varieties of functional insanity, i.e., insanity without a known organic cause, but, unlike French psychiatrists who saw in them different expressions of the same pathology (to be related to the same organic or other cause, when knowledge of it developed), Kraepelin was of the opinion that different terms reflected different essences and that, therefore, these were each a pathology *sui generis*—different, first and foremost, in their causes (though nothing was known about these when he was writing). The authors of *MDI* stress their dependence on Kraepelin. On the first page of the 2007 edition they write:

> derived from the work of Kraepelin, the "great classifier," our conception encompasses roughly the same group of disorders as the term manic-depressive illness in European usage. . . . Kraepelin built his observations on the work of . . . European psychiatrists who . . . had catalogued abnormal human behavior into hundreds of classes of disorder. More than any other single individual, Kraepelin brought order and sense to this categorical profusion. He constructed a nosology based on careful description, reducing the categories of psychoses to two: manic-depressive illness and dementia praecox, later renamed schizophrenia.
>
> It is to Kraepelin, born in the same year as Freud, that we owe much of our conceptualization of manic-depressive illness. It is to him that we owe our emphasis on documenting the longitudinal course of the illness and the careful delineation of mixed states and the stages of mania, as well as the observations that cycle length shortens with succeeding episodes; that poor clinical outcome is associated with rapid cycles, mixed states, and coexisting substance abuse; that genetics is central to the pathophysiology of the

disease; and that manic-depressive illness is a spectrum of conditions and related temperaments.

Kraepelin's model consolidated most of the major affective disorders into one category because of their similarity in core symptoms; presence of a family history of illness; and, especially, the pattern of recurrence over the course of the patient's lifetime, with periods of remission and exacerbation and a comparatively benign outcome without significant deterioration.[5]

A cloud of confusion hangs over this preliminary presentation: its elements are not logically connected. To begin with, a definition of manic-depressive illness à la Kraepelin cannot be attempted without at the same time defining schizophrenia, because both are dependent on being distinguished from the other illness in the same—psychotic—category. The fact that no clear definition of schizophrenia exists makes the possibility of a clear definition of mdi highly unlikely; whatever are the core symptom similarities between major affective disorders. It is not, in fact, that mdi is affective that distinguishes it from schizophrenia, according to Kraepelin, but, as the authors of *MDI* stress, its comparatively benign outcome without significant deterioration—the essence of schizophrenia lying in its malignant outcome and degenerative quality. The question, however, arises, how can one speak about even a relatively benign outcome of a disease, characterized, like schizophrenia, by a pattern of recurrence over the course of the patient's lifetime? One cannot, and, indeed, Kraepelin did not emphasize the chronic character of mdi, because this would not help to distinguish it from *dementia praecox*. The stress on the course and, particularly, outcome of a psychotic disease—which is what, for Kraepelin, distinguished schizophrenia from mdi—implies a relative unimportance of its symptoms (beyond the symptom of psychosis), including the affective quality of mdi. Insistence on the family history of illness as an element of the definition further complicates the issue. We would not characterize a coronary heart disease as anything but a coronary heart disease whether or not there is history of coronary heart disease in the patient's family. Family history may be a sign of presumed cause of the illness (and Kraepelin believed that psychotic illness was essentially genetic), but it cannot diagnose it. In fact, such diagnosis, in the absence of 100 percent certainty that mdi is genetic and the knowledge of the specific gene(s) that cause it, is tantamount to hypostatizing such certainty and, therefore, to circular (tautological and scientifically illegitimate) reasoning. In the absence of a clear definition—which the very principles of Kraepelin's nosology make impossible—diagnosis of mdi cannot be accurate, and we can neither understand nor cure this disease.

And yet, this is what the psychiatric establishment is expected to do and, even more incongruously, is believed to be doing. The category mdi includes two of "the big three" of contemporary psychiatry (the third being schizophrenia)—major depression and bipolar (depressive) disease, and, at least in terms of its economic burden, major depression, undefined and misunderstood as it is, alone represents the greatest single public health problem in modern society.[6]

It is trying to be constantly faced by a blatant logical contradiction—which is what Kraepelin's separation of psychoses into *dementia praecox* and mdi on the basis of course and outcome is—and so, similarly to the case of schizophrenia, the blatancy of the contradiction in the approach to mdi was camouflaged by the shift of emphasis from outcome to presenting symptoms, specifically, the abnormality of affect. Similarly to the case of schizophrenia, this unconscious flight from the most jarring logical problems without any attempt at their solution (a logical whitewashing, in fact), created other logical problems. Now, after more than a hundred years of research—and practice—within this logically faulty framework, our "knowledge" of the subject represents such a tangled knot of contradictions that nothing but a radical surgery in the style of Alexander could untie it and allow our understanding to advance.

Since, before the Kraepelinian revolution in classification, all forms of psychotic illness without a known organic cause were considered as expressions of the same pathological condition, distinguished mostly by the degree of their severity as reflected in the patient's subjective feeling and functional impairment, thinking about mdi for a long period developed together with ideas about schizophrenia. Thus it was Bleuler, again, who first attempted to resolve some of the contradictions within the nosology of his illustrious predecessor. While keeping Kraepelin's distinction between two types of psychotic illness, Bleuler reintroduced the idea of a continuum on which mdi and schizophrenia occupied different positions, mdi closer to the beginning, and schizophrenia to the end, with numerous intermediary states that did not allow for a qualitative separation between the two. A "patient's location on the spectrum depended on the number of schizophrenic features he demonstrated."[7] At the same time, Bleuler was the first to use the term "affective illness" in regard to mdi. This was not because schizophrenia presented without affective abnormality (this was, according to Bleuler, one of its central features), but because, in comparison with schizophrenia, in mdi a disturbance in mood was "the predominant feature."[8] In Kraepelinian psychiatry (namely, in European psychiatry throughout the period, and in American psychiatry during the post-psychoanalytic—contemporary—period), only Bleuler's identification of mdi as "affective illness" was retained, while both the idea of psychotic continuum and the very important affective elements in schizophrenia were forgotten. Thus Kraepelin's classification of *dementia praecox* and mdi as two separate psychotic diseases, distinguished by course and outcome, reemerged as one that separated between schizophrenia as essentially a thought-disorder and mdi as essentially a mood disorder. In consequence, the abnormality of affect, from a symptom of any psychotic disorder, metamorphosed into the key to the explanation of mdi: psychiatric attention concentrated on mood-regulation.

The subcategories of mdi are distinguished by the type of affective abnormality with which they present. Since mood (very low mood, very high mood, all shades of mood in-between, and change of moods) is an element of normal mental functioning, such abnormality is necessarily only a matter of degree, making it impossible to draw a sharp line between health and pathology. Already this makes diagnosing mdi problematic—a matter of the clinician's subjective feeling and, ultimately, a function of the patient's desire to seek help. The main distinction within mdi, which includes all the recurrent forms of affective illness, is between unipolar and bipolar mood disorder. Unipolar disorder is another name for an abnormally low mood, or depression, which is the most common of major mental illnesses.

Depression

To qualify as a major depression, according to *DSM-IV,* the low mood must persist for at least two weeks, not be provoked by bereavement, and be accompanied by certain behavioral, cognitive, or emotional changes in the patient's routine:

The essential feature of a Major Depressive Episode is a period of at least 2 weeks during which there is either depressed mood or the loss of interest or pleasure in nearly all activities. In children and adolescents, the mood may be irritable rather than sad. The individual must also experience at least four additional symptoms drawn from a list that includes changes in appetite and weight, sleep, and psychomotor activity; decreased energy; feelings of worthlessness or guilt; difficulty thinking, concentrating, or making decisions; or recurrent thoughts of death or suicidal ideation, plans, or attempts.[9]

MDI offers a more informative description of depression:

Mood in all of the depressive states is bleak, pessimistic, and despairing. A deep sense of futility is often accompanied, if not preceded, by the belief that the ability to experience pleasure is permanently gone. The physical and mental worlds are experienced as monochromatic, as shades of gray and black. Heightened irritability, anger, paranoia, emotional turbulence, and anxiety are common.[10]

Numerous quotations from clinicians' and patients' accounts expand on this introductory paragraph. Some of these quotations stress features that are remarkably similar to the presentation of schizophrenia. For instance, a clinician writes in 1953:

General impairment in emotional feeling is another symptom often described by the manic-depressive patient in a depressive episode. In addition to *distortions in sensing impressions, such as a queer, odd or unreal feeling,* the patient may complain of a *universal dulling of the emotional tone.* This symptom, like *the feeling of unreality,* frightens the patient because it tends to alienate him from his environment. Indeed, it is an important constituent of the patient's fear of insanity. It is bad enough not to speak the same language as other people—it is worse not to feel the same emotions.[11]

This sounds very much like the description of schizophrenic *Stimmung* and its "flat affect." A team of mdi experts in 1960 also emphasize the latter: "There is a diminished capacity for normal affective response to sad as well as happy events, a phenomenon which is merely one aspect of a generalized insufficiency of all mental activities. . . . Whatever is experienced seems to be painful. . . . The depth of the affect cannot easily be measured from its outward expression. The silent shedding of tears may be seen in an otherwise expressionless face; another patient will mock at himself and at his complaints with a grim and sardonic but surprising humor or call himself a fraud or a fool: in another a sudden smile or expression of gaiety will deceive the physician about the severity of the underlying emotion."[12]

Other statements lay stress on the slowing down, even paralyzing quality of the experience of depression, affecting both mental activity and behavior. Already Jaspers in 1913 emphasizes "the profound impairment of will," characteristic of depressed patients. At the core of depression lies, he writes, "an equally unmotivated and profound sadness to which is added a retardation of psychic events which is as subjectively painful as it is objectively visible. All instinctual activities are subjected to it. The patient does not want to do anything. The reduced impulse to move and do things turns into complete immobility. No decision can be made and no activity begun." At the same time, patients feel extremely dissatisfied with themselves: they "complain of their inefficiency . . . accuse themselves of much past guilt . . . notions of worthlessness . . ." This self-dissatisfaction is closely associated with profound pessimism, bordering on terror of the future, and the experience of the present as at the very least not worth any effort. This experience is physical, felt by patients "as a sensation in the chest or body as if it could be laid hold of there."

It is also reflected in outward physical appearance and behavior. Campbell writes:

> Depressed mood is often suggested by the bearing, gait or general appearance of the patient. The depressed individual usually walks slowly and reacts sluggishly. He appears to push himself along, as if he were being held back, rather than propelling himself with normal agility. There are no unnecessary movements with the hands or feet, the patient sitting in a languorous but not restful posture. The shoulders sag, the head is lowered and the entire body seems to droop; loosely hanging clothes sometimes suggest the weight loss often present in the melancholic individual. Everyone is acquainted with the tendency of the angles of the mouth to turn down in the saddened person; a smile, when it occurs, must be forced, and even then there is something sickly or distorted in its expression. . . .

The eyes, which normally portray the spark, vitality and curiosity of the personality, are dull and lusterless. In some individuals the eyes have a far-away, unnatural stare, which even the layman recognizes as a mark of extreme preoccupation or mental illness."[13]

The most striking feature of depression, undoubtedly, is "the extraordinarily strong tendency to suicide." Goodwin and Jamison quote Kraepelin: "The torment of the states of depression, which is nearly unbearable, according to the perpetually recurring statements by the patients, engenders almost in all, at least from time to time, weariness of life, only too frequently also a great desire to put an end to life at any price . . ." This desire may continually accompany the whole course of disease, "without coming to a serious attempt owing to the incapacity of the patients to arrive at a decision." But in other cases "the impulse to suicide emerges very suddenly without the patients being able to explain the motives to themselves."[14]

For some reason, obsessive thinking of death, the sense of the absolute necessity to put an end to oneself, is not considered a delusion or a sign of thought disorder in depression. Write Goodwin and Jamison: "By definition, patients with no psychotic depression do not manifest clouding of consciousness, nor do they experience delusions or hallucinations. Suicidal thinking, however, is often of dangerous proportions, and morbidly ruminative and hypochondriacal thinking is common."[15] Psychotic depression, they say, presents itself with the same symptoms as non-psychotic depression, though "usually in worsened form, [and] with the addition of delusions and/or hallucinations." The primary content of depressive delusions is somatic (i.e., hypochondriacal—one believes oneself affected by terrible, incurable bodily diseases), religious, and financial. Bleuler describes:

> In the severer cases delusions are invariably present and may stand in the foreground. At the same time the hallucinations usually but not always increase. . . . The devil appears in the window, makes faces at the patients.
>
> They hear themselves condemned, they hear the scaffold erected on which they are to be executed, and their relatives crying who must suffer on their account, or starve or otherwise perish miserably.
>
> But the delusions especially are never absent in a pronounced case and always as delusions of economic, bodily, and spiritual ruin. The patients

think they became poor, and it does no good to show them their valuables or their balance in the bank; that has no significance for them. Debts are there anyway, or demands are to be expected that will wipe out everything.

This description—minus the devil in the window—could well apply to the psychotic experiences of John Nash.

MDI quotes Kraepelin describing a severe form of psychotic depression:

[a] further, fairly comprehensive group of cases is distinguished by a still greater development of delusions. We may perhaps call it "fantastic melancholia." Abundant hallucinations appear. . . . There are also multifarious delusional interpretations of real perceptions. The patient hears murderers come; someone is slinking about the bed; a man is lying under the bed with a loaded gun; . . . The trees in the forest, the rocks, appear unnatural, as if they were artificial, as if they had been built up specially for the patient, in fact, even the sun, the moon, the weather, are not as they used to be. . . .

Consciousness is in this form frequently somewhat clouded. The patients . . . complain that they cannot lay hold of any proper thought, that they are beastly "stupid," confused in their head, do not find their way, also perhaps that they have so many thoughts in their head, that everything goes pell-mell. . . .

At times more violent states of excitement may be interpolated. The patients scream, throw themselves on the floor, force their way senselessly out, beat their heads, hide away under the bed, make desperate attacks on the surroundings. . . . Serious attempts at suicide are in these states extremely frequent.

This "fantastic melancholia" gradually transforms into the most severe state of psychotic depression, "delirious melancholia," which, Kraepelin says, is

characterized by profound visionary clouding of consciousness. Here also numerous, terrifying hallucinations, changing variously, and confused delusions are developed. . . .

During these changing visionary experiences the patients are outwardly for the most part strongly inhibited; they are scarcely capable of saying a word. They feel confused and perplexed; they cannot collect their thoughts, know absolutely nothing any longer, give contradictory, incomprehensible, unconnected answers, weave in words which they have heard into their detached, slow utterances which they produce as though astonished. . . . For the most part the patients lie in bed taking no interest in anything.[16]

It is clear from the comparison of these descriptions with those of schizophrenia that psychotic depression, in particular in the states of "fantastic and delirious melancholia," cannot be symptomatically distinguished from the latter disease.

And this is how Kay Jamison describes her own experience of depression in *An Unquiet Mind:*

A floridly psychotic mania was followed, inevitably, by a long and lacerating, black, suicidal depression. . . . From the time I woke up in the morning until the time I went to bed at night, I was unbearably miserable and seemingly incapable of any kind of joy or enthusiasm. Everything— every thought, word, movement—was an effort. Everything that once was sparkling now was flat. I seemed to myself to be dull, boring, inadequate, thick brained, unlit, unresponsive, chill skinned, bloodless, and sparrow drab. I doubted, completely, my ability to do anything well. It seemed as though my mind had slowed down and burned out to the point of being virtually useless. [It] worked only well enough to torment me with a dreary litany of my inadequacies and shortcomings in character, and to taunt me with the total, the desperate, hopelessness of it all. What is the point in going on like this? I would ask myself. . . . What conceivable point is there in living?

The morbidity of my mind was astonishing: Death and its kin were constant companions. I saw death everywhere. . . . Everything was a reminder that everything ended at the charnel house. My memory always took the black line of the mind's underground system; thoughts would go from one tormented moment of my past to the next. Each stop along the way was worse than the preceding one. . . .

At the time, nothing seemed to be working, despite excellent medical care, and I simply wanted to die and be done with it. I resolved to kill myself.[17]

Varieties of Bipolar Disorder

In bipolar forms of affective illness, the mood cycles between abnormal lows and highs, depressive states alternating with manic or hypomanic ones, which the authors of *MDI* emphasize. Bipolar states, they stress, are heterogeneous.

> Most studies, particularly those first to use the distinction, did not specify criteria for bipolar beyond indicating a "history of mania." In many studies, bipolar included only those patients with a history of frank mania requiring hospitalization; in others, the bipolar group included patients with milder symptoms (hypomania). Then [in the late 1970s], Goodwin and colleagues at the National Institute of Mental Health suggested that bipolar patients could be classified more meaningfully as either bipolar-I or bipolar-II. They based this recommendation on their studies of hospitalized depressed patients who met criteria for primary major affective disorders; that is, they had no prior history of another psychiatric diagnosis. Bipolar-I patients were defined as those with a history of mania severe enough to have resulted in treatment, usually hospitalization. Such full-blown mania was often accompanied by psychotic features. Bipolar-II patients, by contrast, had, in addition to major depression requiring hospitalization, a history of hypomania—that is, specific symptoms of sufficient magnitude to be designated as abnormal by the patient or the family and to result in interference with normal role functioning, but not severe enough to result in hospitalization.[18]

The reliability of the diagnosis was further reduced in later studies that used the bipolar-I/bipolar-II distinction. While the above-mentioned *NIMH* 1970s Program on the Psychobiology of Depression-Clinical Studies based its recommendations on "observations of hospitalized depressed patients without other psychiatric diagnoses, many of the more recent studies were conducted in patients in whom neither the depressed nor the hypomanic phase was severe enough to require hospitalization and in whom concomitant diagnoses (principally borderline personality disorder and substance abuse disorder) were not uncommon." Thus the category of mdi or "affective illness," first conceived of to better conceptualize severe psychotic disease without a clear organic cause (and so of unknown etiology), came to include, on the one hand, mild mood abnormalities and, on the other, organic mental disorders (namely, ones with a known organic cause), eventually allowing for the classification of mental problems associated with pregnancy, childbirth (puerperal insanity), and menopause under the same rubric. Such "definitional broadening," write the authors of *MDI*, is not universally accepted, some psychiatrists pointing out "that mood fluctuations can be found in many if not most psychiatric disorders and express[ing] concern that the continued broadening of the bipolar diagnosis risks weakening the core concept of bipolar disorder."[19]

A researcher with the most appropriate name, Angst, whose work has spanned many decades, in 1978, "having earlier recognized the problem of the range of meanings that could confuse application of the bipolar-II category, proposed a nomenclature that would account for milder forms of both depression and mania. He divided bipolar patients into Md and mD, with M and D indicating episodes of mania and depression requiring hospitalization, and m and d episodes clearly different from normal but not of sufficient severity to necessitate hospitalization." In other words, Angst has classified bipolar conditions by degrees of severity, from MD (the most severe)—through Md and mD—to (the least severe) md. "More recently," report Goodwin and Jamison, "Angst completed a long-term follow-up study of his original 1959–1963 cohort." As might have been expected, "he concluded that the Md group, compared with their MD counterparts, have a more favorable course and are less likely to require long-term maintenance medication," namely, that a less severe form of the disorder was less severe than the more severe one. "Whatever the level of depressive severity," comment the authors of *MDI*, "bipolar-II patients represent a very important group," specifically because "both family history and pharmacological response data indicate that, while in some respects bipolar-II should be considered an intermediate form between bipolar-I and unipolar, some of the data are consistent with its being a distinct subgroup." Unfortunately, they add, the study of bipolar-II disorder has been plagued by the problem of "the poor reliability of the diagnosis."[20]

Obviously, the consideration of the mild, ill-defined forms of bipolar disorder (under the rubric of bipolar-II) makes bipolar disorder more common than it would have been if the term only applied to its disabling severe form (bipolar-I). This, in turn, makes bipolar disorder a greater public health concern and, therefore, a problem whose study deserves greater public funding. The authors of *MDI* view this as "most significant." "Most significant," they write, "contemporary data necessitate revision of the more traditional view of bipolar as substantially less common than unipolar illness." Studies which consider "cyclothymia [mood fluctuation between highs and lows, which does not impair normal role performance], bipolar-II, and bipolar-I together" find "the incidence of bipolar disorder [to be] approximately equal to that of unipolar illness—that is, [accounting] for 50 percent of major affective illness."[21] Here we enter a realm that can only be compared to Alice's Wonderland. Cyclothymia is at most a minor illness. According to the *DSM-IV*, it explicitly does not meet the criteria for a major affective illness of any kind. Bipolar-II disorder, as Goodwin and Jamison emphasize, is a mild form of mdi, which only according to some definitions meets the criteria for Major Depressive Episode and never meets the criteria for Major Manic Episode, that is, even in its severest expression only meets the criteria for the unipolar affective disorder. Where does the conclusion that bipolar disorder accounts for 50 percent of the incidence of major affective illness come from? Nothing but utter conceptual confusion which feeds on itself and grows ever more confusing can account for it.

Mania

The term "bipolar" suggests that mania is an affective condition opposite to depression, that is, if depression implies low spirits, mania implies high spirits. In common parlance, "high spirits" signify joy, just as "low spirits" signify sadness. As is clear from the clinical and personal accounts of depression quoted above, "sadness" does not begin to describe it: not only is the experience of an entirely different order of intensity, generality, and hold on the person (no outside stimulus, such as the laughter of a child, frolicking kitten, physical pleasure, can penetrate it), but it is also qualitatively different from sadness, connoting an altogether different complex of emotions—meaninglessness of existence, sense of unreality, self-loathing, mental lethargy, so central in depression, are not distinguishing characteristics of sadness. Similarly, there is very little that is actually joyful in the highs of a full-blown mania. But very often the two poles of mdi are presented in the literature as "exaggerations of normal sadness and joy."[22]

In the *DSM-IV* criteria for diagnosis of mania, the joyful quality of the mood is not central:

> A Manic Episode is defined by a distinct period during which there is an abnormally and persistently elevated, expansive, or irritable mood. The period of abnormal mood must last at least 1 week (or less if hospitalization is required). The mood disturbance must be accompanied by at least three additional symptoms from a list that includes inflated self-esteem or grandiosity, decreased need for sleep, pressure of speech, flight of ideas, distractability, increased involvement in goal-directed activities or psychomotor agitation, and excessive involvement in pleasurable activities with a high potential for painful consequences. If the mood is irritable (rather than elevated or expansive), at least four of the above symptoms must be present. . . . The disturbance must be sufficiently severe to cause marked impairment in social or occupational functioning or to require hospitalization or it is characterized by the presence of psychotic features. The episode must not be due to the direct physiological effects of a drug of abuse, a medication, other somatic treatments for depression (e.g., electroconvulsive therapy or light therapy) or toxin exposure. The episode also must not be due to the direct physiological effects of a general medical condition . . .
>
> The elevated mood of a Manic Episode may be described as euphoric, unusually good, cheerful, or high. Although the person's mood may initially have an infectious quality for the uninvolved observer, it is recognized as excessive by those who know the person well. The expansive quality of the mood is characterized by unceasing and indiscriminate enthusiasm for interpersonal, sexual, or occupational interactions. . . . Although elevated mood is considered the prototypical symptom, the predominant mood disturbance may be irritability. . . . Lability of mood (e.g., the alternation between euphoria and irritability) is frequently seen.
>
> Inflated self-esteem is typically present, ranging from uncritical self-confidence to marked grandiosity, and may reach delusional proportions. . . .

Grandiose delusions are common (e.g., having a special relationship to God or to some public figure from the political, religious, or entertainment world).[23]

The authors of *MDI* note that the *DSM-IV* notion of mania is rather narrow in comparison to "concepts used 100 years ago and into ancient times," when "mania" referred to "any kind of 'excitement' or agitation." Today, they say, some innovative thinkers suggest we return to this broader concept. Agitation, of course, is not "high spirits"; and following this suggestion may lead to changing the conception of manic condition as a form of affective illness, shifting the focus away from mood. Clinicians and sufferers from mania quoted in the course of the description of mania in *MDI* mention the joyful aspect of the condition, but also stress the deceptive and, ultimately, destructive quality of such experience. Kraepelin, for instance, insists: mood in mania is "very changing, sometimes anxiously despairing ('thoughts of death'), timid and lachrymose, distracted, sometimes unrestrainedly merry, erotic or ecstatic, sometimes irritable or unsympathetic and indifferent." Jaspers adds:

> The feeling of delight in life is accompanied by an increase in instinctual activities: increased sexuality, increased desire to move about; pressure of talk and pressure of activity, which will mount from mere vividness of gesture to states of agitated excitement. The psychic activity characterized by flight of ideas lends an initial liveliness to everything undertaken but it lacks staying-power and is changeable. All intruding stimuli and any new possibility will distract the patient's attention. The massive associations at his disposal come spontaneously and uncalled for. They make him witty and sparkling; they also make it impossible for him to maintain any determining tendency and render him at the same time superficial and confused.[24]

The initial lively interest a manic patient manifests in everything, the multiplicity of associations, and the witty and sparkling appearance create the impression of heightened creativity, and, indeed, bipolar disorder is often praised, even by people affected by it (such as Kay Jamison), for spurring imaginative, specifically artistic, activity. This is true, unfortunately, only of mild hypomania. Mania, for all its excited busyness, is remarkably unproductive, therefore, not creative. Explains Bleuler:

> The thinking of the manic is flighty. He jumps by by-paths from one subject to another, and cannot adhere to anything. With this the ideas run along very easily and involuntarily, even so freely that it may be felt as unpleasant by the patient. . . . Because of the more rapid flow of ideas, and especially because of the falling off of inhibitions, artistic activities are facilitated even though something worthwhile is produced only in very mild cases and when the patient is otherwise talented in this direction.

A particular and, perhaps, most notable expression of the manic excited and unproductive activity is graphomania: "The number of documents produced by manic patients is sometimes astonishing," notes Kraepelin, ". . . the pleasure of writing itself is the only motive." A later clinician, Campbell records in 1953:

> The manic patient may expend a considerable amount of his energy and pressure of ideas in writing. His writing is demonstrative, flashy, rhetorical and bombastic. He insists that the physician must read every word, even though the content is biased, full of repetition, rambling and circumstantial. Capital letters are used unnecessarily, sentences are underscored and flight of ideas and distractability destroy the coherence of the theme. The subject of the manic's writing often pertains to the correction of wrongs, religious tangents, gaining his freedom, institution of lawsuits.[25]

One is inevitably reminded of Matthews and Nash, both paradigmatic schizophrenics—and graphomaniacs.

Like other specific expressions of manic hyperactivity, graphomania is often associated with the inflated sense of self-importance, which, as the "delusion of grandeur," represents a characteristic form of a manic delusion. *MDI* quotes a patient:

> The condition of my mind for many months is beyond all description. My thoughts ran with lightning-like rapidity from one subject to another. I had an exaggerated feeling of self-importance. All the problems of the

universe came crowding into my mind, demanding instant discussion and solution . . . I even devised means of discovering the weight of a human soul . . .

Another patient's experience was similar:

I must record everything and later I would write a book on mental hospitals. I would write books on psychiatric theory too, and on theology. I would write novels. I had the libretto of an opera in mind. Nothing was beyond me. . . . I made notes of everything that happened, day and night. I made scrap-books whose meaning only I could decipher. I wrote a fairy tale; I wrote the diary of a white witch; and again I noted down cryptically all that was said or done around me at the time, with special reference to relevant news bulletins and to jokes, which were broadcast in radio programmes. . . . The major work which would be based on this material would be accurate, original, provocative, and of profound significance. All that had ever happened to me was now worthwhile.

In distinction to affect which, as the above descriptions clearly demonstrate, may be quite similar in mania and depression, the characteristic manic sense of self-importance is indeed the very opposite of the sense of worthlessness characteristic of depression. It is nonetheless important to note the focus on, and the problematization of, the self, which is equally central to both mania and depression, and is also invariably prominent in the presentation of schizophrenia. Another symptom common to mania and schizophrenia, though, in the latter often eclipsed by the elaborate nature of bizarre delusions, which attract most attention, is racing thoughts. This symptom, again, seems to be the opposite of the mental sluggishness characteristic of depression. Yet, again, in fact it is an alternative expression of losing control over one's mental activities, that is, of the impairment of the will. This is described by one patient:

Thoughts chased one another through my mind with lightning rapidity. I felt like a person driving a wild horse with a weak rein, who dares not use force, but lets him run his course, following the line of least resistance. Mad impulses would rush through my brain, carrying me first in one direction

then in another. . . . my mind could not hold on to one subject long enough
to formulate any definite plan.[26]

This loss of control extends to outward behavior as well. *MDI* authors
write: "Particularly dramatic and extreme among the clinical features of
acute mania are the frenetic, seemingly aimless, and occasionally violent
activities of manic patients. Bizarre, driven, paranoid, impulsive, and
grossly inappropriate behavior patterns are typical." They go on to quote
Kraepelin: "The patient cannot sit or lie still for long, jumps out of bed,
runs about, hops, dances, mounts on tables and benches, takes down pictures. He forces his way out, takes off his clothes, teases his fellow patients,
dives, splashes, spits, chirps and clicks."[27]

To the sense of unreality characteristic of depression is opposed the
sense of "heightened awareness" in mania, which, as a patient notes, corresponds also to the "times of strong emotion, and especially [to] moments
of great fear" in normal life, when "we find that we are more keenly aware
than usual of the external details of our world," as if they each acquire a
deeper significance. Another patient remembers about "the preliminary
stage of a manic episode":

The first thing I note is the peculiar appearances of the lights—the ordinary
electric lights in the ward. They are not exactly brighter, but deeper, more
intense, perhaps a trifle more ruddy than usual. . . . All my other senses
seem more acute than usual. . . . My hearing appears to be more sensitive,
and I am able to take in without disturbance or distraction many different
sound-impressions at the same time.[28]

This heightened awareness is also reminiscent of the "apophany" stage of
the schizophrenic prodrome, which coincides with or replaces the feeling
of meaninglessness of reality with the aura of special meaningfulness, so
hard to spell out that it results in "delusional tension" and announces the
descent into the phase of acute psychosis. It is, indeed, remarkable that,
though manic-depressive illness is believed to have always a sudden (rather
than insidious) onset, and not to have a prodrome, here Goodwin and
Jamison refer to "the preliminary stage of a manic episode."

Acute mania is often a psychotic—in the sense of "delusional"—

condition. The delusions, like in schizophrenia, are commonly paranoid and grandiose. In grave cases, writes Kraepelin, they "acquire . . . an elaboration which calls to mind paranoid [i.e., schizophrenic] attacks. His surroundings appear to the patient to be changed; he sees St. Augustine, . . . the Kaiser, spirits, God. . . . The delusions . . . move very frequently on religious territory. . . . He preaches in the name of the holy God, will reveal great things to the world, gives commands according to the divine will." Acute delusional mania may reach the even more "profoundly disturbed" stage of delirious mania, which, *MDI* suggests, is the referent of the concept of "raving maniac." Once more they quote Kraepelin:

> Patients frequently display the signs of senseless raving mania, dance about, perform peculiar movements, shake their head, throw the bedclothes pell-mell, are destructive, pass their motions under them, smear everything, make impulsive attempts at suicide, take off their clothes. A patient was found completely naked in a public park. Another ran half-clothed into the corridor and then into the street, in one hand a revolver in the other a crucifix. . . . Their linguistic utterances alternate between inarticulate sounds, praying, abusing, entreating, stammering, disconnected talk, in which clang-associations, senseless rhyming, diversion by external impressions, persistence of individual phrases are recognized. . . . Waxy flexibility, echolalia, or echopraxis can be demonstrated frequently.[29]

Recent authors quoted echo Kraepelin. It is not surprising that the descriptions of psychotic mania sound so much like the descriptions of schizophrenia, for, as we remember, Kraepelin's distinction between the two psychotic disorders—which *MDI* and the contemporary experts it quotes accept—was not based on the symptomatic differences between them.

The Spectrum Conundrum

The diagnosis of mania is complicated by the common occurrence of "mixed states" (that is, states combining elements of depression and mania) in bipolar disorder and of "atypical depression" (i.e., depression which presents with symptoms of mania) in unipolar depression. This heterogeneity of both the bipolar and unipolar diagnoses, Goodwin and Jamison write, "makes any generalizations difficult to say the least." The distinctions within the mdi category are unclear, which renders dubious their usefulness for treatment. Attempts at further articulation of the existing classification so far seem to have contributed to greater confusion. "Indeed," say the authors of *MDI*, "it has been suggested that bipolar-unipolar differences become clearer when the bipolar-II group is excluded. The most widely replicated studies point to a picture of the bipolar-I depressed patient as having more mood lability, psychotic features, psychomotor retardation, and comorbid substance abuse. In contrast, the typical unipolar patient in these studies had more anxiety, agitation, insomnia, physical complaints, anorexia, and weight loss."[30]

This, of course, brings us back to the idea of mdi as a continuum, leading from unipolar depression through bipolar-II disorder to bipolar-I (just like age two leads via age three to age four, and the differences in development between ages two and four become much clearer, if we eliminate from the comparison age three). More than that, it seems that all of mdi represents only the middle part of the continuum, which also includes on the one end, eating disorders and on the other schizophrenia. Anorexia to a significant extent overlaps with unipolar depression, unipolar depression is indistinguishable from the depressive conditions associated with bipolar II and bipolar-I, hypomanic episodes of bipolar-II overlap, on the one hand, with periods of remission in unipolar depression and differ only in degree from non-psychotic mania in bipolar-I, and psychotic mania is indistinguishable from schizophrenia.

The linear image of continuum leads naturally to its interpretation as a progression along one particular quantitative dimension, and, in the case under discussion, severity of mental impairment suggests itself as this dimension. This interpretation is implied in the concept of manic-depressive spectrum. Goodwin and Jamison credit Kraepelin with the authorship of the idea and quote him:

> Kraepelin . . . was the first to formally posit a continuum between the psychotic and less severe of affective disorders, merging imperceptibly with normality . . . : "Manic-depressive insanity . . . [includes] certain slight and slightest colorings of mood, some of them periodic, some of them continuously morbid, which on the one hand are to be regarded as the rudiment of

more severe disorders, on the other hand pass without sharp boundary into the domain of personal disposition. In the course of the years I have become more and more convinced that all the above-mentioned states only represent manifestations of a single morbid process."[31]

Yet, it is clear that manic-depressive continuum is not a continuum of increasing severity: anorexia kills, major depression, in most cases not at all associated with mania, contributes the great majority of suicides to mortality statistics, it is, without a doubt, the most fatal of mental disorders and on this count alone may be considered the most severe. The authors of *MDI* seem to agree with this. To sum up their chapter on "Conceptualizing Manic-Depressive Illness," they write: "the concept of a manic-depressive spectrum appears to be shaping a new paradigm, much of it extending into the domain of traditional depressive disorders. Indeed, whether one examines bipolar pedigrees . . . , offspring of bipolar . . . , epidemiological samples . . . , or the microstructure of the course of bipolar-I and -II disorders . . . , bipolar illness is dominated by depressive symptomatology. In this respect, bipolar-I and bipolar-II appear to be quite similar. . . . This [i.e., depression] is where a great deal of the disability associated with the illness appears to reside . . ."

Alongside the impossibility to distinguish between unipolar and bipolar disorders within mdi, the "most important" problem facing this diagnostic category remains that of differentiating between mdi and schizophrenia. Time and again the authors of *MDI* stress that the boundary between psychotic mania and schizophrenia is not clear and the psychiatric profession constantly attempts to fill the grey area of their overlap with hybrid, schizoaffective and schizobipolar, diagnostic categories. Most of the psychotic diseases can be distinguished etiologically, on the basis of the organic pathology which causes them, but even genetic research—the most promising of the leads in the search for the organic causes of both schizophrenia and mdi—"indicate that psychosis may be an overlapping feature of bipolar illness and schizophrenia." This, Goodwin and Jamison recognize, makes of particular interest "studies that address the similarities and dissimilarities in the psychotic presentation of the two illnesses," namely, their symptoms. The problem is that functional psychoses, defined as they are only by their symptoms, by definition, have the same manner of presentation in both illnesses, and thus the researchers are faced with a whole lot of similarities and hardly any dissimilarities. As was pointed out in the discussion of schizophrenia, the concept of "psychosis" itself is very ill-defined, and so they attempt to deal with this problem by articulating and modifying this concept *ad hoc.*[32]

For example, "there is no single or comprehensive definition of thought disorder [which, as we remember is one of the aspects of psychosis in schizophrenia, specifically]. Instead, thought disorder has been used as a general phrase to describe problems with the ability to attend to, abstract, conceptualize, express, or continue coherent thought. Deficits in thought and language were at one time described in general terms; today these deficits are defined by specific measures. . . . This increased specificity makes it possible to disentangle, at least in part, disorders of thought from those of language or speech. . . . Much of thought is nonverbal . . ." The authors of *MDI* opt for the noncommittal definition: "thought disorder is not intended to denote a unitary dimension or process; rather, it refers to any disruption, deficit, or slippage in various aspects of thinking, such as concentration, attention, reasoning, or abstraction." They then separate thought disorder from other components of the definition of "psychosis" as it is used in regard to schizophrenia and say: "Certain psychotic features of mania and bipolar depression—delusions and hallucinations—are relevant but not central to the concept of thought disorder." (In fact, the three vaguely defined terms refer to different aspects of psychosis, therefore, while they are related, none is relevant—and certainly not central—to the understanding of the other two.) Then they discuss studies that have attempted to establish "the specificity of thought disorder to the major psychoses—mania and schizophrenia." These studies use the 1985 Thought Disorder Index, which "comprises twenty-three categories of thinking disturbances evaluated at four levels of severity. . . . The least severe level includes vagueness and peculiar verbalizations; the most severe includes thought contamination and neologisms." This is what Goodwin and Jamison conclude:

> Virtually all studies of formal thought disorder in mania and schizo-phrenia . . . have found comparably high levels in both diagnostic groups. In fact, although Resnick and Oltmann (1984) observed more thought

disorder in schizophrenic patients, Harrow and colleagues (1982) found a trend toward greater levels in manic patients. There is, therefore, no indication that thought disorder per se is in any way specific to schizophrenia. This observation is consistent with the evidence for the strong presence in mania, as well as in schizophrenia, of psychotic features, such as hallucinations and delusions. . . . Findings of qualitative comparisons of manic and schizophrenic thought disorder are less consistent, although increased pressure of speech appears to be more characteristic of mania, as are increased derailment, loss of goal, and tangentiality . . . Poverty of speech and other negative symptoms were reported [in 1984] to be more characteristic of schizophrenic thought, although [a 1987 study], using the same scale, did not confirm this finding. More recent studies have found greater poverty of thought, less complexity of speech, and less overall quantity of speech in schizophrenic than in manic patients.

One should not lose sight of the fact that the subjects of these studies were patients diagnosed as manic or schizophrenic and treated for mania or schizophrenia; the slight differences in thought disorder found between the two groups could have reflected the effects of the different medications.[33]

Studies of differences in idiosyncratic and/or bizarre thinking have been equally inconclusive,

With some authors finding higher levels in manic patients and others higher levels in schizophrenic patients. . . . In general, investigators have found that those with mania have more complex speech than those with schizophrenia. . . . Simpson and Davis (1985) made the useful distinction that manic patients appear to be more disordered in thought structure, whereas schizophrenic patients appear to be more disordered in thought content. Jampala and colleagues (1989) argued that manic patients with formal thought disorder may "have a more severe rather than a different condition than manic patients without formal thought disorder . . ." Qualitative differences in thought disorder between mania and schizophrenia are more distinct in the use of combinatory thinking, the "tendency to merge percepts, ideas, or images in an incongruous fashion". . . . Solovay and colleagues (1987), using the Thought Disorder Index, found no significant difference in the quantity of thought disorder in manic and schizophrenic patients, but did note that manic thought disorder was "extravagantly combinatory, usually with humor, flippancy, and playfulness." Schizophrenic thought disorder, by contrast, was "disorganized, confused, and idealistically fluid, with many peculiar words and phrases."[34]

The tabulated findings of all fourteen studies on comparative thought disorder of manic and schizophrenic patients from 1972 to 2002 point every which way and do not offer a possibility to distinguish between the two diseases on this score. Still, "in summary," write Goodwin and Jamison, "although the overall amount of thought disorder does not differentiate manic from schizophrenic patients, qualitative differences do exist. Manic patients are more likely than schizophrenics to exhibit more pressured and complex speech; grandiosity; flight of ideas; combinatory and over inclusive thinking; and a strong affective component to thought that is characterized by humor, playfulness, and flippancy." The experts on mdi are not disturbed by the fact that, for experts on schizophrenia, these symptoms represent the markers of the schizophrenic condition, but they admit that, "the causal relationships among affect, psychomotor acceleration, and the often strikingly different manifestations [which?] of the underlying thought disorders in mania and schizophrenia remain unclear."[35]

Some studies focused on the course of manic thought disorder. One of them, Andreasen, 1984, "observed that most manic patients, unlike schizophrenic patients, demonstrated a reversible thought disorder [showing] nearly complete recovery over time." This observation would have been in accord with the original Kraepelin's distinction of the two psychotic illnesses by their outcome, the prognosis of mania being considerably more positive than that of schizophrenia. But several other studies in the 1980s contradicted Andreasen's results, finding, instead that, in the long run, "manic patients were at least as thought disordered as, if not more so than, schizophrenic patients."

Yet another set of studies investigated differences in linguistic patterns between manic and schizophrenic patients, some of them finding that "total speech deviance and utterance length were greater in manic than in schizophrenic patients." Hoffman and colleagues (1986) "concluded that 'manic speech difficulties were due to shifts from one discourse structure to another, while schizophrenic speech difficulties reflected a basic deficiency in elaborating any discourse structure.'" Ragin and Oltmann's team in 1983 analyzed verbal communication of bipolar and schizophrenic patients, using as a measure of its understandability/bizarreness the ability of normal subjects to guess words deleted from transcripts of patients' speech samples. They found that "depressed speech was the most predictable, schizophrenic the least, and manic somewhere in between."[36]

The comparative analysis of thought disorder in mania and schizophrenia has not been very indicative, to say the least, of the differences between the two separate forms of major psychotic illness. The majority of studies found mania and schizophrenia indistinguishable, while those subtle, qualitative differences that were detected have by and large been suspiciously of precisely the kind one would expect to distinguish the mental disorder of the lower classes (schizophrenia) from that of the educated elite (mdi): poverty vs. complexity of speech, deficiency of thought content and disorganized thought vs. extravagant connections between ideas and images, spiced by humor and playfulness. And yet, confusing as it is, the study of thought disorder, apparently, still is more suggestive of the differences—absolutely necessary to justify the existing organization of psychiatry—between mdi and schizophrenia than that of the frankly psychotic features, such as delusions and hallucinations.

The authors of *MDI* open their discussion of this unpromising area of comparison with a warning: "Problems in the assessment of delusions and hallucinations are many and troublesome."[37] Part of the trouble is that the comparison of mania and schizophrenia along this, par excellence psychotic, dimension inevitably leads to the conclusion that mdi and schizophrenia are one and the same disease, at most distinguishable as stages or degrees of severity. To the extent that mdi is a psychotic disease, and the heavy presence of delusions and hallucinations characterizes it as such, it is schizophrenia, in other words. Indeed some recent investigators have asserted "that the manic syndrome is basically a psychotic condition";[38] this is what schizophrenia is considered to be—mdi, as the reader may remember, in distinction, is believed to be basically an affective disorder. "Some evidence," say the authors of *MDI*, "relates the presence of psychotic symptoms to severity of illness," and, specifically, an association between the severity of the manic syndrome and "schizophrenic features," such as delusions and hallucinations.[39] "While several studies have not found a correlation between psychosis (in mania) and poorer outcome, many more have. [And there is agreement] that mood-incongruent psychotic features [what in schizophrenia discourse is referred to as psychosis with improper affect] predict a less positive course."[40] In other words, psychotic mdi is a more debilitating form of mental disorder than is mdi without psychotic features. Psychotic features are, by definition, schizophrenic. The development of psychotic features in fact turns mdi into the more severe condition of schizophrenia. It is possible to conclude that mdi is but an early, less debilitating stage of schizophrenia.

But hope that mdi and schizophrenia are two separate mental diseases springs eternal, and so Goodwin and Jamison write: "Delusions, like thought disorder, vary widely in severity, fixedness, content, and effect on overt behavior." Apparently, already Jaspers in 1913 and Kraepelin in 1921 thought so. Manic delusions, we are told, "are usually grandiose and expansive in nature, often religious, and not infrequently paranoid," i.e., as we know from the discussion of schizophrenia, precisely like certain schizophrenic delusions. But "they generally can be differentiated from schizophrenic delusions by their tendency to be wish-fulfilling in nature and oriented more toward communion than segregation."[41] Whatever this statement means, it relies on the 1980 study by Lerner. To augment it, Goodwin and Jamison quote Winokur and colleagues, writing in 1969:

> The delusions that are seen in schizophrenia usually last for months or years and are often primary; that is they do not explain a real or disordered perception. They fulfill the definition of a delusion as a fixed, false belief. In mania the delusions are quite different. They are often evanescent, appearing or disappearing during the course of a day, or even during an interview. They also vary with the patient's total state, being more frequent when he is more active; and his flights of ideas become more pronounced and fading as he becomes more quiet. Frequently they are extensions of the patient's grandiosity.
>
> At times the patient can be talked out of his delusion, and at other times he gives the impression that he is only being playful rather than really being deluded. In our group the delusions were often secondary to the patient's

exalted affect. This was especially true of those patients who felt their mood could be described only as a religious experience.

The most subtle and earliest distortions of reality are manifest in the frequent extravagance and grandiose self-image expressed by the patients.[42]

The feature that distinguishes schizophrenic from manic delusions in this statement is their fixity in the former case and fleeting nature in the latter. In what concerns the content of manic delusions ('grandiose self-image and religious feeling'), it is characteristic of schizophrenia. The problem here, apart from the fact that schizophrenia experts would find nothing exceptional in the changing degrees of attachment to their delusions among their patients, is that a delusion cannot be defined as "a fixed false belief" (which, according to the statement, is the nature of delusions in schizophrenia). For champions of the Darwinian idea of the descent of man, the Biblical story of the Creation of Adam is a false belief, this belief has been fixed in the minds of millions of people in the course of several millennia, and this fact does not make these millions delusional. What is false in one culture is often true in another, and it would be at the very least presumptuous to diagnose cultures with fixed beliefs different from ours as schizophrenic. In the absence of a clear understanding what a delusion, as such, is it is indeed impossible to distinguish between delusions characteristic of different groups of delusional patients in any but a quantitative fashion, e.g., as mdi specialists tend to do, to claim that manic patients are less delusional than schizophrenics, and this means, again, reducing the differences between the two diseases to those of degrees of severity within one disease.

In so far as concerns hallucinations, this is, in fact, the conclusion that Goodwin and Jamison reach. Hallucinations, they report, have been observed only in "the most severely disturbed" of the mdi patients. They are considered "the least common of symptoms" of psychotic mdi and "also the first symptoms to disappear during recovery from a manic episode, followed in turn by delusions, flight of ideas, push of speech, and distractability." Goodwin, in "one of the few phenomenological studies," a 1971 study of a sample of twenty-eight patients, of whom seven were bipolar, wrote that "(1) the modality of hallucinations (e.g., auditory or visual) was not consistent from one affective episode to another; (2) patients with affective illness were far more likely than those with schizophrenia to hallucinate only when no other person was there; (3) color was usually normal; (4) the people who appeared in the hallucination were usually of normal size and appearance; (5) the hallucinations were intermittent; (6) they were often in several sensory modalities; and (7) accusatory voices were not specific to affective illness—indeed, they were more common in schizophrenia." Characteristics 3–6 do not distinguish between affective illness and schizophrenia, while 1 is applicable to schizophrenia only if it is examined as a bipolar affective illness (i.e., during depressive and manic episodes), but it is never examined as such. Characteristics 2 and 7 allow for quantitative comparison between schizophrenia and affective disorders and suggest that schizophrenia is a more developed/severe psychotic condition than mdi. Other investigators found that manic hallucinations have more in common with organic psychoses, such as general paresis (caused by the infection of syphilis), on the one hand, and drug-induced conditions, on the other, than with schizophrenia. The study making the latter comparison, noted—somewhat in contradiction to Goodwin's earlier findings—that "manic hallucinations tended to be more of the visual type; strikingly vivid and associated with bright, colorful sensations; and often coupled with intensely pleasurable or ecstatic feelings (similar to psychedelic experiences)." In summary, *MDI* authors write: "Hallucinatory phenomena appear to represent the extreme end of the symptomatic picture [of mdi], being nonexistent in milder forms of depression and mania and most pronounced in the gravest, most delirious states. . . . They appear qualitatively, at least in the few studies in which they have been addressed, to be more similar to organic than to schizophrenic psychoses."[43]

Interim Conclusion

The current state of expert knowledge on the descriptive nature of mdi (what is diagnosed as such) thus does not allow us to distinguish between mdi and schizophrenia. Based on the accumulated literature on mdi—which, as the reader could observe, while having grown immensely, has not changed in its conceptualization in the seventeen years that elapsed

between the first and the second editions of *MDI*, the vast majority of
quotations on what we define as this disease in the second edition citing
publications available in 1990—we must apply to it the conclusions reached
in the previous chapter and approach mdi as a species (or several different
species) of the same, schizophrenia, genera, that is, as varieties of the *disease of the will.* At the same time, we cannot, as researchers advocating the
spectrum concept suggest, regard these varieties as positioned along the
continuum of severity, because the disease *burden* (i.e., years lost to life as
a result of premature death or disability due to the disease) of depression is
significantly heavier than that of schizophrenia, and yet, schizophrenia is
the end-point of the suggested spectrum.

We can, however, place all these species of schizophrenia on the continuum of complexity, in which unipolar depression would be the least
complex disease (which happens also to be the most severe) and schizophrenia the most complex, with bipolar disorder (including mania as well
as depression) occupying the middle range of complexity. In unipolar
depression the will is impaired in its motivating function—one no longer
controls one's thoughts and actions in the sense that one cannot force,
move oneself to think or do whatever one would like to think or do. The
thought is fixed on the ideas of death and futility; the action appears
beyond one's powers. One seems to be stuck in the early (meaningless)
stage of schizophrenic *Stimmung,* when the loss of the acting self is first
dimly perceived through the changed sense of the outside world (referred
to by both schizophrenics and depressive patients as the sense of "unreality"). The mind at this stage remains individualized and one has a definite, in fact acute, sense of self. The relationally constituted self, however,
is misrepresented by the "I of self-consciousness" as worthless and worse,
and, as a result, experienced as painful; it is insufferable to be oneself.
Death naturally appears the only possibility of escape. As in patients diagnosed with schizophrenia, the thinking self in the mind of depressed individuals attempts to assume the functions of the impaired will. It attempts,
specifically, to return meaning to the confused externally and internally
generated experiences by calling their names, as the schizophrenic girl
Renee tried to do, in vain, when confronted by jugs, chairs, and friends
asserting their independent-from-her existence. For this reason, among
other things, such a colossal proportion of poets (especially modern free-

form poets) are depressive: depression breeds free-form poetry, it invites language to make sense of reality which the impairment of the acting self leaves without sense. (For the same reason, bereaved individuals for whom death in our secular world cannot make any sense turn to poetry—reading and writing poetry—for comfort as well.)

In bipolar disorder, in addition to the disabling of the motivating capacity of the will in depression, there is also the impairment of its restraining capacity in mania; one can neither move oneself in the desired direction nor restrain one's thoughts and actions from running in every direction. The transition from depression to mania repeats the course of schizophrenic prodrome towards "apophany," which combines the sense of heightened awareness with ideas of reference and delusions of grandeur. At this point mania can either cycle back to depression or, through delusional tension, develop into acute psychosis with its loss of the sense of self, formal thought disorder, and complete, terrifying disorientation as a result. When not only the content of thought (and speech) is out of one's control, but the structure itself, schizophrenia reaches its ultimate complexity.

It has to be kept in mind that both "psychotic mania" and "psychotic depression," characterized by formal thought disorder, *is* schizophrenia in its acute, full-blown form; the two diagnoses are absolutely indistinguishable and present with precisely the same symptoms. On the other hand, none of the three diagnoses require formal thought disorder: negative symptoms of schizophrenia, most resistant to treatment and observable throughout the course of the disease, are, in fact, characteristic symptoms of manic-depressive illness in its various forms, and Type II schizophrenia, which presents primarily with negative symptoms, cannot be distinguished from mdi. Nevertheless, bipolar disorder (which necessarily implies depression) and unipolar depression differ from schizophrenia in complexity *as* psychotic diseases. It turns out that formal thought disorder, and not delusions, characterizes psychosis in the completeness of its development, i.e., at its final, most complex stage. Delusions reflect only the disorder of thought content; they are present in mania in feelings of grandiosity and exaggerated self-confidence (the characteristic delusions of grandeur), just as in depression they are present in feelings of absolute worthlessness, futility, and suicidal ideation. Given that expert mdi discourse offers us no definition of delusion which could replace the one at which we have arrived in the discussion of schizophrenia in the previous chapter—delusion as inability to separate between subjective and objective realities and as substitution of the internally-generated experiences for the ones originating outside—there is no reason whatsoever not to regard the fixation on death and the pervasive, debilitating sense that life is unbearable in depression as a delusion. Depressive disease, therefore, is always a delusional, thus a psychotic, disorder.

The greater complexity of schizophrenic dysfunction in its paradigmatic, accomplished form—the inability to control not only the contents of thought, and therefore motivation in thought and action (as in its simpler forms of depression and manic-depression), but also the structure of thought itself—is related to the comprehensive nature of the mental impairment, which involves not only the structure of the will—the acting self—but also that of the thinking self, and results in the loss of the sense of self altogether. It is obvious from descriptions above that both the major unipolar depression and the severe bipolar disorder can and do exist in this complex, comprehensive form. The most significant difference between the forms of the schizophrenic disease is the difference between enduring depression and formal thought disorder, i.e., the difference in the character of depression in them. In classical schizophrenia (and varieties of mdi which cannot be distinguished from it), depression forms an intermittent and transient phase in the development toward acute psychosis, which marks the most painful and life-threatening point of the disease. But in major depression, whether unipolar or bipolar, it is not a phase but the illness itself, and it becomes more painful and dangerous the longer it lasts. Moreover, major unipolar depression is naturally irresolvable (in the sense that it contains no inherent mechanism of relief), contrasting with bipolar disorder cycling between the horrors of depression and acute psychosis (thus at the very least changing the nature of the pain), and the actually self-relieving capacity of schizophrenia which reaches the stage of elaborate (thought-content only) delusions. Thus the rare "madness in its pure form" seems to have some redeeming qualities, and it is the most common and, one may say, almost bordering on normality, variety that truly deserves to be called "the cancer of the mind." Quite possibly, the continuum of severity runs in the direction opposite to the continuum of complexity.

The disease of the will: continuum of complexity

Depression	Mania/acute psychosis	Delusional (full-blown) schizophrenia
Loss of positive (motivating) control in action and content of thought	Loss of positive and negative (restraining) control in action and content of thought	Complete alienation of the acting self, loss of cultural individualization, and loss of positive and negative control in action and both content and structure of thought

"Molecular Medicine Revolution" and the Streetlight Method

The conceptualization and, therefore, the understanding of the nature of mdi have not advanced since the days of the "classification revolution" at the turn of the twentieth century. Thus, having applied the conclusions reached in regard to schizophrenia to the recurrently depressive and bipolar species of its genera, I would arguably be justified in ending this chapter here. But I know that, however justified logically, I will not be forgiven for doing so. I would be accused of being ignorant of another revolution—that one occurring at the turn of the millennium and, as I write, keeping us all enthralled by almost daily announcements of its ever more astonishing discoveries. This "molecular medicine revolution" was brought about by the colossal strides in molecular and cellular biology since the 1990s and by the development of remarkable new technologies, such as, among others, neuroimaging. Psychiatry, write the authors of *MDI*, "like the rest of medicine, has entered a new and exciting age" as a result.[44] Surely, the understanding of mdi could not remain unaffected by such advances, it would be argued against me, and only laziness or inability to comprehend their implications (after all, sociologists, as is well known, are not brain surgeons) could explain my unwillingness to dwell on them. Dwell I, therefore, shall, and, to avoid the natural suspicion of misinterpretation owing to lack of specialist knowledge, I shall quote even more extensively from the 2007 manual by Goodwin and Jamison—the one source beyond any such suspicion. If, in the end, the reader would still conclude that mdi is as little understood, as causally unexplained, as far from a cure and the slightest possibility of prevention, as it was when Kraepelin first defined it as a distinct disease entity, this would not be because I have concealed from my audience any of the new biological knowledge acquired on the subject up to this moment. The achievements of the recent biological revolution in psychiatry will be summarized in the words of its participants.

I should emphasize that nothing I shall say below is intended to cast aspersions on, or point to some inherent defect in, this new knowledge or the methods of its acquisition. Showing that it has failed to answer any of the fundamental, important, questions about mdi (just as earlier I showed that it has failed to answer them about schizophrenia), I imply no criticism whatsoever of the sophisticated specialist work done by biologists. Their *biology,* I am certain, is impeccable (and were it faulty, a non-specialist such as myself would not be the one to uncover its faults). In any case, no degree of improvement, were it needed, could make it successful where it failed. The reason for its failure is not *biological,* but *logical.* No increase in the sophistication of the concepts or methods at the disposal of the molecular biologists, no advance in their technology can resolve the problem the root of which is neither biological, nor technical. I am sure that some of this knowledge (for instance, certain recent discoveries in epigenetics, which will be touched upon later) will, in fact, be useful in the treatment of the diseases in question—after the conceptual, logical problems around mdi and schizophrenia are resolved.

The logic behind the current approach of neurobiology and biological psychiatry may be called the "streetlight logic." One adopts it when looking for a lost object—an earring, for instance, a contact lens, or the proverbial needle—under a streetlight, not because the object was lost there, but because the streetlight is there. Obviously, lots of things may be found, when one looks carefully, but not the object one is looking for. It would be silly to blame this on the dimness of the light or the weakness of one's eyesight: the object is not there to be found; under the streetlight, however bright it may be made, is the wrong place to look for it. Goodwin and Jamison tell their readers that the interest in biological psychiatry, the reputation of which suffered from association with Nazism after World War II, and which revived in the late 1960s, "has grown enormously in the past decade as the computer-based and molecular tools available . . . have multiplied exponentially." They stress that "attempts to comprehend the brain's role in mania and depression . . . began in earnest as clinically effective mood-altering drugs began to appear in the late 1950s and early 1960s.

The psychopharmacological revolution fortuitously coincided with the arrival of new techniques that made it possible to characterize neurotransmitter function in the central nervous system."[45] This particular streetlight, in other words, has become so bright as to turn irresistible.

In mdi research, as with schizophrenia, it was first powered by genetics. Goodwin and Jamison open the respective chapter:

> A generation ago, few mental health professionals believed that inherited vulnerabilities could be central to the development of psychiatric illness. Fearing that discovery of a genetic diathesis might cast a stigma on patients and lead to therapeutic nihilism, many clinical observers found social and developmental reasons to explain the inescapable fact that mental illness runs in families.

This seems to suggest that even "inescapable facts" do not of themselves give rise to interpretations, which, instead, may well be shaped by extra-scientific, in this case ideological, considerations. It is not that mental health professionals earlier ignored existing data; they were simply unwilling to interpret them in a certain way. However, the authors continue,

> Gradually, the genetic evidence became too compelling to ignore. Recent advances in the molecular genetics of several neuropsychiatric diseases, particularly the discovery of linkage and association of deoxyribonucleic acid (DNA) markers with the bipolar subtype of mdi, appear to reaffirm the older evidence [that mental illness runs in families]. If, as expected, particular gene variants are definitely implicated in manic-depressive susceptibility, better understanding should follow . . . the new discoveries [to be made] could result in new diagnostic tests and improved treatment methods.[46]

This opening paragraph sets the tone for the rest of the strictly biological discussion in the volume and makes obvious how irremediably confused is the logic on which it is based.

The tone set is that of firm and triumphant belief in that, unlike the ideologically-biased position of mental health professionals a generation ago, current view of the inescapable, but equivocal fact that mental disease runs in families as proof of genetic transmission *will* be supported by research in the nearest future. Goodwin and Jamison are most optimistic about the prospect of more certain diagnosis and better treatment, which such future confirmation *will* make possible.

"*It is our firm belief,*" they write in the chapter devoted to advances in the neurobiology of mdi, "that the impact of molecular and cellular biology—which has been felt throughout clinical medicine—*will have major repercussions* for understanding the fundamental pathophysiology of [mdi] and that *we will see* the development of markedly improved treatments for these devastating diseases."

And again:

Since [1990], there have been tremendous advances in our understanding of both the normal and abnormal functioning of the brain. Indeed, *it is our firm belief* that the impact of molecular and cellular biology—which has been felt in every corner of clinical medicine—*will ultimately* also have major repercussions for our understanding about the fundamental core pathophysiology of mdi and *will lead to* the development of improved treatments.

Regarding genetics they assert:

It is clear that *we are on the verge of truly identifying* susceptibility (and likely protective) genes for bipolar disorder. . . . There is no doubt that knowledge of the genetics and subsequent understanding of their relevant biology *will have a tremendous impact* on diagnosis, classification, and treatment of psychiatric disease.

The long chapter on neurobiology ends with a salvo of optimism:

We are optimistic that the advances outlined here *will* result in dramatically different diagnostic system based on etiology, and ultimately in the discovery of new approaches to the prevention and treatment of some of humankind's most devastating and least understood illnesses. This progress holds much promise for developing novel therapeutics for the long-term treatment of severe, refractory mood disorders, and for improving the lives of millions.[47]

The use of the future tense and subjunctive mood in this scientific text on manic-depressive illness somewhat diminishes the impression of the sobriety which would fit the genre—or the subject. The appeal to trust and repeated invitations to share in the authors' belief in the future in the latest, most comprehensive and in every respect weighty statement of the current state of biological knowledge is as likely to dim admiration for the magnificent science with some measure of frustration, as to spread the boundless optimism which the authors apparently feel. Indeed, a question arises: do they? For the promises that future research *will* confirm the genetic nature of manic-depressive illness, that susceptibility genes for it *will* be discovered and that the result of these future confirmations and discoveries *will* be a useful diagnostic system based on etiology (i.e., understanding of the nature and causes of manic-depressive illness) and, therefore, efficient means of treating and preventing it, actually underscore the very disappointing fact that today (after more than a century of similar promises, "tremendous advances" in molecular and cellular biology and in research technology, and billions of dollars spent) the genetic nature of mdi still has not been confirmed, no susceptibility genes were found, and we still have no useful diagnostic system based on etiology, which would allow us to treat and prevent this disease.

If the tone of discussion disappoints, the logical confusion of the introductory paragraph quoted eliminates every shred of a doubt, if such still remained in the hearts of most credulous believers in the miraculous abilities of people in white overcoats, that the promises of the authors of *MDI* have no grounds. Correlation, as is known, is not causation. The possibility that familial aggregation of mental illness cases is a sign of genetic transmission of psychiatric disorders is only one among a number of possibilities. (As the authors of *MDI* themselves write: "Familial aggregation of disease suggests, but does not prove, a genetic contribution to disease. Environmental factors, such as exposure to toxins or emotionally traumatic family experiences, could in theory also lead to familial aggregation.") So is the (statistical) association of DNA markers with bipolar subtype. What is the basis for the expectation that "particular gene variants are definitely implicated in mdi susceptibility"?[48] Moreover, what is the causal significance of such genetic *susceptibility,* and how are we to make sure that it exists, if, as with schizophrenia, it might be only expressed if the disease is contracted? Similarly to the case with schizophrenia, the genetics of mdi is caught in a vicious logical circle. It may be safely expected to go round and round and round in it, never leading to anything.

"At present," write Goodwin and Jamison in 2007, "the most clinically useful evidence for genetic transmission continues to be the traditional genetic-epidemiological findings of twin, family, and adoption studies." The studies, they say, "demonstrate genetic transmission," but do not "allow one to identify the mode of genetic transmission in recurrent affective disorder. And neither they nor pedigree studies illuminate other important genetic issues: Is there biological heterogeneity? What is the pathophysiological inherited process in an illness? Where on the gene map is the disease locus (or loci)? What are the gene defects?" At this heady time of "molecular medicine revolution," genetic research on mdi is focusing on the search for "a susceptibility gene [trying] to home in on genes with unique features potentially relevant to manic-depressive illness." But, say Goodwin and Jamison, "only when heritability has been firmly established does it make sense to begin looking for the particular genes responsible for this inheritance." The question is a disease heritable, however, they also say, must be preceded by another one, "What is the phenotype, or trait, under study?"[49] In other words, genetic research, from which we expect the better understanding of mdi, depends on such understanding in the first place.

Traditional genetic-epidemiological studies of bipolar illness and major depression, which Goodwin and Jamison list since 1960s, have not produced any new findings after 1990. From the family aggregation studies we now know that having a first-degree relative with major depression triples one's lifetime risk of major depression, but having a bipolar first-degree relative increases the lifetime risk of bipolar disorder by a factor of ten (All the problems related to the definition and the differential diagnosis of the two categories, obviously, should be kept in mind when interpreting these agreed-upon figures). It is believed that twin and adoption studies, as against family aggregation ones, allow researchers to separate the contribution of the genes to the morbid risk from that of the environment. Calculations of (genetic) heritability are based on the twin studies, specifically, since there were only four adoption studies of mdi (with the last one in 1986), and, being inconsistent, they supported a genetic contribution to it only "modestly." Heritability of bipolar disorder, calculated from twin studies, is 0.78, the concordance rate between monozygotic twins being 63 percent. Heritability of major depression, in distinction, is only 0.34, with a MZ concordance rate of 34 percent, though the numbers are higher when only the "highly recurrent" depression is taken into consideration. However, twin studies are based on a remarkably abstract, even vacuous, notion of the nature of human environment and, for this reason, cannot disentangle the genetic and environmental influences. These numbers, in fact, do not measure heritability of mdi at all. Goodwin and Jamison explain the rationale behind twin studies:

> Identical or monozygotic twins are 100 percent genetically the same, whereas fraternal or dizygotic twins share just 50 percent of their genes; yet the two twin types *are assumed* to be no different in the degree to which they share environments. Therefore, any increased similarity in manifestation of manic-depressive illness detected in MZ twins compared with that in DZ twins should be due to the greater genetic similarity of the former.[50]

But this assumption (on which all depends) is wrong. It reduces the entire socio-cultural "environment" to having the same pair of biological parents. Neither parents, nor society at large treat different children in the very same manner: even tall versus short children, or pretty ones versus less pretty ones are likely to have different experiences, not to speak of girls versus boys. This means that the environment of dizygotic twins must be far more heterogeneous than that of monozygotic twins, who, being identical, are, in fact, likely to be treated in close to identical ways. The heritability numbers derived from twin studies, therefore, measure the combined effect of shared genes and shared environment, the comparison offering no possibility to control for the influence of either, and it is quite obvious that when all the influences are to a high degree shared (as in MZ twins), the concordance rate for any of these twins' traits would be significantly higher than it would be when all the influences on them are expected to be different.

Indeed, the significant degree of *dis*cordance between monozygotic twins in mdi (35 percent probability of not being affected by the disease when one's twin is affected), given that both their genetic material and their environment are assumed to be the same, presents a problem for the genetic paradigm. Yet, it is accounted for within the theoretical framework presented in this book, which, stressing the extreme complexity and ever-changing, processual nature of the cultural environment, can never assume identical influences in the case of any two individuals, and expects the mind-forming experiences of even monozygotic twins to be significantly different. The authors of *MDI* explain the 35 percent of MZ discordance as a result of *epigenetic regulation*, but this is just the biologists' way of admitting the influence of the environment without saying anything about it. "In recent years," write Goodwin and Jamison:

> epigenetics—the study of changes to the genome that, unlike mutations, do not alter the DNA sequence—has delineated just how inextricably linked nature and nurture truly are. Epigenetics purports to define the molecular mechanisms by which different cells from different tissues of the same organism, despite their DNA sequence identity, exhibit very different cellular phenotypes and perform very different functions. It is presumed that phenotypic and functional differences are the cumulative result of a large number of developmental, environmental, and stochastic events, some of which are mediated through the epigenetic modifications of DNA and chromatin histones. Epigenetic regulation is thus one of the molecular substrates for "cellular memory" that may help us understand how environmental impact results in temporally dissociated, altered behavioral responses.[51]

In effect, through epigenetics neuroscience is being led to the very point of meeting and connection with the theory of the mind as a cultural phenomenon developed here. As was repeatedly emphasized in Chapter 2, an emergent phenomenon necessarily organizes and adjusts the functioning of its elements, out of which it emerges, to itself, as it were from the top; the mind at every moment is supported by the mechanisms of the brain, which constitute the boundary conditions of the mind's existence, but it is supported by the mechanisms of the brain, already organized in accordance with, and adjusted to the needs of the mind. It is very likely that such organization and adjustment occur by the means of epigenetic regulation. In relation to mental illness, such as schizophrenia and manic-depressive disorders, epigenetic discoveries could indeed have important therapeutic implications. As put by Goodwin and Jamison, "In sum, although considerable additional research is needed, our growing appreciation of the molecular mechanisms underlying gene-environment interactions raise the intriguing possibility that environmentally induced neurobiological changes in early life may be amenable to subsequent therapeutic strategies targeting the epigenome."[52] Of course, this presupposes, on the part of neuroscience, at the very least the recognition that the environment side of the interaction may be as, or even more, complex as that of the genes and must be as carefully studied and analyzed, and the abandonment of the dogma of the essentially organic nature of mental diseases of unknown organic origin. An open-minded approach, admitting the causal role of the environment as an equal possibility that deserves serious consideration, may indeed lead to the identification of relevant epigenetic modifications and the arrest of advanced disease processes through their reversal. The realization of the promise of epigenetic research in the area of human consciousness, normal and abnormal, requires combining two kinds of expertise: the understanding of cellular and molecular biology and the understanding of another empirical reality—culture and the mind. We are still very far from such cooperation, and without it the significance of epigenetics in mdi research remains that of the flavor of the month, no more.

But let us return to the search for the genes responsible for mdi. This search has been given considerable boost by the Human Genome Project. Encouraged by the great success of this undertaking (which, to use earlier proposed analogy, indicated a great improvement in the brightness of the streetlight), and convinced by the family and twin studies (which, as noted above, in no way support such conviction) that the disease is largely (78 percent) genetically inherited, a considerable number within the research community have undertaken to confirm this idea microgenetically. Goodwin and Jamison explain why this turn to the molecular level is taking place:

Beginning in the late 1990s, extensive sequencing of the human genome began to reveal very large numbers of single nucleotide differences, or polymorphisms—called single nucleotide polymorphisms (SNPs) across the genome. These polymorphisms have been found to exist at about 1 of

every 200 nucleotides. This finding suggests that people are about 99.5 percent the same in terms of DNA sequence, and that it is in the 0.5 percent
difference that the factors influencing vulnerability to bipolar disorder lie.
About 10 million SNPs have been identified in the public SNP database; it
is expected that 15 million SNPs should exist, of which about 6 million
should be common. Studies of bipolar disorder that take advantage of this
understanding of SNPs began to appear in 2002.

The authors define human genome by analogy to *Oxford English Dictionary:*
"the genome is a collection of all the genes that can create things in the
human body" just as *OED* is the compendium of "all the words that can
create meaning in English," and write in direct continuation of the quotation above: "As of this writing . . . the word entries have been largely
spelled out. Much work remains to be done, however, particularly in clar-
ifying the function of genes, a task analogous to defining the meanings for
each word entry in the dictionary." The analogy is truly revealing: imagine
the utter uselessness of the *OED*, with all the words in it correctly spelled
and none of them defined. Not surprisingly, the new direction of research
into the mdi genetics has so far led to no particularly interesting results.
"There have been 21 genome wide linkage scans for [mdi]. . . . At least five
bipolar linkage findings . . . have reached genome wide statistical significance in multifamily samples . . . promising though they are, these findings were not replicated consistently . . ."[53]
    Linkage research, however, confirmed the findings of family studies,
already mentioned in the first edition of *MDI,* which suggested "the existence of some shared genetic liability between bipolar disorder and schizophrenia."

> These studies showed an excess of major depression and schizoaffective dis-
> order in the relatives of both bipolar and schizoaffective probands. . . .
> [Studies done after 1990] also suggested shared liability between the two
> disorders.
>   Linkage studies of bipolar disorder and schizophrenia have implicated
> overlapping chromosomal regions that could harbor susceptibility genes
> shared by the two disorders . . . [additional] findings suggest that bipolar ill-
> ness with psychotic features may be a genetically meaningful subtype and that
> this subtype may share some susceptibility genes with schizophrenia. . . .

The hypothesis of etiologic overlap suggests the existence of either psychosis genes (within the oligogenic model) or joint mood and psychosis genes.[54]

The assumption that mdi, like schizophrenia, is likely to be "oligogenic" (which means "polygenic," perhaps with a more hopeful connotation) complicates the search for its genetic basis but also suggests a strategy for its simplification: an attempt to divide the illness into "clinical and biological features . . . that might define more genetically homogeneous subtypes" or endophenotypes. "The term endophenotype," we read:

> is described as an internal, intermediate phenotype (i.e., not obvious to the unaided eye) that fills the gap in the causal chain between genes and distal diseases, and therefore may help to resolve questions about etiology. The endophenotype concept assumes that the number of genes involved in the variations of endophenotypes representing more elementary phenomena (as opposed to the behavioral macros found in the *DSM*) are fewer than those involved in producing the full disease.

So far this reasonable (in the given biopsychiatric framework) strategy has produced no discoveries. "Will an endophenotype strategy lead to a major payoff," ask the authors of *MDI,* usually so optimistic. Its promise is, they believe, great:

> Endophenotypes provide a means for identifying the "upstream" traits underlying clinical phenotypes, as well as the "downstream" biological consequences of genes. The methods available to identify endophenotypes include neuropsychological, cognitive, neurophysiological, neuroanatomical, imaging, and biochemical measures. The information revised in this volume suggests that candidate brain function endophenotypes [are numerous].

And yet

> none of the suggested endophenotypes have been fully validated. Moreover, while it might seem intuitively obvious that the genetics of these candidate endophenotypes will be simpler than that of manic-depressive illness, this has yet to be clearly established.

Regarding the troubling kinship between mdi and schizophrenia, the authors note:

> While the search for predisposing genes had traditionally tended to proceed under the assumption that schizophrenia and bipolar disorder are separate disease entities with different underlying etiologies, emerging findings from many fields of psychiatric research do not fit well with this model. Most notably, the pattern of findings emerging from genetic studies shows increasing evidence for an overlap in genetic susceptibility across the traditional classification categories. It is clear that there is not a one-to-one relationship between genes and behaviors so that different combinations of genes . . . contribute to any complex behavior. . . . It is also critically important to remember that polymorphisms in genes will very likely simply be associated with bipolar disorder or recurrent depression; these genes will likely not invariably determine outcome, but only lend a higher probability for the subsequent development of illness. In fact, genes will never code for abnormal behaviors per se, but rather code for proteins that make up cells, forming circuits, that in combination determine facets of both abnormal and normal behavior. These expanding levels of interaction have made the study of psychiatric diseases so difficult.[55]

The authors of *MDI* stick to their guns, even resisting the conclusion that the traditional model, contradicted as it is by all the evidence, might be wrong and schizophrenia and mdi might be one and the same disease, but they admit that, in general, the results of linkage research, which "has been the major focus of genetic investigation of bipolar disorder since the mid-1980s," have been largely disappointing. "As of this writing," they write in 2007,

> attempts to localize bipolar genes through linkage have had only limited success, as the findings obtained have not converged as consistently as might be hoped on one or a small number of chromosomal regions. The most likely reasons for this are that bipolar illness is a genetically complex disorder . . . and that differing combinations of susceptibility genes may *cause* disease in different groups of people. Though the pace of progress has been slower than expected, the 20 or so genome scans of bipolar illness

conducted today have yielded some strong linkage signals, some of which have been identified in a number of studies. The most promising linkage regions . . . are worthy of further study to clarify whether they do, in fact, harbor bipolar genes. The lack of definitive success in discovering bipolar genes has prompted some investigators to consider other approaches to the problem, including refining the phenotype . . . and rethinking potential genetic mechanisms that may underlie the disease.[56]

In the future, they predict,

Linkage studies, the workhorse of research in bipolar genetics since the late 1980s, will move from center stage as association studies assume a greater role. The chromosomal regions implicated by bipolar linkage studies will be studied using large case-control and trio (case-parents) samples. This shift is occurring because linkage studies can identify the general chromosomal localization of a gene, but only association can truly pinpoint the location of the disease gene and, even more specifically, the location of the particular variant within the gene that is responsible for disease susceptibility. By analogy, think of searching for a needle in 23 enormous haystacks. Linkage is analogous to figuring out which haystack and which general area of the haystack holds the needle. Once that has been accomplished, a more fine-grained approach is needed to sort through the pieces of straw.

This would be an appropriate analogy if it were known for certain that the needle was lost among the twenty-three haystacks. As this is not known, but only ardently believed, we are forced to return to the streetlight one. Think of searching for that needle under the bright streetlight because the streetlight washes a certain area with its luminous light; think of dividing the area under the streetlight into twenty-three regions (to keep the number of regions equal to that of the chromosomes) and further subdividing these into smaller parcels; think of distinguishing some twenty parcels that appear to give off a metallic reflection, with eleven of them being particularly promising (perhaps because on a different occasion when, happening to be reinserting a contact lens under a streetlight and losing it momentarily then and there, someone actually found that lens in a spot that, according to reports, looked similar); think of zeroing in on these eleven promising spots and finding nothing; and then think of remaining undaunted and conceiving a more fine-grained approach: bringing a microscope and examining the spots millimeter by millimeter.

"Once bipolar genes have been discovered," continue Goodwin and Jamison,

> researchers will want to know whether the illness occurs more often when people carrying the susceptibility allele are exposed to particular factors or experiences. A number of environmental exposures that have been suggested as causative factors in manic-depressive illness, whether bipolar or recurrent depressive, such as a loss of a parent at an early age or obstetrical complications, could be assessed to determine whether they increase the risk of illness in conjunction with the risk genotype. For example, the interaction between the short variant of the serotonin transporter promoter polymorphism and stressful life events may play a role in the predisposition to major depressive episodes . . . [57]

We have already met the serotonin transporter promoter polymorphism (gene 5-HTT) in the discussion of research on schizophrenia. It has been the subject of much scrutiny in mdi research as well, and, quite possibly, everything that is to be known about it is known.[58] The constant finetuning of the streetlight mechanism is necessarily producing a wealth of new information; its light is steadily becoming brighter and it is not for lack of diligence of the competent people, or money spent on, searching under it that it fails to illuminate the problem of mdi and turn this information into useful knowledge. 5-HTT, write Goodwin and Jamison,

> is the most heavily studied gene in research on manic-depressive illness because of the importance of serotonin in depression, the central role of 5-HTT in serotonogenic function at the synapse, and the demonstration of a functionally meaningful DNA variation in the promoter region of the gene. The promoter region plays a crucial role in the expression of the gene, and 5-HTT has a stretch of promoter DNA that exists in a short and a long form. The short form has been found to result in decreased levels of gene expression compared with the long form. Four studies of bipolar disorder have found a positive association between the short variant and illness,

while 13 studies have found no significant difference. . . . A meta-analysis of 15 case-control samples found evidence for a significant, though quite small, effect of this polymorphism in bipolar disorder, reporting an odds ratio of 1.13 for having the short versus the long allele among the cases as compared with the controls.[59]

Add to this the fact that the short allele is the normal one, i.e., the allele found in two thirds of the human population, and it is obvious that all these findings (weak even in the estimation of our confident authors) are useless. They suggest the conclusion: "If you've got the regular variant of the human genome—you run the risk of bipolar disorder." Sometimes, such obviously true, tautological, conclusions are meaningful: for example, radical mastectomy is one effective method of preventing breast cancer, based on the truism: no breasts—no cancer. But in most cases the obviously true claim that being alive exposes one to the danger of death, makes no practical sense: it is true that having lungs is a necessary condition for pulmonary tuberculosis and that without a heart one runs no risk of coronary heart disease, but getting rid of these vital organs in order to reduce one's lifetime's probability of their diseases is really not an option. So it is with 5-HTT "the most heavily studied gene in research on manic-depressive illness." And what does it, or any of the yet undiscovered genes or alleles contributing to susceptibility to (i.e., being able to contract) mdi, have to do with the environmental factors or life-experiences? Why does the research into these possibly important factors have to wait for the discovery of bipolar genes, so long expected and, despite all, never found? Why not step from under the streetlight and, while resting from its blinding brightness, consider for a moment, think, where the damned needle could be lost?

So far the association method has not delivered either. And, in any case, Goodwin and Jamison write:

> Proving that a gene—or more specifically a particular gene variant, an allele—is causally related to mdi will require more than simply demonstrating a statistical association between an allele and the disease; an important piece of evidence would be the demonstration that the allele causes meaningful alteration in the structure or expression level of messenger RNA. A number of genes have been shown to have abnormal expression levels in the

prefrontal cortex, hippocampus, or amygdala of bipolar subjects, though none of these findings have yet been replicated. Allelic variation, however, has not yet been shown to correlate with any of these changes. . . .

Ultimate proof of a causal relationship between a gene variant and mdi will depend on investigations that go beyond the study of nucleic acids. Changes in structure and/or function will need to be shown in the protein product of the putative disease gene. Further, the proposed disease allele should result in observable changes in aspects of biochemical pathway processes, in neuronal and/or glial function, in brain region structure or function, and in intermediate phenotype measures. Again, study of the promoter region polymorphism of the serotonin transporter gene provides an example of this kind of study. The short variant was shown to be associated with greater amygdala activation in response to fearful stimuli in a functional magnetic resonance imaging study.

Though pointing to certain caveats, Goodwin and Jamison consider these scanty pickings "reasons for optimism":

There are no genetic tests available at present to provide precise estimates of the risk to children in specific cases. . . . It is possible that the first genes for bipolar disorder have already been discovered, though ultimately proving that a particular gene plays an etiologic role in the illness will require studies that extend beyond DNA to demonstration of the gene's role in a pathogenic pathway. . . .

Despite these reasons for optimism about the future of genetic medicine in mdi, there are also grounds for caution and pitfalls of which to be aware. Because of the possibility that alleles for the illness or any of its subgroups will have only small effects, the use of each individually in genetic testing may be limited . . .

And yet, they also write: "Genetic counseling is a feature of current clinical practice."

In short:

Although we have yet to identify the specific abnormal genes or proteins associated with mdi, there have been major advances in our understanding of the illness, particularly in the bipolar subgroup and in the mechanisms of action of the most effective treatments. These advances have generated considerable excitement among the clinical neuroscience community and are reshaping the views about the neurobiological underpinnings of the disorder.[60]

The excitement of the neuroscience community (apparently, very excitable—perhaps, because of a yet undiscovered gene) is directly proportionate to the sophistication of its research technologies. These technologies, for instance, today allow one to actually see some of the brain mechanisms that support various mental processes. Nobody has doubted the existence of such mechanisms at least for the last hundred years (every event in the mind is obviously supported by the brain), but until recently one could not point to them with a finger. We do not, of course, yet know which particular mental events the events in the brain correspond to (because we know close to nothing about mental events themselves), but we can associate broad classes of occurrences in the brain with broad classes of mental phenomena, such as disease versus health. So, Goodwin and Jamison report that since the publication of the first edition of their text in 1990, there have "truly been tremendous advances" in the understanding of the circuits, and especially cellular plasticity cascades involved in mdi. They write:

> Through functional brain imaging studies, affective circuits have been identified that mediate the behavioral, cognitive, and somatic manifestations of manic-depressive illness. Key areas of these circuits include the amygdala and related limbic structures, orbital and medial prefrontal cortex, anterior cingulate, medial thalamus, and related regions of the basal ganglia. Imbalance within these circuits, rather than an increase or decrease in any single region of the circuit seems to predispose and mediate the expression of manic-depressive illness.

It is to be noted that, in the above formulation, the general function of the circuit mechanism in neuronal processing implies mediation on the cellular level between the information that is processed, in this case, information communicating to the organism the disease, and the organism, thus mediation in the expression of mdi. (Goodwin and Jamison's description presupposes a tripartite division between the disease, the mediating circuits, and the organism.) But the imbalance within the circuits *is* the expression of the disease; just like diseased lung cells would be (not mediate) the expression of tuberculosis and diseased breast tissues would be (not mediate) the expression of breast cancer. Thus it is hard to understand why these brain circuits would *predispose* one to the disease, thereby on their own perverting information they are supposed to process, unless we know that the disease is genetic. Goodwin and Jamison continue:

> Moreover, studies of cellular plasticity cascades in manic-depressive illness are leading to a conceptualization of the pathophysiology, course, and optimal long-term treatment of the illness. These data suggest that, while manic-depressive illness is clearly not a classic neurodegenerative disease, it is in fact associated with impairments of cellular plasticity and resilience.

This fact of the association between mdi and impairments of cellular plasticity (or of the expression of mdi in such impairments) makes the authors declare:

> It is our strong contention that manic-depressive illness arises from abnormalities in cellular plasticity cascades, leading to aberrant information processing in synapses and circuits mediating affective, cognitive, motoric, and neurovegetative function. Thus, manic-depressive illness can be best conceptualized as a disorder of synapses and circuits—not 'too much/too little' of individual neurotransmitter or neuropeptide systems.[61]

Whatever are the relative merits of the "too much/too little" argument, this claim is strictly analogous to suggesting that pulmonary tuberculosis is best conceptualized as a disease of the lungs and breast cancer as an illness of the breasts. One would readily agree with Goodwin and Jamison that it is "unfortunate" that there "has been little progress in developing truly novel drugs specifically for the treatment of manic-depressive illness" based on this discovery.[62] But it is not surprising.

Manic-depressive illness is a very serious disease. Twenty percent of those who suffer from its depressive form commit suicide; in its advanced manic form it is indistinguishable from schizophrenia. Obviously, it results in "abnormalities in multiple systems and at multiple levels" connected to mental functioning. Neuroimaging technology has so far allowed the identification of the following structural brain abnormalities in mdi patients (as compared with healthy controls):

1. Increased lateral ventricular enlargement;
2. Increased cortical sulcal enlargement;
3. Increased third ventricular enlargement;
4. Increased subcortical hyperintensities (in younger and older bipolar, older MDD patients);
5. Frontal and prefrontal volume decreases;
6. Cerebellar volume decreases;
7. Hippocampal volume decreases (in MDD).

Four of these seven findings were confirmed with meta-analyses. The finding that mdi patients and healthy controls have similar global cerebral volumes was also confirmed. "Methodological advances—including new methods of image acquisition, such as DTI, and new image processing techniques, such as the ability to segment images into gray and white matter," write Goodwin and Jamison, "promise to advance structural neuroimaging studies. Limited statistical power related to clinical heterogeneity and small sample sizes in individual studies needs to be addressed, however. This problem is particularly salient with respect to understanding clinical correlates [i.e., symptoms] of structural imaging abnormalities in mood disorder patients."[63]

Functional neuroimaging has also identified a number of abnormalities related to mdi. These abnormalities in brain activity are:

1. Decreased global cerebral activity (in older, more depressed patients);
2. Decreased dorsolateral prefrontal activity;
3. Decreased temporal cortical activity;
4. Decreased basal ganglia activity (in MDD)
5. Variable anterior cingulate and medial prefrontal activity;
6. Increased amygdala activity;
7. Decreased prefrontal phosphomonoesters (in euthymic bipolar patients versus healthy controls and depressed bipolar patients).

Only this last finding was confirmed with meta-analysis.

Contrary to their usual optimism, the authors of *MDI* end their chapter on neuroimaging with a stress on the limitations of this recent research and an emotion rather resembling frustration.[64] They write:

> The cerebral activity studies reviewed here have important limitations, including small sample sizes, varying methodology, and reliance on measures of patterns of activity across cerebral structures rather than assessment of specific neurochemical differences. Their findings need to be combined with emerging data from studies of specific cerebral neurochemistry using specific neurochemical radiotracers and MRS . . . to yield more comprehensive understanding of the nature of the neurobiology of mood disorders.
>
> Methodological advances in MRS studies are beginning to allow in vivo assessment of specific cerebral neurochemistry that is less invasive . . . and more generally available . . . than PET techniques using specific neurochemical radiotracers. MRS studies are limited, however, by relatively poor spatial resolution, and by the ability to assess only a small and in some cases inadequately characterized group of metabolites.
>
> Studies of specific cerebral neurochemistry share important limitations with those of cerebral activity, such as small sample sizes and varying methodology. Technical advances, including new methods of image acquisition . . . , promise to advance neuroimaging studies. As with structural neuroimaging studies, however, limited statistical power related to clinical heterogeneity and small sample sizes in individual studies remains problematic. . . . large collaborative studies and/or standardized designs that facilitate meta-analyses may help address these difficulties. . . .
>
> Despite providing substantial contributions to our understanding of which cerebral structures mediate affective processing in health and mood disorders, neuroimaging has not yet realized its potential to be a clinically relevant tool in the diagnosis and treatment of major mood disorders. Technological innovations to enhance spatial and temporal resolution, decrease or eliminate exposure to ionizing radiation, increase neurochemical specificity, increase availability, and decrease expense are needed if research is to further advance our knowledge of the neuroanatomical and neurochemical substrates of these disorders. As these technical innovations

unfold, it becomes even more important that we put considerably more effort into improved methods for diagnosis and clinical evaluation, including an agreed-upon standard for distinguishing the more recurrent forms of MDD that fall within Kraepelin's concept of mdi. More careful differentiation between state and trait is also needed, as are consensus protocols for assessing the multiple sources of variance in these measures. Given the great promise and expense of these technologies, we can afford to do no less. While it remains to be seen whether such advances will ultimately yield clinical applications to facilitate diagnosis and target treatments more effectively in patients with mood disorders, it is clear that this potential will not be realized unless we invest more effort in standardizing the clinical characteristics of the patients we study.[65]

Thus we are back to square one. When one does not know what it is, specifically, that one wishes to explain, it is logically impossible to explain it. When one is not sure what it is one wants to cure and prevent, it is impossible to cure and prevent it. The explanation, the cure, and the prevention of mdi depend first and foremost on its correct, consistent and comprehensive, conceptualization. We must revisit our notions as to where the needle was lost. And making the streetlight brighter is becoming too expensive.

Epidemiology of Manic-Depressive Illness

It remains to us to consider the epidemiological findings regarding manic-depressive illness. Despite obviously enormous problems connected to the difficulties of conceptualization and logical confusion reviewed above, which are fundamentally identical to those, already discussed, besetting the epidemiology of schizophrenia, these data are extremely suggestive.[66] Particularly interesting data concern distributions by age, race, what may be broadly called "ethnicity," and class. The epidemiological findings reported and discussed in the first and the second editions of *Manic-Depressive Illness* are, by and large, the same, since the great majority of the studies cited were published before 1990, and those that were carried out within the subsequent seventeen years are consistent with them. And yet, there are some changes in the overall picture they paint that stand out if the two editions are compared.

For example, the first edition already suggested, on the basis of research conducted in the 1980s, that in the United States younger birth cohorts (those born in 1944 and later) had lower age of onset and, possibly, higher rates of prevalence, than older birth cohorts. This, in the culturally meaningful idiom, indicated that the burden of manic-depression was increasing in several ways for the baby boomers and later generations. Still, the consensus was that the mean age of onset for bipolar disorder was thirty; while for major unipolar depression it fell between forty and fifty. Goodwin and Jamison then hypothesized that "although this difference may result from faulty memory and inadequate record keeping, among other factors, it is possible that susceptible individuals may now express their phenotype at a younger age."[67] Several large-scale studies, carried out since 1990, in particular the National Comorbidity Survey (NCS) in the early part of the decade and its replication ten years later in the beginning of the new century, made evident the increase in the rates (though the higher rates were explained not as an increase but as a methodological artifact, resulting from the inadequacy of earlier data-collection techniques, which systematically underestimated the true prevalence of affective disorders) and confirmed that manic-depressive illness is (in fact, that it has become) a young adults' disease.[68]

As regards race, in 1990, in the United States, "the most replicated finding [was] a lower incidence rate among blacks," with the average white/black ratio established as 2.4:1. Goodwin and Jamison cited Kolb (1968) saying that "manic-depressive illness was often labeled as a white upper class disorder in the early part of [the twentieth] century," attempted to explain this as a result of a racial bias on the part of earlier researchers, and stressed more recent studies (e.g., the NIHM ECA program, 1981) that found no "significant difference in the prevalence or incidence rates of manic-depressive illness among races." They concluded: "Thus, despite a majority of studies reporting lower rates of manic-depressive illness in blacks than in whites, the data, because of the presence of uncontrolled factors, such as misdiagnosis, cross-class comparisons, and racial biases, yield no clear picture."[69]

The 2007 edition did not devote to race a separate section, but treated it among other "associated factors" under the rubric of "Race/Ethnicity and Cultural Differences." Unfortunately, this was not because of the dimin-

ished significance of race in epidemiological discourse, but because ethnicity and culture are used as substitute terms for it, all three being
understood as biological realities (i.e., in racist terms). The new data discussed in the (half a page long) section, however, suggest the importance
of disregarded *cultural* factors in the differential distribution of manic-
depressive illness. Write Goodwin and Jamison:

> A number of studies have examined racial similarities and differences in the
> prevalence and incidence of bipolar illness. Many factors . . . cloud the
> accurate determination of these rates, including inadequate sampling from
> different socioeconomic groups, cultural differences and consequent prob-
> lems regarding presentation, the misdiagnosis of schizophrenia . . . , and
> possible racial insensitivity among early researchers. These factors must be
> accounted for in such analyses.[70]

They then list three studies that found "equal rates of diagnosis of bipolar
illness among African-Americans and Caucasians," mention the 1981
ECA study that "revealed no significant difference . . . among the races,"
and note that "the NCS [1994], on the other hand, indicated that African-
Americans had significantly lower rates of mania than Caucasians." This
means that in 2007, too, the finding that the rates of mdi differ among
different populations of the U.S. nationals, with African Americans, specifically, being less at risk than Americans of other origins, remains well
replicated. Immediately after the above-quoted sentence, however, *MDI*
authors say: "There is also some evidence that African Caribbean and
African individuals are less likely to have experienced a depressive episode
before the onset of first mania, and more likely to have more severe psychotic symptoms during their first mania, relative to Caucasian Europeans"
obviously uniting the three very distinct *cultural* groups by the color of
their skin, i.e., the genetic material they hold in common, and attributing
the differences in the rates and course of mdi in these groups versus
"Caucasians" to this "racial" heritage.[71] These differences—which, it must
be noted, are different: comparative rates of illness among African
Americans, and unusual course of illness among African Caribbeans and
Africans—however, may as well be attributed to the specific cultural experiences of African Americans as distinguished from white Americans, and

specific cultural experiences of Caribbeans and Africans as distinguished from Europeans. (For example, this can be attributed, as was suggested in regard to similar differences between cultures observed in the WHO international study of schizophrenia, to the possibility that the disease presenting so differently from the Euro-American classical pattern among other populations is not the same disease at all.)

This interpretation is supported by the immediate continuation of the passage under analysis, as Goodwin and Jamison write:

> In the study of the Cross-National Collaborative Group, the rates among two Asian samples (Taiwan and Korea) and the Hispanic sample (Puerto Rico) were compared with those among the primarily Caucasian samples from Edmonton, Canada; West Germany; and Cristchurch, New Zealand. The Asian samples clearly showed the lowest rates of bipolar disorder. . . . Moreover, the Asian sites (Taiwan, Korea, Hong Kong) generally showed the lowest rates for all psychiatric disorders.[72]

Again, the only thing that unites these Asian populations with the previously discussed populations of African origin is that their genetic endowment is different from that of the Caucasians (and the inclusion of a linguistically-defined group, Hispanics, among non-Caucasians throws an additional dose of confusion into this already troubling mix). But, the biologistic (racist) interpretation to the contrary, the reported data insistently point to the association of manic-depressive illness, just like of schizophrenia, with the Western, Europe-derived, culture. Something exposes the people in it to far higher rates of psychotic diseases of unknown organic origin, than any other population on earth. Still, the *MDI* authors press the point (though opening their concluding paragraph with a surprising remark):

> In general, the newer epidemiologic data are consistent with the results of earlier studies in indicating no strong association between race/ethnicity and bipolar illness, with the possible exception of the unexplained lower rates of many psychiatric disorders in Asian countries. Too few Asians were included in the ECA and NCS to study the consistency of this finding among Asians living in the United States. Such data could aid in understanding

whether low rates of bipolar disorder are intrinsic to Asian people [!] or affected by environmental factors.[73]

The lower rates of mdi among African Americans in comparison to other Americans cannot be explained by differences between cultures characterizing entire societies, but they certainly can point to what precisely, in societies of the kind to which the American society belongs, elevates (or creates) the risk of such diseases. Epidemiological data collected under the rubric of class help to explore this issue—and explain the resistance of African Americans to this disease. In the first edition of *MDI,* Goodwin and Jamison preface the presentation of the consistent association of mdi with the upper social classes by pointing to the many reasons why these data are suspect:

> Studies of social class and manic-depressive illness have been hampered, and the interpretation of data has been made difficult, by two major types of methodological problems: diagnostic bias (and diagnostic over-inclusiveness) and treatment bias. . . . For example, upper and middle class people are more likely to be diagnosed as manic-depressive, whereas lower class individuals, especially among poor urban black populations, are more likely to be diagnosed as schizophrenic (often mistakenly so), and are consequently treated as such. Minorities generally are underrepresented in these studies as well. Further, criteria for social class vary across studies. Some authors have used the system of Hollingshead and Redlich (1958), others used occupation alone or parental social class, and still others used only educational achievement.[74]

They remark on the lack of "a significant downward social drift in individuals with manic-depressive illness," which distinguishes them from schizophrenics, who are downward drifters. This makes the claim that lower class individuals, especially poor blacks, are more likely to be diagnosed as schizophrenic dubious, however widely believed, and adds to the fact that misdiagnosis as schizophrenic could not account for the lower rates of mdi among African Americans or among lower class individuals in general, even if such class bias did exist, because the rates of mdi, wherever the statistics are available, exceed those of schizophrenia by a factor of ten. In the end, they nevertheless conclude:

> With the methodological considerations in mind, it appears that the majority of studies report an association between manic-depressive illness and one or more measures reflecting upper social class. . . . *none found a significantly lower than expected rate of illness associated with indices of upper social class* (defined by educational status, occupation, economic status, or parental social class.) Thus, considered in its entirety, the literature is highly suggestive of an association.[75]

A table lists all the main findings of all the studies on mdi and social class, conducted between 1913 and 1989.[76] They are consistent: poverty, specifically (low economic class) is shown to be a protective factor, and mdi is most widespread in the middle (professional, managerial) social class.[77] Obviously, the data are drawn predominantly from Western modern societies. An earlier literature review quoted (Bagley, 1973) sums up: "The studies reviewed suggest that there is some support for the view that some types of 'depression' and upper class economic position are related. The finding seems to hold in several cultures, and in different points in time in the present [twentieth] century." Though the definition of depression, notes Bagley, "has often been unclear in many studies," there is evidence that the finding applies to "psychotic" depression and to "the classic manic-depressive psychoses in particular."[78]

Goodwin and Jamison are baffled and refuse to accept the consistent association between upper social classes and mdi as a fact: "two main types of arguments have been advanced," they write, "to explain the *hypothesized* greater incidence of manic-depressive illness in the middle and upper social classes." But what is under discussion is not a hypothesis, but a constantly replicated finding which is actually contrary to the implicit hypothesis that the burden of depressive illness should be heavier in the lower classes. It is precisely because these findings go against this implicit hypothesis (conjecture or intuition) that they are so counter-intuitive. The first argument makes a certain sense to *MDI* authors, because they insist that manic illness, in particular, is connected to creativity (thus containing a side-benefit). "Some authors," they write, "suggest that a relationship exists between certain personality and behavioral correlates of affective (primarily bipolar) illness and a rise in social position. . . . In fact, many features of hypomania, such as outgoingness, increased energy and intensified sexuality, and heightened productivity, have been linked with increased achievement and accomplishments." But "the second *hypothesis* posits that *manic-depressive illness is secondary to the stresses of being in or moving into the upper social classes*." Of it they declare: "This hypothesis is implausible because it assumes that, compared with lower classes, there is a special kind of stress associated with being in the upper social classes, one capable of precipitating major psychotic episodes. Further, it ignores genetic factors and evidence suggesting that parental social class is often elevated as well [i.e. the hypothesis that mdi is a disease of the upper classes *ignores* that it is related to the upper social classes]."[79]

The seventeen years that elapsed between the two editions of the magisterial text fail to bring any relief from this cognitive dissonance, and in 2007 edition, Goodwin and Jamison reiterate:

> In the first edition of this text, we reviewed more than 30 early studies of the association between social class and manic-depressive illness published between 1913 and 1989. We discussed in detail the considerable methodological problems involved in virtually every one of the studies but were impressed, nonetheless, by the overall association between bipolar illness and one or more measures reflecting upper social class. . . .
>
> . . . it is likely that most of the earlier associations between bipolar disorder and higher social class had to do with diagnostic practices and inaccuracies in the concept. Upper- and middle-class people were more likely to be diagnosed as bipolar, whereas lower-class individuals, especially the urban poor, were (and still are) more likely to be diagnosed as schizophrenic (often mistakenly so) and consequently treated as such. Criteria for social class also varied widely across studies. Nonetheless, these investigations remain interesting for their span over many decades, their historical significance, and their great range across countries and cultures.

This phrasing and emphasis on "historical significance" naturally lead one to think that recent studies consistently contradict the thirty early studies. But, write Goodwin and Jamison immediately following this statement,

Most newer studies have failed to find a significantly lower than expected rate of bipolar disorder associated with indices of upper social class (educational status, occupation, economic status, or parental social class). In both ECA and the NCS, lower educational level was not found to be associated with an increased risk of bipolar disorder. The NCS found an association between rates of bipolar illness and lower family income; it is unclear, however, whether the latter is a direct consequence of the illness or a trigger for its onset [especially since a later study (Tsuchiya et al., 2004) found] that higher parental educational level and greater parental wealth were associated with an elevated risk for bipolar disorder, but that the patients themselves were more likely to be unemployed and less well educated.

Granted that the language is very confusing—one could simply say that most newer studies have confirmed the association of mdi with upper social classes—but the truth outs despite the hedging. To explain the obstinate data, the *MDI* authors revert to the first, genetic, argument above: It may be, they say, "that milder forms of the illness on occasion lead to high achievement, but that the illness expressed in offspring of successful individuals is of a more severe nature."[80]

The conclusion one must derive from the existing epidemiological studies, which supports the hypothesis of this book, is that the majority of manic-depressive patients, like the majority of schizophrenics, come from the upper classes. This, of course, is perfectly consistent with the finding of the lower rates of mdi among African Americans and explains it: African Americans have a lower risk of the illness, because they are concentrated in the lower classes; this is a class, not a race, thing. Class is a cultural and historical, not a biological, phenomenon: as African Americans increasingly move into the upper classes, the rates of mdi among them may be expected to increase. This conclusion is further supported by another set of findings, which Goodwin and Jamison are discussing in the first edition under the rubric of "Cross-Cultural Findings" and in the second one under "International Studies"; it concerns Jewish populations.

Studies carried out among Jews have been "perhaps the most quantified" of the cross-cultural studies of the incidence of manic-depressive illness. *MDI* authors report the findings, but do not comment on them; these findings, however, are not that straightforward and deserve comment.

Studies of Jewish populations have been carried out in Israel, in Britain, and in the USA and Canada. In Israel, Miller (1967) found that affective psychosis was far less common in Sephardic Jews (i.e., Jews of African or Asian origin and in 1967 likely born in Africa and Asia, because the immigration of these groups to Israel only started in the 1950s) than in Ashkenazi Jews (ones of European or American origin). The 1975 study of Gershon and Liebowitz replicated this, finding that the rate of mdi among Ashkenazis was twice as high as that among Sephardi Jews. "However," say Goodwin and Jamison, "Halpern (1938) and Hes (1960), in their studies of Jewish subpopulations in Palestine/Israel, did not find the incidence of affective psychosis particularly high among Jews compared to other cultures."[81] They treat the Jewish population in this instance as if it were one culture, while it is obvious from their own citations above that it contains at the very least two different cultures, one African/Asian (traditional), another European/American (modern), and nothing said about the differences within this culturally-mixed population suggests that general rates among Jews should be "particularly high" in comparison to non-Jewish populations (Muslim and Christian). Evidently, "culture" substitutes in this *MDI* discussion for "race," or genetically-defined population. Immediately following the above quotation, Goodwin and Jamison report on the 1962 North-American study by Malzberg, who found that "Jews in New York and Canada were significantly more likely than Gentiles to have manic-depressive psychosis, a finding Cooklin and colleagues (1983) replicated in London."[82] It is notable that the latter study was published with the subtitle "Is manic-depressive illness a typically Jewish disorder?"—a suspicion likely entertained by Goodwin and Jamison, given their biological idea of "culture." But the data clearly point away from biology. Instead, they point consistently to the likelihood that manic-depressive illness is a disease of modern societies and that, within modern societies, it is a disease of the upper classes. That is why in Israel during the first decades after the founding of the state Ashkenazi Jews were far more at risk than Sephardi ones. And that is also why, while there was no difference between the rates of mdi among the Jews of Palestine/Israel and other populations in 1938 and 1960 (now Israel is lagging far behind the United States in this respect, but is, probably, still very much ahead of any African country), Jews of New York or Canada are far more likely than Gentiles to have this illness: in New York and Canada they are concentrated in the upper classes, and in 1938 and 1960 studies, rates of mdi in Palestine/Israel were examined for the Jewish society in general, without controlling for class.[83]

The causal explanation of the psychotic illnesses under discussion here, which turn out to be one disease existing in several forms, boils down to the nature of experiences of the upper classes of modern societies and is to be sought in the cultural history of these classes. A most important point in this context is that these classes did not exist before modernity; they have no equivalent in other types of societies. Therefore, their experiences, and the diseases created by these experiences, did not exist. The agent of disease in this case is the product not of evolution but of history, it is not our genetic makeup but our cultural environment that makes us vulnerable.

Self-Loathing versus Loss of Self

One more question remains to be considered before, at last, we turn our attention to history. The overwhelming majority of sufferers from functional psychoses classed as schizophrenia and mdi in fact suffer from the most fatal of these—depression. Like the diagnoses of schizophrenia and mania, depression refers to a disease of the will: it is, like the others, an impairment of a particular aspect of the self—the agency or the acting self. The impairment of the acting self necessarily disorganizes the overall self structure, affects the sense of self and thus creates the so-called "I-problems." The chief "I-problem" in depression, as contrasted to mania and full-blown schizophrenia, is not the loss of self, however, but self-loathing. Neither does the depressed person lose his or her mind; the culture in the depressed person's brain remains individualized, and acutely individualized throughout the course of the illness. The process of the mental disease, so aptly called by Bleuler "schizophrenia," to which the three generally recognized varieties belong, is the process of the mind's disintegration. Schizophrenic thinking, say the experts, is "unanchored," "unhinged." It is deindividualization that unhinges it. What arrests the commenced disintegration of the depressed person's mind, what keeps his or her thinking so obviously and immovably anchored, so obviously individualized and focused on the self it rejects?

Of course, since depression and acute psychosis are stages of the same process, in which the former precedes the latter, the probability of developing depression is greater than the probability of reaching the stage of acute psychosis, and this should already in some part explain why depression is so much more common than schizophrenia (and bipolar-I disorder). At the same time, this higher probability of an earlier stage cannot on its own explain the duration of major depression, which is, undoubtedly, what makes it so unbearable and life-threatening. It is likely that something— a specific feature absent among those who develop formal thought disorder—holds the process back at the depressive stage. I suggest that this something is the developed but malformed, contradictory identity, the relationally-constituted self that contains too many—and some mutually-exclusive—possibilities. While being born to two déclassé parents, preoccupied to the point of obsession with appearing as if they still belonged to the superior position once occupied by their families (as happened to John Nash) is recognizable as a pattern in our society, but very rare (thus making rare the difficulty to form *any* identity, which is likely to be the effect of such accident of birth on the unlucky child), finding oneself bombarded by contradictory cultural messages and overwhelmed with choices is an exceedingly and increasingly common modern experience. It is, therefore, not surprising that the period of adolescent moratorium among us often lasts into one's early forties, that so many spend their youth in frequently futile searching for oneself, that what one finds is as likely to be unsatisfactory as gratifying, and that, when it is gratifying, one is rarely secure in that the self one has found is one's to keep. Modern society is inherently anomic and problems with identity are endemic to it. We are all exposed to the "virus" of depression, the cultural agent that carries the disease, and are, probably, as likely to catch it in a mild form, as we are to get a runny nose or a headache due to the common cold. Certain environments, such as college, for instance, which render the multitude of identity choices we have salient, make the virus particularly active and let it affect more people, as do circumstances that actually offer more possibilities, such as upper class background. In the end, the great majority of us reconcile with the identities reflecting the choices we have made; acquire responsibilities which reinforce these identities and, thankfully, limit our freedom to choose again; and settle into a life livable enough even when not happy.

But a significant and probably growing minority catches the virus and develops the severe form of depression.

The probable increase in the rates of the manic-depressive illness consistently reflected in the ever-improving statistical studies makes it unlikely that the reason the majority escapes and the minority succumbs to the disease is organic vulnerability or diathesis, since such vulnerability itself would have been spread in the population at a certain stable rate. The reason, rather, must be the increasing probability of triggering events—events that problematize one's identity, *specifically undermining one's sense of social status*—in the lives of the minority and the absence of such events in the life of the majority. It is remarkable that obviously traumatic experiences (torture, rape, being witness to the murder, torture, rape of loved ones and similar acts of violence—that is, experiences capable of producing post-traumatic stress syndrome) do not trigger mdi. The most striking example of this is the relative rarity of functional mental disease (mdi or schizophrenia) among the survivors of the Holocaust.[84] Suicide among them is rather common as is deep, overwhelming, entirely understandable sadness, and a sense of worthlessness of life after such indescribable and unforgettable suffering, but, clearly, there is nothing delusional in the horrible memories with which they must live; their rejection of life is situational and reflects no mental pathology. Events that trigger depression, rather, are of the kind that to most observers would appear trivial: moving to a new environment in which the kid that had been considered the smartest in the environment left is no longer considered the smartest, or, on the contrary, in which one is suddenly being considered the smartest, or in which norms of status ascription are generally different; being rejected in love, or not accepted to one's preferred college during early admissions, or unexpectedly becoming the object of love of an exceptional or higher-status person; later in life, getting or not getting a particularly desired, responsible position, etc. These are events that trigger self-examination, undermine the unstable, vague, contradictory identity, actively disorient the potentially disoriented (because affected by the general anomic situation) person, and initiate the process of mental disintegration, to begin with impairing the will. They are non-obviously traumatic, and are, therefore, usually disregarded.

These triggering events are also accidental. The majority of people with malformed identity (due to anomie) will meet with no accidents. Most of them, by definition, would be average and not considered the smartest kids either in the original or in a new environment; most would live their whole lives in environments with very similar norms; most would have no shocking heart-breaks in love; would not aspire or get appointed to especially responsible or prestigious positions, would not know great failure or success, etc. They would live their lives peacefully, carrying the virus of depression in themselves, but rarely if ever after the trying teenage years made aware of their vulnerability. The risk of contracting a major depression or mdi, in this respect, is similar to that of having a car accident. All of us who drive or ride in cars are vulnerable, but to most of us accidents will not happen. The increase in the numbers of cars implies the growing risk of having an accident. Similarly, increasing mobility, geographical and social, i.e., increasing availability of choice and the growing proportion of highly individualized, not average, biographies in the population would necessarily increase the probability of depression-triggering events. The only way not to be vulnerable to car accidents is to keep away from cars under all circumstances. The only way not to be vulnerable to depression (and all other forms of schizophrenia) is to have a clear, unshakable identity—the old principle of "know thyself." The development of such identity in modern, anomic society is a matter of education.

Discomforts of Conforming to the Unconformist Society: The Unquiet Mind of Kay Jamison

We are fortunate to have a recent description of a case of manic-depression at least as widely recognized as Sylvia Nasar's biography of John Nash, and though not as detailed, written by "one of the foremost authorities on manic-depressive illness"—the personal memoir of Kay Redfield Jamison, *An Unquiet Mind*. Subtitled "A Memoir of Moods and Madness," the 1995 book, a national bestseller, according to Oliver Sacks, a major authority on the subject himself, "stands alone in the literature of manic-depression for its bravery, brilliance and beauty." It has earned Dr. Jamison a MacArthur Fellowship—a most prestigious award, only slightly inferior to the Nobel Prize, brought praise for "the gutsy way she has made her disease her life's work," and was declared "invaluable . . . , at once medically knowledgeable,

deeply human, and beautifully written . . . always unashamedly honest."[85]
Thus, though, unlike full-blown schizophrenia, almost always acutely psychotic and/or in disagreement with the surrounding society ("bizarre") in
its elaborate delusions at the moment of diagnosis, manic-depressive illness, which mostly cycles between episodes of major depression, mild
mania (or hypomania) and absolute lucidity and is likely to be diagnosed at
the depressive and not thought-disordered phase, is rather often a subject
of autobiographical writing, it would be wrong not to focus on this particular memoir, written by a famous psychologist.

As in the earlier analysis of the case of John Nash, in my attempt to
explain causally the manic-depressive illness of Kay Jamison, I shall rely
entirely on the evidence the book provides and present it to the extent that
this is reasonable in regard to space in the author's words, not mine. Mine
here will be only the argument, and whenever Jamison's own commentary
on facts will be in agreement or disagreement with it, I shall refer to such
agreements and disagreements to prevent confusion as to the provenance
of the interpretation.

When Dr. Jamison wrote *An Unquiet Mind,* she was forty-nine years old
and had been suffering from manic-depressive illness "for more than thirty
years." The reason behind her decision to write it at this stage was that she
was "tired of hiding, tired of misspent and knotted energies, tired of the
hypocrisy, and tired of acting as though I have something to hide." This
decision was not an easy one. Beginning the project, Jamison "had many
concerns about writing a book that so explicitly describes my own attacks
of mania, depression, and psychosis, as well as my problems acknowledging the need for ongoing medication. Clinicians have been, for obvious
reasons of licensing and hospital privileges, reluctant to make their psychiatric problems known to others." "These concerns are often well warranted," she wrote in the *Prologue,* "I have no idea what the long-term
effects of discussing such issues so openly will be on my personal and professional life," but concluded: "whatever the consequences, they are bound
to be better than continuing to be silent."[86] The book, the reader infers,
therefore, was therapeutic, relieving some of Dr. Jamison's suffering, and
we can rejoice with her that her particular concerns were not at all justified, on the contrary. Yet we have here, certainly, a serious matter for concern: how many psychiatrists and clinical psychologists are mentally ill

themselves, specifically suffering from the "psychiatry's big three"? How many of them keep this hidden? How many are in treatment (whether openly or not) and refuse to take medication? According to Jamison, her choice of profession was motivated by a "personal, as well as professional, interest in the field" of clinical psychology, and, given the number of other clinicians with mental troubles who are mentioned, the book creates an impression that this is common.[87]

The Course of the Disease

Jamison's own trouble began when she was around seventeen years old. Her description of the onslaught is classic for mdi and at the same time, not surprisingly, bears a strong resemblance to the experiences of the schizophrenic prodrome. She writes:

> I was a senior in high school when I had my first attack of manic-depressive illness; once the siege began, I lost my mind rather rapidly. At first, everything seemed so easy. I raced about like a crazed weasel, bubbling with plans and enthusiasms, immersed in sports, and staying up all night, night after night, out with friends, reading everything that wasn't nailed down, filling manuscript books with poems and fragments of plays, and making expansive, completely unrealistic, plans for my future. The world was filled with pleasure and promise; I felt great. . . . I felt I could do anything, that no task was too difficult. My mind seemed clear, fabulously focused, and able to make intuitive mathematical leaps that had up to that point entirely eluded me. . . . they elude me still. At the time, however, not only did everything make perfect sense, but it all began to fit into a marvelous kind of cosmic relatedness. . . .
>
> I did, finally, slow down. In fact, I came to a grinding halt. Unlike the very severe manic episodes that came a few years later and escalated wildly and psychotically out of control, this first sustained wave of mild mania was a light, lovely tincture of true mania; like hundreds of subsequent periods of high enthusiasms it was short-lived and quickly burned itself out: tiresome to my friends, . . . exhausting and exhilarating to me . . . ; but not disturbingly over the top. Then the bottom began to fall out of my life and mind. My thinking . . . was tortuous. I would read the same passage over

and over again only to realize that I had no memory at all for what I just had read. Each book or poem I picked up was . . . [i]ncomprehensible. Nothing made sense. . . . It was very frightening.[88]

It is only in retrospect that Jamison would diagnose young Kay's experience of enjoyable ebullience in which everything appeared so wonderfully meaningful and connected as the polar opposite of the depression that replaced it and thus a phase of the manic-depressive illness. This "mild mania," "a light, lovely tincture of true mania," was, obviously, at worst hypomania and might not deserve to be regarded as a form of illness at all, were it not for the exaggerated sense of meaningfulness (the apophany so close to the state of delusion—which, of course, in itself is not a symptom of schizophrenia) so soon followed by the terrifying sense of meaninglessness. Indeed, it is depression that makes Kay ill and arouses her suspicions that something is terribly wrong with her, even though for years, even after she receives a PhD in clinical psychology, she would not be able to connect her own experiences with the diseases for which she treats her patients.[89] Her description of the experience of depression makes starkly evident the sense of badly impaired will, the loss of the acting self, while the thinking self observes this with its eye of the (outside) observer:

my mind has turned on me: it mocked me for my vapid enthusiasms; it laughed at all of my foolish plans; it no longer found anything interesting or enjoyable or worthwhile. It was incapable of concentrated thought and turned time and again to the subject of death: I was going to die, what difference did anything make? . . . I was totally exhausted and could scarcely pull myself out of bed in the mornings. . . . I wore the same clothes over and over again, as it was otherwise too much of an effort to make a decision about what to put on. . . . I dragged exhausted mind and body around a local cemetery, . . . sat on the graves writing long, dreary, morbid poems, convinced that my brain and body were rotting, that everyone knew and no one would say. Laced into the exhaustion were periods of frenetic and horrible restlessness; . . . For several weeks, I drank vodka in my orange juice before setting off for school in the mornings, and I thought obsessively about killing myself. . . . I knew something was dreadfully wrong, but I had no idea what. . . . It was impossible to avoid quite terrible wounds to both my mind and heart—the shock of having been so unable to understand what had been going on around me, the knowledge that my thoughts had been so completely out of my control, and the realization that I had been so depressed that I wanted only to die—and it was several months before the wounds could even begin to heal. . . . I aged rapidly during those months, as one must with such loss of one's self, with such proximity to death . . . [90]

Dr. Jamison is remarkably self-observant and sensitive in her descriptions of her own and others' experiences of manic-depressive illness. Her descriptions of her own experiences are undoubtedly honest and her descriptions of the others' symptoms are obviously accurate—they are descriptions of the classic, characteristic expressions of the disease. Thus throughout the book the reader is presented with the unwitting testimony of striking similarities between mdi and schizophrenia. Were *An Unquiet Mind* a memoir of schizophrenia, it would certainly contain descriptions of additional symptoms and experiences, which might well take the greater part of the book (this, among other things, is one reason why Nasar's biography of Nash is so much bigger than Kay Jamison's autobiographical essay), but all the symptoms and experiences that are the focus of this memoir of living with manic depression would be there as well. For example, when a freshman in college—the time which, for Kay, "was, for the most part, a terrible struggle, a recurring nightmare of violent and dreadful moods," when she "felt as though only dying would release [her] from the overwhelming sense of inadequacy"—she took an upper-division psychology course in personality theory, during which the participants were asked to write down their responses to Rorschach cards, which were then handed to the instructor. "He read aloud from a sort of random selection; midway through," writes Jamison, "I heard a recital of somewhat odd associations, and I realized to my great horror that they were mine. . . . a few of them were simply bizarre. . . . Most of the class was laughing, and I stared at my feet in mortification." Kay was convinced that, "being a psychologist, [the professor] could see straight into [her] psychotic underpinnings." She was lucky, however: instead, "he said that in all his years of teaching he had never encountered such 'imaginative' responses to the Rorschach." "It was my first lesson," Jamison says, "in appreciating the complicated, permeable boundaries between bizarre and original thought."[91]

According to the experimental psychologist Louis Sass, responses to Rorschach so strikingly imaginative as to impress observers as bizarre are almost exclusively characteristic of schizophrenics (whose imaginative freedom, indeed, is considered "pathological"). The episode described by Jamison occurred before the landmark 1972 study which established that the majority of people diagnosed with schizophrenia in the United States would be classed as manic-depressive in Britain, and, in fact, Jamison comments that "[at] that time, in clinical psychology and psychiatric residency programs, psychosis was far more linked to schizophrenia than manic-depressive illness."[92] What was the impressionable professor of personality theory thinking, when he caught sight of Kay's "original" responses and what was on her mind when she supposed that he was aware of her "psychotic underpinnings"? Did she suspect she was schizophrenic?

This similarity of experiences and symptoms in mdi and schizophrenia is especially clear in the description of Jamison's first major manic episode, which turned psychotic and, at last, led her to seek professional help. This happened in 1974, when, at the age of twenty-eight, she joined the UCLA Psychiatry Department as an Assistant Professor. It was after this psychotic episode that she was diagnosed as suffering from manic-depressive illness. The description is remarkably illuminating and calls for comment at numerous points. To begin with, Jamison does not shy away from calling her condition "madness":

> There is a particular kind of pain, elation, loneliness, and terror involved in this kind of madness. When you're high it's tremendous. The ideas and feelings are fast and frequent like shooting stars, and you follow them until you find better and brighter ones. Shyness goes, the right words and gestures are suddenly there, the power to captivate others a felt certainty. . . . Sensuality is pervasive and desire to seduce and be seduced irresistible. Feelings of ease, intensity, power, well-being, financial omnipotence, and euphoria pervade one's marrow. [In addition to resembling the apophany of the early stage of schizophrenia and common to it delusion of grandeur, this experience is reminiscent of the experience of being in love—which is by no means pathological. "Financial omnipotence," which is emphasized throughout the memoir as an essential ingredient suggests that the experience is characteristically Western—it is hard to imagine a member of a

traditional society, even if manic, believing oneself financially omnipotent.] But, somewhere, this changes. . . . ideas are far too fast, and there are far too many; overwhelming confusion replaces clarity. Memory goes. . . . Everything previously moving with the grain is now against—you are irritable, angry, frightened, uncontrollable, and enmeshed totally in the blackest caves of the mind. . . . madness carves its own reality.

It goes on and on, and finally there are only others' recollections of your behavior—your bizarre, frenetic, aimless behaviors—for mania has at least some grace in partially obliterating memories.[93]

Does the patient, if so, recollect the early pleasant experiences of the manic episode correctly? What if mania is like labor, causing the sufferer to forget the actual suffering and replacing it with memories appropriate to the event—joy of giving life in the case of labor, exaggerated high spirits in the case of mania?

In the aftermath, Jamison muses: "What then, after the medication, psychiatrist, despair, depression, and overdose? All those incredible feelings to sort through. . . . Then, too, are the bitter reminders—. . . . Credit cards revoked, bounced checks to cover, explanations due at work, apologies to make, intermittent memories (what did I do?), friendships gone or drained, a ruined marriage. And always, when will it happen again? Which of my feelings are real? Which of the me's is me? The wild, impulsive, chaotic, energetic, and crazy one? Or the shy, withdrawn, desperate, suicidal, doomed, and tired one? Probably, a bit of both, hopefully much that is neither."[94] This is not the loss of self, as in complete schizophrenia, but a certainly destabilizing confusion as to what this self is. Reality is what we experience. Good or bad, this is what there is. The mind—and the self—is a process, not a static system. When one experiences mania, the self is impulsive, chaotic, and crazy. When mania gives way to depression, the self is shy, withdrawn, desperate, suicidal, doomed, and tired. A manic-depressive self is always a sick self out of control; this is what there is. And, naturally, one does not want to be that self.

When Kay Jamison experienced this fateful episode that led to her diagnosis, she was "almost entirely free of serious mood swings for more than a year." She did not expect them to return. "Feeling normal for any extended period of time," she writes, "raises hopes that turn out, almost invariably, to be writ on water."[95] Now she was noticing something alien taking possession of her: "My mind was beginning to have to scramble a bit to keep up with itself, as ideas were coming so fast that they intersected one another at every conceivable angle." She explains this feeling of unregulated, out-of-control culture processing, the only way she imagines how, as a problem in the brain: "There was a neuronal pileup on the highways of my brain, and the more I tried to slow down my thinking the more I was aware that I couldn't." In the meantime, her mind—the customized version of culture processed in her brain to assure her adaptation—points her, that "I" that she constantly mentions, unconscious of it, to where the source of the problem lies. The language itself that she uses—the incessant repetition of first-person pronouns in regard to obviously heterogeneous referents, as in the above quotation—is trying to help her. Her enthusiasms were going into overdrive, she says, but there often was "some underlying thread of logic" in them that she did not at the time recognize, "some prescience and sense in those early days of incipient madness."

For example, she got

> into a frenzy of photocopying [and made numerous copies of a poem by] Edna St. Vincent Millay. . . . The Millay poem, "Renascence," was one I had read as a young girl, and, as my mood became more and more ecstatic, and my mind started racing ever and ever faster, I somehow remembered it with utter clarity and straightaway looked it up. Although I was just beginning my journey into madness, the poem described the entire cycle I was about to go through: it started with normal perceptions of the world (. . .) and then continued through ecstatic and visionary states to unremitting despair and, finally, reemergence into the normal world, but with heightened awareness. Millay was nineteen years old when she wrote the poem, and, although I did not know it at the time, she later survived several breakdowns and hospitalizations. Somehow, in the strange state I was in, I knew that the poem had meaning for me; I understood it totally.[96]

The chaos in manic Kay's mind is soon reflected in the chaos in her apartment—very much like in the case of John Nash.[97] Her behavior resembles his in numerous respects. Jamison writes:

I kept on with my life at a frightening pace. I worked ridiculously long hours and slept next to not at all. When I went home at night it was to a place of increasing chaos. Books, many of them newly purchased, were strewn everywhere. Clothes were piled up in mounds in every room, and there were unwrapped packages and unemptied shopping bags . . . There were hundreds of scraps of paper as well . . . , forming their own little mounds on the floor. One scrap contained an incoherent and rambling poem. . . . There were many such poems and fragments, and they were everywhere.

It is certain that were Kay, by definition—and at the core of her relationally-constituted self—not a "scientist," but a "poet," let's say, like Lowell, these poems would now be published in a collection and, who knows, perhaps discussed as models in creative writing classes. As it happened, her mania, for all its incessant activity, was totally unproductive, as it mostly is. Following the recognized phases of schizophrenic *Stimmung* (fragmentation, mere being of things, then their super-meaningfulness and back again), it rapidly spiraled out of control:

My awareness and experience of sounds in general and music in particular were intense. . . . I heard each note alone, all notes together, and then each and all with piercing beauty and clarity. I felt as though I were standing in the orchestra pit; soon, the intensity and sadness of classical music became unbearable to me. I became impatient with the pace, as well as overwhelmed with emotion. I switched abruptly to rock music. . . . Soon my rooms were further strewn with records, tapes, and album jackets. . . . The chaos in my mind began to mirror the chaos of my rooms; I could no longer process what I was hearing; I became confused, scared, and disoriented. . . .

Slowly the darkness began to weave its way into my mind, and before long I was hopelessly out of control. I could not follow the path of my own thoughts. Sentences flew around in my head and fragmented first into phrases and then words; finally, only sounds remained. One evening I stood in the middle of my living room and looked out at a blood-red sunset. . . . Suddenly I felt a strange sense of light at the back of my eyes and almost immediately saw a huge black centrifuge inside my head. I saw a tall figure in a floor-length evening gown approach the centrifuge with a vase-sized glass tube of blood in her hand. As the figure turned around I saw to my horror that it was me and that there was blood all over my dress, cape, and long white gloves. I watched as the figure carefully put the tube of blood into one of the holes in the rack of the centrifuge, closed the lid, and pushed a button on the front of the machine. The centrifuge began to whirl.

Then, horrifyingly, the image that previously had been inside my head now was completely outside of it. I was paralyzed by fright. The spinning of the centrifuge and the clanking of the glass tube against the metal became louder and louder, and then the machine splintered into a thousand pieces. Blood was everywhere. . . . I looked out toward the ocean and saw that the blood on the window had merged into the sunset; I couldn't tell where one ended and the other began. I screamed at the top of my lungs. . . . my thoughts . . . had turned into an awful phantasmagoria, an apt but terrifying vision of an entire life and mind out of control. I screamed again and again. Slowly the hallucination receded. I telephoned a colleague for help . . . [98]

I would like to draw your attention to the numerous cast of characters in this chilling passage. There is Kay's mind, which, to begin with, is Kay, but then becomes separate from her and escapes her control, so that she no longer can follow her own thoughts; then there is Kay—the being she refers to as "I"—the watcher, the observer, the one who keeps on processing the stimuli from inside and outside, who is paralyzed by fright and, in the end screams and calls for help. There is the figure in the long gown and white gloves, holding a tube of glass; this figure is observed by Kay and, to Kay's horror, turns out to be Kay, too, "me"—thus (a declension of) "I"; there is the obviously biological machine, which the figure who is fearfully watched by Kay and frighteningly turns to be Kay operates—against Kay's will, Kay has no will, the figure which is also Kay is out of Kay's control. When the figure with blood on her hands which, according to Kay's observations, begins its existence in Kay's head, steps outside, Kay no longer can tell the difference between inside and the outside; she becomes delusional. But her "thinking I" continues clear-eyed, keeping the record for Kay to tell her story over twenty years later.

The colleague Kay called—a man she was dating, while separated from her husband, obviously a psychiatrist with physician privileges—told her that he believed she was suffering from manic-depressive illness and had to see a (less personally involved) psychiatrist. Before she would schedule an appointment, he, "on a very short-term, emergency basis" prescribed her lithium, still a rather unfamiliar drug for use in cases of mania, as well as the true-and-tried-in-schizophrenia thorazine, and some barbiturates. Unquestionably, he succeeded in calming her down and ending the state of acute psychosis in which she was immediately previous to phoning him. Though in a dulled form, the psychotic episode, however, continued. After filling her first lithium prescription, she bought twelve snakebite kits—all the pharmacy where the purchase was made had in stock. She writes of the event:

> The pharmacist, having just filled my first prescription for lithium, had smiled knowingly as he rang up the sale for my snakebite kits and the other . . . bizarre purchases. . . . He, unlike me, however, appeared to be completely unaware of the life-threatening problem created by rattlesnakes in San Fernando Valley. God had chosen me, and apparently only me, to alert the world to the wild proliferation of killer snakes in the Promised Land. Or so I thought in my scattered delusional meanderings. . . . I was doing all I could do to protect myself and those I cared about. In the midst of my crazed scurrying up and down the aisles of the drugstore, I had also come up with a plan to alert the Los Angeles Times to the danger. I was, however, far too manic to tie my thoughts together into a coherent plan.[99]

Were it not for the latter disability, Kay's conduct would exactly parallel that of delusional but no longer acutely psychotic Matthews with his concern for the British interests, given the discovery he made of the French agents' assault on them—but, with her "thinking I" sharply focused on her mental process, and her mind, therefore, remaining individualized, she is unable to form an elaborate delusion.

This first time she was psychotically manic, writes Jamison, was "the most dreadful" she had ever felt in her entire life:

> Although I had been building up to it for weeks, and certainly knew something was seriously wrong, there was a definite point when I knew I was insane. My thoughts were so fast that I couldn't remember the beginning of

a sentence halfway through. Fragments of ideas, images, sentences, raced around and around in my mind like the tigers in a children's story. Finally, . . . they became meaningless melted pools. Nothing once familiar to me was familiar. . . . My energy level was untouched by anything. . . . Sex became too intense for pleasure, and during it I would feel my mind encased in black lines of light that were terrifying to me. My delusions centered on the slow painful deaths of all the green plants in the world— vine by vine, stem by stem, leaf by leaf they died, and I could do nothing to save them. Their screams were cacophonous. Increasingly, all my images were black and decaying.

At one point I was determined that if my mind—by which I made my living and whose stability I had assumed for so many years—did not stop racing and begin working normally again, I would kill myself. . . . I gave it twenty-four hours. But, of course, I had no notion of time, and a million other thoughts . . . wove in and raced by.[100]

An Unquiet Mind is a memoir, not a theory. It recounts an experience without attempting to provide an explanation for it. And yet, Dr. Jamison's explanation of Kay's madness is clearly and repeatedly stated. Manic-depression, she says again and again, "is an illness that is biological in its origins [even though it] feels psychological in the experience of it"; it is Kay's "exquisitely vulnerable genes" which are ultimately responsible for her descent "into florid madness": she is certain that "manic-depressive illness is hereditary." There is a credo-like intonation to her assertions: "I believe, without doubt, that manic-depressive illness is a medical illness."[101] But, as we already know from both the 1990 and 2007 editions of the authoritative manual for clinicians Jamison co-authored, there was by the time she wrote *An Unquiet Mind* (1995), and there is still not a shred of evidence to support these assertions. However, Jamison's reminiscences about her childhood and adolescence, which she treats as a stylistic back-drop to the centerpiece of the illness experience, and numerous side-remarks she makes almost unconsciously while telling this centerpiece story, provide excellent evidence for the causal explanation suggested here. The cause of Kay's madness was a malformed, conflicted identity—itself a result of the multiplicity of choices she was faced with and contradictory

messages she received from her privileged, open, anomic environment—
the split relationally-constituted self, whose most desired parts would not
be realized, contradicting the girl's ideal self-image, making her forever a
disappointment to herself, afraid to be found out by others, always insecure and at fault, trying to pass for Kay Redfield Jamison, a fraud.

The Background

Kay Jamison was born into the family of a career Air Force officer, a
Colonel, who "was first and foremost a scientist [a meteorologist] and only
secondarily a pilot." The Air Force was a subject of family discussion and
an object of loyalty and pride. When Kay would remind her father, teas-
ingly, that the Navy and the Army were both older than the Air Force, he
would respond on cue that the Air Force was "the future. Then he would
always add: And—we can fly." She writes on the second page of her introductory chapter:

> This statement of creed would occasionally be followed by an enthusiastic
> rendering of the Air Force song, fragments of which remain with me to this
> day, nested together, somewhat improbably, with phrases from Christmas
> carols, early poems, and bits and pieces of the Book of Common Prayer: all
> having great mood and meaning from childhood, and all still retaining the
> power to quicken the pulses.
>
> So I would listen and believe and, when I would hear the words "Off we
> go into the wild blue yonder," I would think that "wild" and "yonder" were
> among the most wonderful words I had ever heard; likewise, I would feel
> the total exhilaration of the phrase "Climbing high, into the sun" and know
> instinctively that I was a part of those who loved the vastness of the sky.[102]

She knew precisely where she belonged and was happy with her identity.

Despite frequent moves, characteristic of military families, Kay's parents, especially her mother, who believed this her responsibility, "kept life
as secure, warm, and constant as possible" for their three children, of
whom Kay was the youngest. Kay's mother, she writes, had "the type
of self-confidence that comes from having been brought up by parents

who not only loved her deeply and well, but who were themselves kind, fair, and generous people." Kay's maternal grandfather was, like her father, a scientist—a college professor of physics, her grandmother—a proper professor's wife. "By no means an intellectual, . . . she joined clubs instead. . . . both well liked and a natural organizer, she unfailingly was elected president of whatever group in which she became involved . . . a gentle but resolute woman, who wore flowered dresses, buffed her nails, set a perfect table, and smelled always of flowered soaps. She was incapable of being unkind, and she was a wonderful grandmother." Brought up by such parents, Kay's mother

> was a popular student in both high school and college. Pictures in her photograph albums show an obviously happy young woman, usually surrounded by friends, playing tennis, swimming, fencing, riding horses, caught-up in sorority activities, or looking slightly Gibson-girlish with a series of good-looking boyfriends. The photographs capture the extraordinary innocence of a different kind of time and world, but they were a time and a world in which my mother looked very comfortable.

These would have to be, to situate the reader historically, 1930s and early 1940s, with the country still in the Great Depression and the world hung over the abyss of the most colossal catastrophe in the history of Western civilization, which makes it quite remarkable that Jamison continues:

> There were no foreboding shadows, no pensive or melancholic faces. No questions of internal darkness or instability. Her [mother's] belief that a certain predictability was something that one ought to be able to count upon must have had its roots in the utter normality of the people and events captured in these pictures, as well as in the preceding generations of her ancestors who were reliable, stable, honorable, and saw things through. Centuries of such seeming steadiness in the genes could only very partially prepare my mother for all of the turmoil and difficulties that were to face her once she left her parents' home to begin a family of her own.[103]

The somewhat Lamarckian interpretation aside, this description shows clearly that one can live in the world and yet not be of it and that what is happening inside the self is often far more important than what is going on outside.

There were very clear rules and expectations that applied in the world of the military families, of which Kay's mother was explicitly made aware. She told her daughter, for instance, of the tea to which the wife of her husband's commanding officer invited her.

> [L]ike the women she had invited to tea, [she was] married to a pilot. Part of her role was to talk to the young wives about everything from matters of etiquette . . . to participation in community activities on the air base. After discussing these issues . . . , she turned to the real topic at hand. Pilots, she said, should never be angry or upset when they fly. Being angry could lead to a lapse in judgment or concentration: flying accidents might happen; pilots could be killed. Pilots' wives, therefore, should never have any kind of argument with their husbands before the men leave to go flying. Composure and self-restraint were not only desirable characteristics in a woman, they were essential.

Both Kay and her mother appreciated what being a part of this environment offered them and believed that it was worth some gratitude. Kay wrote:

> There was a wonderful sense of security living within this walled-off military world. Expectations were clear and excuses were few; it was a society that genuinely believed in fair play, honor, physical courage, and a willingness to die for one's country. True, it demanded a certain blind loyalty as a condition of membership, but it tolerated, because it had to, many intense and quixotic young men who were willing to take staggering risks with their lives. And it tolerated, because it had to, an even less socially disciplined group of scientists, . . . most of whom loved the skies almost as much as the pilots did. It was a society built around a tension between romance and discipline: a complicated world of excitement, stultification, fast life, and sudden death, and it afforded a window back in time to what nineteenth-century living, at its best, and at its worst, must have been: civilized, gracious, elitist, and singularly intolerant of personal weakness. A willingness to sacrifice one's own desires was a given; self-control and restraint were assumed.

Limited imagination is a blessing; it prevents one from seeing what one does not want to see. The problem was that the privileged, closed, secure world of the Air Force scientists did not limit the imagination of its denizens enough. It was, after all, a privileged, closed, and secure world in a prosperous, widely open, and unstable United States of America, which was abundant with choices and incessantly suggested to everyone that the choice one has made might not have been the very best choice available. This society bred the expectation, regarded as a god-given right, to have one's cake and eat it too. And so this is how Kay's mother told the story of the commanding officer's wife's advice to her daughter:

> As my mother put it later, it was bad enough having to worry yourself sick every time your husband went up in an airplane: now, she was being told, she was also supposed to feel responsible if his plane crashed. Anger and discontent, lest they kill, were to be kept to oneself.[104]

As a result, despite "centuries of steadiness in the genes," Kay's mother did not see things through. Her husband changed his jobs, became depressed, the going got tough, and she divorced him. She had her own self to take care of, after all, and her own life to live.

In the halcyon days before all this was to happen, however, it was Kay's choices that were uppermost on her parents' minds. Several were available and the parents kept them wide open. Since the military "clearly put a premium [i.e. gave prestige and approbation to] on well-behaved, genteel, and even-tempered women," the obvious choice was to become such a woman—a military wife, like her mother. Another was to become, like her father and grandfather, a scientist. This was a more prestigious option, and, at twelve, Kay had settled on that. Because of the hospital at Andrews Air Force Base, medicine was eminently available as the science on which a twelve-year-old could try her hands. Her parents, Jamison writes, "fully encouraged" her interest:

> they bought me dissecting tools, a microscope, and a copy of Gray's Anatomy; . . . its presence gave me a sense of what I imagined real Medicine to be. The Ping-Pong table in our basement was my laboratory, and I spent endless late afternoons dissecting frogs, fish, worms, and turtles; only when

I moved up the evolutionary ladder in my choice of subjects and was given a fetal pig—whose tiny snout and perfect little whiskers finally did me in—was I repelled from the world of dissection.[105]

Thank goodness for the little pig: what we see before us is a child contentedly depriving creatures (some of them evidently sentient) of life because she believes that this is what proper medical scientists do. Her interest in medicine is not a product of a natural sympathy for the suffering or of a keen intellectual desire to understand a particular problem; it is a self-imposed interest in a particular, highly prized, identity.

It is clear that this identity soon eclipsed the other choice for Kay—becoming a military wife; she learned to think about that option as limiting and undignified. She tells us:

So I was almost totally content: I had great friends, a full and active life of swimming, riding, softball, parties, boyfriends, summers on the Chesapeake, and all of the other beginnings of life. But there was, in the midst of all of this, a gradual awakening to the reality of what it meant to be an intense, somewhat mercurial girl in an extremely traditional and military world. Independence, temperament, and girlhood met very uneasily in the strange land of cotillion. Navy Cotillion was where officers' children were supposed to learn the fine points of manners, dancing, white gloves, and other unrealities of life. It also was where children were supposed to learn, as if the preceding fourteen or fifteen years hadn't already made it painfully clear, that generals outrank colonels who, in turn, outrank majors and captains and lieutenants, and everyone, but everyone, outranks children. Within the ranks of children, boys always outrank girls.

One way of grinding this particularly irritating pecking order into the young girls was to teach them the old and ridiculous art of curtsying. It is hard to imagine that anyone in her right mind would find curtsying an even vaguely tolerable thing to do. But having been given the benefits of a liberal education by a father [NB: not by a mother] with strongly nonconforming views and behaviors, it was beyond belief to me that I would seriously be expected to do this. I saw the line of crisply crinolined girls in front of me and watched each of them curtsying neatly. Sheep, I thought, Sheep. Then it was my turn. Something inside of me came to a complete boil. . . . it was one too many times watching girls willingly go along with the rites of submission. I refused. . . . within the world of military custom and protocol—where symbols and obedience were everything, and where a child's misbehavior could jeopardize a father's chance of promotion—it was a declaration of war. . . . Miss Courtnay, our dancing teacher, glared. I refused again. She was, she said, very sure that Colonel Jamison would be terribly upset by this. I was, I said, very sure that Colonel Jamison couldn't care less. I was wrong. As it turns out, Colonel Jamison did care. However ridiculous he thought it was to teach girls to curtsy . . . , he cared very much more that I had been rude to someone. I apologized, and then he and I worked on a compromise curtsy, one that involved the slightest possible bending of knees . . . [106]

What is to be particularly noted in this torrential passage is the centrality of social status in the young girl's experience of the world, her "painful" awareness that generals outrank colonels: at fourteen she is shot through, mentally electrocuted, as it were, by envy, inspired by the expectation of equality and the right to not ever be outranked by anyone. She has made up her mind to be a medical scientist, and as such, far superior to military wives who would willingly submit to the humiliation of a curtsy. But her parents, including her strongly nonconforming father, keep all her choices open for her. They have not made up their minds as to what she should become and do not deprecate the image of a "well-behaved, genteel, and even-tempered woman." They are offended by Kay's behavior. The expectations of her privileged environment are not entirely clear. She learns that she has been a disappointment to her parents. Her choices are already too many.

A determined girl, she sticks to the one she made at twelve. The interest in scientific medicine, we read, for some years plays a very important role in the development of Kay's sense of self.

Doctors at the hospital at Andrews Air Force Base, where I volunteered as a candy striper, or nurse's aide, on weekends, . . . took me and my interests very seriously. They never tried to discourage me from becoming a doctor, even though it was an era that breathed, If woman, be a nurse. They took me on rounds with them and let me observe and even assist at minor surgical procedures. I carefully watched them . . . held instruments, peered into wounds, and, on one occasion, actually removed stitches from a patient's abdominal incision.

I would . . . bring books and questions with me: What was it like to be a medical student? To deliver babies? To be around death? I must have been particularly convincing about my interest on the latter point because one of the doctors allowed me to attend part of an autopsy. . . . I stood at the side of the steel autopsy table, trying hard not to look at the dead child's small, naked body, but being incapable of not doing so. . . . Eventually, in order to keep from seeing what I was seeing, I reverted back to a more cerebral, curious self, asking question after question, following each answer with yet another question. . . . Initially it was a way of avoiding the awfulness of what was going on in front of me; after a while, however, curiosity became a compelling force in its own right. I focused on the questions and stopped seeing the body. As has been true a thousand times since, my curiosity and temperament had taken me to places I was not really able to handle emotionally, but the same curiosity, and the scientific side of my mind, generated enough distance and structure to allow me to manage, deflect, reflect, and move on.[107]

So here we have the teenager Kay, the future doctor, almost completely inured from sympathy for others, determinedly self-centered, a long way to constructing herself, contentedly and even proudly, as a scientist, a person of superior intelligence. And then her life drastically changes.

When Kay was fifteen, Colonel Jamison retired from the Air Force and became a scientist with the Rand Corporation. The family left the walled-in world in Washington, DC, in which it was so easy for Kay to feel superior and to rebel, and moved to the far more open, fiercely competitive playing fields of California's self-made people. It was 1961—the good old days— but, Jamison writes: "everything in my world began to fall apart." For a starter, she understood that the environment of traditional military families that she taught herself to despise was, without the slightest effort on the part of her new peers—children of "the industry," i.e., the film business, rich people, corporate attorneys, businessmen, or highly successful physicians—despised by them as well. This confirmation of her natural instinct did not sit well with her; she realized that she was different, and not different in a superior way:

For a long time I felt totally adrift. I missed Washington terribly. I had left behind a boyfriend, without whom I was desperately unhappy; he was blond, blue-eyed, funny, loved to dance, and we were seldom apart during the months before I left Washington. . . . I also had left behind a life that had been filled with good friends, family closeness, great quantities of warmth and laughter, traditions I knew and loved [?], and a city that was home. More important, I had left behind a conservative military lifestyle that I had known for as long as I could remember. I had gone to nursery school, kindergarten, and most of the elementary school on Air Force or Army bases; my junior and senior high schools in Maryland, while not actually on bases, were attended primarily by children from military, federal government, or diplomatic families. It was a small, warm, unthreatening, and cloistered world. California, or at least Pacific Palisades, seemed to me to be rather cold and flashy. I lost my moorings almost entirely, and despite ostensibly adjusting rapidly to a new school and acquiring new friends . . . I was deeply unhappy. . . . I was furious with my father for having taken a job in California instead of staying in Washington. . . . In Washington, I had been a school leader and captain of all my teams; there had been next to no serious academic competition, and school work had been dull, rote, and effortless. Palisades High School was something else entirely . . . it took a very long time to reestablish myself as an athlete. More disturbing, the level of academic competition was fierce. I was behind in every subject that I was taking, and it took forever to catch up; in fact, I don't think I ever did. On the one hand, it was exhilarating to be around so many smart and competitive students; on the other hand, it was new, humiliating, and very discouraging. It was not easy to have to acknowledge my very real limitations in background and ability.

Later, Jamison will explain her mental trouble, her feeling of dis-ease, of illness, of losing oneself, of not knowing who she was and where she fit in the world, by her "exquisitely vulnerable genes"—because, as we know, it is established wisdom since Kraepelin, that manic-depression is a biological problem. She needs this explanation psychologically: it is her elaborate delusion that she shares with so many sufferers, and elaborate delusions are therapeutic, they are a powerful coping mechanism provided by the sick mind. But, intellectually, this explanation is not needed; it is, in fact, altogether redundant. The explanation of Kay's misfortune is emerging in front of our very eyes from her biography: its root is in her privileged, prosperous background, in the choices for self-creation that it offers, in the absence of responsibilities and limits—of objectively-existing difficulties. She has too much: too much freedom, above all. Her life is made too good—that's why it turns so bad.

Pay attention, she does not appreciate her father's freedom of choice, wants his options closed, is angry with him for making the choice that interferes with her idea of who she is. Yet, California does not pressure girls into curtsying: it is a rebel country quite willing to accommodate someone mercurial who prides herself on her own independence. Everything is open in California: "Everyone seemed to have at least one, sometimes two or even three, stepparents, depending on the number of household divorces. My friends' financial resources were of astonishing proportions." And they were not even blond and good-looking in the Air Force sort of way. Writes Jamison:

> I also learned for the first time what a WASP was, that I was one, and that this was, on a good day, a mixed blessing. As best I could make out, having never heard the term until I arrived in California, being a WASP meant being mossbacked, lockjawed, rigid, humorless, cold, charmless, insipid, less than penetratingly bright, but otherwise—and inexplicably—to be envied. It was then, and remains, a very strange concept to me. In an immediate way all of this contributed to a certain social fragmentation within the school. One cluster, who went to the beach by day and partied by night, tended toward WASPdom; the other, slightly more casual and jaded, tended towards intellectual pursuits. I ended up drifting in and out of both worlds, for the most part comfortable in each. . . . The WASP world provided a tenuous but important link with my past; the intellectual world, however, became the sustaining part of my existence and a strong foundation for my academic future.[108]

Sustained, however, Kay was not: however comfortable she felt in this split new world of hers, in which she also says one page above, she was deeply unhappy, she did not belong, and while believing that a strong foundation was built for her, decided upon at twelve, academic future, she was primed for the future of a life-long manic-depressive illness. The only way for her to stop its onslaught that had already begun at that point was to take account of her mental experience: to understand what was the meaning of WASPdom, and of its new marginality, in her identity; what was she pressuring herself to do, why did she want to mold herself into a scientist; what were her interests, actually; what was *in* her interest—but, of course, she could not do so, and nobody could do this for her. And so it went from bad to worse, and worse, and worse, without ever swerving from the hell-bent course on which too much misunderstood freedom so often does set a life.

As we already know, within a year of moving, Kay would already struggle with her manic-depression. She was not alone. Her two closest friends, "both males—attractive, sardonic, and intense—were a bit inclined to the darker side as well, and," she writes:

> we became an occasionally troubled trio, although we managed to navigate the more normal and fun-loving side of high school as well. Indeed, all of us were in various school leadership positions and very active in sports and other extracurricular activities. While living at school in these lighter lands, we wove our outside lives together in close friendship, laughter, deadly seriousness, drinking, smoking, . . . engaging in passionate discussions about where our lives were going, the hows and whys of death, . . . and vigorously debating the melancholic and existential readings—Hesse, Byron, Melville, and Hardy—we had set for ourselves. We all came by our black chaos honestly: two of us, we were to discover later, had manic-depressive illness in our immediate families; the other's mother had shot herself through the heart. We experienced together the beginnings of the pain that we each would know, later, alone. In my case, later proved rather sooner than I might have wished.[109]

Such social experiences are, obviously, not genetic. Kay's father, in the meantime, unrecognized by his new scientific environment for what Jamison calls "ingenious but disturbingly idiosyncratic [reasoning which] had absolutely nothing to do with the meteorology research that he was being paid to conduct," medicated his black depressions with alcohol; this was not genetic either. But facts do not speak on their own; their tongues must be loosened before they are able to communicate to us their message. Thus one goes on believing in whatever one wishes to believe.

At eighteen, Kay had "reluctantly" started college at UCLA. "It was not where I wanted to go," she writes:

> For years I had kept in the back of my jewelry box a red-enamel-and-gold University of Chicago pin that my father had given me; . . . I wanted to earn my right to wear it. I also wanted to go to the University of Chicago because it had a reputation for tolerating, not to say encouraging, non-conformity, and because both my father and my mother's father, a physicist, had gone there for graduate school. This was financially impossible. My father's erratic behavior had cost him his job at Rand, so, unlike most of my friends—who went off to Harvard, Stanford, or Yale—I applied to the University of California.[110]

College was already "a terrible struggle," for her, "a recurring nightmare," since, by that time, she had become ill, and oscillated between black depressions and manias, during which she would throw herself, as so many do in their attempt to escape from their private hell, into all sorts of political and social causes ("everything from campus antiwar activities to slightly more idiosyncratic zealotries, such as protesting cosmetic firms that killed turtles in order to manufacture and sell beauty products"), over-spending money (which people who have no money never do, no matter how they feel), and enrolling in seven instead of five classes, which she then did not attend or barely passed. At the age of twenty, life offered her some reprieve: she took a year off to study at the University of St. Andrews in Scotland. Jamisons, apparently, were of Scottish ancestry, and Kay's brother and cousin, who—quite possibly for this reason—studied in Britain at the time, suggested that she join them: this was another option for her, and an unproblematic one, to define who she was. It worked to perfection, not because she felt Scottish and reconnected to her ethnic "roots," but because in this pleasantly but actually foreign environment she was defined—and fully accepted—as an American, which gave her time to rest from her incessant and self-destructive self-making. Scotland was not the place where her life was, she did not belong there, definitely—she did not have to fit in in any way, did not have to compete for an appropriate spot under its charitable Northern sun. For once, she could focus out of herself. "St. Andrews," she writes,

> provided a gentle forgetfulness over the preceding painful years of my life. . . . For one who during her undergraduate years was trying to escape an inexplicable weariness and despair, St. Andrews was an amulet against all manner of longing and loss, a year of gravely held but joyous remembrances. Throughout and beyond a long North Sea winter, it was the Indian summer of my life.[111]

She does not account for the obviously and totally non-biological way this cultural context lulled her "vulnerable genes" to sleep.

And then it was home back again. There, Kay realized that she did not have it in her to become a medical scientist. She could not do it. She was not what she believed she was. "It had become clear to me over time that my mercurial temperament and physical restlessness," she wrote, "were going to make medical school—especially the first two years, which required sitting still in lecture halls for hours at a time—an unlikely proposition." In any case, she thought that she learned best on her own. She loved research and writing, but "the thought of being chained to the kind of schedule that medical school required was increasingly repugnant" to her. Luckily, at St. Andrews she discovered William James's *Varieties of Religious Experience* and was now fascinated by psychology. She began working for an attractive, moody professor of psychology, who liked her very much, and this helped her to "make up [her] mind to study for a PhD in psychology."

While she was in graduate school, "almost everyone" Kay "knew was seeing a psychiatrist." Kay, however, had other choices. "It quickly came down to a choice," for her, she writes, "between seeing a psychiatrist or buying a horse." Because Kay was not like "almost everyone" in California: she came from a WASP military family, in which ladies rode horses; it was not at all unreasonable to suppose that being what she was, at one point at least, supposed to be might solve her problems. Unfortunately, she did not love the animal and did not actually like riding. She had to acknowledge, she says, "that I was a graduate student, not Dr. Dolittle; more to the point, I was neither a Mellon nor a Rockefeller. I sold my horse, as one passes along the queen of spades, and started showing up for my classes at UCLA."

Graduate school proved less trying than college:

> It was a continuation, in some respects, of the Indian summer I enjoyed in St. Andrews. Looking back over those years with the cool clinical perspective acquired much later, I realize that I was experiencing what is so coldly and prosaically known as a remission—common in the early years of manic-depressive illness and a deceptive respite from the savagely recurrent course that the untreated illness ultimately takes—but I assumed I was just back to my normal self.[112]

She adds, incongruently for either a PhD student in psychology, specializing in moods, or for an eminent psychologist that she had become since: "In those days [early 1970s] there were no words or disease names or concepts that could give meaning to the awful swings in mood that I had known."

She got married, participated in Vietnam War protests, was "painfully intense, rail thin, and, when not moribund, filled to the brim with a desire for an exciting life, a high-voltage academic career, and a pack of children." She had a rather clear ideal image of herself, in other words: a person of a superior social status, famous intellectual, and an accomplished woman in more traditional respects, somewhat like her mother and grandmother. It is remarkable that these dreams were completely self-centered: there was no intellectual problem that particularly piqued Kay's curiosity, nothing and nobody in the vast and densely populated world outside of her that genuinely interested, impassioned, or provoked her sympathy. She had started off studying experimental psychology, "especially the more physiological and mathematical sides of the field"—this corresponded closely to her not-entirely-given-up idea that she was a medical scientist after all; but midway switched to clinical psychology. "Most of my real education," Jamison writes, "came from the wide variety and large number of patients that I evaluated and treated during my predoctoral clinical internships." (One wonders how many are the clinicians such as her—severely mentally ill themselves, by the nature of their disease acutely and exclusively self-centered and, as a result, lacking sympathy—lacking the ability for sympathy—for the outside world and patients whom they treat.) Her own ordeal was only reaching its first high point:

> The rites of passage in the academic world are arcane and, in their own way, highly romantic, and the tensions and unpleasantries of dissertations and final oral examinations are quickly forgotten in the wonderful moments of sherry afterward, admission into a very old club, parties of celebration, doctoral gowns, academic rituals, and hearing for the first time "Dr.," rather than "Miss," Jamison. I was hired as an assistant professor in the UCLA Department of Psychiatry, got good parking for the first time in my life, joined the faculty club posthaste, and began to work my way up the academic food chain. I had a glorious . . . summer, and, within three months of becoming a professor, I was ravingly psychotic.[113]

The coincidence of the psychotic onslaught with something that outwardly looks as an achievement and self-realization is very common, because it is the realization of the wrong, undesired, and extremely insecure self. After so much and such painful striving, Kay Jamison became something she did not want to become; she was not what she had believed she was; she was a failure. The very paraphernalia of her new status, which she stresses—the "Dr.," and the gown, and becoming a member of an old club—that should be soothing and self-gratifying, are a proof of that: she is neither a medical scientist, nor a lady-equestrian, nor a mother of children, and because she is interested only in status and not in any specific problem in psychiatry, being appointed an assistant professor at the Department of Psychiatry at UCLA (the wrong university to start with) is not meaningful to her. Her mind had let her down completely: it cannot provide her existence with meaning.

As we follow Kay Jamison in her experience of manic-depressive illness, confusion and deep dissatisfaction with identity emerges as the central theme in it, although, clearly, Jamison is not fully conscious (not self-conscious) of that and wishes to stress other aspects—in particular, her struggle with medication. Her feelings are those of "embarrassment" and "fear," "I was confused and frightened and terribly shattered in all of my notions of myself," she writes, "my self-confidence, which had permeated every aspect of my life for as long as I could remember, had taken a very long and disquieting holiday." Her therapy begins and for the first time this clinician imagines what it is to be a mental illness patient.

> I realized that I was on the receiving end of a very thorough psychiatric history and examination; the questions were familiar, I had asked them of others a hundred times, but I found it unnerving to have to answer them, unnerving not to know where it all was going, and unnerving to realize how confusing it was to be a patient.

Kay Jamison was becoming capable of sympathy. Were this pressed on her, shifting her mental focus from her own ailing self onto the phenomena of the outer world, this could be the beginning of the cure. As it happened, she was given another choice of identity, and, in her exhaustion, has accepted it. Her psychiatrist, she writes,

> made it unambivalently clear that he thought I had manic-depressive illness and I was going to need to be on lithium, probably indefinitely. The thought was very frightening to me . . . but all the same I was relieved: relieved to hear a diagnosis that I knew in my mind of minds to be true. . . . I was bitterly resentful, but somehow greatly relieved.[114]

She knew now who she was—a plaything of a grand biological influencing machine, of "exquisitely vulnerable genes" (which, as a side effect, also made for creativity, touching the ones it chose with fire), a victim, no longer responsible before anyone on earth, including herself, for what she made of herself, no longer responsible for herself—what a relief. Now she can rest. She will be in therapy forever.

She had also decided that this is who she always was: a mad woman. Lithium, in this sense, endangered her identity. "Why did it take having to go through more episodes of mania, followed by long suicidal depressions, before I would take lithium in a medically sensible way?" she asks herself, and answers:

> In my case, I had a horrible sense of loss for who I have been and where I have been. It was difficult to give up the high flights of mind and mood, even though the depressions that inevitably followed nearly cost me my life.

My family and friends expected that I would welcome being "normal," be appreciative of lithium, and take in stride having normal energy and sleep. But if you have had stars at your feet and the rings of planets through your hands, are used to sleeping only four or five hours a night and now sleep eight, are used to staying up all night for days and weeks in a row and now cannot, it is a very real adjustment to blend into a three-piece-suit schedule, which, while comfortable to many, is new, restrictive, seemingly less productive, and maddeningly less intoxicating. People say, when I complain of being less lively, less energetic, less high-spirited, "Well, now you're just like the rest of us," meaning, among other things, to be reassuring. But I compare myself with my former self, not with others. Not only that, I tend to compare my current self with the best I have been . . . when I have been mildly manic. When I am my present "normal" self, I am far removed from when I have been my liveliest, most productive, most intense, most outgoing and effervescent. In short, for myself, I am a hard act to follow.[115]

But there is nothing to regret in Dr. Jamison's manias: her manic self, as she herself stresses, was only "seemingly" more productive. Nothing of any value remains from Kay's manic episodes, nothing that has done anything good or in any way contributed to anyone or anything in the world. Yet, it is only such contributions to the world that can make life meaningful, and life that is not meaningful is misery.

She incessantly reverts back to shreds of her lost identities. It is, for example, extremely important to her that people with whom she associates look right—that they have the recognizable external characteristics of WASP military families. The very first thing she says about her psychiatrist, a central person in her life, is that he was "tall, good-looking." Her trust in him undoubtedly rests on these particular good looks. Her memory of their first meeting is centered on them: "I have next to no memory of what I said during that first session, but I know it was rambling, unstrung, and confused. He sat there, listening forever, it seemed, his long six-foot-four-inch frame spread out from chair to floor, legs tangling and untangling, long hands touching, fingertip to fingertip." Looks are also what she concentrates on in talking of her brother—her chief protector and probably the central presence in her life. A PhD in economics from Harvard (the family is extremely intelligent and academically successful—this must be stressed) he is the first one to arrive to help her sort out the practical mess left by her terrible manic episode. She is tremendously lucky to have such a caring, responsible brother and is fully aware of her luck, writing:

> He is . . . a fair and practical man, generous, and one who, because of his own confidence, tends to inspire confidence in others. . . . During the time of my parents' separation, and subsequent divorce, he had put his wing out and around me, protecting me to the extent that he could from life's hurts and my own turbulent moods. His wing has been reliably available ever since . . . whenever I have needed a respite from pain or uncertainty, or just to get away, I have found an airplane ticket in the mail, with a note suggesting I join him someplace like Boston or New York, or Colorado, or San Francisco. Often, he will be in one of these places to give a talk, consult, or take a few days off from work himself; I catch up with him in some hotel lobby or another, or in a posh restaurant, delighted to see him—tall, handsome, well dressed—walking quickly across the room.[116]

And if he were short, or not well dressed, or the restaurant were not posh— she would not be delighted to see him?

She is also very concerned with self-presentation. Some of her problems with lithium are caused by this concern. She writes:

> I have been violently ill more places than I choose to remember, and quite embarrassingly so in public places ranging from lecture halls and restaurants to the National Gallery in London. . . . When I got particularly toxic I would start trembling, become ataxic and walk into walls, and my speech would become slurred; this resulted not only in several trips to the emergency room . . . , but much more mortifying, make me appear as though I were on illicit drugs or had had far too much to drink.[117]

She creates for herself a set of rules for self-presentation, while on medication:

> *Rules for the Gracious Acceptance of Lithium into your Life*
> Clear out the medicine cabinet before guests arrive for dinner or new lovers stay the night.

Remember to put the lithium back into the cabinet the next day.

Don't be too embarrassed by your lack of coordination or your inability to do well the sports you once did with ease.

Learn to laugh about spilling coffee, having the palsied signature of an eighty-year-old, and being unable to put on cuff links in less than ten minutes . . .

And so on. She is also trying cerebrally, laboriously to teach herself sympathy through comparison: "Be patient when waiting for this leveling off. Very patient. Reread the Book of Job. Continue very patient. Contemplate the similarity between the phrases 'being patient' and 'being a patient.'"[118]

Her stress is on the self as others see it, as it shows. She is particularly hurt by not *looking* as attractive a personality as she believes she is. "I had become addicted to my high moods," she writes, "I had become dependent on their intensity, euphoria, assuredness, and their infectious ability to induce high moods and enthusiasms in other people. . . . I found my milder manic states powerfully inebriating and very conducive to productivity. I couldn't give them up." But there is also something else entirely in her regret: "More fundamentally, I genuinely believed—courtesy of strong-willed parents, my own stubbornness, and a WASP military upbringing—that I ought to be able to handle whatever difficulties came my way without having to rely upon crutches such as medication." Her problem is not that she has lost her former, mildly manic, exciting, productive self, but that she cannot lose the self that was supposed and failed to emerge. She is chained to that failed self. At the core of her disease lies self-loathing; the essence of her depressive experience, it is self-loathing that drives these depressions suicidal. Unlike full-fledged schizophrenics, she cannot separate from her self (none of her selves!), she remains, relentlessly, self-centered. And she does not want to be that worthless self, she feels it does not deserve to live. She describes her emotions after a suicide attempt:

Both my manias and depressions had violent sides to them. Violence, especially if you are a woman, is not something spoken about with ease. . . . The aftermath of such violence, like the aftermath of a suicide attempt, is deeply bruising to all concerned. And, as with a suicide attempt, living with the knowledge that one has been violent forces a difficult reconciliation of totally divergent notions of oneself. After my suicide attempt, I had to reconcile my image of myself as a young girl who had been filled with enthusiasm, high hopes, great expectations, enormous energy, and dreams and love of life, with that of a dreary, crabbed, pained woman who desperately wished only for death and took a lethal dose of lithium in order to accomplish it. After each of my violent psychotic episodes, I had to try and reconcile my notion of myself as a reasonably quiet-spoken and highly disciplined person, one at least generally sensitive to the moods and feelings of others, with an enraged, utterly insane, and abusive woman who lost access to all control of reason.

What pains her most is that:

These discrepancies between what one is, what one is brought up to believe is the right way of behaving toward others, and what actually happens during these awful black manias, or mixed states, are absolute and disturbing beyond description—particularly, I think, for a woman brought up in a highly conservative and traditional world. They seem a very long way from my mother's grace and gentleness, and farther still from the quiet seasons of cotillions, taffetas and silks . . .

For the most important and shaping years of my life I had been brought up in a straitlaced world, taught to be thoughtful of others, circumspect, and restrained in my actions. We went as a family to church every Sunday, and all of my answers to adults ended with a 'ma'am' or 'sir.' The independence encouraged by my parents had been of an intellectual, not socially disruptive, nature. Then, suddenly, I was unpredictably and uncontrollably irrational and destructive. This was not something that could be overcome by protocol or etiquette. God, conspicuously, was nowhere to be found. Navy Cotillion, candy-striping, and *Tiffany's Table Manners for Teenagers* could not, nor were they ever intended to be, any preparation or match for madness. Uncontrollable anger and violence are dreadfully, irreconcilably, far from a civilized and predictable world.[119]

But a match for madness is precisely what Navy Cotillion and *Tiffany's Table Manners* were, only Kay Jamison, like so many others in our free and prosperous society, was given the choice, in fact encouraged, to disregard and despise them. Curtsying was not more humiliating, or oppressive of girls, than any social ritual that symbolizes belonging to a group—i.e., recognizing one's self as a part, above all, a part, of something larger, more important and more enduring than oneself. But the availability of the option to make oneself into a person of superior, more admired, status—a medical scientist, let us say, rather than a military wife—can easily make it appear humiliating. Generals should outrank colonels, because they are generals—this is good for all of us—and everyone, but everyone should outrank children. That the awareness that this is so is painful for so many of us is a tragedy of our society. Equality is not a God-given right; when experienced as such, it is a curse: one has to earn the right to be equal to those who have earned it earlier. It is not that a girl from a military family should not have the choice to become a medical scientist, of course: she should have such a choice, but for the right reason—because she has a genuine interest in medical science, and not in order to be a medical scientist; what we, as a society, should prevent, is giving our children the choice to be self-centered.

An Unquiet Mind is a very frightening book, far more frightening than Kay Jamison imagines. It is, obviously, written during a lucid period, and very clearly when she is not depressed. There is a saving grace to bipolarity: one is not always depressed. A clinician, Dr. Jamison also uses her writing ably as self-therapy, what with the influencing machine delusion and the belief that manic-depressive illness is genetically connected to creativity, but, in the end, she knows that these are delusions and, though, from time to time soothing, do not cure her deep malady. Despondently, she returns to the trouble with her identity:

> These fiery moods . . . had made me impatient with life as it was and made me restless for more. But, always, there was a lingering discomfort when the impatience or ardor or restlessness tipped over into too much anger. It did not seem consistent with being the kind of gentle, well-bred woman I had been brought up to admire and, indeed, continue to admire.[120]

My analysis of *An Unquiet Mind* may seem, at places, harsh. But I want to stress that it implies no moral judgment, just a diagnosis of a terrible, indeed terrible, affliction. With its strident emphasis on equality of result, our open, limitless society, which offers us more and more choices for self-definition, forces very many of us to focus exclusively on the self, deprives us of interest in the world outside, destroys our natural ability for sympathy, and thus makes millions desperately ill. For the sake of the sufferers such as Kay Jamison we should turn our attention just a bit away from the undoubted biological reality of this illness and onto the culture that causes it.

III

HISTORICAL

5

The Cradle of Madness

The sixteenth century in England was a time of colossal transformations. The graves of feudal lords slain on the one side and the other in the War of the Roses contained not only these mortal remains: a whole world lay buried in them. Rigor mortis, paradoxically, was a central characteristic of that, now dead, world in its life: for it was the world of the society of orders—a stony social structure, as imposing as that of a fortified castle towering over the countryside, with its thick walls, deep dungeons, and narrow windows letting in just enough light to enable its in-dwellers to follow their assigned ways. It was built on the secure foundation of the unchanging word of God, once and for all revealed in the Holy Scriptures, which everyone was obliged to obey, but few were allowed to know, and even fewer to interpret. No part of this rigid world would change position vis-à-vis the others, nothing moved, and everyone was kept to one's place: it was as stable as a human world can be—not, perhaps, as stable as a castle, but eminently stable in comparison to the world that came to replace it. Now it was dead, and the stability was gone.

The birth of the new world that came into being with the new dynasty and the new aristocracy, which stepped into the void left by the slain lords who fought to such bitter ends for the rights of Lancasters and Yorks, could only be compared to a volcanic eruption of Earth's early days. This world itself was to prove a volcano. Constantly but unpredictably active, it would forever swallow aging formations and disgorge new ones and swallow them again, it would never rest still. In its bowels steely characters were tempered and softer mettle melted, and its brightly burning fires illumined humanity as it never had been illumined before. In their glow it appeared beauteous. This new world was named "modern," and the light which would guide souls in it was no longer Holy Scripture, but the new, radically humanistic perspective which history dubbed "nationalism."

The Cradle

The cardinal feature of nationalism—which necessarily follows from the principle of popular sovereignty and underlies every other aspect of the national reality, including the fundamental egalitarianism of the national membership—is its secularism. Popular sovereignty, which is the essence of the idea of the nation as elite, makes God defunct; with God defunct, man becomes the ruler of the universe. There emerged a completely new understanding of man (according to the first English Renaissance, Sir Thomas Elyot's, *Dictionary*—a sexless and ageless concept, "a liuing creature with the capacitie of reason, subject to death: a manne, a woman, a chylde"[1]) as an agent, a self-governing and dignified state, the individual responsible for and capable of shaping one's own destiny. Human life acquired a new—and supreme—value: the death of children untouched by sin was no longer a cause for celebration as augmenting the population of angels, but now represented death at its most senseless. In general, death was stripped of the sacred significance—which made it almost attractive— bestowed on it by Christianity: man was no longer dust and worm, and death was not the return of the soul to its Maker on High, the portals to the better and eternal life, but the end, incomprehensible and unacceptable, of the only existence this extraordinary double being, a body and a spirit at once, could have. The change in the meaning of life and death changed the nature of the existential experience—what moved men and women, what made them suffer or content, the essence of suffering and contentment, human desires and fears, the general character of their emotions and ways of thinking—all this was new.

This radical transformation was felt in England already in the early sixteenth century. The "modernization" of English (the addition of countless neologisms, reconceptualization of existing words, and invention of new morphological constructions)—under way by its third decade, at the latest, reflected the fact. There existed no language to describe and express the new existential experience before: coming to grips with the new life, therefore, involved creating it. What we know as modern English—one, and not the earliest one, of modern vernaculars—is, in fact, the lingua franca of modernity. It encoded the new view of reality, enabling everyone who spoke it to experience life in the new way. Henceforth translation from English changed the nature of experience in communities of other languages as well. Modern reality thus arrived in the rest of the world as translation from English.

This process of the "modernization" of English language, thinking, and experience was complete by 1600, certainly by 1610, when the King James Version of the English Bible was published. From that point on speakers (and writers) of English communicate with us directly, we share the same understanding, live in the same world, our fundamental values (by which I, obviously, do not mean political ideologies, but rather conceptions of man-in-universe and the meaning of human life) are the same. This is so even in regard to those late sixteenth- and seventeenth-century thinkers who must still be considered religious. The "Holy Mr. Herbert," that unusual in the period "godly and painful [painstaking] divine," included in the *Temple,* his collection of devotional poetry, the poem "Man," which was addressed to God, and read:

> My God, I heard this day
> That none doth build a stately habitation,
> But he that means to dwell therein.
> What house more stately hath there been,
> Or can be, than is man? To whose creation
> 　All things are in decay.

"Man," he continued, was "every thing and more," "all symmetry, full of proportion," for him ("for us," Herbert said) the winds blew, fountains flowed, the earth and heaven themselves and "all things" existed, rendering service to his (our) mind or "flesh." Herbert concluded:

> Oh, mighty love! Man is one world, and hath
> 　Another to attend him.

Since then, my God, thou hast
So brave a palace built, O dwell in it,
That it may dwell with thee at last!
Till then, afford us so much wit,
That, as the world serves us, we may serve thee,
    And both thy servants be.[2]

These last lines sound very much as a reminder, even an admonition to the Almighty, urging him to honor his responsibilities toward the magnificent house He built to inhabit—man (and become, as it were, at last, a responsible house owner).

Donne's *Holy Sonnets* express similarly mixed feelings: an immense pride in being human and a deep frustration with human mortality:

I am a little world made cunningly
Of elements, and an angelic sprite;
But black sin hath betrayed to endless night
My world's both parts, and O, both parts must die.

Something is amiss, in fact illogical and unacceptable, with Providential plan:

Thou hast made me, and shall thy work decay?
Repair me now, for now mine end doth haste;
I run to death, and death meets me as fast,
And all my pleasures are like yesterday . . . [3]

Shakespeare, a generation ahead of Donne and Herbert, no longer questions God, but not because he still accepts His will. In fact God is altogether absent from the work of this greatest modern poet. His sonnets are not "Holy." The world constructed in them is impersonal, it is ruled by Time, something akin to the eighteenth century idea of Nature, our idea of natural forces. Preoccupied as he is obsessively with the duality, temporality, and "sad mortality" of human existence, he nevertheless insists that immortality, physical and spiritual, is possible and within human powers. This view of immortality is dramatically different from the Christian idea

of the immortality of the soul; it is our view: physically, one lives on in
one's children, spiritually in the creations of one's mind. Thus immortality—
such as there is—becomes every person's own responsibility. One should
take care not to "consume [oneself] in single life," "to be Death's conquest
and make worms [one's] heir." But, if one has children: ". . . what could
Death do if thou shoudst depart / Leaving thee living in posterity?" A very
great poet can do more: stop time itself, giving eternal life both to oneself
and objects of one's love. Supreme confidence in human *authorship*, supreme
self-confidence, sounds throughout the sonnets:

> But thy eternal summer shall not fade,
> Nor lose possession of that fair thou owest;
> Nor shall Death brag thou wander'st in his shade,
> When in eternal lines to time thou growest;
> So long as men can breathe, or eyes can see,
> So long lives this, and this gives life to thee (Sonnet 18);
>
> Yet, do thy worst, old Time: despite thy wrong,
> My love shall in my verse ever live young (Sonnet 19).

And more and more.[4]

Shakespeare is a genius; this—even more than religious faith in the
cases of Donne and Herbert—makes him an exception. The keenness of
his imagination is responsible for the play of light and shadow in his least
ambivalent panegyrics to humanity. He realized that to be human in a
godless world (as in a world with an imperfect God) was a tragedy, and
remembered this, even as he marveled at man's powers and gloried in his
dignity. In early modern England, however, the sense of tragedy was limited to men of genius and troubled believers, while the celebration of man's
virtues was a general phenomenon. Minds less profound, whose divine
spark—every man's property and distinguishing characteristic—was but a
firecracker to Shakespeare's lustrous flame, and whose hearts, as a result,
were lighter, rejoiced innocently in their human selves. Never again, in
fact, the mere fact of being human was sung with such unclouded cheerfulness. A very popular broadside ballad, set to music by William Byrd in
1588, offers an example of this universal self-satisfaction:

My mind to me a kingdom is;
Such present joys therein I find
That is excels all other bliss
That earth affords or grows by kind.

No princely pomp, no wealthy store,
No force to win the victory,
No wily wit to salve a sore,
No shape to feed a loving eye;
To none of these I yield as thrall.
For why? My mind doth serve for all.[5]

The word "mind," which does not appear in the last medieval English-Latin dictionary *Promptorium Parvulorum* of 1499, became a near synonym of the "soul" and was used almost as frequently. Shakespeare's concordance, for instance, lists over two pages of "mind" against two-and-a-half pages of "soul." Elyot's *Dictionary*, the first to define the word "nation," among others, translated as "the sowle" the Latin *anima*, but commented on *animus* (rendered as "the mynde, the wyl,") that "sometime it is put for the soule," explaining in regard to *mens, tis,* that it represented "the byghest and chiefe parte of the mynde." The two words were only near synonyms, because the mind clearly belonged to, and originated with, man, while the "soul," figuring prominently in the religious services, did not allow one to lose sight of its connection to God. Still, the near equation of the two terms could not fail to secularize the concept of the soul, just as it could not help but further elevate the idea of man.

This exhilarating realization of one's humanity—as much a function of the new, secular vision of nationalism as was national identity itself—must have represented a central element in the early modern Englishmen's self-understanding, reinforcing the sense of being English. Nationality implied the new concept of the human being as an autonomous agent, an author and creator in one's own right, a meaningful, beautiful, complex world unto oneself—a godlike, dignified image and an identity in which one justifiably could take pride. Above this uplifting foundation of humanity and Englishness, an individual's identity was left for the individual to construct. The social structure—to the extent it existed in the world in which nothing stood still—now resembled nothing less than a stone castle (indeed a rollercoaster would be a better simile) and no longer could restrain—or direct—one's movements, leaving its human components free to wander from place to place. Both the secularism and egalitarianism of the new, nationalist, image of reality that served as its cultural foundation empowered men (and, to a lesser extent, women) to choose their social positions. Neither God's will nor one's birth limited these choices. Thus, travelers before, moving inexorably to the eternal Beyond, mortal men had acquired the status of permanent residents, even citizenship, on earth, and became travelers in society. They set their own destinations in life and more often than not traveled alone, leaving behind families of their origins, pulling out roots without regret. The system of social stratification, the chief mechanism of social traffic control, was opened, no impenetrable dividers existed between any of its sectors, there was none, in principle, that could not be reached from any of the others; one was in charge of one's own itinerary. Social maps existed, but they were numerous, ambivalent, and lent themselves easily to various interpretations. As one's social position could be legitimately changed, it did not teach with whom one belonged, what one's expectations from life were, and how far the sphere of one's activity extended, or, rather, its lessons could be forgotten or kept, depending on one's wishes. The individual became master of his (sometimes her) own life and was free to create oneself. It was impossible to lose one's humanity and Englishness (therefore fundamental equality to all other Englishmen): this double dignity of nationality was one's to keep. This meant one could only move up: add to this dignity, become equal to the best. The possibilities were breathtaking. Indeed, the word that sixteenth-century Englishmen selected for thinking about them—to aspire—alluded to the sensation.

The verb itself, in this sense of "upward desire," was used already in the late fifteenth century, although the *OED* finds only one instance of such an early use, John Fortescue's proposition that man's "Courage is so Noble that Naturally he aspireth to hye things and to be exaltyd." All the derivatives of "aspire," however—"aspiration," "aspiring," and "aspirer"—were products of the sixteenth, mostly late sixteenth century, "aspiration" being first used by Shakespeare.[6] The experience, it was discovered, was a pleasant one, and Elyot, in his *Dictionary* added to its physically uplifting quality a morally elevating and even specifically intellectual dimension (consistent with his definition of man as, first and foremost, a rational being), translating *aspiro* as, among other senses, "to gyue all my studye and wytte to optayne a thynge."

On the whole, aspiring, whether as a disposition, an act, or an experience, retained its original dignified connotations; when Bacon in *The Advancement of Learning* characterized humanity as "aspiring to be like God in Power," he certainly was not commenting on man's inexcusable hubris. Several other words were similarly reconceptualized, their semantic field broadened with new forms, to reflect the newly realized possibilities and scope of human creativity and, in particular, the individual's ability to make oneself. The verb "to achieve" acquired a new meaning of gaining dignity (status)—or a symbol of dignity—by effort, as in Shakespeare's: "Some are born great, some atchieue greatnesse." From this were derived "achievement" (as in "great Achieuements done By English"), "achiever," and "achievance" (as in "noble actes and atchieuances,").[7] Like the neologisms "betterance" and (the noun) "bettering," referring to improvement by human action, the latter was not much used after the early seventeenth century, but "achievement" and "achiever," like the verb "to better," in the sense of "bettering oneself" or being "bettered" by someone, were permanent additions to the vocabulary. So was "success," originally a neutral term meaning any outcome of an attempt and reconceptualized as equivalent to only "good success," and its derivatives, "successful" and "successfully."

It should be stressed that the new vocabulary emerged together with the new experience. It was created in order to capture it, and thus reflected and constructed it at the same time. This means that people did not aspire before, did not achieve anything, did not better themselves, and did not succeed. I am not saying that they created different "discursive artifacts," finding themselves in the same situations, living through the same emotions, but representing them differently, calling them different names. No. A vast new area was annexed to meaningful (i.e., human) life, a new existential dimension, and modern English both mirrored and was an instrument of its formation. What we are witnessing in tracing these concepts to their sixteenth-century beginnings is the emergence of entirely new semantic space—new areas of meaning and experience—semantic space that is central to our lives today.

It is because this space itself was new that the position of ambition—its core concept—was equivocal. "Ambition" was an old word, derived from Latin and used, however rarely, in the Middle Ages, for an eager desire, among other things, specifically of honor, and for ostentation and pomp. It was a negative term. In the middle of the fifteenth century, for instance, it was as a matter of course included among "Vicis [such] as pride, ambicioun, vein glorie." When Elyot translated *ambitio* in his Latin-English *Dictionary*, he ascribed to it this familiar meaning: "inordynate desyre of honour or auctoritie." But in the sixteenth-century ambition was everywhere and it became difficult to consider it "inordinate." The opinion was revised. The word would often carry its connotations of self-aggrandizement and sin—as it still often does. In 1593, in *Christ's Tears over Jerusalem*, Thomas Nashe defined it as "any puft up greedy humour of honour or preferment," the fallen Cardinal Wolsey in Shakespeare's *Henry VIII* of 1613 advised Cromwell: "I charge thee, fling away Ambition, By that sin fell the Angels." As often, however, it would be neutral, becoming a synonym for desire, a strong wish. Bacon argued that there were ambitions of all kinds: ambition could be "of the meaner sort" or altogether "foul," to quote Shakespeare in *Henry VI, I* and *II*—the desire for status for its own sake, the ambition of social "climbers" (yet another one of the sixteenth-century concepts), was such. In distinction, "the Ambition to prevail in great Things" was as great as the particular "thing" in which one wished to prevail. Far from being a sin, it could be "divine," it was the virtue of a soldier and could be a virtue in other pursuits. It became necessary to introduce the word with a qualifier, as "success" was introduced in "bad" versus "good" success prior to the sixteenth century, and it was the qualifier that determined one's attitude to the emotion.[8]

Whether it was a sin or a virtue, base or noble, as an emotion ambition was intense, and this intensity was its essential quality. It is in connection with ambition that the word "passion" began to acquire its current meaning of intense, overpowering emotion, a sovereign, authentic movement of the soul or the mind. This change reflected the growing recognition of the sovereignty of the mind as the constitutive element of the self, thus the sovereignty of the self—vis-à-vis God, in the first place, but also vis-à-vis society—which was the cardinal implication of the new English view of reality and defined the new English experience. Ambition was one of the two central examples of such sovereignty. It came from within oneself; it was an inner drive. The identification of ambition as a passion, however (and it could not be otherwise), arose from the earlier, widespread at the time, meaning of "passion"—suffering in the sense of being a passive and powerless object of an action of some external power. For ambition would brook no restraint not only from the outside; an overpowering emotion, it overpowered the self from whence it came. If one had it, one could not resist it.

The passion of ambition—a super-emotion, so to speak—gave a direction (thus sense of order, thus meaning) to life to which society refused to give direction and was a source of myriad other emotions: excitement, hope, sense of inspiration. A realized ambition brought one feelings of gratification, self-satisfaction, confidence, pride, intense joy. But, alas, even in England of the sixteenth century, which equated "success" with "good success," not all among the thousands of competing ambitions were realized, and frustrated ambition, as well as failure that followed in the wake of success, gave rise to passion in yet another earlier sense of the word, that of pain. Ambition was the main cause of the characteristic suffering of the age. We catch a glimpse of the depths of despair into which one could be plunged from the anonymous lyrics of a song by John Dowland (the composer "whose heavenly touch upon the lute" Shakespeare compares to "the deep conceit passing all conceit" of his favorite poet, Spencer), even when they are unaccompanied by the mournful melody.[9]

> Flow, my tears, fall from your springs!
> Exiled for ever, let me mourn;
> Where night's black bird her sad infamy sings,
> There let me live forlorn.
> Down vain lights, shine you no more!
> No nights are dark enough for those
> That in despair their lost fortunes deplore.
> Light doth but shame disclose.
> Never may my woes be relieved,
> Since pity is fled;
> And tears and sighs and groans my weary days
> Of all joys have deprived.

From the highest spire of contentment
My fortune is thrown;
And fear and grief and pain for my deserts
Are my hopes, since hope is gone.
Hark! you shadows that in darkness dwell,
Learn to contemn light
Happy, happy they that in hell
Feel not the world's despite.[10]

That these were lyrics of a song means that they were better known than any poem that existed only in print. That they were put to music testifies to the certainty that the sentiment they expressed would find widespread sympathy among the audience. Ambition was the inner compass one used in the ceaseless social travels in search of one's own identity. From within it drove one to aspire and achieve, always aspire for and achieve the same thing: an individual identity with even more dignity than was implied in one's national identity and humanity. One did not rest until one found one's proper social place—the place; often one would never rest. And burning in hell was better than losing the place one had gained. With it one lost oneself.

The defense against threats—or experience—of a thwarted ambition was love.

When in disgrace with fortune and men's eyes,
I all alone beweep my outcast state,
And trouble deaf Heaven with my bootless cries,
And look upon myself, and curse my fate,
Wishing me like to one more rich in hope,
Featur'd like him, like him with friends possess'd,
Desiring this man's art, and that man's scope,
With what I most enjoy contented least;
Yet in these thoughts myself almost despising,
Haply I think on thee,—and then my state
(Like to the lark at break of day arising
From sullen earth) sings hymns at heaven's gate;
For thy sweet love remember'd such wealth brings,
That then I scorn to change my state with kings.[11]

I must pause here and make a special announcement, so counterintuitive and shocking is what one is about to read: Ladies and gentlemen, love too was invented in sixteenth- century England. Yes, there was the story of Abelard and Eloise. This means that the capacity for what we call "love" existed. So did the capacity for aspiration and ambition, for any mental experience characteristic of a particular culture—be it reading, writing, enjoying the taste of a particular delicacy, such as fried tarantulas or pork rinds, aspiring, or falling in love—can be experienced only on condition that the capacity for such experience exists within human nature itself. But the existence of a capacity, while it can explain exceptional cases of deviance (such as was the unique and, therefore, tragic story of Abelard and Eloise), cannot account for a virtual universalization in a particular period and society of what was earlier a deviant experience.[12]

"Love," like "ambition," was an old word which, unlike "ambition," was commonly used before the sixteenth century. Its general meaning was similar to that of the original concept of eros in Hesiod—an ecstatic, self-transcendent, desire (for which, ironically, sixteenth- century English substituted "ambition" in its neutral sense). It is because of this general meaning that "love" could be used to express both the lofty sentiment of Christian love and even the divine love of God itself (*agape, caritas, eros* as used in Christian theology) and the base because carnal, essentially sinful, sexual lust. The sixteenth century English concept of love—which is our concept—was dramatically different. While it implied the very opposite attitude to sex from the one that characterized Christian thinking, it retained clear sexual connotations (which grew in importance in the next several hundred years and in some of "love"'s peregrinations in translation). Thus the connection of love to lust seems obvious. But the other older usages were completely eclipsed, becoming so foreign to us that learned dissertations are required to convince our contemporaries that they ever existed.[13]

The new, as it came to be known later "romantic," love was the other central expression of the sovereignty of the self—the ultimate passion, in fact, in the sense of its authentic and free expression, the supreme movement of the sovereign human spirit. As such, it, no less than ambition, reflected the new, national, image of reality and was a creation of nationalism. Shakespeare who, more than any other single individual, was responsible for encoding this new view of reality in the English language, making it the integral part of language itself (and therefore enabling anyone who spoke it to share in the new experience), according to the *OED*, was the first to define love as a passion. He did so in 1588 in *Titus Andronicus.* Spencer followed suit in 1590 in *Fairie Queene;* and then, two years later, Shakespeare did this again in *Romeo and Juliet*—the paradigmatic story of love as it has been understood in the modern age, in which he, in effect, constructed its ideal type.[14]

There are 131 instances of the word "passion" in Shakespeare, used mostly in its original sense of "suffering." But it is certain that *Romeo and Juliet,* in which it appears only three times, all in the modern sense and specifically in connection to love, presented the one interpretation which Shakespeare's contemporaries awaited and which became the foundation of the modern view of human nature. The dedication in the first folio edition of the great poet's work in 1623, "TO THE MEMORIE of the deceased Author Maister W. Shakespeare," singles out *Romeo and Juliet* as the example of passion:

> . . . This Booke,
> When Brasse and Marble fade, shall make thee looke
> Fresh to all Ages . . .
> . . . eu'ry Line, each Verse
> Here shall reuiue, redeeme thee from thy Herse.
> ·
> Nor shall I e're beleeue, or thinke thee dead
> (Though mist) until our bankrout Stage be sped
> (Impossible) with some new straine t'out-do
> Passions of Iuliet, and her Romeo; . . .

In the world of constant change true love was unchanging, once-in-a-lifetime passion. "Love is not love," said Shakespeare (admitting to the multiplicity of interpretations the word allowed),

> Which alters when it alteration finds,
> Or bends with the remover to remove:
> O no; it is an ever-fixed mark,
> That looks on tempests, and is never shaken;

· ·

Love alters not with [Time's] brief hours and weeks,
But bears it out even to the edge of doom.[15]

But, not being fickle, it was uncontrollable, free from extraneous compulsion and oblivious of social norms. Because love was the ultimate passion, that is the most authentic expression of man's very essence in fact, the social arrangements that contradicted it became, by definition, inauthentic—false, wrong, morally abhorrent.

Like ambition, love made it possible for the free and therefore rootless modern individual, whom the society around would not define, to find one's proper place and to define oneself. To use the vulgar tongue of social science, it was an identity-forming device. This, above all else, explains the tremendous importance of this emotional complex in our lives. Moreover, in distinction to ambition, which led the searcher by a circuitous way, made an obstacle course by the myriads of simultaneous, crisscrossing and overlapping searches of others, which demanded unceasing effort on one's part, and never guaranteed the result, love required no effort whatsoever ("God join'd my heart to Romeo's," says Juliet)—it happened to one, one fell into it. Thus it led to the discovery of one's true identity directly, filling life with meaning and at once reconciling one to all of it, even the inevitability of death. The supreme and truest expression of the sovereign self, it was, in effect, a miracle, for which one was in no way responsible. What made it an expression of the self nevertheless was the immediate recognition of the true love's object, the One, that particular her or him who was one's destiny and yet, paradoxically, was most freely chosen. One's identity, one's true self, was found in that other person and what he or she saw in one. (In fact, one had to give oneself up, lose oneself in another, in order to find oneself and realize what that self was.)

This is the central theme of *Romeo and Juliet*.[16] The lovers, though "star-crossed," fall in love at first sight and immediately recognize both the finality of their choice, despite the fact that social conventions and the identities they were assigned by social conventions forbid them to love each other, and its profound difference from any other attachment. "Did my heart love till now?" asks Romeo on encountering Juliet, "forswear it, sight!" and then, learning that she is a Capulet, exclaims: "O dear account! My life is my foe's debt." (The proof, however, that what he feels for Juliet is, indeed, love—and not "loving hate," "heavy lightness," "bright smoke," and "cold fire," all those other meanings of "love" applicable to his pining for Rosaline—is that Juliet returns his feelings; true love is reciprocal.) Juliet's reaction to their first meeting is similar. A dutiful daughter, just hours ago ready to marry, sight unseen, the man proposed to her by her parents, she tells the nurse: "Go, ask his name: if he be married, / My grave is like to be my wedding-bed." When the nurse informs her, she muses: "My only love sprung from my only hate! . . . / Prodigious birth of love it is to me, / That I must love a loathed enemy." There is a sense of a higher duty in the idea of love: true love's call must be answered no matter what one's other obligations—or the consequences—are.

The dialogue in Act two, Scene one, makes the rejection of all identities derived from life before love explicit.

> O Romeo, Romeo! wherefore art thou Romeo?
> Deny thy father and refuse thy name;
> Or, if thou wilt not, be but sworn my love,
> And I'll no longer be a Capulet. . . .
> 'Tis but thy name that is my enemy;
> Thou art thyself though, not a Montague.
> What's Montague? It is nor hand, nor foot,
> Nor arm, nor face, nor any other part
> Belonging to a man. O, be some other name!
> What's in a name? that which we call a rose,
> By any other name would smell as sweet;
> So Romeo would, were he not Romeo call'd,
> Retain that dear perfection which he owes
> Without that title;—Romeo, doff thy name;
> And for that name, which is no part of thee,
> Take all myself.

Juliet, speaking unaware that Romeo listens to her, expresses a wish where Christ commands those seeking eternal life to follow him, abandoning their mothers, fathers, children, and earthly possessions; but, inspired by love, her wish is a command, and, just like Jesus, she gives all of herself in exchange. "I take thee at thy word," responds Romeo,

Call me but love, and I'll be new baptiz'd;
Henceforth I never will be Romeo.

He relinquishes his old identity, finds his authentic self, his soul, in fact: "it is my soul that calls upon my name," he says in Scene two, when Juliet bids him to return as he is about to leave her garden. Finding his soul, Romeo changes his religion: he'll be new baptized. (So does Juliet, telling Romeo: "thy gracious self . . . is the god of my idolatry.") When she asks, alarmed, who is it overhearing her confession of love for him, he answers:

> . . . By a name
> I know not how to tell thee who I am:
> My name, dear saint, is hateful to myself,
> Because it is an enemy to thee;
> Had I it written, I would tear the word.

Juliet herself denies her mother and her father, all her kin, because from the moment of being touched by love she belongs with Romeo only. Her reaction to the news of Tybalt's death and Romeo's banishment attests to this self-transforming change of allegiance:

> My husband lives, that Tybalt would have slain;
> And Tybalt's dead, that would have slain my husband:
> All this is comfort; wherefore weep I, then?
> Some word there was, worser than Tybalt's death,
> That murder'd me: I would forget it fain;
> But, O, it presses to my memory
> Like damned guilty deeds to sinners' minds:
> Tybalt is dead, and Romeo is banished.
> That banished, that one word banished,
> Hath slain ten thousands Tybalts. Tybalt's death
> Was woe enough, if it had ended there:
> Or, if sour woe delights in fellowship,
> And needly, will be rank'd with other griefs,—
> Why follow'd not, when she said Tybalt's dead,
> Thy father or thy mother, nay, or both . . . ?

For his part, falling in love with Juliet, Romeo finds—or, rather, recovers—his authentic and sovereign self, the self-created self that he owes to no one but himself. Mercutio, meeting Romeo on the morrow of his garden dialogue with Juliet, exclaims: "now art thou Romeo; now art thou what thou art, by art as well as by nature." Both lovers also find through love their "home": similarly to the *patria* of the ancients—the dwelling place of the ancestral spirits—their home is wherever the loved one is. Banishment is worse for Romeo than death, he would not see mercy in the duke's commutation of the death sentence into exile: to him "exile hath more terror in his look . . . There is no world without Verona walls, [B]ut purgatory, torture, hell itself. . . . Heaven is here [W]here Juliet lives . . ." He would kill himself and is stopped only by Friar Lawrence's remark: "And slay thy lady, too, that lives in thee . . . ?"

Love saturates life with meaning to such an extent that life without love becomes absolutely meaningless and not worth living. Life with love, on the other hand, is worth any and all the grief it can bring otherwise. (This thought, again, is repeated in the sonnets, Sonnet 66, perhaps, offering the most poignant expression of the redemption of modern life through love:

> Tir'd with all these, for restful death I cry,—
> As, to behold desert a beggar born,
> And needy nothing trimmed in jollity,
> And purest faith unhappily forsworn,
> And gilded honour shamefully misplac'd,
> And maiden virtue rudely strumpeted,
> And right perfection wrongfully disgrac'd,
> And strength by limping sway disabled,
> And art made tongue-tied by authority,
> And folly (doctor-like) controlling skill,
> And simple truth miscall'd simplicity,
> And captive good attending captain ill;
> > Tir'd with all these, from these would I be gone,
> > Save that, to die, I leave my love alone.)

By the same token love makes death acceptable and, as an end to meaningless life from which love has been taken, meaningful too: death is also redeemed by the life in which there is love. Suddenly everything makes perfect sense again, just as it was in a universe ruled by God, and harmony is restored to the discordant world centered on Man. *Romeo and Juliet,* despite its tragic ending in the deaths of both young lovers just days after their union, despite the deaths of friends and relatives (Mercutio, Tybalt, Paris, Lady Montague), the grief and sorrow, caused by their desire to be together, and the general havoc it wreaks in the social structure—despite the well-remembered fact that "never was a story of more woe / Than this of Juliet and her Romeo"—despite all this, *Romeo and Juliet* is a triumphant affirmation of the new human world and its self-sufficiency. In a sense quite different from presenting the ideal type of love, it is the ideal love story and a story of ideal love. Given Shakespeare's unique ability to make reality out of vague intimations of the collective imagination his words captured, the tragedy has been received not as a cautionary tale, but as an irrefutable proof that love that justified death was what life was essentially about, and for five centuries it has formed the substance of our innermost dreams, the hope to find it—"the star to every wandering bark" indeed—sustaining us all through all our tossing on the seas of modern experience, kept restless by the unceasing volcanic activity underneath.[17]

The love between Romeo and Juliet was sexual love between a man and a woman. Defining sexual love between a man and a woman as the ideal type of love and as the exemplary passion purified sexual love, forever clearing it from the association with sin. But the association of true (or "romantic") love with sex, which the contemporary American interprets as natural and naturally suggesting sexual attraction as the source and foundation of love, was quite accidental for the culture which created the concept. The 154 Shakespeare sonnets are emphatic on the point that love is a marriage of minds, not of bodies. In fact, the great love poet had very little to say of sex that was good, his disapproval of that natural activity being at least equal to that of the preachers of abstinence in the days of yore. Even in their writings on the subject it would be hard to find anything comparable in the explicitness of condemnation and revulsion to the following lines:

Th'expense of spirit in a waste of shame
Is lust in action; and till action, lust

Is perjur'd, murderous, bloody, full of blame,
Savage, extreme, rude, cruel, not to trust;
Employ'd no sooner, but despised straight;
Past reason hunted; and no sooner had,
Past reason hated, as a swallow'd bait,
On purpose laid to make the taker mad:
Mad in pursuit, and in possession so;
Had, having, and in quest to have, extreme;
A bliss in proof,—and prov'd a very woe;
Before, a joy propos'd; behind, a dream:
    All this the world well knows; yet none knows well
    To shun the heaven that leads men to this hell.[18]

The unrivalled importance of love in the modern life cannot be explained by the fact that it delivered sex in a new package (adding to its legitimacy when sanctioned by marriage also the legitimacy by association with the ultimate expression of the authentic self). No, love suffused with meaning the life that was rendered meaningless by the withdrawal of God and the bewildering openness of the social structure in which one did not know where to turn to simply know what one was and how one was supposed to live. It was more akin to the exemplary male friendships of antiquity (those of the Dioscuri Castor and Pollux or of Orestes and Pylades), which allowed one person to find his *alter ego* in the other, than to any sexually driven relationship or emotion.

Though the ideal type of love was that between a man and a woman, love was, obviously, possible between persons of the same sex: most of Shakespeare's sonnets are dedicated to a male love. (One should pause before taking this as a proof of a homosexual attraction, as Americans tend automatically to do, if only because this is such a distinctive national tendency: rather than see sex where it does not exist, a Russian, for instance, is likely not to see it where it is evidently present. Generally, one should beware equating erotic desire with sexual attraction lest one reduces the spiritual being that is man to the level of reptiles, fish, and insects, since by now we have learned that mammals and even some birds are certainly capable of deep attachments that are not materially motivated.) The love of which Mrs. Katherine Philips wrote in the middle of the seventeenth century was a friendship between women, which clearly had nothing sexual about it: it was a union of souls, joined together, like those of Romeo and Juliet, by higher forces:

> But neither chance nor compliment
> Did element our love:
> 'Twas sacred sympathy was lent
> Us from the choir above . . .

Like Romeo's and Juliet's, the souls of the two female friends dwell in each other's breast:

> Our changed and mingled souls are grown
> To such acquaintance now,
> That if each would resume their own,
> Alas! We know not how . . .
> We have each other so engrossed
> That each is in the union lost. . . .

The two beings become one and the identity of each receives its affirmation in the other:

> Inspired with a flame divine,
> I scorn to court a stay;
> For from that noble soul of thine
> I ne'er can be away.
> But I shall weep when thou dost grieve;
> Nor can I die whilst though dost live. . . .
> All honor, sure, I must pretend,
> All that is good or great:
> She that would be Rosania's friend
> Must be at least complete . . .

Finally, repeating yet another central theme in *Romeo and Juliet*, through love, the two women are reconciled to death:

Thus our twin souls in one shall grow,
And teach the world new love,
Redeem the age and sex, and show
A flame fate dares not move:
And courting death to be our friend,
Our lives, together too, shall end.[19]

Mrs. Philips was quite representative of her historical time and place (which includes sex, among other things). She was a Puritan, but whatever zeal characterizes her poetry, it was not religious. Rosania was not her only true love, she had another—her "first and dearest child," Hector, born to her after seven years of marriage and dead within forty days. She was inconsolable: here, too, religion was of not much use. She vowed to abandon poetry and, though a mother once more, did not survive him much, dying at thirty-two. Many a woman would find true love—and her self—only in motherhood and the love of a child: this, far more than the increased value of human life and significance of the individual, explains why modern society places children on such a pedestal. Moreover, the deep need for finding meaning in one's life—the reason for being on this earth at this time—and for the affirmation of self soon led Englishmen to expand the concept of such self-affirming love further and include in it dumb creatures, cats and dogs. Our concept of animals as pets and the idea of dog as a man's best friend derive directly from the search for self-definition in a culture that left the individual (a concept it constructed) free to construct it on one's own. Most modern languages do not have a special category for pets within the general designation of domestic animals. Derived from a Scottish and North English agricultural term for a lamb (or kid) taken into the house and brought up by hand, the word "pet" was, in Scotland, first applied metaphorically in early sixteenth century to spoiled children and then to animals, "parroquets, monkeys, peacocks, swans," kept for entertainment or home adornment, rather than a utilitarian purpose such as hunting mice and protection. In England it seems to have arrived in the seventeenth century and since the eighteenth century was used as a synonym for "favorite," a term of endearment. (Esther in Dickens's *Bleak House,* for instance, calls Ada her "pet.") The first instance of the word's application to a dog, cited by the *OED*—interestingly, in connection to "amorous passions"—is in Steele's *Tattler* in 1710.[20] A little later we find a love poem dedicated to a cat—not a joke, but a sincere and serious poem, worshipful in its expression of a powerful, ecstatic, emotion for another spiritual being, capable of moral judgment and of goodness, a possessor of a soul. This is Christopher Smart's "My Cat Jeoffry" from *Jubilato Agno:*

> For I will consider my Cat Jeoffry.
> For he is the servant of the Living God duly and daily serving him. . . .
> For if he meets another cat he will kiss her in kindness.
> For when he takes his prey he plays with it to give it a chance.
> For one mouse in seven escapes by his dallying.
> For when his day's work is done his business more properly begins.
> For he keeps the Lord's watch in the night against the
>   adversary. . . .
> For he counteracts the Devil, who is death, by brisking about the
>   life. . . .
> For he will not do destruction if he is well-fed, neither will he spit
>   without provocation. . . .
> For the English Cats are the best in Europe . . .
> For I bless the name of the Lord Jesus that Jeoffry is better. . . .
> For he is docile and can learn certain things . . .
> For he can jump from an eminence into his master's bosom.
> For he can catch the cork and toss it again.
> For he is hated by the hypocrite and miser.
> For he is good to think on . . . [21]

It is our need for self-affirming love, thus nationalism that led us to see a fellow being, a companion, in a dumb creature with a tail and four paws (It is remarkable, indeed, that English national pride finds its way into the panegyric to Jeoffry!). I am not aware of equally early published expressions of love for a dog, but it is clear that no other species of animal has been as ready to respond to the call of true love as that one. We have used dogs selfishly and thoughtlessly, very often cruelly, as live tools and weapons since time immemorial—thousands of years after, in their absolute goodness, they had adopted us, weak and as capable of evil as of good, as their special charge. Finally, we have come to appreciate their unique ability to give all of themselves. The retirement of God and the refusal of our free and open society to define us made us turn to dogs, among others, in search of the self, and, lo and behold, nowhere it proved easier to find.[22]

The ideal type of true ("romantic") love found its *locus classicus* in *Romeo and Juliet*. The word "love," therefore was generally reserved for a passionate, essentially spiritual, but by association sexual, relationship between a man and a woman that naturally expressed itself in marriage. Like Christian marriage, it was supposed to happen once and to last a lifetime—"till death do us part." But, while sex (only accidental to love), apparently, was good as cheap in the England of the sixteenth century as gentlemen and as it is today (though it must be said that in the sixteenth century one often had to pay dearly for it—women quite commonly dying young in the agony of childbirth and many of the best men rotting alive of the uncharitably named "French pox," syphilis), love was a miracle and miracles happened rarely.[23] Thus, inevitably, there was a tendency to lower the standards, to compromise, make the dream of love at least to some extent realistic. This led to the confusion of true love with false, the readiness to see true love in purely sexual passion (therefore treated with more indulgence than by Shakespeare) and discern it in unrequited attachment. True love was in the nature of the Protestant calling, which American Puritans took to mean that, if one was not sufficiently successful in one line of work, one was perfectly justified in turning to another, since the first one, clearly, could not have been a real calling.[24] Similarly, believers in true love, convinced that it happened only once in a lifetime and was unchanging, found no problem in a succession of love objects, to each of which one could be at different times equally passionately drawn, for, evidently, past loves that waned could not be true. The rarity of love also led to the deviations from the ideal type itself, which steadily increased with time, in particular in the course of the twentieth century in America. It led to increasing acceptance both of love relations without marriage—"love on trial" so to speak—and of homosexual relations; it also led to dramatically increased dependence on pets. In the final analysis, ambition, despite the fact that it required hard work, proved to be a far more reliable way to establishing identity than love which relieved one of responsibility but allowed one no control over the realization of one's dreams and therefore over one's self-realization.

At a later stage, as it traveled in translation, love acquired various national characteristics. Different cultures focused on different aspects of this powerful emotional complex and developed national ideal types of it. Ultimately heuristic devices and explicit cognitive constructions, these ideal types, like the original English one, are found mostly in works of art, especially literature. But, while uncommon in their pure form in actual experience, they, like *Romeo and Juliet,* have obviously influenced common experience. All modern societies accepted love as a passion—an authentic and sovereign expression of human nature, but some stressed its freedom from convention, and therefore, the freedom of the self—the Russian, as well as Anglo-American, ideal type was of this kind; while others saw it as a dark natural force which the self could not resist and which subjugated the self. In French, for instance, love was interpreted as an essentially sexual concept and as, particularly, a man's passion. "Passion," moreover, in this context retained a very strong earlier connotation of suffering. Whatever the reasons for such interpretation, a man passionately in love, which is experienced as sexual bondage and which destroys all his previous relationships, undermines his position in society, changes him as a person, and ultimately wrecks his life, became a French literary trope, though it was most compellingly presented on the operatic stage. Three of the greatest French operas, to which one finds no parallel anywhere else—Bizet's *Carmen,* Massenet's *Manon,* and Saint-Saëns' *Samson et Dalila*—have as their subject the desperate plight of a man in love;[25] "Tu n'avais eu qu'a paraitre / Qu'a jeter un regard sur moi / Pour t'emparer de tout mon etre, / O ma Carmen! / Et j'etais une chose a toi," sings José in what is perhaps the most erotic aria in all of the operatic repertoire just before he gasps, as if giving up the ghost, "Carmen, je t'aime." Making him a thing in the hands of the woman, an inanimate object, deprived of spirit and will—this is what the passion of love does to a man!

The man-in-love—Don José, Chevalier Des Grieux, Samson—has as his counterpart a woman who embodies the power of sexual desire itself, a sort of sexual magnet that draws the man in spite of himself; *femme fatale* is a peculiarly French concept. For her part, the woman may—and is likely—to suffer from the sexual passion as well, but not because, like the man, she is also in love. She suffers because of the destructive nature of such passion itself. Hard-hearted Carmen is killed, the softer Manon dies from exhaustion, Dalila escapes their fate only because she feels no passion; she only pretends it. But the starkest example of a woman destroyed by sexual passion is, of course, Marguerite Gautier of *La Dame aux Camélias*. Red and white, the camellias of the title are not exquisite flowers whose rare beauty matches that of the lady; they shamelessly advertise red, menstruation, white, Marguerite's availability for sex. No other work of modern art paints sex as so pitilessly carnal. It is a tragic and morbid affair, the other face of death. No scene in literature drives the point home as brutally as the exhumation of the girl's decomposed body. There is no escape, life itself is just sickness and dying, and the more passionately it is lived, the more ravaging the sickness and the swifter is death. It is telling that all this emphatic carnality entirely disappears in Verdi's—Italian—operatic rendition of Dumas' novel, the beautiful *La Traviata*. The French story is sanitized of sex, it becomes a spiritual and uplifting tale of a wronged, misled, but pure in heart maiden, sacrificing herself for the sake of her beloved's good name and his virginal sister's future. We cry when Violetta dies of consumption, her virtue triumphing, though recognized too late by her simpleminded lover and his father—and cringe when Marguerite's face, eaten by death, glares at us from her open grave.

No, this is not the kind of emotion that would express itself in marriage. Marriage, in this framework, remarkably, is best when it is dispassionate. As an ideal type it is a bourgeois institution, i.e., rational, strictly organized, and obedient to social conventions, though why should such sedate qualities be associated with cities—the obvious epicenters of the modern earthquakes—is not entirely clear. Of course, the bourgeoisie in France has been traditionally disparaged as a class—first by the aristocracy of the old regime, then by Marxism. The result of this disparagement, in the present context, has been that the institutions its members were believed to value were rejected by the intellectuals who created and were most influenced by literary tropes, and thus, in distinction to the Anglo-American world, love remained dissociated from marriage.

Nothing can be more different from the French ideal type than the Russian one, embodied in the third of the three great literary traditions of the modern world. Tolstoy's *Anna Karenina* is its archetypal expression, though one meets with it in the works of every Russian author of renown, from Pushkin and Lermontov in the early nineteenth century to Kuprin and Pasternak a century later. In the Russian tradition, love is understood primarily as the woman's passion and it is purely spiritual. The woman realizes herself in love—it is certainly the authentic and sovereign expression of her spiritual self, her soul—and she realizes herself in bodily self-sacrifice. That is, rather than losing her spiritual self in another and recovering it reflected and affirmed in the English manner, she gives to the man she loves her body in sex—this is the way sex enters the Russian concept of love. This sexual giving of herself is a sacrifice, because, though she gives herself freely, she does it without pleasure. Sex satisfies no desire in her— she is, essentially, an asexual being—but only serves to satisfy man's desire. Love, again, is closely linked to suffering: the woman suffers and expects to suffer from sex, both physically (the act is at best not entirely revolting to her and then there is the possibility, almost certainty, of pregnancy and childbirth) and spiritually, because man's love is too sexual to be true, and when his desire is satisfied he is likely to be unfaithful. She does not hold this against him: men cannot help it—they are deceived by sexual desire to think that they are, in fact, in love, such is their nature.[26] Both the physical and spiritual suffering is precisely what makes love so important. Suffering is the preferred Russian form of self-affirmation, in general, and a woman's identity can be affirmed only through it. The heart-wrenching descriptions of labor pains in Russian literature, from the fatal childbed of Lisa in *War and Peace* and the nearly fatal one of Anna in *Anna Karenina* to Tonia's agony in *Doctor Zhivago,* all watched in helpless contrition by the men for whom these women sacrifice themselves (and so different from the naturalistic yet detached depiction of the complicated labor in, for instance, Zola's *Nana*), make the analogy with the Passion on the Cross obvious.

The call of love cannot be disobeyed: it is a supreme value. No true woman will leave it unanswered: in this she would perjure her soul. Neither can marriage be made a condition for the woman's self-sacrifice, this would be tantamount to prostitution—real, because spiritual, prostitution in distinction to the merely surface prostitution of the body. This, in the nineteenth century, when the ideal type is constructed, is extremely problematic: love marriage may be the ideal, but in practice women marry young and they marry much older men whom they do not love—thus they prostitute their bodies. They chance to fall in love when they are already married, and then, not to prostitute their soul, they must commit adultery. Adultery is likely to destroy their world, deprive them of their good name and social and economic position, cause their expulsion from the community. Moreover, love puts them in danger of being torn apart spiritually between equally powerful conflicting moral obligations, the duty to answer its call and the one they owe not to their husband, which is clearly outweighed by the love obligation, but to their children. For, though, unlike in England, the love of a child cannot be interpreted as true love (in Russia only the love between a man and a woman qualifies for that), motherhood is also an authentic expression of the woman's self, achieved in suffering through self-sacrifice, and a supreme value within the modern Russian culture. Karenina's throwing herself under the train is the logical resolution of this otherwise irresolvable conflict and the inevitable conclusion of combining the structural realities of early marriage to an older man as the only way to maintain a woman's social position and economic security or man's inescapable sexuality with cultural ideals of love and motherhood as the supreme values in a woman's life. It is independent of the specific plot and can only be avoided by accident. This is what makes this great novel so tragic.

There is something of making virtue out of necessity and finding joy in suffering in the Russian ideal of love. The woman's identity that is affirmed in love and, significantly, childbirth is her identity as a woman, not as a person. The English word "man" is translated by two Russian words, *chelovek*, which means "a living being, capable of reason, subject to death," as in the original Elyot's definition, and *muzhchina*, "an adult human male"— the meager meaning of "man" in American English today. A phrase "she is a real/wonderful/terrible man (*chelovek*)" makes perfect sense in Russian.[27] One's personal identity in Russia depends primarily on friendship, which was the form in which the original English concept and experience of love migrated to Russia, and Russians remained much more faithful to the ideal, than the descendants of the sixteenth century English, who eventually sexualized it out of recognition. The concept of *alter ego* is readily understandable to a Russian. Russian friendships are intense, intimate and physically close without any hint of sex, and expected to be for life. They are not exclusive: one can have several close friends, though the relationship with the "best friend" has a special significance. One is supposed to stand by one's friends whatever the cost; that this cultural injunction is taken seriously is amply demonstrated in the Russian history of the nineteenth as well as the twentieth centuries. The abandonment of a friend in need, even under the direst of circumstances, is unforgivable. The harsh politics of modern Russia—both in its Imperial and in its Soviet forms—while, like pre-modern societies, offering the individual sufficient help for the construction of an identity, allowed few possibilities for authentic self-expression, made a necessity in the modern world, and friendship became a vital emotionally-liberating alternative to the otherwise ruthlessly regimented life. One of the Russian equivalents for the contemporary English "honey" or "darling," used between close friends, lovers, mothers and children, is "my soul," a term of endearment which virtually disappeared from English—*dusha moia* (or, with a suffix, *dushen'ka*—"dear soul"). This is, most likely, a trope, spoken without thought and thus quite insignificant, only a pentimento of an idea. But in this way language keeps the memory of forgotten understandings.

All this, however, was to happen much later. In late sixteenth-century England, love, as defined by Shakespeare in *Romeo and Juliet* and the sonnets, was the governing passion if only because happiness was virtually impossible without it. It should no longer come as a surprise that happiness became possible only in the sixteenth century and that the only place in which, for some time, it was possible was England. Neither the concept nor, therefore, the experience existed before. It was, like love, ambition, and success, a product of the national—fundamentally secular and humanistic—image of reality. Students of happiness, which is gaining popularity as an academic subject, always forget that one cannot access any cultural phenomenon by translation backwards. Guided by the worthy sentiment, ingrained in every society considering itself Western since World War II, that all men are created equal, they assume the uniformity of human experience and aspiration (which, the readers of this chapter know, could not be experienced before the sixteenth century) throughout the ages, and, sure enough, find happiness or at least desire for happiness everywhere. But the fact is that no language before modern English had a word for it—therefore it could not be even desired—and there was no word for it, because happiness in a world ruled by transcendental forces of whatever variety was inconceivable.

All the words that we today translate as "happiness"—from the *eudemonia* of the ancient Greeks to the *bonheur, felicita, Glück,* and *schastie* of contemporary modern vernaculars—were originally synonyms of "good luck" and connoted the benevolence of fate. To experience *eudemonia* or *bonheur,* therefore, meant to be subject to such benevolence, to be "blessed"; this was a statement of fact not a description of a subjective state of being. In the framework of the Greek understanding, *eudemonia,* in fact, could not be experienced at all, because easy and honorable death was among its most important ingredients, if not its definitive characteristic, and the fact whether someone was or was not subject to the benevolence of fate, whether one was or was not favored by the gods, could only be established after one quit this vale of tears.

The problem with luck is that there is no justice in it. It is wholly unpredictable and, good or bad, always unexpected. Nothing we do can influence it, it is up to forces we cannot control in any way whether to bestow it on us or not, and because it is so entirely out of our hands, we cannot blame ourselves for not being lucky. One fundamental tradition of Western civilization rejected the idea of luck, opposing to it a view of the world predicated on the concept of justice. Under the influence of Jewish monotheism, the priceless gift the reception of which by the surrounding cultures must be dated to some time in the sixth century BC—the period corresponding to the first, Babylonian, redaction of the Bible—the concept of *eudemonia* changed. The notion of the covenant made human reality to some degree controllable. If people behaved, God, one assumed, did not play dice with the universe. Man, though incomparably the weaker, junior partner, in however minute degree could now affect the course of history and became responsible for his personal fate. This new perspective allowed the conception of *eudemonia* in this life and its interpretation as an actual experience. Since the time of Socrates it would be interpreted first and foremost as the acceptance of mortality, on the reconciliation to which the existential experience of a thinking man in a large part depended. To prepare one for death was the task of philosophy; its advice, roughly, was to live a life, which, while free of actual suffering to the extent that was possible, would be so devoid of enjoyment that one would not regret leaving it when time comes—a sort of nirvana: enjoy nothing and you will not be losing anything worth keeping when you die. This kind of life was the "good life," and living such a life was *eudemonia*. This is the basis of the misconception that happiness is the goal of philosophy.

The interpretation of *eudemonia* as the experience of "good life" understood primarily as absence of fear of death—a specific kind of suffering— was reinforced and at the same time further modified in the Christian thinking. "Good life" acquired the meaning of faith, in particular, the absolute faith in eternal life, which often sought to express itself actively as *praxis pietatis*.[28] Therefore Christian felicity (a derivative from Latin for "luck"—*felix*) could be found in martyrdom, an especially painful death one chose to demonstrate how free of fear one was—the strength of one's faith, or, when such swift ascent to salvation was no longer possible, in hermitage, monastic practice, and various forms of asceticism. Later, when Protestantism removed one's ultimate fate from human control and made it a matter of luck again, thereby creating the psychological need in the certitude of salvation, the felicity was experienced in *unio mystica*—the mystical union with Christ—achieved most expeditiously through bodily suffering in which one could identify with the Lord's Passion.

After considering the early Christian concept of "happiness" (which was nothing of the sort) an historian is apt to jump straight into the eighteenth century and its belief in "the pursuit of happiness" as one's inalienable right.[29] But, of course, to be believed in, such an idea of happiness had first to be conceived. The English word, derived from "hap"—chance or luck, and rare before, came into general use in the second half of the sixteenth century. *Promptorium Parvulorum* of 1499 does not have it, but translates "happe" as *Fortuna* and "happy" as *fortunatus, felix*. Elyot's *Dictionary* does not have "happiness" either but under "Fortuna," translated as "fortune," lists "Fors Fortuna, good fortune or chaunce. Fortunate insulae, the fortunate ilandes, be so callyd of the abundaunce of fruites, of whiche Strabo writeth. Fortunatim, fortunately. Fortunatus, fortunate. Fortuno, to make prosperous, to augment with good fortune."[30] Luck here is secularized and made near synonymous, specifically, with material wealth or prosperity. The *OED*, which not very informatively defines "happiness" as "the quality or condition of being happy," cites as first instance John Palsgrave's French/ English glossary of 1530, *L'Éclaircissement de la langue françoyse*, equating "happynesse" and *prosperité*. It next cites Shakespeare's *Two Gentlemen of Verona*, however, "With me partaker in thy happinesse, / When thou do'st meet good hap," where happiness means good luck. The second definition of "happiness" in the *OED* is "the state of pleasurable content of mind, which results from success or the attainment of what is considered good." The first instance cited is from Spencer's *Ruines of Time*, 1591: "Like beast [that] hath no hope of happinesse or bliss"; the second is from Shakespeare's *Cymbeline:* "To sowre your happinesse, / I must report The Queene is dead." The two citations seem to suggest that the state of pleasurable content of mind they refer to is prolonged, rather than momentary, and that it neither is a matter of luck in the sense of pre-Socratic *eudemonia* nor of freedom from the fear of death in its post-Socratic sense, for beasts, on the one hand, like men, may be favored by gods and, on the other, unlike men, do not consider death a problem. Something new, clearly, is emerging here. What it is is suggested by the *OED*'s fourth sense of the much older word "happy," first used in 1525. "Happy" in this sense refers to "having a feeling of great pleasure or content of mind, arising from satisfaction with one's circumstances or condition; also in weakened sense: glad, pleased." This, obviously, is not a way to characterize a martyr torn by lions, a monk engaged in the mortification of the flesh, or a deceased man who lived and died without suffering excessively.

In distinction to pre-Socratic eudemonia, which could not be experienced at all, the new English—and our—happiness was conceived of as a living experience. In distinction to the Christian felicity, which, in an attempt to escape one kind of suffering often led to another and had to be bought at the price of enjoyment, this experience was conceived of as a pleasant one. Unlike luck, which could be good and bad and which was unpredictable, happiness was purely good and could be pursued. Unlike faith, which was always a gift to which none was entitled, it was a natural, thus inalienable right. In short, happiness had nothing in common with the phenomena whose names were used to translate this utterly novel English experience into other languages. Of course, human beings, like animals, had been familiar with the sensations of joy and pleasure prior to the sixteenth century: our brains were producing endorphins before we were endowed with culture, and when this happened we invented words to relate to these sensations. But, while joyful and pleasant, happiness was a far more complex and significant emotional phenomenon. The new English word referred to an existential condition, a lasting, profound, fully conscious feeling of satisfaction with one's circumstances, indeed—with oneself-in-the-world, the sense that one's life fit one like a glove. This implied that one experienced existence as meaningful, that one felt there was a reason for one's being here and now, and that, above all, one knew who and what one was—namely, had a firm and satisfactory identity. This was not a given in an open secular society. With man as the supreme lawmaker life was not justified from the outside, it had to be justified. It was not all good, it had to be believed that it can and must be all good. The concept of "happiness," which made possible the experience, was the answer to this new psychological need created by the culture (symbolic system) of nationalism. Happiness became the purpose of human existence.

In an open secular society, which left one free to construct one's identity, the bed one slept in was very much the bed one made. Good luck would help and bad might interfere with one's designs, but one was the architect of one's happiness, supposed to choose and then build one's life. This, again, placed the responsibility squarely on one's shoulders, but the reward one could reap was more than worth it. Not only was happiness a lasting joy, not only was it fully conscious, namely experienced as it were doubly—as a vague pleasurable emotion and as articulated thought (involving, therefore—for we must believe neuroscience—both the amygdala and the frontal cortex, and producing heretofore inconceivable amounts of endorphins), but there was an "umph" in it, that most joys and pleasures of the past lacked. It was the "umph" of triumph—because happiness was an achievement. Like a great artist, one would be eager to acknowledge the sources of one's inspiration and feel genuine gratitude to people and animate an inanimate universe. But, in the final analysis, one had no one to thank for it but oneself—for recognizing the true love, for persevering in ambition despite attendant anxieties and frustrations, above all for being one's own maker. For it all boiled down to the construction of identity—self-definition, self-expression, self-realization. Through passions—ambition and love foremost among them—one expressed, discovered, and realized one's authentic and sovereign self. Happiness was the realization of this self-realization.

Well might Miranda of *The Tempest* exclaim of the world created in sixteenth-century England: "How beauteous mankind is! O brave new world!" For it was new, and brave, and beyond all compare beauteous indeed. If anyone of us today—wherever that may be—feels the thrill of ambition, it is because sixteenth-century English defined it as "upward desire." If any of us loves, or dreams of true love, it is because from this cradle of modernity and out of their hands we received the gift of self-affirmation through (unreserved) self-transcendence. If any of us is happy, it is because they invented happiness.

The sixteenth century in England was the first century of the world as we know it. It gave us so much that we are, so much of what we now consider the inner capacities and needs of the human nature: love, ambition, happiness, the dignity of man.

It also gave us madness.

Of Madness

In 1961 two books were published, one in France and one in the United States. Both proved to be extremely influential in the area of discourse on mental illness, profoundly affecting the way general public understood it and drastically changing, in effect creating a new field in, the literature on the history of psychiatry. These books were Michel Foucault's *Folie et déraison: Histoire de la folie à l'âge classique* and Thomas Szasz's *The Myth of the Mental Illness*.[31] Their styles were as different as could be expected from a French *philosophe* who regarded philosophy as a form of poetry and an American-trained psychiatrist who used language, for the lack of a simpler alternative, as a tool for taking clinical notes. But their arguments were quite similar. Both thought that mental illness was a social construction, lacking biological reality and nevertheless interpreted as a medical problem, either in the interest of the ascendant bourgeoisie which wished to confine so called "madmen" or "fools"—socially disruptive elements insensitive to its value—in a sphere apart (Foucault) or of the overzealous psychiatric profession desirous of the broader recognition in medicine where it was a newcomer and bent on controlling deviant behavior (Szasz). This "medicalization," according to both writers, was a modern trend, taking place most conspicuously in "the age of reason," i.e., the eighteenth and nineteenth centuries, and reflected in the emergence and establishment of psychiatry. In Foucault's opinion, it had a grievous impact on the experience of the numerous marginal individuals, whose extravagances earlier societies would tolerate with good humor, but who were now defined as carriers of a terrible, possibly contagious disease, and thus virtually excluded from the community. In the view of Szasz, it discredited and psychologically disabled maladjusted but perfectly healthy people, making them incapable of dealing with events of normal life and preventing them from taking responsibility for their own actions.

In the academic circles, Foucault's version of the argument, sympathetic to the distress of the socially excluded "mental patients" and stressing the complicity of the society at large in their exclusion, has been by far the more popular of the two, but both texts, irrespective of their moral stand, encouraged the shift of attention from mental illness itself to attitudes to mental illness, thereby effectively redefining the subject as a constructed reality and opening a broad venue, in place of an extremely narrow one that existed before, through which historians and other social scientists could participate in the discussion about it.[32] Since then contributions of a historical and sociological nature, as well as those hailing from literary and feminist and gender theory, to the study of the social context of mental illness proliferated. An extensive literature resulted from this new work, its authors, comfortable with the assumption that discursive artifacts are, in any case, the only thing that we could know and that is worth knowing, subscribing to either the weak or the strong version of Foucault's and Szasz's constructivist approach. In the former case, they have either accepted current biological ideas regarding the nature and causation of the phenomenon of mental illness itself, or professed agnosticism in regard to it (rendering, as it were, unto science what the authority of science demanded) while in the latter, they believed that there was no such thing at all. Thus scholars in this very active community which concentrated around mental illness in a sense intentionally refrained from attempting to understand it and—in case they did more than "theory" to begin with and engaged in research—from drawing conclusions from their findings.

It was fortunate for the practitioners of the new socio-historical approach that much of it was indeed theory, because history (on which all areas of social and cultural study depend for their data) offers no foundation for the work of its founding fathers. Neither psychiatry nor the modern society in general or its "age of reason," specifically, could be credited with the creation of the concept of mental disease that has existed since time immemorial. The rich vocabulary of early psychiatry, originally derived from the medical literature of Ancient Greece and used by physicians throughout the Middle Ages, makes this abundantly clear. The constructivist argument is similarly unsupported by simple logic. The brain, after all, is a part of the body and, insofar as they affect the brain, numerous physical conditions must produce mental symptoms. How could such symptoms not be considered mental illness, especially at a time when any illness was defined almost exclusively by symptoms, is hard to fathom.

That illness was so defined, again, is evident from the language. The most general terms of medical discourse, such as "pathology," "illness," and "disease," obviously originally have none but the clinical significance, focusing, as these three do, specifically on the personal, subjective experience of suffering. The concept "pathology," for instance, derives from Greek for "suffering" (*pathos*), even though the knowledge (*logos*) to which it commonly refers today is not the knowledge of suffering, but rather that of an objective morbid condition underlying it. It is true that quite often the sense of the word "pathology" becomes limited to such objective morbid condition, leaving out the suffering associated with it altogether. In general, though, it implies a causal relationship between the two: an objective material condition causing the subjective experience.[33] The concepts of "disease" and "illness," of course, also derive from words for negative subjective experience, feelings of discomfort: disease as opposed to ease, illness as opposed to wellness. In their case, too, the emphasis on the objective morbid condition, supposedly causing these feelings, replaces the original emphasis on suffering. In contemporary discourse, both "disease" and "illness" commonly refer to objective—namely, material—medical conditions. An historian or a sociologist, however, must look at the root of a concept and cannot be guided in one's interpretation by the current meaning alone.[34] The word "insanity" (with its numerous traditional subcategories), etymologically an equivalent of "illness" or "disease," meaning simply a condition of un-health, but referring specifically to "mental illness" and "mental disease," in accordance with the ancient principle of *mens sana in corpore sano*, also assumes physical causation of mental dysfunction. In contrast to "pathology," "disease," and "illness" (and their equivalents in other languages), however, the initial referent of "insanity" is not the subjective experience of suffering, but observable behavioral irregularities presupposing an unsound mind which is not in control. To claim, therefore, that mental illness is a myth or a social construction of recent centuries is incongruent with all that we know about the history of medicine. At most we can argue that medicine itself became increasingly materialized, shifting the focus of study from subjective experience to underlying bodily conditions. But this, again, though very pronounced today, began long before either modernity in general, or the modern medical specialty of psychiatry, came into being.

The New Semantic Field

All this, however, is not to say that nothing new happened to mental disease with the emergence of modernity or that psychiatry was but a continuation under a new name of the traditional medical preoccupation with mental illness. In the sixteenth century a new form of mental disease appeared in England. We know that it was new, because none of the many existing terms for mental disorders seemed sufficient to capture it and a new word—in fact, an entire vocabulary charting a new semantic field— was created to do so. It was called, most famously, "madness" and was essentially different from all the numerous forms of mental distress known before. What distinguished this new trouble from the familiar varieties, in the first place, was that it felt more like a curse than a medical trouble. While the old diseases, mental and physical, were temporary, either accidental or related to a particular stage in life (such as pregnancy or old age, for instance), and ended after a short duration in a cure or death, the new illness was chronic: it appeared to be a permanent, existential condition which first affected one at a relatively young age and then lasted the lifetime. The most common synonym of "madness" was indeed "lunacy" (another new word), which underscored the repetitive, ever-returning character of the new illness, relating it to the pernicious influence of the moon. This was a traditional lay explanation for all sorts of erratic periodic behavior, but not only. Astrology, in a way, was a precursor of genetics. Like the latter today, it formed a part of common consciousness and thus was, among other things, also a necessary element of physicians' intellectual equipment, the stars, of which the moon was central, being considered a prime influence on the individual's life chances, including health. Eminent physicians of the sixteenth century took lunar influences seriously. Thomas Vicary, who attended to both Henry VIII and Elizabeth, wrote, for instance: "the brain hath this property that it moveth and followeth the moving of the moon . . . and this is proved in men that be lunatic or mad . . . and also in men that be epulentic [epileptic?] or having the falling sickness, that be most grieved in the beginning of the new moon and the latter quarter of the moon."[35] The most famous writer on madness in its first century, Robert Burton, who was not a physician himself, in *The Anatomy of Melancholy* seconded the opinion of Paracelsus that no physician could "either understand the cause or cure of any disease, either of this, or gout, nor so much as toothache; except he see the peculiar geniture and scheme of the party affected," unless, that is, he knew under what stars, etc., etc., the patient was born. Whether the lay opinion led or followed the expert one, it concurred: "Madmen act their gambols to the full of the moon."[36]

The chronic character of madness, in distinction to the previously known forms of mental disease, made mental disorder a legal issue almost as soon as madness was first observed. The first legal provision in England for mentally disturbed individuals—referred to, specifically, as "madmen and lunatics"—dates back only to 1541.[37] Simultaneously, and, again, for the first time in history, mental disorder was perceived as a specific social or public health problem, which required a special, publicly regulated solution. Traditionally, mentally sick people, if indigent, were cared for, alongside with other "impotent poor", such as orphans, aged, and physically disabled, in "hospitals" or charity houses, by religious organizations. In England of that period monasteries were dissolved, but the care of the poor and sick as an undifferentiated mass continued. The mentally ill, however, no longer belonged to this mass; they came to constitute a separate category of people who had a claim on public support. This claim was based on the nature of their suffering, not on their lack of resources. The first specialized public hospital in the current sense of the word, i.e., as a medical institution, was a hospital for the insane—Bethlehem, or Bedlam. It was made the property of the city of London in 1547. According to the 1598 report made by the inspection committee of its board of governors, it had twenty inmates, all kept in single rooms (or, rather, cells—an arrangement very different from charitable dispositions of the disabled in other groups) of whom only six were charity cases, the other fourteen being private—that is, paying—patients. The chief officer of Bedlam was, at least intermittently a physician, and this became a permanent arrangement in 1618, when King James had appointed one of his private court physicians to the mastership of the hospital. It is ironic that this Dr. Hilkiah Crooke, while a bona fide Doctor, "skilful in the practice of medicine," was also a real crook, apparently more true to his name than his title.[38]

The new condition was also noticeably more common than all the other mental diseases taken together.[39] Since 1561 the annual income, settled at thirty-four pounds in 1555, was considered insufficient to meet the expenses of Bedlam, and from 1575 on the hospital was expanding constantly, first demolishing the church and the chapel of the ancient priory of St. Mary of Bethlehem, on the site of which it was founded and whose name it assumed, and replacing them with "houses" for its patients, then, once and again, building various additions. In 1632, with an annual income increased to above 277 pounds and thirty inmates, it was still unable to meet the demand. The London population was growing quite rapidly, but not by 50 percent in thirty-four years between 1598 and 1632, which does suggest that madness was from the first adding unexpectedly large numbers of sufferers to otherwise mentally ill.[40]

In the course of the sixteenth century the word "madness" and various derivatives and compounds of "mad" and "lunatic" entered common discourse. Multiple idiomatic expressions incorporating "mad" and "madness" augmented this emerging vocabulary. Medical men might not have been the first to notice the new phenomenon, but they were quick to challenge the lead of the legal and municipal authorities and appoint themselves as the experts on the subject. Attempts to familiarize the novel reality the new vocabulary recognized began almost as soon as it appeared and it took the form of medicalization of madness, its assimilation to the known forms of mental disease. Thus the new, chronic, and rapidly spreading form of mental disorder brought insanity in general into focus. The word "insanity" (or later abandoned "insanie") entered English at that time, and by the end of the century legal texts, too, were treating madness and lunacy as its form, as, for instance, did Swinburne in his 1590 *Testaments:* "Madfolkes and Lunaticke persons, during the time of their furor or insanitie of minde, cannot make a testament." Such assimilation, undoubtedly, affected the subsequent understanding of madness, but the new affliction with its accompanying vocabulary with equal necessity changed the existing medical views of mental disease.

Of the new expressions, "madness" was by far the most significant addition to the English vocabulary. The first use of the adjective "mad," is dated by the *OED* to about the year 725, as that of the synonymous "wood," both meaning "foolish" and "unwise." "Wood" appears to be more common; it is specifically applied to rabid animals ("wood dog") and, as a metaphor, to people behaving like rabid animals, that is to conduct—in modern parlance—"going beyond all reasonable bounds; utterly senseless; extremely rash or reckless, wild; vehemently excited"; "extremely fierce or violent, ferocious; irascible, passionate"; "violently angry or irritated; enraged, furious." One finds such employment of "wood" as late as the novels of Walter Scott, though in 1828 *Craven Glossary,* having defined "wood" as "mad, rhyming with food," advises: "this word is rarely used."[41] In the sixteenth century "mad," as it introduced into the English language an entirely new semantic field, replaced "wood" for whatever "wood" suggested earlier. Perhaps most revealingly as regards the nature of the new mental ailment, in the process folly was left outside the semantic field of madness.

There were several aspects to this separation. The word "folly" (like the French *folie*), which was semantically cognate to the Old English root of the neologism "madness," meant deficiency of understanding or stupidity, but also lewdness, wantonness (as in *folles filles*—prostitutes), and even wickedness, evil, mischief, and harm. It was an ethical concept, a term of moral judgment, and implied disapprobation and disgust.[42] Both "lunacy" and "madness," in contrast, were generally nonjudgmental (though occasionally in the later part of the sixteenth century "mad" and "fool" would be used as synonyms), most commonly referred to the subjective experience, rather than behavior, and, when depicting behavior, stressed its abnormal affect—specifically affect that was not under one's control—such as extreme excitement or extreme sadness, rather than its ethical significance. The individual who was lunatic or mad, in distinction to a fool, was a victim, rather than agent and instigator of the condition. Unlike folly, lunacy or madness was a misfortune, not a character flaw. The moralization of folly was one consequence of its exclusion from the semantic field of madness. The other was its equation with idiocy.

Idiocy was a mental dysfunction but not a disease, in the sense that it caused no dis-ease to its subjects. Idiots were not intelligent enough to realize that there was a demerit in not being intelligent enough and to take offence at being regarded as such. They were neither frightened nor humiliated by their condition and did not struggle against it. Like animals or little children, they were defenseless and easy victims of cruelty and neglect and had to be protected from suffering. But the condition itself, unlike madness, was not tragic. As a synonym of "idiocy," "folly" became the very opposite of "madness." The contrast between the two concepts, and the mental conditions they signified, was expressed very clearly in the end of the seventeenth century by Locke in *An Essay on Human Understanding.* "In fine," he wrote,

> the defect in naturals[fools], seems to proceed from want of quickness, activity, and motion, in the intellectual faculties, whereby they are deprived of reason, whereas madmen, on the other side, seem to suffer by other extreme. For they do not appear to me to have lost the faculty of reasoning, but having joined together some ideas very wrongly they mistake them for truths . . . as though incoherent ideas have been cemented together so powerfully as to remain united. . . . herein seems to lie the difference between idiots and madmen. That madmen put wrong ideas together, and so make wrong propositions but argue and reason right from them. But idiots make very few or no propositions, but argue and reason scarce at all.[43]

This insistence on the overactive and quick intelligence in madness—"the other extreme" from the dullness of folly (which suggests that Locke was referring to psychosis characterized by delusions and, specifically, to what we would recognize as schizophrenia today) was lost on much of modern psychiatry. But already in the sixteenth century the only way folly and fools figured in discussions of mental disorders was as a name for congenital idiocy which found itself on the opposite end of the scale of mental defect from madness and lunacy.

In *Promptorium Parvulorum* of 1440, the two adjectives "mad" and "wood" were still treated as interchangeable: "madd, or wood, amens, demens, furiosus." The neologism "madness" reflected this attitude. In Old English, according to the *OED*, the adjective "mad" appeared once in the compound "madmod," signifying "folly." The 1440 *Promptorium Parvulorum*, which is *OED*'s first instance of the new noun, defined "maddenesse" as English rendition of the Latin *amencia* and *demencia*.[44] The great sixteenth-century dictionaries, Elyot's 1538 *Dictionary* and Cooper's 1565 *Thesaurus*, stressed the connection of both the noun and the adjective to animal distemper—Elyot defining rabies as "madnesse of a dogge" and Cooper, in the translation of "*furibundus*," offering the examples of "*canis furibundus, a madde dogge*" and "*taurus furibundus, a madde bull*." The popularity of the newly introduced (madness) and reintroduced after long disuse (mad) terms, however, had to do with humans.

Something was abnormal in the long familiar experience of mental affliction, something that could not be accounted for by the old terms of *amencia* and *demencia*, and the ancient medical learning inherited with them. From 1495 the word "madness" began to appear systematically in discussions of mental disease. The first such use was in the reprinting, that year, of the fourteenth-century translation of Bartholomaeus Anglicus's *De proprietatibus rerum*, a "compendium of information for monks".[45] The original translation presented madness as a general category, distinguishing two varieties of the illness, mania and melancholia: "these passions ben dyuers madnesse that hyghte Mania & madnesse that hyghte Malencolonia." The amended 1535 version limited the use of "madness" only to mania (more in line with the equation of "mad" and "wood" or "furious"), translating the same paragraph thus: "Madnes is infection of the formeste celle of the heed, with privacion of imaginacion, lyke as melancolie is the infection of the middell celle of the heed, with privacion of reason. . . . these passions ben divers after the diversitee of the hurt of theyr workings: for by madnesse that hyghte Mania principally the imaginacion is hurte." The traditional medical interpretation of mental disease, clearly, was organic.[46]

In general, however, translations of medical texts, which in the sixteenth century, as the above example demonstrates, displayed a great deal of poetic license, show greater awareness of the novelty of the word, and the inchoateness of the concept "madness." For instance, the rendition of *The Touchstone of Complexions* . . . by a Dutch physician Levinus Lemnius, *englished* by Thomas Newton in 1576, omits madness altogether in a long list of mental diseases while introducing the subject: "The proper and peculiar place, assigned and allotted for the Memory, is the Brayne, the mansion & dwelling house of wit and all the Senses: which being affected, or by any distemperature discrased, all the functions and offices of Nature are semblably passioned: insomuch that . . . there steppeth in place, Sottage, forgetfulness, amazednesse, dotage, foolishness, lack of right wits, doltishness & idiocie." Later, however, when Lemnius suggests shaving as a preventive measure, the translator adds to the roster a variety so unmistakably English as to eliminate any possibility of its being equivalent to any foreign term, and therefore phenomenon. "[F]or the redresse of certayne diseases of the head," he says, "losse of right witts, feeblenes of brayne, dottrye, phrensie, Bedlem madnesse, Melancholicke affections, furie and franticke fitts, Physitions deeme it the beste waye to have the hayre cleane shaven of."[47] But "Bedlem" was at that time the only specialized mental asylum in the Western world; the handful of its "mad" patients and their affliction was a uniquely English reality, as yet unfamiliar to other European nations.

The hospital and its inmates make appearance in spiritual texts of the period as well, which consider madness in a very different light, as does, for instance, the 1572 translation of *Of Ghostes and Spirites Walking by Nyght*, a 1570 treatise about hallucinations and delusions by a Swiss divine Lewes Lavater. There the translator writes: "Madde men which have utterly loste the use of reason, or are vexed by Gods permission, with a Divell . . . doo marvelous thinges, talke of many visions and divers other matters. Theyr sight deceiveth them, in somuche as they mistake one man for an other: which thing we see by experience, in Bedleme houses where mad and frantike men are kepte." In a laudable effort to ensure a more accurate understanding of the translated text the specific experience is generalized and the singular institution is made plural.[48]

Religion, needless to stress, was a very important epistemological system in the framework of which madness was discussed and defined. To begin with, even the body was subject to the will of God, and there was a widespread though vague feeling that the connection of some mental diseases to the diseases of the body was less definite than of others. Some of the physicians who dealt with the subject were also divines, and many divines who were not physicians participated actively in the discourse. Andrew Boorde, who studied medicine at Montpellier and was a bishop of Chichester, was able to combine religion and medicine in his understanding. In 1552 he published *The Seconde Boke of the Brevyary of Health, Named the Extravagantes,* which distinguished several kinds of madness. One of them was the disorder of Demoniackes, defined as follows: "Demoniacus or Demoniaci be the latin wordes. In greke it is named Demonici. In Englyshe it is named he or they the which be mad and possessed of the devyll or devils, and theyr propertie is to hurt and kyll them selfe, or else to hurt and kyll any other thynge, therefore let every man beware of them, and kepe them in a sure custody." A similar "infirmytie," however, came "from a corrupte bloude in the head." It was called "mania"; Boorde explained: "Mania is the greke. In Latin it is named Insania, or Furor, In Englishe it is named a madnes or woodnes like a wylde beast . . ." The treatment suggested in this case was only a little different from the sure custody prescribed for Demoniacs' spiritual affliction. "[K]epe the pacient from musynge and studieng," advised Boorde, "and use myrth and mery comunication, and use the pacient so that he do not hurt hym selfe nor no other man, and he must be kepte in feare of one man or an other, and if need requyre he must be punished & beaten . . ."[49] In the sixteenth century at issue often—in connection with behavior that religious opinion considered witchcraft and, increasingly, with offences that raised the question of legal responsibility—was not the wellbeing of an individual body, but the right of the community, in self-defense, to separate it from the soul. It is clear that in such cases the medical interpretation, as inhumane as it was, by our standards, was certainly preferable.

Both the life-saving virtue of the medical view and its limitations in regard to madness were manifest in the case of Peter Berchet, "a lunatic" and "a deranged Puritan."[50] In 1573, Berchet, a law student, stabbed Sir John Hawkins, a very firm Protestant, whom he mistook for Sir Christopher Hatton, an advisor to the Queen and also a Protestant, accused by Berchet of being "a wylfull Papyst [who] hindereth the glory of God." The incident taking place at the time of increasing Puritan agitation, Elizabeth wished Berchet to be questioned under torture to reveal the names of co-conspirators she suspected. On the testimony of two of his fellow students, however, Berchet's examiners became convinced that he was not a political/religious extremist, but, rather, suffered from "nawghtye mallenchollye," i.e., was stark mad. The description of his condition bears an uncanny resemblance to the paranoid schizophrenia of John Nash.

The distemper expressed itself in "very strange behavior" at the Middle Temple, which his friends attributed to overmuch study and which, shortly before the attack on Hawkins reached a stage we would consider psychotic. "He rarely slept and would pace up and down in his room, striking himself upon his breast, throwing his hands in the air, filliping with [snapping] his fingers and speaking softly to himself . . . while alone in his chamber, [he] would walk up and down reciting biblical verses and rhymes to himself, then suddenly he would race to the window. With a pointed diamond that he wore in a ring on his little finger, he would scrawl one of his own compositions upon the glass," when asked by a friend whether he was all right, he responded that "there was 'a thing at his hart wich noe man in the world showld knowe' and . . . would throw his hands in the air and use other 'frantic gestures'." To distract him, his friends took Berchet to a wedding in the country, where he proceeded to inform the bride that "she was another man's daughter, and that she had been born in London. Staring into her eyes while pounding his hands upon the table, Berchet declared that he had 'seene the verrye same eyes but not the same face,'" punctuating his "outrageous monologue . . . with unspecified but insulting gestures." Before his departure from the house of the friend with whom Berchet and his fellow students stayed in the country, he "for no apparent reason beat a young boy . . . sent to his room to build a fire" and then "came out of his room, filliping his fingers and talking very strangely, saying in a loud voice, 'watche, shall I watche hark, the wynd bloweth, but there is neither rayne, wynd, nor hayle, nor the Deuyll hym self that can feare me, for my trust is in thee Lord.'" On the way back to London his companions thought that his "head was verrye muche troubled," among other things, he "galloped away from the party, dagger in hand, determined to kill some crows that had offended him." In London, one of Berchet's friends warned him that, if he continued behaving so, "his position at the Temple would be jeopardized. Berchet reproached [the friend] and maintained that he had 'a thing at my hart which them nor anye man alyue shall knowe.' The day that Berchet performed the fateful act, he and a fellow student . . . had attended a lecture given by Puritan zealot Thomas Sampson. The lecture seemed to provide Berchet with a necessary inspiration to attack Hawkins, for later the same day [another friend] observed Berchet by peering at him through the keyhole of his room door and heard him, as he filliped with his fingers, remark, 'shall I doe it and what shall I doe it? Why? Then I will doe it.' Running quickly toward the Temple gate, Berchet hesitated for a brief moment, repeated the same words, then dashed into the Strand where he confronted Hawkins."

The outraged Queen, as mentioned above, wished Berchet to be both questioned under torture and executed immediately. Instead, following the testimony of his friends, he was committed to the Lollards Tower for his heretical beliefs, where the Bishop of London promised him that, if he recanted, he would live. Berchet recanted and was transferred to the Tower, apparently for an indefinite term of imprisonment under relatively humane conditions, to judge by the fact that the room was kept warm and had light enough, allowing his personal keeper to stand comfortably and read his Bible by the window. At this, however, Berchet took umbrage, promptly killing this innocent with a piece of firewood supplied by the charitable state. Thus, in the end, he was executed—not because his original, and, from the viewpoint of the authorities, graver, crime was attributed to madness (which, in fact, could save him), but because his madness could not be contained.

The trial of William Hacket, Edmund Coppinger, and Henry Arthington for inciting the people of London to overthrow Queen Elizabeth was among the first to call on medical men as experts and employ insanity defense as a matter of legal procedure. Hacket's declarations to the effect that he was God's confidant and "the King of Europe" as well as his utterly ineffectual directives to his two followers (whom he appointed "The Lords messenger of mercy" and "The Prophet of Gods judgements [sic] to the whole world"), all almost calculated to lead to the conspirators' immediate apprehension, create the impression that, at least in his personal case, such defense was justified. Richard Cosin, a Doctor of Law and a Member of Parliament, who published an account of the trial in 1592, was not convinced. In stating his objections to "the calumniations of such as affirme they were mad men," he offered a careful classification of mental disorders which gives a modern reader an idea of what representatives of the legal profession thought of madness in the end of the sixteenth century. Cosin wrote:

> In wants of understanding and reason there are noted divers degrees, . . . that is to say: Furor sive Rabies: Dementia sive Amentia: Insania sive Phrenesis: Fatuitas, Stultitia, Lethargia, & Delirium. And albeit the three first (by sundry writers) be sometimes confounded & taken for one . . . : yet . . . they are for the most part thus properly termed and distinguished by the best writers.
>
> Furor . . . an entire and full blindness or darkening of the understanding of the mind, whereby a man knoweth not at all, what he doeth or sayth, and is englished madnes or woodnes . . .
>
> Dementia . . . A passion of the minde, bereaving it of the light of understanding: . . . when a mans perceivance and understanding . . . is taken away, and may be englished distracted of wit, or being beside himselfe . . .
>
> Insania is . . . A kind of Inconstancie voide in deede of perfite soundnes of minde, yet such, as that he which hath it can observe and doe the common offices of his life amongs men, in some reasonable and tolerable sorte: such be all they, whome commonly wee terme either franticke, braine-sicke, cracked-witted, cocke-braines, or hare-brained men, being not altogether unapt for civill societies, or voide of understanding . . . : albeit they have many strange conceites, toying fancies, and performe sundry, rash, undiscreete, mad, and foolish parts . . .
>
> Fatuitas is the want of wit and understanding, wherewith natural fooles are possessed: But Stultitia is that follie which is seene in such, as albeit they be but simple and grosse witted, yet are not to bee accounted very Idiotes, or Naturals . . .
>
> A Lethargie is a notable forgetfulness of all things almost, that . . . commeth by some blowe, sickenes, or age.
>
> Delirium is that . . . which we call dotage: when a man, through age or infirmitie, falleth to be a childe againe in discretion . . .

It is only the two first conditions, says Cosin, that is, "Furor," "englished madnes or woodnes" and "Dementia," "englished distracted of wit," that can be used in insanity defense.

What is striking about this long excerpt in the context in which it is considered here is the extensive terminology of mental disease and the abundance of cognate vernacular words among which "madness" stands out in its equivocation and (still, in the end of the sixteenth century) novelty. To Cosin, a man who, obviously, weighs his terms and does not use them lightly, it both means something additional to "woodness" and to "folly" and does not. If it is just another, less familiar, word for furor or rabies, whether meant literally or figuratively, then why use it at all? But the fact is that "calumniators" affirmed the three men in question not furious or rabid, but mad.[51]

Sir Thomas Elyot, the author of the *Dictionary*, who, as befits a Renaissance man that he was, among other important works, also produced, in 1539, "the first manual of popular or domestic medicine in the vernacular," explored a different side of the semantic field of madness in his discussion of "affectes and passions of the mynde."[52] The gravity of such afflictions which "not onely annoye the body, & shorten the lyfe, but also . . . appaire and somtyme lose utterly a mans estimation[. A]nd . . . bringe a man from the use of reason, and sometyme in the displeasure of almighty god" discouraged their comparison to a condition of a sick dog or bull. Among mental passions (i.e., forms of suffering) Elyot emphasized not fury, recklessness, or extreme excitement to which classical medicine referred by the terms "furor" and "mania" (and which the friends of Peter Berchet saw as elements of his "nawghtye mallencholie"), but the "dolour," "sorowe," or "hevynesse of mynde," which "darkeneth the spirites, letteth the use and judgement of reason, and oppresseth memorye," a condition that we today would undoubtedly recognize as "depression" or even "depressive psychosis." Neither did he attribute this illness to "melancholic humors" (although he mentioned them), which most physicians of his time would do, but to traumatic psychological experiences, specifically death of children and—*nota bene*—disappointed ambition. "By hevynesse deth is hastened," wrote Elyot, "it hydeth vertue or strengthe, and hevynesse of harte boweth downe the necke. This is so puissant an ennemye to nature and bodily helth, that to resiste the malyce and violence thereof, are required remedies, as well of the holsome counsayles founded in holy scripture, and in the bokes of morall doctrine, as also of certayne herbes, fruites, and spyces, havynge the propretie to expelle melancolyke humours . . ." Somewhat inconsistently with the above description of the effects of depression, he then offered the following counsel, founded on holy scripture and clearly more modern "morall philosophie":

> If deathe of chylderne be cause of thy hevyness, call to thy remembrance some . . . whose lyves either for uncorrigible vices, or unfortunate chances, have ben more grievous unto theyr parents, than the death of thy children, ought to be unto the: consideringe that deth is the discharger of al griefs and myseries, and to them that dye well, the first entrie in to lyfe ever-lastynge.
>
> The losse of goodes or authoritie doo greve none but fooles, which do not marke diligently, that lyke as neyther the one nor the other doth always happen to them that are worthy, so we have in dayly experience, that they falle from him sodeynly, who in increasynge or kepynge theym semeth most busye.
>
> Oftentymes the repulse frome promotion is cause of discomforte, but than consyder, whether in the opinion of good men, thou art demed worthy to have such advauncement, or in thyne owne expectation and fantasy . . ."[53]

"Know thyself," he advised in other words, "measure thy ambition by thy worth, and do not let misfortunes which do not reflect on who you are in truth depress you."

The idea that madness was precisely the heaviness of soul of which Elyot spoke in 1539 was already around: "Gife I be sorrowfull and sad, Than will they say that I am mad," one reads in an undated poem from between 1500 and 1520 by the Scottish poet Charles Dunbar.[54] It is so obvious to us that depression is the typical mental disease that it is hard to comprehend how late this notion is, and how novel in the sixteenth century, was the experience. "Melancholy," which became the word for depression in the seventeenth century was but slowly acquiring this meaning. Originally it referred to one of the cardinal humors, or fluids, of the body, believed in classical medicine to determine both physical and mental health of a person. "It is a thing most freely agreed upon in Phisike," wrote Andre du Laurens, the royal physician in Paris in a 1597 discourse, translated into English in 1599, "that there are foure humours in our bodies, Blood, Phlegme, Choler, and Melancholie; and that all these are to bee found at all times, in every age, and at all seasons to be mixed and mingled together within the veins, though not alike much of every one . . . if blood doe abound, we call such a complexion, sanguine; if phlegme, phlegmatic; if choler, cholerike; and if melanchole, melancholike. These foure humours, if they doe not too much abound, may very easily stand with the health of the partie . . ." Melancholy, in particular, was in some ways the best humor to have in excess, for melancholics, according to du Laurens, were "accounted as most fit to undertake matters of weightie charge and high attempt. Aristotle in his Problemes sayth, that the melancholike are most wittie and ingenious . . . and when this humour growth hot, by the vapours of blood, it causeth as it were, a kinde of divine ravishment, commonly called Enthousiasma, which stirreth men up to plaie the Philosophers, Poets, and also to prophesie."[55]

By the time the book was published in France, in England the word "humor" was rapidly losing its ancient medical connotation—for which a reader of Shakespeare can indeed find numerous examples—and the concept of melancholy, therefore, was redefined as well.[56] The transformation, suggest Hunter and Macalpine, started at least half a century earlier, with the publication in 1547 and 1550, "among the earliest medical books written in English by a practicing physician" of Christopher Langton's *A very brefe treatise, orderly declaring the principal partes of phisick* . . . and *An introduction into phisycke, with an universal dyet*. In these treatises Langton argued that "the perturbations, and sudden motions of the minde" could as powerfully affect the bodily humors, as the latter were believed to affect the mind, and it was this that marked "transition towards the modern figurative sense of 'humour' as in 'ill-humoured.'" As regards melancholy, Langton still considered it to be an organic substance, therefore it does not figure in his vivid description (in the first volume) of depression, which he called simply "sorrow" and which was one of four "affections of the mynde" that could "make great alteration in all the body" and for that reason "ought not to be neclected of the phisition": "feare, Joy, angar and sorrow." Of these sorrow, clearly, presented the most serious medical problem: fear, anger, and joy were all of short duration, and, though they could change one's pulse and temperature, "sorrow," wrote Langton, "is an affection with the which ye hart as though it were smitten, is drawn together, and doth tremble and quake, not without great sense of payne: and so lyttel by lyttel whiles the sorow goeth not away, the strength of the hart, is quite overthrowen, and the generation of spirites is letted, by means whereof, the lyfe is utterly extinct: such a cruell scourge is sorrow unto man." It was its chronicity, in particular, that distinguished sorrow from other mental "affectes."

Apparently, unlike anger, fear, and joy, sorrow could be caused by bodily humors, in which case it was one of the varieties of madness—the sad madness, as demonstrated by examples from classical sources. The 1550 *Introduction into phisycke* stated: "If melancholye it selfe, without the admixtion of other humours be burned, than it maketh hym sad and solitarye, as Bellerophon, whyche as Homer sayeth, beying full of sorowe and care, forsoke all companye, and wandered in desolate feyldes solitarye al alone." In distinction, "Democritus madness was somewhat more pleasaunte, whyche laughed always at mennes folyshnes, whereby he prolonged hys lyfe an hole hundred yeres. Empedocles was so outeragious madde, that he lepte alyve in to the burnynge fyer of the hyl Ethna, but Sophocles madnes was much sweter, the whyche dyd ease the incommodities of olde age, with making of verses. Marius whan he was madde, fantasied nothing but fyghtynge. But Lucullus beying madde, was mery, full of game and sporte."[57]

It may be difficult to find a *DSM* equivalent to the life-prolonging and enhancing madness of Democritus, Sophocles, or Lucullus, or understand in which sense, given that it made people merry and increased their sense of wellness and ease, it could be considered a disorder demanding the attention of a physician. But it is clear that melancholic madness (or depression) was an organic disease.

The nature of madness, which no medical text of the period could afford to neglect, remained obscure throughout the sixteenth century, though it appears that most commonly it was identified with mania. Of course, mania was often referred to as "melancholia," as in the case of Berchet's "nawghtye" disease or other cases of "furious melancholy." Moreover, a "melancholic" was "like a huge vessel on the rolling sea. . . . .either hoist up to the ridge of a main billow or else hurried down to the bottom of the sea valley," in other words, madness was a bipolar disorder.[58] Still, however slowly, "melancholy," was becoming identified with depression, often in its psychotic mode, and as such was considered a most serious mental disease, even when those affected by it, in the language of the medic concerned, were not "mad." It is important to note that there was no term for depression in classical medicine, and that, therefore, English physicians who so well described it had to come up with new terms. Today's understanding of depression was too narrow for the sixteenth-century view of it. The author of an authoritative textbook, much used to the middle of the next century, the 1583 *Methode of phisicke, conteyning the causes, signes, and cures of inward diseases in mans body from the head to the foote*, Philip Barrough wrote of madness: "Mania in Greeke is a disease which the Latines do call Insania and furor. That is madnes and furiousness. They that have this disease be wood and unruly like wild beastes. It differeth from the frenesie, because in that there is a fever. But Mania comes without a feaver. It is caused of much bloud, flowing up to the braine ..." ..." Of melancholy, in distinction, he wrote:

> Melancholie is an alienation of the mind troubling reason, and waxing foolish, so that one is almost beside him self. It cometh without a fever, and is chiefly engendered of melancholie occupying the mind, and changing the temperature of it ... The most common signes be fearfulness, sadness, hatred, and also they that be melancholious, have straunge imaginations, for some think them selves brute beastes [or] vessels of earth, or earthen pottes, therefore they withdrawe themselves from them that they meet, lest they should knocke together. Moreover they desire death, and do verie often ... determine to kill them selves, and some feare that they should be killed. Many of them do always laugh, and many do weep, some thinck them selves inspired with the holie Ghost, and do prophecy uppon thinges to come ... [59]

A modern day psychiatrist would likely construe such "alienation of the mind" as schizoaffective disorder or even paranoid schizophrenia.

Others interpreted "melancholy" as something akin to the eighteenth-century "nervous exhaustion" or to neurasthenia, as it was originally, before being integrated in the diagnosis of depression which proved to be more popular, defined by George Beard. In scholars, it was specifically expressed in susceptibility to mental breakdown. Thomas Cogan, a physician and head master of a grammar school, was aware of that and strongly advised his charges against "studying in the night." "All wearinesse is hurtfull to health," he taught, "wearinesse of the bodie is evill, but wearinesse of the minde is worse." As a prophylactic he, like many of his contemporaries, suggested music and, which was original, also scalp massage and rubbing of teeth: "Diligent students . . . must applie themselves earnestlie to reading and meditation for the space of an houre: then to remitte a litle their cogitation, and in the meane time with an Ivorie combe to kembe their heade from the foreheade backewardes about fourty times, and to rubbe their teeth with a course linnen cloth."[60]

Still others pointed to melancholy's attacks on menopausal women. This was particularly important because it was this unfortunate class of humanity that was most commonly—and increasingly so at the time in question—accused of witchcraft. Reginald Scot, Justice of the Peace and Member of Parliament, the English counterpart of the celebrated Johann Weyer, argued in 1584 that the disease turned many of its victims delusional, likely to believe the "impossible" accusations against them, and making them often into willing accomplices of their persecutors. "[T]the force that melancholie hath," he insisted,

> and the effects that it worketh in the bodie of a man, or rather of a woman, are almost incredible. For as some of these melancholike persons imagine, they are witches and by witchcraft can worke wonders, and doo what they list: so doo other, troubled with this disease, imagine manie strange, incredible, and impossible things. . . . what is it that they will not imagine, and consequentlie confesse that they can doo; speciallie being so earnestlie persuaded thereunto, so sorelie tormented, so craftilie examined, with such promises of favour, as wherby they imagine, that they shall ever live in great credit and wealth?[61]

One does not have to be "melancholike" to confess to impossible things under torture, such confessions—as those of us who paid some attention to the twentieth century know very well—have been successfully secured even in the most rational of times. A person might also be cajoled into agreeing to quite unlikely propositions, without necessarily losing one's wits, by promises of reward. Self-delusion, a sincere belief that one is a powerful witch, is, of course, very different and does suggest a mental disease. In the nineteenth century such convictions received the name of "mania of ambition" or "delusions of grandeur" and soon after were included among the classical symptoms of schizophrenia.

The first treatise by an English physician on mental disease was called *A treatise of melancholie*.[62] This 1586 work by Timothy Bright, also an Anglican priest and the inventor of modern shorthand, was a first in many respects. It was the first to declare psychiatry the foremost medical specialty, stating that "Of all other practise of phisick, that parte most commendeth the excellency of the noble facultie, which not only releeveth the bodily infirmity, but after a sort even also correcteth the infirmities of the mind." It was the first to draw attention explicitly, yet in a matter-of-fact fashion, as if what was said was nothing new, to the proliferation of mental dysfunction in sixteenth-century England, "the dayly experience of frenzies, madnesse, lunasies, and melancholy." Above all, it was the first to focus on and offer a systematic analysis of the new form of mental illness—melancholy, which Bright equated with madness. In their comment on this text Hunter and Macalpine point to the fact that Bright distinguished two kinds of melancholy that was "similar to present-day classification of depression into reactive where the patient knows what depresses him although he cannot throw it off, and endogenous where no precipitating psychological cause is evident and which for this reason is sometimes presumed to be caused by some organic or biochemical disturbance." Bright, they argue, "made the distinction partly on clinical grounds but also to meet the theological contention that mind equated with immortal soul was incorruptible and not susceptible of disease. There was no objection to allowing the body to produce 'Perturbations and afflictions of the minde,' but where this was not so he attributed 'the mindes apprehension' to the 'heavy hande of God upon the afflicted conscience'— expressed in modern terms depression and anxiety due to guilt feelings." The intention behind this comment might have been to account for the religious interpretation of melancholy caused by the "conscience of sinne" ("reactive depression" in the parlance of 1963), perhaps seen as out of place in this truly important medical text. But it prompts one to question whether Bright actually believed in the somatic (humoral) explanation of "endogenous depression" he proposed. In any case this medic and divine was critical of judging "more basely of the soule, than agreeth with pietie or nature" and taking "all manner affection thereof, to be subject to the phisicians hand, not considering herein any thing divine, and above the ordinarie events, and naturall course of thinges," thus esteeming "the vertues them selves, yea religion, no other thing but as the body hath ben tempered, and on the other side, vice, prophanenesse, & neglect of religion and honestie,. . . . nought else but a fault of humour." Such an approach to the mind (which today would be called "neuroscientific" and which dramatically gained in popularity twenty to thirty years after the publication of Hunter's and Macalpine's priceless sourcebook) was, in Bright's view, an "absurde errour."[63]

By the time Bright wrote, "the word Melancholie" was already taken "diverslie" and, as he stressed, was subject to much confusion. "It signifieth," he argued, "either a certayne fearefull disposition of the mind altered from reason, or else humour of the body, commonly taken to be the only cause of reason by feare in such sort depraved. This humour is of two sorts: naturall, or unnaturall . . . these two . . . do ingender diversitie of passions, & according thereunto do diverslie affect the understanding, & do alter the affection, especially if by corruption of nature or evill custome of manners the partie be over passionate." This passage that, despite the characteristic spelling, seems to use English words with which we are well familiar nevertheless requires careful translation. As argued earlier, in 1586 English was in the throes of dramatic development and accelerating conceptual transformation which both reflected and was reflected not only in a massive creation of neologisms (it is remarkable how many first instances in today's vocabulary date to the late sixteenth century), but also in the very way life was experienced, one's empirical reality. The concepts with which Bright operated, and which he constructed as he employed them, are not necessarily the concepts we would use the same words to express; they are not even the concepts he always uses the same words for, a word may carry two completely different meanings (one old and one new) in the same sentence. It is important to keep in mind, for instance that "natural" means "organic" or "belonging to the body" and that, therefore, "unnatural" means "belonging to the spirit," "mental," and "supernatural," rather that what would be a common sense of the word today "abnormal" or "inhuman"; "corruption of nature," similarly, means "organic disease," not "moral abomination."[64] Consequently, "humor" is already employed in two different ways: in the traditional medical sense, and in the figurative sense of mental disposition. So is "passion"—the original and still dominant in the

1580s meaning of the word is "suffering," but it is clear that this is not the sense attributed to the term in the phrase "over passionate." Here, instead, Bright unconsciously introduces the modern concept of passion as a powerful, uncontrollable, authentic movement of the soul.

Of the natural (or endogenous) melancholy Bright writes:

> We doe see by experience certaine persons which enjoy all the comfortes of this life . . . yet to be overwhelmed with heavines, and dismaide with such feare, as they can neither receive consolation, nor hope of assurance, notwithstanding ther be neither matter of feare, or discontentment, nor yet cause of daunger, but contrarily of great comfort, and gratulation. This passion being not moved by any adversity present or imminent, is attributed to melancholie the grossest part of all the blood, either while it is yet contained in the vaines: or aboundeth in the spleen . . . surcharged therwith for want of free vent . . . [65]

That spleen "is to Malencolie Assigned for herbergerie" we read in English as early as Gower. "The spleen or mylte," explains Elyot in *The Castel of Healthe*, "is of yl juice, for it is the chamber of melancholy." This, however, does not imply that it is associated with heaviness of heart, fear, and groundless discontentment. In fact, during the period in question, the common association was of spleen with laughter and gayety. Already quoted Andrew Boorde, in his *Breviary of Health*, wrote: "A spleen . . . doth make a manne to laughe." So did Shakespeare, in *Love's Labors Lost* of 1588, then again in 1596 in *The Taming of the Shrew*, and once more in the *Twelfth Night* in 1601.[66] But Shakespeare also used "spleen" to signify the modern idea of passion, (which the word "passion" itself, as we saw above and in Bright, was only beginning hesitantly to convey); in fact, it was his preferred term for that.[67] This was a rare case in which Shakespeare's choice of words did not carry the day. "Passion" came to designate what the great poet meant by "spleen," while the "English spleen"—that national characteristic, that uniquely English property, which foreigners observed with astonishment and, in times of conceptual need, would borrow without translating— which by the second half of the seventeenth century became the vernacular term for melancholy in the sense of madness, in general, and endogenous depression, in particular, evolved out of the thinking of medical men, of whom, clearly, Bright was the foremost. This, as we shall see, profoundly affected the conception of mental illness in the next two hundred years.

Bright had anticipated the future thinking on the subject of madness and helped to form it in many ways. He wrote in continuation of the passage that suggested the connection of depression with spleen:

> Of all partes of the body, in ech perturbation, two are chiefly affected: first the brayne, that both apprehendeth the offensive or pleasaunt object, & judgeth of the same in like sort, and communicateth it with the harte, which is the second part affected: these being troubled carie with them all the rest of the partes into a sympathy, they of all the rest being in respect of affection of most importance. The humours then to worke these effectes, which approch nigh to naturall perturbations grounded upon just occasion, of necessity, alter either brayne or hart . . . if both partes be overcharged of humour, the apprehension & affection both are corrupted, and misse of their right action, and so all thinges mistaken, ingender that confused spirite, and those stormes of outrageous love, hatred, hope or fear, wherewith bodies so passionate are here and there, tossed with disquiet . . .

In mental disease, he thus gave us to understand, the body and the soul alternately affect each other: even when the ultimate cause of an illness is organic, i.e., when it proceeds from the imbalance of "humours," the effects of such a physical disturbance become indistinguishable from "naturall perturbations grounded upon just occasion," i.e. from purely mental afflictions of troubled consciousness or "reactive depression" (in this case "natural" means "obvious"), and it is this proximate cause that now affects the brain and the heart, which, in turn, interfere with perception and correct emotional reaction to environmental stimuli, throwing the individuals who suffer from such humoral disorder ("bodies so passionate") into despair. Bright's list of the forms this despair takes, "that confused spirite, and those stormes of outragious love, hatred, hope or feare," also deserves attention.[68]

Holding the Mirror Up

The *Treatise of Melancholie* was "the most representative thesis upon melancholy and insanity of the Elizabethan period."[69] It was precisely at the time of the book's composition, 1580s, that melancholy became "epidemic." It "continued for several decades. For some time melancholy men were so numerous in London that they constituted a social type, often called malcontent."[70] The "epidemic" seems to have been confined to the upper classes and affected, in particular, the intellectuals, whose numbers at that time expanded rapidly, learning being the necessary component of upward mobility. "Under Elizabeth," writes Lindsey Knights, "there had been a considerable increase of educational activity, with a consequent heightening of men's expectations. Even before the close of the sixteenth century there were more than a few who could find no definite place in the existing organization of the state . . . Contemporaries were well aware of the danger of over-education and thwarted ambition."[71] Naturally, mental trouble formed a central subject in the literature of the period—"as every student of the Elizabethan period knows. . . . Among poets, Breton, Daniel, and Campion were perhaps particularly mindful of the pathology of melancholy; among pamphleteers, Nashe in *The Terrors of the Night* drew an acute picture of the terrifying apparitions of 'fuming melancholy.'"[72] But all late Elizabethans— Camden, Chapman, Green, Harvey, Sidney, Spencer—wrote about it. This was the time of the very first bloom of what was to become one of the world's greatest literary traditions, and so, however many these writers were, it was a very small group: we know all its members by name. But this small group was, clearly, stricken by the new and incurable malaise: melancholy was "the prevailing mood with intelligent writers."[73]

From the first years of the seventeenth century, however, the preoccupation with the subject spread to the stage, so that "the great majority of the [period's] allusions to melancholy, in addition to the comparatively more important pathological studies of insanity, are quite significantly found among the dramatists, particularly in the works of Marston, Shakespeare, Tourneur, Webster, and Ford." It was the "democratic circumstance of his profession," thinks Robert Reed, which made him sensitive to the interests of the audiences, that prompted the playwright to focus so on mental disease, which suggests that by the early seventeenth century the audiences have developed such interests. That they did so, apparently, some twenty years later than those who wrote for them, in turn justifies the inference that the disease was rather rapidly percolating down through the urban population.

The use of madness on the Jacobean stage, writes Reed in the book specifically devoted to this subject, was "abnormally extensive." This was not a completely new phenomenon.

> In the latter part of the Elizabethan period, beginning with Kyd's Hieronimo, at least six well-known madmen trod the boards of the early English theaters. But as yet there was no strong indication that the portrayal of madness had become an end in itself; that is, a theatrical attraction apart from its usefulness to story and plot construction. . . . Consequently, the use of madness in drama before the time of *Hamlet* remained comparatively infrequent . . . there was no consistent effort to introduce it upon the stage. . . . Beginning with *Hamlet,* or about the year 1601, the deliberate and frequent use of insanity upon the English stage becomes increasingly apparent; more often than not, as in the 'Bedlam' scenes of *The Honest Whore* and *Northward Ho,* it was used to produce a purely theatrical spectacle.[74]

Madmen were also "quite apparently intended" as a metaphor for "human disillusionment"; they were "made to comment repeatedly on the instability of man's society," and allowed the Jacobean playwright "to express in unusually artistic terms his misgivings about the world in which he lived."[75] But the average Jacobean playwright understood madness mostly as violent mania or complete loss of reason (instead of melancholia in the sense of depression), was more likely than not to take feigned insanity for the real thing, and considered it, as did Fletcher in *The Mad Lover,* a fashion as much as (or rather than) a disease. Despite such obvious deviations from Bright's *Treatise,*

> a reasonably careful analysis of the Jacobean playwrights' pathological studies, particularly those of Shakespeare, Webster, Massinger, and Ford, indicates not only an interest in, but a professional knowledge of, contemporary psychiatry. A natural humor, usually melancholy or choler, is first of all presented; then, with the occasional exception of studies in 'love-melancholy,' some kind of devastating shock is prepared; finally, as the result of shock working upon the already aggravated humor, the unfortunate character is driven insane . . . Even Shakespeare, despite his great interpretative genius, appears markedly indebted to the current Elizabethan psychology; the undertones were Shakespeare's, but the broad outlines of

his pathological studies . . . were obviously influenced by the Elizabethan theories of mental disease.

Still, in Reed's opinion, Shakespeare had an exceptional "insight into human nature" which made his characters fit the framework of modern, namely 1952, psychology as well.[76]

Shakespeare, of course, was not an average playwright, and it is quite significant that he was the first, in *Hamlet*, to include a serious study of mental pathology in a play written for the stage. He was also the first to introduce numerous idiomatic expressions that continue to shape the way we think on the subject until today (among them, as it happens, a name for a specific form of melancholic madness, which was to become very common—"love-sickness," only later to be referred to as "love-melancholy").[77] Moreover, alone among his contemporaries, he deeply sympathized with all his mad protagonists and did not use madness for dramatic effect. But, for the first generation of professional psychiatrists in the United States in the 1840s, his contribution in this respect towered above that of all the rest, in the first place, because of the clinical accuracy of his many descriptions, which is nothing less than incredible. "The more we read Shakespeare," wrote Dr. Amariah Brigham (physicians, it seems, read Shakespeare in his time as a matter of course), "the more we are astonished; not so much at his wonderful imagination, but at the immensity and correctness of his knowledge."[78] Shakespeare's knowledge of insanity, apparently, was "great and varied" and "his views respecting it—its causes and treatment, were far, very far in advance of the age in which he lived." This made the great dramatist, in the doctor's opinion, "as great a mystery as any case of insanity—as singular an instance of variation from the ordinary standard of mental manifestation."

Two and a half centuries after Shakespeare, the first generation of American specialists on mental disease, whose theories left Elizabethan humoral disquisitions far behind, knew of it no more than he did and were painfully aware of that. Indeed, in the understanding of mental phenomena "of a pathological kind," they considered him—and only him—greatly in advance not only of the notions of his own, but even of "perhaps the present times."[79] They were all clinicians and had the proof of the validity of his insight daily in front of their eyes. "Where did Shakespeare obtain his minute and accurate knowledge of insanity?" they asked, of its causes, varieties, and treatment? Something he may have learned from books; but far more, we believe, from his own observation. He must have seen individuals affected with the various forms of insanity he has described; heard their histories and marked their conduct and conversation, or he could not have been so minutely correct.

The insane he has described . . . may now be found in every large Asylum[:] Macbeth, much of the time conversing rationally, and manifesting a most noble nature, and at other times clutching imaginary daggers, or screaming, terrified by the ghosts of the departed. . . . Hamlet; the well-bred gentleman and scholar, once the "glass of fashion and the mold of form; the observed of all observers;" whose conversation is now often instructive and interesting, but who, at other times is overwhelmed with imaginary troubles, that cause him to exclaim more frantically than Hamlet, and to our terror, "oh, that the Everlasting had not fixed his canon against self-slaughter." . . . King Lear, in a paroxysm of wrath, at some trivial occurrence, but much of the time venting all his rage upon his relations and friends, for abuse of him; and then occasionally in good humor, and conversing with much apparent satisfaction with some demented or half-idiotic patient, whom he considers a "Philosopher and most learned Theban." . . . Ophelia; past cure, past hope, with her pure mind in fragments, playing on the piano and singing songs of Moore . . .

Shakespeare must have seen Lear, and Hamlet, and Ophelia; no reading would have enabled him to have given such complete and minute histories of them, as cases of insanity. With him, however, . . . a little observation no doubt, would suffice. One visit to the Bedlam Hospital, would teach him much; for, what on other minds would have made no impression, or been immediately forgotten, was by Shakespeare treasured up, even as to the most minute particulars, and when he wished, every look, word, or action of the patient, and every idea he heard advanced by the attendants, he was able to recall.[80]

A colleague of Brigham wrote similarly:

That knowledge of insanity which is obtained by the special study of the phenomena in the galleries of a hospital, is confined to medical men, and is used for scientific rather than literary purposes. The opportunities afforded to the poet and novelist for studying this disease, are confined to the few cases that meet their observation in the ordinary walks of life, and most of whom possess an order of intellect not particularly interesting in its best estate. To seize the traits of insanity thus observed, and weave them into the tissue of a character which, with all its aberrations, shall still manifest, to a certain degree, its natural consistency and congruity, the insane bearing the impress of the sane, and each in harmony with the other, . . . —this is the work of the master mind.

Such a mind was Shakespeare's . . . His success . . . is to be attributed to that distinguishing faculty of his mind, of deducing with wonderful correctness general principles of character from the narrowest possible range of observation. . . . It is not to be supposed, however, that he was guided solely by intuition. He unquestionably did observe the insane, but he observed them as the great comparative anatomist of our age observed the remains of extinct species of animals—from one of the smallest bones, reconstructing the whole skeleton of the creature, reinvesting it with flesh and blood, and divining its manners and habits. By a similar kind of sagacity, Shakespeare, from a single trait of mental disease that he did observe, was enabled to infer the existence of many others that he did not observe, and from this profound insight into the law of psycological [sic] relations, he derived the light that observation had failed to supply.[81]

The expertise of the asylum doctors, which made them appreciate in Shakespeare an authority on their subject, may have been too new to determine the spelling of "psychology" ("psycology," "pschychology," and "psychology" were all tried), but, by the same token, they have not yet become specialized enough to stop reading—and thinking deeply—outside their field. Their broad knowledge suggested comparisons, which not only threw light on the dark recesses of their patients' minds, but, as we see here, enabled them to recognize the nature of genius. In science as in literature, the quotation above seems to suggest, genius was the imaginative ability to reach correct conclusions from but a little data, to perceive the whole picture from a few elements by understanding its organizing principle.

Because they have not yet acquired professional blinders and saw things as they were, rather than as they were presented by the reigning theory (no theories reigned in American psychiatry in its early days), it is especially valuable to read Shakespeare through the eyes of these first superintendents of insane asylums, and more informative than would be doing so through the eyes either of psychiatrists of later generations or those of literary theorists informed (or misinformed) by their views. By the end of the sixteenth century, madness as a form of human suffering was noticeably spreading in England, thus becoming, necessarily, a foundation for increasing number of social processes. Focused as he was on the inner springs of man's life, it is not surprising that Shakespeare introduced mental disease into all four of his great tragedies, whose heroes were leaders of men, and "that it was with him a favorite subject of contemplation."[82] Out of this psychiatric legacy two works attracted particular attention of the first American asylum officers: *King Lear* and *Hamlet*. It is worth our while to read them with the running commentary by Dr. Isaac Ray, the superintendent of the Butler Hospital for the Insane in Providence, RI.

To American psychiatrists of the 1840s *King Lear* represented a paradigmatic case of acute mania—i.e., florid psychosis, "that form of mental disorder in which the mind becomes, at last, completely unsettled," the play depicting the origin, development, and the end of the manic episode.[83] Although brought on by the behavior of his elder daughters, the king's madness might have been expected: Lear is already unwell in the beginning of the play, and, in the absence of the actual trigger, his trouble would have been developed by another exciting cause. It is the Earl of Kent who first suggests this, when the old king—in the very first scene of act one—divides his kingdom and disinherits his favorite child for being honest. At Kent's advice, "in thy best consideration check this hideous rashness," the king flies into a rage, Kent is banished, the King of France leaves in dismay with Cordelia, and the kingdom is divided between Goneril and Regan. The sisters' dialogue with which scene one ends makes it clear that they have been aware of Lear's strange behavior for some time and are unwilling to excuse it.

> GON. You see how full of changes his age is; the observation we have made
> of it hath not been little: he always loved our sister most; and with what
> poor judgment he hath now cast her off appears too grossly.
> REG. 'Tis the infirmity of his age, yet he hath ever but slenderly known
> himself.

GON. The best and soundest of his time hath been but rash; then must we look to receive from his age not alone the imperfections of long-engrafted condition, but therewithal the unruly waywardness that infirm and choleric years bring with them. . . . Pray you, let us hit together: if our father carry authority with such dispositions as he bears, this last surrender of his will but offend us.

When we next meet Goneril in scene three, her father had just struck her gentleman for chiding of his fool. She reacts angrily:

By day and night he wrongs me; every hour / He flashes into one gross crime or other, / That sets us all at odds. I'll not endure it . . . Idle old man / That still would manage those authorities / That he hath given away!— Now, by my life, / Old fools are babes again; and must be us'd / With checks as flatteries . . .

Dr. Ray thinks Goneril and Reagan "heartless," but not evil. They are ordinary people, i.e., self-centered and self-interested, not particularly sensitive to others and not sympathetic to others' suffering, not naturally grateful or sincere, considering expressions of gratitude good form and sincerity a sign of stupidity. They believe their father's generosity their due, especially as he, in their opinion, is unfit to rule in any case, and feel imposed upon by his demand that they pay for their freely given inheritance by taking care of him and keeping his retinue. Irritated to the limits of her patience (which could be expected of any ordinary human being whose life is disrupted by an elderly parent in the stage of incubation of a mental disease, remarks our physician attending from beyond the Atlantic and a gap of 250 years), Goneril becomes reproachful. And Dr. Ray writes:

were Lear not already ill, he would have acknowledged the justice of the reproof. As it is . . . he attributes the whole of it to her, flies into a passion, pours upon her head the bitterest curses, upbraids her with the vilest ingratitude, and forthwith proclaims his wrongs to the public ear. Like most cases of this kind in real life, it would have, to a stranger, the appearance of a family quarrel springing from the ordinary motives of interest or passion, but where, really, the ill regulated conduct resulting from the first influences of disease, provokes restrictions more or less necessary and appropriate, that become exciting causes of farther disorder. Another life-like touch is given to the picture, in Lear's attributing all his troubles to filial ingratitude . . . In fact, nothing is more common than for the patient when telling his story, to fix upon some event, and especially, some act of his friends, as the cause of his troubles, which occurred long subsequently to the real origin of his disorder, and might have had but an accidental connection with it.

To Lear's daughters, he continues, their conduct "may not have appeared like unmitigated ingratitude towards a father who had loved and cherished them . . . but to be founded on provocation that seemed to justify their behavior . . . It is fearful to think how often the case of Lear and his daughters is paralleled in actual life . . ."

As it happens, Goneril, in her heartless ordinariness and misunderstanding of her father's condition, propels him to the next stage of his disease. Possibly, he begins to doubt his identity, "Does any here know me?—This is not Lear: / Does Lear walk thus? speak thus? / Where are his eyes? / Either his notion weakens, his discernings / are lethargied.—Ha! Waking? 'tis not so.—/ Who is it that can tell me who I am?" Certainly, he can no longer listen to reason. When the Duke of Albany, Goneril's husband, protests ignorance of what provoked Lear's outburst, which happens to be true, the old king accuses him of lying. At the same time he is becoming aware that his mind is not right. "O most small fault," he cries to Goneril,

> How ugly did'st thou in Cordelia show! / Which, like an engine, wrench'd my frame of nature / From the fixed place; drew from my heart all love, / And added to the gall. O Lear, Lear, Lear! / Beat at this gate, that let thy folly in / And thy dear judgment out!" [A stage direction indicates: "striking his head." And, as he leaves Goneril's court, he pleads] O, let me not be mad, not mad, sweet heaven! / Keep me in temper: I would not be mad!

Regan surpasses her sister in cruelty. Forewarned by Goneril, she leaves her house where Lear expects to be comforted for what he suffered in his

elder daughter's home, retires to Gloster's castle and there puts Lear's messenger in the stocks. The old king is smitten by this affront and can hardly
believe it: "They durst not do't. / They could not, would not do't; 'tis worse
than murder, / To do upon respect such violent outrage . . ." This makes
him physically ill. The symptoms may be those of an impending heart
attack, but the diagnosis would satisfy a psychoanalyst. "O, how this mother
swells up towards my heart!" exclaims Lear, "Hysterica passio,—down,
thou climbing sorrow, / Thy element's below!" and then again: "O, me, my
heart, my rising heart!—but, down!" Humiliations to which he is subjected
are too much for him. When both his daughters insist that they would willingly take care of him, but don't wish to support his retinue in which he has
no need, he explodes: "O, reason not the need"; it is not his body, but the
respect of his person that they deny him. He flies into a rage, then begs: "I
pr'ythee, daughter, do not make me mad," tries to keep himself from
bursting into tears, flies into a rage again, finally exclaims, addressing the
one forever loyal—and completely unable to protect him—creature by his
side, his fool "O, fool, I shall go mad," rushes out, and goes mad.

Act three opens with the scene on the heath during the storm. A gentleman, met by Kent, answers his question, where's the king?

> Contending with the fretful elements; / Bids the wind blow the earth into
> the sea, / Or swell the curled waters 'bove the main, / That things might
> change or cease; tears his white hair . . . / Strives in his little world of man
> to out-scorn / The to-and-fro conflicting wind and rain. / This night, wherein
> the cub-drawn bear would couch, / The lion and the belly-pinched wolf /
> Keep their fur dry, unbonneted he runs, / And bids what will take all.

Kent interposes: "But who is with him?" to which the gentleman replies:
"None but the fool; who labours to out-jest / His heart-struck injuries."
We then see Lear and the Fool. Lear adjures the forces of nature—
addressing them in all seriousness—to destroy whatever in the world
makes man "ingrateful," his daughters' ingratitude becoming a fixed idea
with him as the source of all evil. He reasons with the elements:

> I tax not you, you elements, with unkindness; / I never gave you kingdom,
> call'd you children; / You owe me no subscription: then let fall / Your

horrible pleasure; here I stand, your slave, / A poor, infirm, weak, and despis'd old man:—/ But yet I call you servile ministers, / That will with two pernicious daughters join / Your high-engender'd battles 'gainst a head / So old and white as this. O! O! 'tis foul!

All this time the Fool, like a dog who feels without understanding the full measure of his master's distress, is scampering around, trying to distract Lear's attention with his silly jokes and ditties. "My wits begin to turn," says Lear, but, when Kent suggests they seek cover in a hovel nearby, still feels enough sympathy and responsibility for that defenseless creature, entirely dependent on him, as to suggest: "Come on, my boy: how dost, my boy? Art cold? / I am cold myself. . . . / Poor fool and knave, I have one part in my heart / That's sorry yet for thee."

Kent leads them to the hovel and urges Lear to enter. Lear answers, reasonably:

> Thou think'st 'tis much that this contentious storm / Invades us to the skin: so 'tis to thee / But where the greater malady is fix'd, / The lesser is scarce felt. Thou'dst shun a bear; / But if thy flight lay toward the roaring sea, / Thou'dst meet the bear i' the mouth. When the mind's free / The body's delicate: the tempest in my mind / Doth from my senses take all feeling else / Save what beats there—Filial ingratitude! [returning to his fixed idea] / Is it not as this mouth should tear this hand / For lifting food to't?—But I will punish home:—[getting enraged again] / No, I will weep no more. In such a night / To shut me out!—Pour on; I will endure:—/ In such a night as this! O Regan, Goneril!—/ Your old kind father, whose frank heart gave all,—/ [And here he stops himself, sensing a point of no return] O, that way madness lies; let me shun that; / No more of that . . .

Still reluctant to enter, he remembers the Fool and interrupts himself in midphrase: "But I'll go in.—/ In, boy; go first [to the Fool].—You, house-less poverty,—/ Nay, get thee in." Here we have Dr. Ray's commentary:

> Unable as the insane are to perceive their own insanity, yet this apprehension of its approach so frequently repeated by Lear usually occurs during its incubation. While still able to control his mental manifestations, the patient

is tortured with anticipations of insanity, but when he actually becomes so insane, that the most careless observer perceives the fact, then he entertains the most complacent opinion of his intellectual vigor and soundness. And yet this is one of the nicer traits of insanity which the ordinary observer would hardly be supposed to notice. But Shakespeare was no ordinary observer . . .

In the hovel they encounter Edgar, the framed and persecuted son of the Earl of Gloster, disguised as a madman. Earlier (in act two, scene three) Edgar decides to feign madness to escape his enemies: "I will preserve myself," he says

and am bethought / To take the basest and most poorest shape / That ever penury, in contempt of man, / Brought near to beast: my face I'll grime with filth; / Blanket my loins; elf all my hair in knots; / And with presented nakedness outface / The winds and persecutions of the sky. / The country gives me proof and precedent / Of Bedlam beggars, who, with roaring voices, / Strike in their numb'd and mortified bare arms / Pins, wooden pricks, nails, sprigs of rosemary; / And with this horrible object, from low farms, / Poor pelting villages, sheep-cotes, and mills, / Sometime with lunatic bans, sometime with prayers, / Enforce their charity.—Poor Turlygod! Poor Tom!

In addition to giving us a picture which is worth a thousand words of the absolute, heart-wrenching misery of the deinstitutionalized mentally ill, quieted down by the judiciously administered whipping and starvation and released, often with the license to beg, into the community—Toms o'Bedlam—Edgar, in deciding on his disguise, underscores the commonness of madness in England of his creator's time. Toms o'Bedlam must be a normal part of the landscape to offer a fugitive the best means to avoid attention.

On seeing Edgar, Lear immediately takes to him. His own mental affliction makes the old King recognize in him a comrade in misfortune. "Did thou give all to thy daughters," he asks with sympathy, "And art thou come to this?" Edgar's gibberish serves to confirm the king in his mad supposition. He goes on, vehemently:

What, have his daughters brought him to this pass?—/ Couldst thou save nothing? Didst thou give 'em all? / . . . Now, all the plagues that in the pendulous air / Hang fated o'er men's faults light on thy daughters! [Kent interposes: He hath no daughters, sir. And Lear replies:] Death, traitor! Nothing could have subdu'd nature / To such a lowness but his unkind daughters.—/ Is it a fashion that discarded fathers / Should have thus little mercy on their flesh? / Judicious punishment! 'twas this flesh begot / Those pelican daughters.

Edgar continues to do his best in making no sense at all, which provokes Lear to call him a "noble philosopher," "learned Theban," and "good Athenian" and prompts him to strike a conversation on urgent questions such as "What is the cause of thunder?" Later, in the farmhouse, where he is led by Gloster, he imagines sitting in trial over Goneril and Regan, in which Edgar plays the role of a "most learned justicer." At this advanced stage, even his fool appears to Lear a "sapient sir." (When the imaginary Goneril is arraigned, the Fool, always willing to play along with his master and always sincere, exclaims: "Cry you mercy, I took you for a jointstool.") The imaginary court allows the imaginary Goneril to escape. The king then changes Edgar's employment, saying: "You, sir, I entertain you for one of my hundred; only I do not like the fashion of your garments: you will say they are Persian; but let them be changed."

The scene on the heath between Lear, Edgar, and the fool inspires a long set of professional comments from our attending American physician:

No less a genius than Shakespeare's would have ventured to bring together, face to face, three such difficult characters,—one actually mad, one falsely pretending to be so, and the third a fool; . . . yet who can finish this scene, without feeling that he has read a new chapter in the history of mental disease . . . ? . . . Thus far the progress of Lear's insanity is represented with the closest fidelity to nature. It is not more different from the disease as daily observed, than Lear's moral and intellectual constitution, when in health, was different from ordinary men's. At every interview reason has seemed to have lost somewhat of its control; the mental excitement has been steadily increasing, until now having reached its height, he is singing, dancing and capering through the fields, fantastically decorated with weeds and flowers, looking, acting and talking like a madman. His perceptive organs are deceived by hallucinations, and his discourse . . . is full of incoherence and incongruity. . . . he is now what is called raving. In the representation of this condition, we have another instance of Shakespeare's unrivalled powers of observation. To ordinary apprehension, the raving of a maniac, is but an arbitrary jumble of words and phrases between which no connecting threads can be discerned. But in fact, discordant and heterogeneous as they may appear, they are nevertheless, subjected to a certain law of association, difficult as it may be frequently to discover it. . . . In consequence of the cerebral excitement, impressions long since made—so long perhaps as to have been forgotten previous to the attack—are so vividly and distinctly recalled, that they appear to be outward realities . . . the impressions are actually considered to be what they appear, and the patient thinks and discourses about them as such. In his mind's eye he sees sights, and in his mind's ear he hears sounds, imperceptible to others, and this is the source of much of our difficulty in discovering the object and the relevancy of his remarks. . . . past scenes and associations are recalled in all their original freshness, suggesting thoughts to which he alone possesses the clew [sic]. The images raised in the mind by this morbid excitement, are also rapidly changing, thus giving to the thoughts that phantasmagoric character by which they are so distinguished in mania. They seem to be suggested and associated very much as they are in ordinary dreaming in which the mind is occupied with impressions previously made, and uncontrolled by that regulating principle necessary to give them logical sequence and cohesion. In sleep the person we are addressing, for instance, unaccountably changes into some other; the scene in which we are engaged suddenly vanishes away, and another appears in its place; the powers of memory are endowed with an energy seldom witnessed in the waking state; the relations of space, of time . . . are . . . embroiled; the living and the dead, the near and remote, wisdom and folly, stand side by side, and no sense of the strange combination is perceived. We may strive perhaps, to believe it a dream, but with some few exceptions, we strive in vain. Precisely so it is in mania which may, with some propriety, be designated as dreaming with the senses all open . . .

Another source of our difficulty in discovering the filiation of the maniac's thoughts, has been generally overlooked. . . . The maniac, being

restrained by no sense of propriety or fitness of things, expresses every
thought that enters his mind, . . . is governed by no principle of selection.
In the sound mind . . . a considerable portion of the thoughts never find
utterance in words, being suppressed from their want of connexion with
one another, or their irrelevancy to the subject in hand. Every one must be
aware how often, in the course of ordinary conversation, thoughts start up
having the remotest possible connection with anything already said—so
remote indeed as to defy any one but himself to discover it. Any person who
should utter every thought that arose in his mind, in the freest possible
conversation, would most certainly be taken for a fool or a maniac. . . . we
readily see how there should always be some method in madness, however
wild and furious it may be; some traces of that delicate thread which though
broken in numerous points, still forms the connecting link between many
groups and patches of thought. It is in consequence of Shakespeare's knowledge of this psycological [sic] law, that in all his representations of madness,
even though characterized by wildness and irregularity, we are never at a
loss to perceive that the disease is real, and not assumed.

It is different with most writers, he continues: they share the popular misconceptions of madness and, in their misunderstanding, imagine mad talk
as purely meaningless. Thus their representations of madness at best
resemble attempts at feigning it (such as Edgar's), both because those who
feign it share the same misunderstanding and because, if they are unusually astute, they know what those whom they mean to deceive expect.
Lear's behavior when "stark mad," in distinction to such ignorant depictions, still shows the workings of the same mind, deformed, fissured, and
contorted as if seen through a broken lens, but still the same mind. He,
says Dr. Ray, "is solely occupied with images formed under the influence
of the intense excitement of the internal perceptive organs" and so first
imagines himself in a battle, then in sports; something suggests a thought
of Goneril, this leads to the white beard, flattery of courtiers, his seeing
through it. Gloster's recognition of the king's voice near Dover bring back
Lear's experiences of his kingship and they, step by understandable step,
move him to discourse cogently on the vices of contemporary society. His
thoughts are out of control of his will; his mind is sick, but not weak: and,

as Edgar notes, matter and impertinency mix in his talk and there is reason in his madness.

Shakespeare's treatment of Edgar's feigned madness, equally accurate in Dr. Ray's opinion, serves to underscore "the real madness of Lear." Juxtaposing the actual disease and the pretense of it, Shakespeare not only makes unmistakable his understanding of mental illness, but also demonstrates his awareness of the common misconception of its nature. The character of the Fool, which shows that the sixteenth-century poet's "observation of mental impairment was not confined to one or a few of its forms" and that, in regard to idiocy as well he "knew what is not generally known even now," is also used as a contrast to Lear. (In this context it is worth noting, as does Winfred Overholser, a psychologist writing another century later, that Shakespeare used fools, but not madmen, for comic relief.[84]) Indeed, Shakespeare drew a sharp distinction between natural folly, or idiocy, and madness. The former made one less human, in the sense of obliterating some of the characteristics that distinguished man from animals (though not in the sense of being "worse" or even "worse off" than human: fools knew no malice and were immune to humiliation), while the latter was an emphatically human reality: the disease peculiar to man and tied inseparably to human social experience and relations.[85]

The madness of the Prince of Denmark necessarily brings us back to the question of feigned madness. Hamlet's derangement has been often—for a long period, universally—regarded as feigned.[86] The sage Dr. Johnson, otherwise an astute observer of insanity, in fact, saw in "the pretended madness" of Hamlet a "cause of much mirth." Most of those who subscribed to this diagnosis until the twentieth century were literary critics. Dr. Ray disputed even the textual reasons for it:

> Aside from [Hamlet's] own intimation after meeting the ghost, that he might "put an antic disposition on," it is difficult to conceive of any foundation for this opinion. . . . this notion has been handed down . . . from one critic to another . . . in the very face of the fact, that Hamlet's insanity which is supposed to be assumed for the purpose of concealing his plans, immediately excites the apprehensions of the king, and leads to his own banishment from the state. True, it is supposed to answer another purpose—

that of enabling him to break off his attachment with Ophelia, which the dread mission he had to perform forbade him any longer to entertain. But the necessity of this step is unsupported by a single proof. No intimation of it is given in the course of the play, and it has no foundation in the nature of things.

The play offered, he insisted, "the most faithful delineation of a disordered mind," with Hamlet's condition "often manifested under circumstances that forbid the idea of simulation." Nothing but insufficient knowledge of the nature of mental disease could account for the critics' interpretation; and, although, in years previous to his essay, psychiatry garnered sufficient authority to oppose it, "it could not be expected that the deductions of science would universally prevail against critical theories." Hamlet's madness could not be reconciled with popular prejudice, which the critics shared.

> They . . . are reluctant to attribute so sad and humbling an incident as madness to such a noble and elevated character. His profound speculations on the purposes of life and his solemn questioning of its meaning, the pertinency of his replies, the exquisite wit and wisdom of his discourse, the sagacity and forecast displayed in his plans, the true nobility of his nature,— all forbid the idea of madness. These persons embrace the popular error of regarding madness as but another name for confusion and violence, overlooking the daily fact that it is compatible with some of the ripest and richest manifestations of the intellect.[87]

"In plain terms," he concluded, "Shakespeare's science of human nature is more profound than that of his critics." Not only did Hamlet's insanity display all the pathological and psychological symptoms of the condition "in wonderful harmony and consistency," it furnished the only explanation for otherwise inexplicable conduct and for "the leading principle of the play." It explained, most notably, how a character otherwise so resolute and quick in action, turns vacillating and indecisive precisely when it comes to his self-imposed duty as the avenger of his father. If "he evinces great infirmity of purpose in regard to the great mission assigned to him," says Dr. Ray, "it is because a will sufficiently strong and determined by nature, has been paralyzed by mental disease. . . . While his whole soul is occupied with the idea of revenge, he is ever finding excuses for postponing the moment of execution,—constantly turned from his purpose by the merest whim, and justifying his conduct by reasons too flimsy to satisfy any but a disordered intellect. Such is the nature of insanity,—to talk, but not to act; to resolve, but never to execute; to support the soundest projects for action, by the most imperfect performance." He adds in a footnote: "It is, perhaps, not generally known how common is this effect of insanity, to enfeeble the resolution and break the force of will, and that to an extent that would be incredible were it not a matter of frequent observation."

Hamlet's madness differs from Lear's: rather than express itself in acute mania, it takes the form of depression. He shows signs of it from the start, with his first appearance in the play. The Queen, his mother, remarks on the unusual duration and power of his grief: "Thou know'st 'tis common,— all that live must die, / . . . Why seems it so particular with thee?" He responds:

> Seems, Madam! nay, it is; I know not seems. / 'Tis not alone my inky cloak, good mother, / . . . Nor the dejected 'havior of the visage, / Together with all forms, modes, shows of grief, / That can denote me truly: these, indeed, seem, / For they are actions that a man might play: / But I have that within me which passeth show; / These but the trappings and the suits of woe.

Already then he is weary of life and entertains thoughts of suicide:

> O, that this too too solid flesh would melt, / Thaw, and resolve itself into a dew! / Or that the Everlasting had not fix'd / His canon 'gainst self-slaughter! O God! O God! / How weary, stale, flat, and unprofitable / Seem to me all the uses of this world! / Fie on't! O fie! 'tis an unweeded garden / That grows to seed; things rank and gross in nature / Possess it merely.

("Shakespeare has here evinced his usual fidelity to nature, in attributing to Hamlet sentiments that are entertained by almost every person whose insanity is accompanied by melancholy views," comments Dr. Ray.) This consideration of the ephemeral value of everything in life leads the prince to think of his mother's unseemly haste in remarrying: it has been but two months since his father's death and already a month since the Queen's remarriage to his uncle. It is this that rankles Hamlet most: the impropriety of his mother's conduct—it is not how it should have been, if one believed in love and the possibility of finding it in a woman. But Hamlet is in love: he loves Ophelia; his father's death and his mother's remarriage so soon after it undermine much more of his world than immediately meets the eye.

Already depressed severely enough to become suicidal, Hamlet meets the ghost of his father. Horatio who has seen the ghost before is suspicious lest the apparition lure the prince away from his friends and then "assume some other horrible form, / Which might deprive your sovereignty [Hamlet's self, mind, that is] of reason, / And draw you into madness?" That a shock may drive one mad is, apparently, a common notion. But Hamlet wouldn't be deterred: life is already without value for him and he is not afraid for his immortal soul. Besides, though he may not know it, he is already mad. The ghost, who turns out to be an honest one, that is, the true ghost of Hamlet's father, appraises Hamlet of the "foul and most unnatural murder," committed by his uncle, who at once dispatched his father "of life, of crown, of queen," sending him to face his judgment unabsolved and thus making it impossible for his soul to rest in peace, demands revenge, but urges him not to taint his mind or let his soul contrive anything against his mother. Hamlet resolves and swears to obey, even recording this in his notebook. His friends then find and question him about the interview. Hamlet's answers, his "wild and whirling words" are diagnosed by Ray as "the excitement of delirium,—the wandering of a mind reeling under the first stroke of disease." They may also reflect an agitation quite understandable under the circumstances: a person in the best of mental health would be profoundly shaken by the meeting with the ghost of a beloved and mourned father, even without being told that the father was murdered by the uncle who is now married to one's mother and holds the father's position, or by such a revelation, even if not made by a ghost.

The conclusion of Hamlet's conversation with his friends about the ghost is perfectly lucid. His mentioning the possibility that he might "put an antic disposition on," which has so often been interpreted as proof of Shakespeare's intention to have his hero feign madness, is certainly a proof of his lucidity at this moment and would be so, even if "antic" were used, as it probably was, without any reference to madness.[88] He enjoins his friends never to speak about what they saw to anyone. When Horatio exclaims, that "this is wondrous strange!" Hamlet answers:

> There are more things in heaven and earth, Horatio, / Than are dreamt in your philosophy. But come;—/ Here, as before, never, so help you mercy, / How strange or odd soe'er I bear myself,—/ As I, perchance, hereafter shall think meet / To put an antic disposition on, / That you, at such times seeing me, never shall, / With arms encumber'd thus, or this head-shake, / Or by pronouncing of some doubtful phrase, . . . / Or such ambiguous giving out, to note / That you know aught of me:—this not to do, / So grace and mercy at your most need help you, / Swear.

They swear, and he says: "The time is out of joint:—O cursed spite, / That ever I was born to set it right!"

Hamlet's condition does, however, deteriorate after that. We know this from Ophelia's report of his visit to her, as she is "sewing in her chamber":

> Lord Hamlet,—with his doublet all unbrac'd; / No hat upon his head; his stockings foul'd, / Ungarter'd, and down-gyved to his ancle; / Pale as his shirt; his knees knocking each other; / And with a look so piteous in pur-port / As if he had been loosed out of hell / To speak of horrors,—he comes before me . . . He took me by the wrist, and held me hard; / Then goes to the length of all his arm; / And with his other hand thus o'er his brow, / He falls to such perusal of my face / As he would draw it. Long stay'd he so; / At last,—a little shaking of mine arm, / And thrice his head thus waving up and down,—/ He rais'd a sigh so piteous and profound / That it did seem to shatter all his bulk / And end his being . . .

This visit, in the course of which Hamlet says not a word, is immediately interpreted by Polonius as love-madness: the explanation seems natural, especially since he had commanded his daughter to repel Hamlet's advances, and Ophelia dutifully obeyed. Could he have feigned it? Dr. Ray thinks not. And, indeed, even if appearing in front of a girl whose chastity he cherishes with his stockings ungartered would be consistent with a character such as this, unless genuinely mad, Hamlet would have to be a consummate actor to make himself pale as his shirt. It is not, as we know, Ophelia's sudden coldness that made him mad, but the fact that the diagnosis makes perfect sense to both the father and the daughter, and later to the Queen and, to some extent, the King as well, is indicative of the frequency with which it must have been met in 1602.[89] And that Shakespeare believed that love-madness was real and common and a disastrous disease is proven by his decision to make Ophelia, blameless but blaming herself for driving Hamlet mad, succumb to and die from it.

The King and Queen commission Rosencrantz and Guildenstern, he to get to the root of Hamlet's distemper, she to help him. Hamlet suspects that these old schoolmates of his were especially sent for, but describes his condition honestly to them, without any silliness and exaggerations necessary to make his madness obvious to the uninitiated, which is what he would have done, if it was feigned. In fact, while he feels ill, he says openly that he does not believe he is mad:

> I have of late,—but wherefore I know not,—lost all my mirth, forgone all custom of exercises; and, indeed, it goes so heavily with my disposition, that this goodly frame, the earth, seems to me a sterile promontory; this most excellent canopy, the air, look you, this brave o'erhanging firmament, this majestical roof fretted with golden fire,—why, it appears no other thing to me than a foul and pestilent congregation of vapors. What a piece of work is man! How noble in reason! . . . the beauty of the world! The paragon of animals! And yet, to me, what is this quintessence of dust? Man delights not me; no, nor woman neither . . . my uncle-father and aunt-mother are deceived . . . I am but mad north-north-west when the wind is southerly I know a hawk from a handsaw.

"A most faithful and vivid picture is this," runs Dr. Ray's commentary,

> of a mental condition that is the precursor of decided insanity. . . . In Hamlet the disease has not yet proceeded so far as to prevent him, in his calmer moments, from recognizing and deploring its existence, though he mistakes its character. Like every other person in his condition, he is very far from considering himself insane, and indeed there is no reason why he

should. He entertains no delusions; persons and things appear to him in their customary relations; and for the most part he well sustains his character as a man and a prince. His unwonted excitability of temper, his occasional disregard of some minor propriety of life, the cloud which envelops all outward things, depriving them of their worth and beauty,—in the eyes of the world, these do not constitute insanity, and are not incompatible with the most perfect integrity of intellect. Why then should he suppose himself insane, or beginning to be so? Such a mistake is very natural to the patient . . .

And yet, Hamlet is already in the grip of the disease. His duty weighs heavily on him, yet, inexplicably, he cannot make himself act: his will is paralyzed. Passion displayed by a traveling actor arrived at Elsinore on his request for a demonstration makes him doubt himself, consider himself a coward, finally argue himself into believing his procrastination necessary because the ghost, after all, could have been a fake and his version of the events needs to be confirmed:

O, what a rogue and peasant slave am I!/Is it not monstrous that this player here,/But in a fiction, in a dream of passion,/Could force his soul so to his own conceit/That from her working all his visage wan'd . . . And all for nothing! . . . What would he do,/Had he the motive and the cue for passion/That I have? He would drown the state with tears,/And cleave the general ear with horrid speech; Make mad the guilty, and appal the free;/Confound the ignorant, and amaze, indeed, /The very faculty of eyes and ears. Yet I,/A dull and muddy-mettled rascal, peak,/Like John-a-dreams, unpregnant of my cause,/And can say nothing; no, not for a king/Upon whose property and most dear life/A damn'd defeat was made. Am I a coward?/Who calls me villain?breaks my pate across?/Plucks off my beard and blows it in my face?/Tweaks me by the nose? Gives me the lie i' the throat,/As deep as to the lungs? who does me this, ha?/'Swounds, I should take it: for it cannot be/But I am pigeon-liver'd, and lack gall/To make oppression bitter; . . . Why, what an ass am I! . . . A scullion! Fie upon't! foh! [He resolves to make the players play something like the murder of his father before his uncle—to observe whether he would flinch; then he would know that the ghost was telling the truth.] The spirit that I have seen/May be the devil: and the devil hath power/To assume a pleasing shape; yea, and perhaps/Out of my weakness and my melancholy,—/As he is very potent with such spirits,—/Abuses me to damn me: I'll have grounds/More relative than this:—the play's the thing/Wherein I'll catch the conscience of the king.

Excited by the prospect, he loses the power over himself, his emotional reactions become inadequate and he no longer controls what he says. His thoughts, in the famous soliloquy, again turn to suicide. In this state he meets Ophelia, sent to ascertain that what he suffers from is indeed "the affliction of his love," a task she hopes to accomplish by returning his gifts and thus provoking him to reassert his feelings. Instead, within a moment he grows suspicious (for, in his madness, he loses nothing of his keen intelligence) erupts in anger against the falseness of the entire world, and rather peremptorily sends her to a nunnery. Poor girl, clearly very much in love herself with the handsome, charming prince, "the expectancy and rose of the fair state, the glass of fashion and the mould of form, the observ'd of all observers" and so much above her station in life, is overwhelmed with the change in his affections and crushed with guilt: "And I, of ladies most deject and wretched/That suck'd the honey of his music vows,/Now see that noble and most sovereign reason,/Like sweet bells jungled, out of tune and harsh;/That unmatch'd form and feature of blown youth/Blasted with ecstasy: O, woe is me . . ." This will eventually drive her mad too.

When, after the king storms out during the play, proving the ghost true, and he is summoned to his mother, Hamlet attempts his utmost to control himself: "O heart, lose not thy nature; let not ever/The soul of Nero enter this firm bosom:/Let me be cruel, not unnatural:/I will speak daggers to her, but use none." He needs all the power remaining to his will to keep this resolve, especially after the additional shock of discovering spying Polonius in her room and killing him. His mother is unaware of her second husband's crime and is herself uneasy about her quick remarriage: she recognizes the truth in Hamlet's lacerating words and pleads with him: "O, speak to me no more; . . . no more, sweet Hamlet." And at this moment his thinking turns delusional: he sees the ghost of his father where, unlike in Act one, there is no ghost and talks to him. The Queen, observing her son hallucinating, concludes: "Alas, he's mad!" Hamlet hears the ghost remind him that his quarrel is not with his mother, who, rather, deserves his gentleness and protection, and asks, obligingly: "How is it with you, lady?" The Queen returns, terrified: Alas, how is't with you?/That you do bend your eyes on vacancy,/And with the incorporal air do hold discourse?/ Forth at your eyes your spirits wildly peep,/And as the sleeping soldiers in the alarm,/Your bedded hair, like life in excrements,/Starts up and stands on end. O gentle son,/Upon the heat and flame of thy distemper/Sprinkle cool patience. Whereon do you look?" Hamlet is convinced that the ghost is real and answers: "On him, on him! Look you, how pale he glares! . . ." then turns to the ghost and begs: "Do not look upon me;/Lest with this piteous action you convert/My stern effects . . ." He cannot believe that his mother does not see and hear the ghost as well as himself. There is no suspicion at all in him that he may be hallucinating; instead, he is certain that it is she who is delusional, her bad conscience blinding her to reality:

> *Queen:* This is the very coinage of your brain: This bodiless creation ecstasy/ Is very cunning in. *Hamlet:* Ecstasy!/My pulse, as yours, doth temperately keep time,/And makes as healthful music: [he offers, quite reasonably and in accord with the prevailing medical theory] It is not madness/That I have utter'd; bring me to the test,/And I the matter will re-word; which mad-ness/Would gambol from. Mother, for love of grace,/Lay not that flattering unction to your soul,/That not your trespass, but my madness speaks. . . . Confess yourself to heaven; Repent what's past . . .

"O Hamlet, thou have cleft my heart in twain," says the Queen: she has just seen the proof of her son's far-gone madness; she is a loving mother: obviously, she is heart-broken. But he takes it for a sign of the repentance he demands. He gives her some more good advice, grows softer: "I must be cruel only to be kind." And then he asks her to reveal to the king that he is only pretending madness, but is not mad in fact.

The last two acts of this magnificent play offer us no new clinical mate-rial insofar as Hamlet is concerned. We see him again blame himself for inaction and worthlessness, again lose control over his conduct in public and give way to an emotional outburst in the course of which he further insults Laertes, which he then sincerely regrets, begging Laertes to attri-bute it to his madness, his not being himself. Dr. Ray finds this attribution strange, for it is exceptionally rare for a delusional patient to recognize his madness, and yet, Shakespeare is never wrong in his descriptions of mental pathology. It is likely, however, that Hamlet's apology to Laertes reflects not at all such recognition, but, rather, his conscious use of the widespread opinion that he is mad (which he earlier asked his mother to affirm and spread). In the end, it seems, we find Hamlet in a lucid interval.

Both Lear and Hamlet die, and, in general, the format of a play would not allow emphasis on the most distinctive characteristic of madness—its chronicity. Was Shakespeare aware that there was a difference between madness and other forms of mental disease or was it, by the end of the sixteenth century already obscured by its assimilation into medicine? Early American psychiatrists believed that he shared their notion that "insanity is a disease of the brain" which could be cured by medical means[90]—an opinion which would not be strange at all in Shakespeare's time, if one considered madness as one of its forms, since this was the prevailing medical view, the universal application of which to all forms of the disease already Bright felt called upon to dispute. However that may be, it is extremely important that asylum superintendents of the 1840s found in Shakespeare what they saw in their clinical practice. Mental disease that they in the great majority of cases attempted to treat and contain in their hospitals was the madness he represented in his plays. It was not triggered by an observable physical disease (though physical symptoms such as rapid pulse or paleness could accompany it), and was radically different from natural folly or idiocy. It rarely affected intelligence, but deranged people's thinking, confused their emotions, and disordered their behavior. They could not control their reactions, flying into rage at the slightest provocation or without any, and sinking in the depths of despair, and they could not make themselves act: their will was impaired. They would lose the ability to distinguish between mental images and outward reality, both being equally visible, audible, and real to them, and sometimes would not know who they were or mistake themselves. At other times they might become dimly, or starkly, aware of the reality of their situation—aware, that is, that their selves were disintegrating—and this would add to their distress. Suffering was there at all times, which nothing could ease. They felt inadequate, detested themselves. Life would lose all attraction to them, become unbearable, and they would long for death. Mania, depression, delusion, all at once or one after another, swirling in some macabre dance, this is what madness was. And well might one call it a disease—for it was agony.

It is also clear that Shakespeare regarded madness as a common enough aberration to juxtapose the truly mad Lear to Edgar pretending to be mad and both to the Fool, to have both Hamlet and Ophelia succumb to it, and to justify his frequent attention in other plays. It was an abnormality that was by his time becoming quite normal in England; the quip in *Hamlet* (Hamlet's being sent to England because madness is "no great matter there" and "there the men are as mad as he") can be taken as evidence that Shakespeare, at least, thought so. It was, in fact, becoming the character-istic form of suffering, and he believed it to be related to the current state of society. The time, as Hamlet put it, was out of joint. The instability of social relations, the unpredictability of personal ties which nothing seemed to hold together and which, therefore, rendered everyone insecure and unable to gain a firm foothold in society—in other words, anomie—are at the root of both Lear's and Hamlet's tragedies (as they are, too, in *Macbeth* and *Othello*). Remarkably, the one true villain, the one evil person in both (in distinction to the many ordinary people who are simply not good)— Edmund in *King Lear* and Claudius, Hamlet's uncle, in *Hamlet*—is the product and the beneficiary of an anomic society. It is the self-made man, acutely conscious of his natural equality to those above him, whose place he ambitiously craves, and resentful of the social conventions that hold him to his place. He would not be so bound: resourceful, intelligent, and self-confident, but characteristically not particular about his choice of means, he breaks these conventions. Unprincipled ambition is not the cause of madness in either *King Lear* or *Hamlet*, but in *Macbeth*, for instance, it is, and, whether or not this passion for self-realization is directly respon-sible for unhinging men's minds, it is always indirectly involved in this, for it is in a society which encourages ambition that madness thrives. Love thrives there too; it also must be free of social conventions and is focused on the self. Is it a wonder, then, that so often madness begins in it? The characteristic disease of the age, connected to its two governing passions and to the very nature of its society, madness is a factor whose interference in the course of human action an historian would be wise to suspect. Acutely attentive to historical forces, Shakespeare clearly considered it one. Both *King Lear* and *Hamlet* offer proof of this. It is Lear's madness that leads to the war between Britain and France; it is the madness of Hamlet that, in the final analysis, delivers Denmark into the hands of Fortinbras.

Early American psychiatrists, of course, were not aware of the historical implications of Shakespeare's treatment of madness. They did not know about the tremendous revolution which occurred in England in the sixteenth century, as a result of which God was banished and man enthroned in his position. At least insofar as they were concerned, He was safely back in nineteenth century's America and presided over history. They could not regard the human mind as the seat of historical forces. Thus they could not appreciate Shakespeare's contribution to psychiatry fully. The fact that they were full of appreciation, nevertheless, allows us to treat his representations of mental disease in plays as clinical descriptions of it, which, since we have no clinical material dating to the late sixteenth century, is of no small importance. But Shakespeare's work provides evidence of much more than the existence in England of the sixteenth century of precisely the kind of mental disorders that were observed in nineteenth-century United States. It provides evidence that this kind of mental disease—madness—was a remarkable and yet unstudied, therefore recent phenomenon, that, however common already, it was spreading further, and that it was somehow correlated with other recent changes in the existential experience brought about by nationalism. Of course, we have plenty of other evidence for this: the changes in vocabulary; the introduction of legal provisions for the insane; the foundation and constant expansion of Bedlam; the growing preoccupation with madness in legal, religious, and especially medical discourse; the "epidemic" among Elizabethan intellectuals and the "abnormally extensive" use of insanity on the Jacobean stage.[91] But, were Shakespeare not to focus on madness, all these data would have been palpably insufficient. Shakespeare was, unquestionably, the greatest genius of the age, thus its keenest observer, capable of perceiving and assessing the true significance of the least conspicuous phenomena. Moreover, the purpose of his work, as he told us himself, and specifically of his work for the stage, was "to hold, as 'twere, the mirror up to nature" and show "the very age and body of the time his form and pressure"—i.e. the understanding of his society. His neglect of, paying less attention to, or even different timing of his dramatic preoccupation with, madness would have been jarringly inconsistent with the rest of our case. The fact that the subject occupied him to the extent that it did and that it came to occupy him more in the last two decades of his life, after he had already considered at length national commitment and pride (in his historical plays, such as *Richard II, Henry IV,* and *Henry V*), ambition (in *Richard III, Julius Caesar*), and the new idea of love (in *Romeo and Juliet*) strengthens and completes this case, making it, in effect, incontrovertible. Shakespeare thus provides us not simply with important additional evidence, but with evidence that is crucial.

The View from Oxford, 1621–1640

The case for the recency of madness, and therefore its historical nature, may be complete, but we still must complete the presentation of its first century, which cannot be done without at least a brief consideration of the longest and most famous book on the subject—*The Anatomy of Melancholy* by Robert Burton. First published in 1621, though augmented through the next five editions before Burton's death in the eventful year of 1640, it was tremendously popular in the seventeenth century and is known, if only by name, even to psychiatrists of our own day. In a way, it was the *DSM-IV* of its time. It was encyclopedic, containing all the conceivable information on its subject (even the comparison to the collectively authored *DSM* cannot do justice to the breadth of its one author's learning), and yet not informative, for the possession of all the knowledge contained in it would not make one understand melancholy any better than before one acquired this knowledge. At the same time, unlike the *DSM,* it was full of interesting insights and most entertaining trivia, and, for all of its half-a-million words, was so well written, that it remains a good read almost four centuries after it first appeared in print.

Melancholy, according to Burton, was the disease, which subsumed almost all mental disorders, with the possible exception of natural folly (because, according to Erasmus, among others, fools were "'free from ambition, envy, shame, and fear; [and] neither troubled in conscience, nor macerated with cares'"[92]), and a large number of physical ailments. This being so, and Burton's method being to quote or, at least, cite all the instances in which the word "melancholy" or any of the numerous illnesses he subsumed in it were used by ancient or contemporary authors, the amount of material he assembled was prodigious. Obviously, "madness" and "lunacy"—which were frequently employed alongside "melancholy" in contemporary English literature (of which Burton in particular relied on Timothy Bright)—were included in his extensive vocabulary. He sometimes subsumed madness, in this case equated with mania, under melancholy, but more often equated the two terms, "melancholy" and "madness," and thus found examples of the latter throughout history. His sources were predominantly Latin, and he translated as "madness" *insania, furor, phrenesis, stultitia, insipientia, amentia,* and so on and so forth, quite indiscriminately. In one instance even *morbo* is rendered as "mad."[93] And yet, though the world had ever been plagued by madness, Burton believed that the world of his day was especially affected. Democritus of old had good reason to laugh at the madness of his age; but, wrote Burton who chose the penname of "Democritus Junior,":

> Never so much cause of laughter as now, never so many fools and madmen.
> 'Tis not one Democritus will serve turn to laugh in these days; we have now
> need of . . . one jester to flout at another, one fool to flare at another: a great
> stentorian Democritus. . . . For now the whole world plays the fool; we have
> a new theatre, a new scene, a new comedy of errors, a new company . . .
> where all the actors are madmen and fools, and every hour change habits,
> or take that which comes next. He that was a mariner to-day, is an apoth-
> ecary to-morrow; a smith one while, a philosopher another; a king now
> with his crown, robes, scepter, attendants, by and by drove a loaded ass
> before him like a carter, etc. . . .
>
> How would our Democritus have been affected to . . . see a man roll
> himself up like a snowball, from base beggary to right worshipful and right
> honorable titles, unjustly to screw himself into honours and offices; another
> to starve his genius, damn his soul to gather wealth, which he shall not
> enjoy, which his prodigal son melts and consumes in an instant.
>
> To see an hirsute beggar's brat, that lately fed on scraps . . . and for an old
> jerkin ran of errands, now ruffle in silk and satin, bravely mounted, jovial
> and polite, now scorn his old friends and familiars, neglect his kindred,
> insult over his betters . . .

To see a scholar crouch and creep to an illiterate peasant for a meal's meat; a scrivener better paid for an obligation; a falconer receive greater wages than a student; a lawyer get more in a day than a philosopher in a year, . . . him that can paint Thais, play on a fiddle, curl hair, etc., sooner get preferment than a philologer or a poet. [Clearly, our Oxford man knew a thing or two about this!] . . .

To see wise men degraded, fools preferred. . . . To see horses ride in a coach, men draw it; dogs devour their masters; towers build masons; children rule; old men go to school; women wear breeches; sheep demolish towns, devour men, etc. And in a word, the world turned upside downward.[94]

This upside-down world, indeed, produced madmen a-plenty and fully justified Burton's decision to anatomize the problem, his "chief motives" being: "the generality of the disease, the necessity of the cure, and the commodity or common good that will arise to all men by the knowledge of it."[95] The anatomy was divided into three parts. The first of these, 314 pages in length, following the 125 pages of front matter, dealt with the many varieties of melancholy, their equally numerous causes, and their symptoms. The broad classes included three kinds of melancholy "proper to parts," such as "melancholy of the head alone," "hypochondriacal, or windy melancholy," and "melancholy of the whole body." Their causes and symptoms alike were divided into general and particular to the kinds. All the symptoms were, in turn, broken into those of the body and those of the mind, general symptoms of the body being "ill digestion, crudity, wind, dry brains, hard belly, thick blood, much waking, heaviness and palpitation of heart, leaping in many places, etc.," and particular, "headache, binding and heaviness, vertigo, lightness, singing of the ears, much waking, fixed eyes, high colour, red eyes, hard belly, dry body; no great sign of melancholy in the other parts" for head melancholy; "wind, rumbling in the guts, belly-ache, . . . belchings, . . . etc." for hypochondriacal one; and "black, most part lean, broad veins, gross, thick blood, their hemrods commonly stopped, etc." for the melancholy of the whole body. The symptoms of the mind were far more numerous. Some were "common to all or most" and included "fear and sorrow without a just cause, suspicion, jealousy, discontent, solitariness, irksomeness, continual cogitations, restless thoughts, vain imaginations, etc." Others were "particular to private persons," that is, specific factors involved in their genetic makeup, such as celestial influences and humoral constitution related to them, and upbringing. The stars under which one was born would have a special effect on the heart in one case, on the brain, liver, spleen, stomach, etc. in others, thus making one of the four humors predominate, as well as affect its condition (its being "adust," for instance, or not). A sanguine melancholic would then be "merry still, laughing, pleasant,, meditating on plays, women, music, etc."; a phlegmatic would be "slothful, dull, heavy"; a choleric afflicted with melancholy would be "furious, impatient, subject to hear and see strange apparitions"; while a melancholic melancholic would become "solitary, sad, [and would believe being] bewitched, dead, etc." One's upbringing and social condition would add to this: "ambitious thinks himself a king, a lord; covetous runs on his money; lascivious on his mistress; religious hath revelations, visions, is a prophet, or troubled in mind; a scholar on his book, etc." All these were but general mental symptoms of melancholy; "the three distinct species" displayed particular ones. Patients suffering from the head melancholy would experience "continual fear, sorrow, suspicion, discontent, superfluous cares, solicitude, anxiety, perpetual cogitation on such toys they are possessed with, [and] thoughts like dreams." Hypochondriacal melancholy would make one "fearful, sad, suspicious, discontent, anxi[ous], lascivious by reason of much wind, [cause] troublesome dreams [and] fits." Melancholy "over all the body" would turn the mind "fearful, sad, solitary, [make one] hate light, averse from company, [and would also cause] fearful dreams." To these were added symptoms of melancholy specifically in females, and among them, in nuns, maids, and widows, as well as some explanations of particularly interesting symptoms, such as "why [melancholics] are so fearful, sad, suspicious without a cause, why solitary, why melancholy men are witty, why they suppose they hear and see strange voices, visions, apparitions, why they prophesy, and speak strange languages; whence come their . . . prodigious fantasies." The section on symptoms concluded with the consideration of the prognostics of melancholy. It was rather good if one had scabs, itch, or rash, if one had black jaundice or if the hemrods opened voluntarily. By contrast, being too thin or hollow-eyed held a bad prospect. "Inveterate melancholy" was incurable, "if cold, it degenerate[d] often into epilepsy, apoplexy, dotage, or into blindness; if hot, into madness, despair, and violent death." Melancholy was, indeed, "grievous above all other diseases," and mental disease, in general, was more grievous than those of the body.

The etiology of such a disease was a question of utmost importance. Burton divided the general causes of melancholy, in the first place, into natural and supernatural ones. The supernatural causes proceeded directly or indirectly either from God or from the devil, the latter often acting through lesser evil spirits who were numerous, or employing magicians and witches. The natural causes could be primary, i.e. related to one's stars, or secondary, i.e. related to everything else; these were, in their turn, divided into "congenite or inward" and "outward or adventitious." The congenital causes, remarkably, in addition to old age and temperament (that is, humoral constitution), included biological heredity, parents transmitting the disease to their children, while the "outward or adventitious" causes were further subdivided into "evident, outward, remote, adventitious" and "contingent, inward, antecedent, nearest." This second category concerned cases in which the body worked on the mind, and melancholy was caused by a preceding infectious disease, such as pox (syphilis), or any other organic malady. The category of evident outward causes was more complicated. To begin with, it consisted of two subcategories of its own: the larger one of necessary causes, and the smaller one of causes that were not necessary, which included traumatic experiences in early childhood, improper education, "terrors, affrights, scoffs, calumnies, bitter jests, loss of liberty, servitude, imprisonment, poverty and want, [and] a heap of other accidents." The very large category of necessary causes comprised three capacious compartments pertaining to 1) "diet offending" causes; 2) retention and evacuation, climate, exercise, and patterns of sleep; and 3) passions and perturbations of the mind. The first two, most detailed, could be of interest to any twenty-first-century nutritionist and philosophically inclined personal trainer, but it will serve our purposes to note the passions and perturbations of the mind alone. Burton divided those that were relevant to melancholy into irascible and concupiscible ones. Irascible passions were sorrow; fear; shame, repulse, and disgrace; emulation, hatred, faction, and desire of revenge; anger; and discontents, cares, and miseries. The concupiscible passions included, in the first place, "vehement desires, ambition"; covetousness; love of pleasure, gaming in excess; desire of praise, pride, vainglory; love of learning and study in excess (the consideration of which in the book contained a twenty-seven-page-long digression on the misery of scholars).[96]

"Envy so gnaws many men's hearts," Burton wrote, citing a number of sources out of his vast reservoir, "that they become altogether melancholy." He quoted verbatim from St. John Chrysostom, who surely knew what he was talking about, "As a moth gnaws a garment, so doth envy consume a man," adding "for so long as an envious wretch sees another man prosper . . . he repines and grieves . . . He tortures himself if his equal, friend, neighbour, be preferred, commended, do well; . . . and no greater pain can come to him than to hear of another man's well-doing; 'tis a dagger at his heart. . . ." After John Chrysostom's day no society offered as many reasons to so grieve and repine as Robert Burton's England, for in no other society so many people considered themselves equal. Emulation was a species of envy, or competition motivated by envy, and again some sage ancient offered a thought for Burton to emulate in English: "Whosoever he is whom thou dost emulate and envy, he may avoid thee, but thou canst neither avoid him nor thyself; wheresoever thou art, he is with thee, thine enemy is ever in thy breast, thy destruction is within thee, thou art a captive, bound hand and foot, as long as thou art malicious and envious, and canst not be comforted." Burton commented: "Every society, corporation, and private family [he meant, in England] is full of it, it takes hold almost of all sorts of men, from the prince to the ploughman. . . . 'Tis a sluggish humour not to emulate or to sue at all . . . but when it is immoderate, it is a plague and a miserable pain. What a deal of money did Henry VIII and Francis I, King of France, spend at that famous interview! And how many vain courtiers, seeking each to outbrave other, spent themselves, their livelihood and fortunes, and died beggars!"[97]

Though irascible and concupiscible passions constituted different categories of perturbations of mind, yet they were "as the two twists of a rope, mutually mixed one with the other, and both twining about the heart." The worst of them all but one, and "an especial cause of melancholy" was the concupiscible passion of ambition—"that exorbitant appetite and desire of honour . . . a proud covetousness, . . . composed of envy, pride, and covetousness, a gallant madness." There was no way to assuage this "great torture of the mind," this desire could not be sated, and "commonly they that, like Sisyphus, roll[ed] this restless stone of ambition [were] in per-petual agony." Every success, every achievement only spurred one to aspire still higher, one would "climb and climb still, with much labour, but never make an end, never at the top. A knight would be a baronet, and then a lord, and then a viscount, and then an earl, etc.; a doctor, a dean, and then a bishop; . . . first this office, and then that." If one failed, one found one-self "in a hell on the other side; so dejected, that he is ready to hang him-self, turn heretic, Turk, or traitor in an instant"—this, too, was a straight road to madness. It appeared indeed that "there could be no greater plague: both ways," wrote Burton, "hit or miss, he is distracted so long as his ambi-tion lasts, he can look for no other but anxiety and care, discontent and grief in the meantime, madness itself or violent death in the end."

And yet, there was a greater plague than ambition, a plague so much greater and both so noxious a cause and so fatal a symptom of melancholy that to it alone Burton had devoted the entire third part of his colossal book. This was love. True, Burton's definition of love was very broad. Given his method—to find and string together every use of the word, whatever it meant—this could not be otherwise. The varieties of love he discussed were, by necessity, as numerous as all the other varieties in his encyclopedic work and included, quite indiscriminately (although usually separated in sections and subsections), love of thy neighbor (as in Christian charity) and love of thy neighbor's wife (as in unlawful lust); love before marriage, and conjugal love; and such different concepts and feelings as the modern understanding of (romantic) love; the Greek eros; the medi-eval knightly ideals, the Christian one as well as the Islamic *ilishi*, regarding which Burton relied on Avicenna; the purely sexual desire; friendship, patriotism, and concern for the common good; and the love of God. All these loves could cause "love-melancholy" (though the love melancholy caused by the love of God was referred to as "religious melancholy"). More specifically, however, the diagnosis was applied to men's love of women, called "heroical love" before marriage and often "jealousy" after. It could do no other but drive men mad, because it was madness itself; those who happened to contract it were mentally ill by definition. Burton wrote:

> heroical, or love-melancholy, is more eminent above the rest, and properly called love. The part affected in men is the liver, and therefore called

heroical, because commonly gallants, noblemen, and the most generous spirits are possessed with it. His power and extent is very large, and in the twofold division of love, fileis and eros, those two Veneres which Plato and some other make mention of, it is most eminent, and [par excellence] called Venus, as I have said, or love itself. Which although it be denominated from men, and most evident in them, yet it extends and shows itself in vegetal and sensible creatures, those incorporeal substances (as shall be specified), and hath a large dominion of sovereignty over them. His pedigree is very ancient, derived from the beginning of the world, as Phaedrus contends, and his parentage of such antiquity, that no poet could ever find it out.[98]

Heroical love, therefore, was erotic love; among men only the upper classes seemed to be susceptible to this disease, yet it held sway over vegetal and sensible creatures, and even affected incorporeal substances. It was vain to seek clarity in such a complicated matter, and clarity was not this great scholar's forte. The stone well that would never loose a drop of the Hebrew Proverbs, he was the paradigmatic collector and repository of information, not one to find meaning in it. The prognostics of love were dispiriting. "Whether love may be cured or no, and by what means, shall be explained in his place;" wrote our systematic Oxonian, "in the meantime, if it take his course and be not otherwise eased or amended, it breaks out into outrageous often and prodigious events." So furiously does it rage in one's mind, that they make one forget all honesty, shame, and common civility. "For such men ordinarily as are thoroughly possessed with this humour, become *insensati et insani* . . . beside themselves, and as I have proved, no better than beasts, irrational, stupid, headstrong, void of fear of God or men, they frequently forswear themselves, spend, steal, commit incests, rapes, adulteries, murders, depopulate towns, cities, countries, to satisfy their lust. 'A devil 'tis, and mischief such doth work, / As never yet did Pagan, Jew, or Turk.'" Burton quotes from Robert Tofte and adds: "The wars of Troy may be a sufficient witness." But, clearly, for him they are not, and he goes through thirteen more footnoted literary testimonies before arriving at one that requires no reference and must be known to him from experience or hearsay: "Go to Bedlam for examples. It is so well known in every village, how many have either died for love, or voluntarily made away themselves, that I need not much labour to prove it."[99]

Nor is there a reference against the distich at the end of the page:

Who ever heard a story of more woe,
Than that of Juliet and her Romeo?

Did our anatomist not know whom he was misquoting? This is possible: in 1621 Shakespeare was dead and the folio that would bring him back to life as literature not yet published: the bookish Burton thus did not have a source. Or was the footnote so uncharacteristically omitted because the words that express the spirit of the age want no attribution? Whatever the reason, this little subtracted from his overwhelming scholarship and did not at all lessen its effect. The quickening understanding of madness towards which Timothy Bright was edging in his analytical *Treatise* and the clarity achieved by Shakespeare in his dramatic studies of it were lost, drowned in the torrent of Burton's relentless erudition. And with this lasting blessing psychiatry, born though not yet christened, was sent on its long way towards the ever-increasing misinterpretation of the devastating disease it was called into being to cure.

6

Going International
The Spread of Madness in Europe

English Extravagances and Irish Baile

In the second half of the seventeenth century the word "spleen" became the vernacular English term for melancholy in the sense of endogenous depression, though it did have numerous synonyms, such as "vapours," "hysteric fits," and the "hyp" or "hypo." The disease itself, "finally, because of its extraordinary prevalence in England," writes Cecil A. Moore, came to be regarded as "the English malady."[1] It is possible that some began to affect it, even if they did not suffer from it in fact, as a national characteristic, the quality that made them what they were. In 1664, a court official and occasional playwright William Killigrew in one of his plays, *Pandora*, remarked that the condition was "call'd the spleen of late, and much in fashion." But in 1690, Sir William Temple, a keen observer, admitted dejectedly: "Our Country must be confess'd to be . . . the Region of Spleen": striking a depressed pose could not explain the waste of ever growing number of lives obviously attributable to this peculiar mental illness.[2] By the turn of the eighteenth century, constant increase in insanity became one of the central problems in England: it was spreading and getting out of control.

Throughout the eighteenth century, this increase was reflected in legislation; in the establishment of numerous private and public asylums all over the country, where a few decades earlier Bedlam alone was sufficient for ministering to the needs of the afflicted and their families; in the ubiquity of madness in literature. "Perhaps the most striking aspect of literary England in the second half of the eighteenth century," according to some, "is how many of its best writers themselves became insane."[3] The madness of the poets, in particular, corresponded to the change in the nature of poetry itself, the abandonment of discipline and craftsmanship, the use of blank verse—of course, not universal and which would become much more pronounced in our own time. Samuel Johnson noticed the trend and disapproved of it, believing it willed, and failing to recognize that the unhappy authors bore no responsibility for, and knew not, what they were doing. He remarked acidly regarding the poet William Collins that he "puts his words out of the common order, seeming to think, with some later candidates for fame, that not to write prose is certainly to write poetry."[4] Poets writing in English have continued to go mad ever since: it is hard to find one among those who have achieved fame who has had no brush with one or another variety of schizophrenia. Their remarkable vulnerability to mental disease became a badge of the profession.[5] Wordsworth, himself one of the milder cases, wrote: "We Poets in our youth begin in gladness; / But thereof come in the end despondency and madness." This predisposition was believed to be universal, and, in the nineteenth century, the father of French psychiatry (or of psychiatry in general, according to the French), Philippe Pinel, was quoted in support of this claim. But it was not universal: there were only a few madmen in one of the three greatest poetry traditions of the nineteenth and twentieth centuries—the Russian; and while French and German poetry also supplied examples of the puzzling association, it was definitely more characteristic of the Anglophone world. (Pinel's assertion that "certain professions conduce more than others to insanity," which he based on the registers of Bicêtre, finding in them "many priests and monks . . . many artists, painters, sculptors and musicians: some poets extatized by their own productions" was interpreted in England—by the author of an influential textbook, no less—to mean that "among the educated classes of patients admitted to Bicêtre, no instances of insane geometricians, physicians, naturalists, or chemists are to be found, while priests, poets, painters, and musicians occur in great numbers." But in his first memorandum on madness Pinel specifically mentioned investigators, geometers, and engineers among the "diverse groups [who] pay an almost annual price to the hospice for the insane.")[6]

It must have been this peculiar association of madness and poetry in English which gave rise to the popular among English-speaking psychiatrists and psychologists view that manic-depressive illness, specifically, is just another expression of genes responsible for exceptional creativity, which implied in a "too much of a good thing" type of argument that the more creative one is, the more one is likely to suffer from manic-depressive illness. It is certainly both more logical and more consistent with the available evidence, however, to conclude the opposite: the more disturbed one is in the mind, the more likely one is to turn to language, abstaining oneself and letting it fix, and fixate, one's unhinged world. In this sense, what explains the striking similarity between schizophrenic thought and language and modern poetry (so meticulously documented by Louis Sass) is the fact that this particular (usually formless) form is a function, a creation, of mental disease. It is, at its root, a symptom, an expression of madness, a desperate "I am" sign—indeed so often made by our "leading poets":

> "I am! Yet what I am who cares or knows? / My friends forsake me like a memory lost, / I am the self-consumer of my woes; / They rise and vanish, an oblivious host, / Shadows of life, whose very soul is lost, / And yet I am . . ."[7]

Of course, mentally ill poets, while very remarkable, were a tiny drop in a much larger bucket. In the eighteenth century, as in the sixteenth, madness still disproportionally affected the educated (thus upper) classes. George Cheyne, in his famous 1733 treatise on "nervous diseases of all kinds," *The English Malady,* singled out people "of the better sort" as particularly hard hit ("[t]hese nervous Disorders being computed to make almost one third of the Complaints of the People of Condition in England") and offered a number of explanations of this peculiarity, such as "the Inactivity and sedentary Occupations of the better Sort (among whom this Evil mostly rages)."[8] The opinion of leading historians of psychiatry to the contrary, Cheyne was engaging in no social construction in calling madness the English malady. Neither was he guilty of embellishing the nature of "nervous" disorders in question by associating them with "the better Sort": patients who most commonly sought help from medical men such as him were, without doubt, "People of Condition."[9] More than seventy private asylums operated in England in the course of the eighteenth century, and "most of private asylums catered to wealthy clients." These were exclusive establishments—"residence[s] of a limited number of Ladies and Gentlemen of the Upper and Middle Classes," whose proprietors prided themselves on ministering to (often only) "persons of distinction."[10] Nathaniel Cotton's private madhouse (for this is how these asylums were called in the insensitive England of those bygone days) in which the poet William Cowper was confined, for example, anticipated Boston's McLean Hospital—the exclusive club for Harvard men gone mad—being "known as the Collegium Insanorum, perhaps because it contained so many educated and literary persons."[11] An eighteenth-century physician interested in diseases of the mind could easily limit one's patients to the rich and famous and be regarded (like Henry Maudsley was a century later) as "very much the aristocrat's alienist." For this—the earliest—medical specialization was a money-making one even before it was called "psychiatry."[12] It certainly was a magnet for talent, medical and other, attracting it from abroad as well as home. The Dutchman Bernard Mandeville (the author of *The Fable of the Bees*, and so famous, rather, as a philosopher and a political economist, but a physician by profession) established his practice in London as the most appropriate place for someone interested in mental disorders and in 1711 published there his *A Treatise of the Hypochondriack and Hysterick Passions, Vulgarly call'd the Hypo in Men and Vapours in Women*. The subject was of personal interest to him: he lived in constant fear of having contracted syphilis (the chances were great) and was a self-diagnosed hypochondriac. His was one of 112 books on madness published in England in the hundred years between 1700 and 1800.[13] Given all this, it is remarkable that the ever-increasing numbers of British psychiatrists de facto for a long time had no professional identity. The guild which was to become in the twentieth century (1971) the Royal College of Psychiatrists only organized in 1841.[14]

As we saw, the upper classes continue to be disproportionately affected by schizophrenia in all its forms, and throughout the nineteenth century it had not been yet considered bad form to comment on this vulnerability. An American noted in 1815 that, even though "the qualifications required for acknowledged insanity are by no means easily attained in England, where a greater latitude is granted for whims, fancies, and eccentricities, than in other countries," "madness appears to be fatally common in Great

Britain," "the higher ranks" and "the rich [being] particularly . . . most exposed to this calamity." A Frenchman, Jean Bernard, abbé Le Blanc, having spent seven years in England, acquired a broader picture, however, and thus commented in his letters already in mid-eighteenth century on the mental disposition of the farmers as well. They were, he said, unquestionably better off, from the material point of view, than their counterpart group in France—French peasants. "However, in the midst of this plenty, we easily perceive that the farmer is not so gay here, as in France; so that he may perhaps be richer, without being happier. The English of all ranks have that melancholy air, which makes part of their national character. The farmers here, shew very little mirth, even in their drunkenness; whereas in France, the farmers in several provinces drink nothing but water, and yet are as gay as possible." It is quite stunning that this comment was made less than forty years before the French Revolution. Still, Le Blanc, too, found the people of condition more affected by the national disease, which, like Cheyne, he attributed to inactivity and too much wealth. And then he summed up the French point of view: "This cheerfulness, which is characteristic of our nation, in the eye of an Englishman passes almost for folly; but is their gloominess a greater mark of wisdom? And folly against folly, is not the most cheerful sort the best? At least if our gaiety makes them sad, they ought not to find it strange if their seriousness makes us laugh." For the native son, Bryan Crowther, who in the early years of the nineteenth century insisted that madness was "rapidly becoming prevalent among all orders of society" this was, obviously, no laughing matter. In 1807, according to a report of a Parliamentary Committee the great majority of insane individuals in custody were pauper lunatics in workhouses. A dramatic change must have occurred within the preceding seventy years, for a 1732 Account of Workhouses mentioned only two insane persons. The 1807 report indeed inaugurated a century-long trend of legislation regarding care of the mentally ill from the lower social strata. An Act for the Better Care and Maintenance of Lunatics, or the County Asylum Act of 1808, "by which counties were encouraged to build public insane asylums, to be paid for with local taxes" was the first of twenty such Acts of Parliament passed in the nineteenth century.[15]

In addition to trickling down the social hierarchy and flooding the heretofore immune to it lower classes, madness was spreading throughout the English society in two other ways. It was spreading through age groups, increasingly affecting younger people: already in 1798 John Haslam (Matthews' attending physician in Bedlam), in *Observations on Insanity*, noted that the age of onset at the time was earlier than was the rule before. It was also spreading geographically from its original concentration in the south of the country and the Midlands northward. A truly new stage in its career was achieved, however, when the English malady reached Ireland and turned international. Since 1750s and in the course of the nineteenth century Ireland vied with England for the title of the maddest nation of all. "There was something different about baile, the Gaelic madness," the authors of *The Invisible Plague* comment. "Whatever was happening elsewhere was happening more frequently in Ireland."[16]

The Invisible Plague makes it quite clear that the history (and historiography) of this competition was directly connected to the development of Irish national consciousness. Varieties of schizophrenia, apparently, became noticeable in Ireland during the so-called Protestant Ascendancy after the Battle of Boyne in 1690—an arrangement which severely limited the rights of Irish Catholics, non-conformist Protestants, and members of other religions, privileging only the members of the established churches: the Church of England and the Church of Ireland. Catholics, who were a majority, were particularly resentful of this situation, which, providing the initial inspiration for Irish nationalism, made Catholicism a central element of this new, essentially secular, consciousness. Insanity, however, in Ireland, as in England and later elsewhere, first affected the elite, thus Protestants, and the rates among the better off—and better educated—remained disproportionately high throughout. A census of the insane, carried out in 1851, found that the most prosperous Irish counties, in the region of Leinster, with larger farms, higher land values, and "higher proportion of traders, shopkeepers, and publicans than any other province," had insanity rates at least three times higher than the poorest ones, consisting mainly of subsistence-oriented plots, such as Connaught, which, the census authors stated, in fact exhibited "a remarkable immunity" from mental disease. The census also supported the conclusion "with respect to the more educated class being more liable to mental affliction than the unenlightened."[17]

The unusual concentration of mentally ill among the upper classes, obviously, only meant that madness was less common, not that it was not common, among the underprivileged. The English malady was quickly becoming the Irish one. Already in 1731, when Jonathan Swift bequeathed "the little Wealth he had/To build a House for Fools and Mad," he, in his own words, "show'd by one satiric Touch/No nation needed it so much."[18] But in the ten-year period after the nationalist uprising of 1798 a "vast increase of insanity" in Ireland was observed, "a sudden and fearful addition to the number of insane," and the physician to the Cork workhouse, William Hallaran, who also ran a small asylum for paying patients, asserted as "an incontrovertible fact" that "from year 1798 to 1809, the number of insane had advanced beyond the extent of any former period." A report to the House of Commons in 1815 suggested that "in Ireland, the necessity of making some further provision for insane persons appears to be more urgent even than in this part of the United Kingdom," i.e., England. The next stage in the development of Irish nationalism, spearheaded by Daniel O'Connell's Catholic movement in the following decades coincided with a further spurt in the rates of insanity. The *Dublin Review* called it "a mental contagion . . . —an actual plague—which is caught by one mind from another." "This disease," it asserted in 1841, "is increasing every day to a most alarming degree."

So it went until the publication in 1894 of the Special Report on Insanity by the Irish Lunacy Commissioners. The report questioned and effectively put an end to the discussion of the singular prevalence and increase of this mental disease in Ireland. The authors of *The Invisible Plague*, who mention nationalism in no other chapter of their book, but the one dealing with Ireland, write:

> The 1894 Special Report on insanity was fundamentally a political document, not a scientific one. Irish nationalism was on the rise following the land reform battles of the 1880s; the Gaelic League had been founded in 1893, the Irish Republican Brotherhood was increasing its activities, and most important, British Prime Minister Gladstone had just introduced Home Rule Bill. The United Irish League and Sinn Fein would follow, leading Ireland to a confrontation with its English overseers. . . . It was within this political context . . . that the Irish Lunacy Commissioners were obligated to address questions of Ireland's insanity rate. During the 1870s and 1880s, summaries of the annual reports of insane asylums in England,

Scotland, and Ireland were published seriatim in the *Journal of Mental Science,* including comparative insanity rates for the three countries.[19] The Irish rates were invariably higher than the other two countries.[20] It had become common knowledge in England, as well as in other countries, that insanity was particularly endemic to Ireland. That would not do for the new Ireland, the emerging Ireland, the Ireland that hoped to throw off its colonial English masters. Having as much insanity as England was acceptable, but having more was not. The 1894 Special Report therefore concluded that "the seeming preponderance of insanity in Ireland as compared with England is fictitious, and depends entirely upon the greater accumulation in Ireland occasioned by the lower death-rate in that country, and (possibly) the lower rate of discharge of the unrecovered."[21]

Very similar arguments were voiced at the same time in England. The politically correct position in regard to the statistics (consistently recording troubling increase in the already very high rates of insanity), which was promoted by the government as well as the young but already supremely confident in its efficacy psychiatric establishment, was that the data must be faulty. Accepting the reported rates of insanity and the suggestion that it was on the increase obviously threw doubt on the powers of the new profession, which was one reason its leading members considered them unacceptable. But a more general reason, and the one likely foremost in the mind of government officials, such as the head of the parliamentary Lunacy Commission, Lord Ashley, who displayed a particular distrust of numbers, was that, with Morel's theory connecting insanity to hereditary degeneration gaining popularity in France, the English malady was becoming a blight on the national character. That such it was, was already argued in the 1820s by "one of the most well-known private madhouse keepers of the early nineteenth century,"[22] George Man Burrows, when the dominant position was that insanity rates reflected the level of development, or civilization, of a nation and their increase, therefore, could be regarded in a positive light. Burrows thought that, "increasing insanity would be a national scandal and therefore it should not be true." "As the respective exciting causes vary," he wrote, "so likewise must everywhere the number of lunatics. But does it thence follow that insanity must be increasing? A conclusion so humiliating cannot be entertained without the most painful reflections; nor, if it be really so, can the consequences be indifferent, even in a national point of view." This was really so, but later in the century it became more difficult to connect mental disease to civilization (among other things, because of the ascendancy of biological thinking), which led to the reinterpretation of the fact as only "a terrible possibility" one could "entirely dispute," "a melancholy theory [that] would unsettle our belief in the onward progress of mankind [and] shake the very foundation of our faith."[23] We have seen similar tendency to consider facts contradicting one's wishful thinking as unproven hypotheses in the scientific practice of our day in previous chapters.

Across the English Channel

In the eighteenth century, however, the connection between madness and civilization still appeared sufficiently convincing to allow British patriots to carry the burden of the English (and Irish) malady with pride. Until the very last years of that century, mental disease of the kind was as yet observed nowhere on the European Continent, and its salience in England—which for Continental observers stood for all of the British Isles—added mightily to the country's fascination in its visitors' eyes. It was particularly fascinating to the French. As René Doumic noted a century ago: *"Aux premières années du XVIIIe siècle, un événement considerable se produisit en France: la découverte de l'Angleterre. Notre XVIIe siècle monarchique, catholique, poli et lettré, n'avait éprouvé qu'une aversion mêlée d'un peu de pitié pour un pays déchiré par les discords civiles et religieuses, et il ne ce souciait guère de connaître ni les idées, ni les moeurs, ni les usages d'un people qu'il se représentait comme plongé en plein barbarie."* But after the revocation of the Edict of Nantes and the Glorious Revolution in England, he says, everything changed.[24] Of course, by 1700 England had accomplished its meteoric rise from cultural, political, and economic marginality to undisputed European dominance, and some astute Frenchmen, recognized the threat that this posed to France and watched it closely. Some were aware of this already in the "monarchical" seventeenth century, Antoine de Montchrétien, the father of political economy, being perhaps the first to point to England as the model in 1615. Colbert's efforts to encourage the subjects of the Sun King to follow the example of their insular neighbors in commerce and trans-Atlantic colonization proved that England was more than an object of aversion and pity for that great minister as well. The transformation of the Bicêtre prison into a public hospital for men, with a ward specifically for the insane, inexplicable without bringing into consideration the fame of Bedlam in London, and the foundation of the *Académie des Sciences*—four years after the formation of the Royal Society and without the long grassroots activity which prepared the way for the English institution—demonstrated that Colbert's respectful interest for things English, if unusual, was not unique.[25] But in the eighteenth century this respectful interest became common.

According to Moore, the writer who did most "to spread an ill report of the English among Continental readers" was a Frenchman, Abbé Prévost. He lived in England when his periodical *Pour et Contre* (1733–1740) began to appear in Paris; it was devoted to a large extent to the depiction of *les extravagances angloises,* responsible for the stereotype of the Englishman *idolâtre de sa tristesse.*[26] But, obviously, the stereotype was not of his creation. By Prévost's time, England had been long known as the land of the melancholy mad, and, coincidentally, it was in 1733, the year *Pour et Contre* began its publication, when George Cheyne came out with his famous treatise on "nervous diseases of all kinds" *The English Malady,* thus justifying the title:

> The Title I have chosen for this Treatise, is a Reproach universally thrown on this Island by Foreigners, and all our Neighbours on the Continent, by whom nervous Distempers, Spleen, Vapours, and Lowness of Spirits, are in Derision, called the ENGLISH MALADY. And I wish there were not so good Grounds for this Reflection. The Moisture of our Air, the Variableness of our Weather, . . . the Rankness and Fertility of our Soil, the Richness and Heaviness of our Food, the Wealth and Abundance of the Inhabitants (from their universal Trade) the Inactivity and sedentary Occupations of the better Sort (among whom this Evil mostly rages) and the Humour of living in great, populous and consequently unhealthy Towns, have brought forth a Class and Set of Distempers, with atrocious and frightful Symptoms, scarce known to our Ancestors, and never rising to such fatal Heights, nor afflicting such Numbers in any other known Nation.[27]

From the start madness, depression, or spleen was the aspect of the English experience that the French observers found particularly puzzling, because it seemed to contradict all their notions of human nature. The author of 1715 *Remarques sur l'état d'Angleterre,* possibly the earliest of the eighteenth-century travelogues to appear, George-Louis Le Sage, apparently concluded: "Surely, the people of England are the most unhappy people on the face of the earth—with liberty, property, and three meals a day."[28] It was all the more difficult to understand since, for the most part, these observers did not speak English and their British friends, who did speak French, in describing and explaining this experience to them, had to resort to a language which at the time lacked the vocabulary to do so. Therefore, very often, the word "spleen" did not appear in its early descriptions and interpretations in French and no specific term at all was used to describe the complex emotion to which it referred—as if it were unspeakable. Not being able to speak English, French interpreters of spleen were limited to observations of its outward expressions. The gloomy appearance of the English became proverbial with them, but what struck them even more—and indeed was more striking—was the extraordinary, in the modern world unprecedented, frequency of suicide in England. Every eighteenth century Francophone commentator on England noticed and tried to account for it. The first of these was a Swiss traveler Beat Louis de Muralt who visited England in 1694–95 and whose *Lettres sur les Anglois et les François et sur les voyages,* though published only in 1726, set the model for all the subsequent French visitors, including Abbé Prévost, as well as Voltaire and Montesquieu.

The English, thought Muralt, were people of extremes: distinguished from all others by their excellent *bon-sense,* they were more likely than members of other nations to lose it altogether, this was evident from the number of people among them who killed themselves and that of unequal marriages. They were violent in their desires, intolerant of the least obstacle, and absolutely contemptuous of death. Public executions were as frequent in London as at any other respectable European capital of the day, but nowhere else did one see the condemned men joke minutes before their death and otherwise show themselves—apparently without any effort—insensible of the prospect. "All this doesn't happen among other peoples," he commented; it demanded an explanation. By way of one he suggested: "Of course, you know that the English take their own lives as calmly as they give them up: it is not unusual here to hear of persons of both sexes who dispatch themselves, as they say, most often for reasons which we would think trifling: men, perhaps, because of cruelty or infidelity of some pretty maiden, and women because of men's indifference." Love, indeed, in England, according to Muralt, was understood and experienced very differently from France or any other country with which he was familiar. "True, when they fall in love, they do so violently: love among them is not a weakness of which they are ashamed; it is a serious affair, which must result either in success, or in losing one's mind or life. Last year, in fifteen days, three maidens hung themselves because of love troubles, and I believe that the English who told me so were less surprised by the act, than by the circumstance that two of these maidens committed it because of Irishmen, whom they hold in contempt and regard as incapable of loving and being loved."[29]

Whatever the English thought about emotional potential of Irishmen, they agreed that love had a totally different significance for themselves and for the French. Thomas Arnold, a most respected eighteenth-century expert on the English malady, was the author of a 1782 *Observations on the Nature, Kinds, Causes, and Prevention of Insanity, Lunacy, or Madness*. In it he, too, discussed, "whether insanity prevails more in England than in other countries," saying: "Insanity, especially of the melancholy kind, has been commonly supposed to prevail so much more in this island than in any other part of Europe, that it had acquired among foreigners the denomination of the English disease." He believed that there was some foundation for such supposition and was, sadly, certain that instances of insanity were at his day "amazingly numerous in this kingdom;—probably more so than they ever were in any former period." Arnold drew a particular comparison between England and France in this respect, France being England's chief rival for world dominance, and connected the relative immunity to madness among the French to the clearly inferior features of their national psyche. Their incapacity for true love was among these. Love, Arnold explained, "with them, is almost wholly an affair of art;—it has more of fancy than passion; and is rather an amusement of the imagination, than a serious business of the heart."[30] It is remarkable that the very same year as Arnold's *Observations*, Chauderlos de Laclos's novel about the French attitude to love, *Les liaisons dangereuses*, was published to great acclaim in Paris: on the whole, it corroborated Arnold's opinion, but also made clear that things were beginning to change: for the victim of the main protagonists' artful games, Mme de Tourvel, love had become a business of the heart serious enough to drive her mad, just as would have happened across the Channel.

Arnold also thought the French showed their lack of seriousness in regard to the other two common causes of the English malady: religion and ambition. The former in France being chiefly superstition, and "pardon for sins of all sorts and sizes [being] so easily obtained," religious melancholy on the grand English scale was not to be expected there, and as to "the desire, and prospect, of acquiring riches . . . there can be but little hope of attaining riches in a land of slaves, where the bulk and strength of a nation is depressed . . . being subject to the will of an absolute monarch." So, England—"the happy land of liberty"—was left quite without competition, insofar as melancholy madness was concerned, from the country which was its most serious competitor in every other sphere, and had to be "depressed" (as we would put it) alone.

In the meantime, Muralt happily chatted in 1695 about the English unreasonableness:

In the past people mostly hanged themselves; now the thing to do is to cut one's throat. Speaking of which, an extraordinary incident occurred recently, because, though tragic, it made the whole city laugh. A Frenchman, who long lived in England, and believed to be transformed into an Englishman, in an emotional turmoil, decided to kill himself. He chose, as might be expected, the fashionable kind of death, and went so far as to cut himself with a razor; but, terrified of the sight of his own blood and immediately losing the desire to die, he called for surgeons, who failed to save him: he expired in their hands, and amidst jokes the English like to make— they who proceed in the matter with determination, and do not turn back.

Muralt thought that these examples would suffice, could not help adding more, but then concluded:

However this may be, it's a pity that this folly or furor is so widespread among them, and regarded as sensible even by serious people. He was tired of life, he left it, said one of them when told that his only son drowned himself in the Thames. To this extent it is ordinary for them to calmly part from life. . . . True, they are careful to enjoy it before, forgetting business and other distractions: such is the English *scavoir vivre*, which implies more than knowing how to well end a visit.[31]

"He was tired of life, he left it," this was as far as Muralt's psychological explanation of the bizarre penchant of the English for killing themselves went. Neither "spleen" nor "madness" nor "melancholy humor" figured in it. He had a smattering of English, apparently enough to attend numerous plays during his visit and to be familiar with Sir William Temple's views on the comparative merits of the English drama and the concept of "humour" the latter defined in the 1690 essay "Of Poetry." It was, indeed, Muralt who introduced the word *houmour* into French. He did not like the concept but admired and, on one of his very few trips from London, visited *Chevalier Temple* at his country home. They conversed in French, of course. Sir William had some things to say about spleen; in fact, "Of Poetry" contained an important passage on the subject, immediately following the discussion of "humour": "with all this, our country must be confessed to be what a great foreign physician called it, the region of spleen, which may arise a good deal from the great uncertainty and many sudden changes of our weather in all seasons of the year. And how much these affect the heads and hearts, especially of the finest tempers, is hard to be believed by men whose thoughts are not turned to such speculations." Unfortunately, no French speaker could understand what this meant. The passage was translated into French as "Il faut avouer, que notre pays est, comme l'appellent les médecins étrangers, la région de la rate . . ."[32] Even half a century later, as we learn from the 1743 edition of the *Dictionnaire de Trévoux, rate* still meant the very opposite of the English spleen, and, what complicates matters still further, so, by necessity, did *mélancolie*—the black bile that resided in the organ it referred to. The *Dictionary* explained: "Les Anciens ont cru qu'elle [la rate] êtoit le réservoir de l'humeur mélancholique, & pour cela quelques uns l'ont appellée l'organe du ris [the organ of laughter], d'ou vient qu'on dit de ceux qui se réjoissent, qu'ils s'épanouissent la rate. . . . On dit s'épanouir la rate; pour dire, se réjouir. [And, quoting Molière]: 'Il faut qu'enfin j'éclate, / Que je lève la masque, & décharge ma rate.'"[33]

Like Muralt, French observers proper could not, and did not bother, to understand the psychology behind the exceptional frequency of suicides in

England, but—at this age of youthful and optimistic materialism, they were certain that underneath it lay some physical illness and found its meteorological explanation most reassuring. Montesquieu, very much like Temple, blamed the English climate, writing in *The Spirit of the Laws*, that it corroded the body and prevented it from functioning; the mind had nothing to do with people killing themselves: ". . . the machine . . . is tired; the soul feels no pain, only a certain difficulty of existence." Voltaire commented on that: "In connection to the influence of climate Montesquieu examines . . . why the English kill themselves so frequently. 'It's, he says, the effect of an illness . . . ' Les Anglais, en effet, appellent cette maladie spleen, qu'ils prononcent splin, ce mot signifie la rate. Nos dames autrefois etaient malades de la rate . . . Les Anglais ont le splin ou la splin, et se tuent par humeur."[34] One can only wonder what he meant by "spleen." As to which peculiarity of the English climate had that lamentable effect on the English physique, he explained this in a draft of an unfinished addition to his philosophical—or English—letters. Voltaire related in it how he arrived in London on a beautiful spring day in the midst of some popular festivities. In Greenwich, where he stopped, in a joyous crowd he recognized a number of gentlemen to whom he had letters of introduction, and these gentlemen received him most cordially and showed every sign of happiness at having him among them. Nothing prepared the philosopher for what happened next:

> The next day, in a dirty, badly furnished, badly served, and badly lit café, I found most of these gentlemen, so affable and good-humoured last afternoon; none of them recognized me; I tried to strike a conversation with them, receiving no response . . . I took the liberty to ask, with a vivacious look which seemed to them very strange, why were they all so sad: one responded grimly that the wind was Easterly. Another gentleman arrived at the moment and coldly announced: "Molly cut her throat this morning. Her lover found her dead in her room, with a bloody razor by her side." This Molly was a young girl, beautiful and very rich, who was planning to marry the man who found her dead. All these gentlemen were Molly's friends, and received the news without blinking an eye. One of them only asked what happened to the lover; he bought the razor, said coldly someone. On my part, terrified by so strange a death and the indifference of these gentlemen, I

couldn't refrain from asking what forced an apparently happy maiden to end her life by such cruel means; I was simply told that the wind was Easterly.

Bewildered and upset, Voltaire went to the Court, "inspired by the beautiful French notion that the Court is always gay. All there was sad and mournful, including ladies in waiting. People melancholically discussed Easterly wind. . . . the climate was already affecting me and, to my astonishment, I could not laugh. A famous Court physician, to whom I communicated my surprise, said that this was not surprising, that things would be worse in November and March; that then people hanged themselves by the dozen; that almost everyone was really ill during these months, with a black melancholy oppressing the entire nation: because then, he said, Easterly wind is constant. This wind is the bane of our isle. Even animals suffer from it and look all exhausted. People robust enough to keep their health with this damned wind, lose at least the good humour. Everyone looks gloomy and is disposed to desperate acts. It was precisely during Easterly wind that Charles I lost his head and James II his throne."[35] Was there a need for deeper reasons why Englishmen, who endured Easterly wind for years, killed themselves by the dozen, when this sinister force of nature caused dumb beasts to lose countenance and a French philosopher, after just one day on the cursed island, all his mirth?

Ennui

The history of ennui represents a short chapter in the history of depression and its becoming eventually a widespread experience in the West. When the French public first became conscious of the "English malady," a fundamentally foreign experience for it, in the eighteenth century, the French experience of ennui provided the chief vehicle for its interpretation. When the English experience of depression finally reached France after the Revolution and became French as well, ennui was equated with spleen.[36]

The French word *ennui* has proven untranslatable—when speakers of other languages wish to make use of the concept, they have no choice but to borrow it. Such inseparable connection between a word (necessarily in a particular language) and its meaning may be more common than one suspects, but whatever the commonness of the phenomenon, it suggests something quite troubling in regard to the nature of humanity. What it suggests is that speakers of different languages, that is, members of different cultures, even if closely related and belonging to the same civilization, may differ in their emotional experiences—that not only the names they give to their feelings, but their feelings themselves, may be different. If only the French have a word for the feeling of ennui, it must mean that only the French have experienced it on a regular basis, and that for others the experience itself, not only the word, is foreign, and, as a result they must use a foreign word to express it. But, if this is so for ennui, this, clearly, can be so, as this book has argued, with ambition, love, happiness, or madness.

The word *ennui,* as appropriated in English, is defined by the *Oxford English Dictionary* thus: "the feeling of mental weariness and dissatisfaction produced by want of occupation or by lack of interest in present surroundings or employments." It entered the vocabulary of refined intellectuals in the eighteenth century, signifying something very close to "boredom." Bishop Berkeley used it in this sense in 1732 ("They should prefer doing anything to the ennui of their conversation") and Lord Chesterfield in 1758 ("In less than a month the man, used to business, found that living like a gentleman was dying of ennui"). Its first use occurs in John Evelyn's memoirs in 1667, but the signification is unclear, Evelyn simply listing *ennui* among other French concepts (such as *naïveté* and *bizarre*) to express which fully English has "hardly any words." Still, this demonstrates a considerable knowledge of the neighboring culture on the part of the great diarist, for the French notion itself is quite vague and rare in the seventeenth century. The word is old, derived from Latin *noxia,* meaning physical hurt or damage, but neither Jean Nicot's *Thresor de la langue françoyse* of 1606, nor—more important—the first, 1694, edition of the *Dictionnaire de l'Académie Française* include it. The *Dictionnaire de Trévoux* of 1743 defined it as "chagrin, fâcherie, tristesse, déplaisir," and as equivalent to "fastidium, taedium, odium, moestitia, agrimonia" in Latin, quoting, among others, M. Scudéry, "l'ennui n'est autre chose qu'une privation de tout plaisir, causé par je ne sai quoi de dehors qui importune"; "en amour, ennui signifie une tendre douleur"; and "si cette femme se couchoit sans être assurée d'un divertissement pour le lendemain, elle mouroit d'ennui, de la seule peur de s'ennuyer," as examples. It also quoted Racine: "Hélas! M'enviez-vous dans l'état ou je suis,/La triste liberté de pleurer mes ennuis?" The *Dictionnaire de L'Académie Française,* fourth edition of 1762, but slightly augmented this definition, stating: "ENNUI. s.m. Lassitude, langueur, fatigue d'esprit, causée par une chose qui déplaît par elle-même, ou par sa durée, ou par la disposition dans laquelle on se trouve. . . . Il signifie aussi généralement, Fâcherie, chagrin, déplaisir, souci." The fifth edition expanded on this further (I emphasize the additions): "ENNUI. s. m. Lassitude, langueur, fatigue *ou inaction* d'esprit, causée par une chose qui déplaît par elle même, ou par sa durée, ou par *le défaut d'intérêt,* ou par la disposition dans laquelle on se trouve," adding, most significantly, "On dit, *L'ennui de la vie,* pour, Le dégoût de la vie," and then repeating the text of the previous edition verbatim: "Il signifie aussi, généralement, Fâcherie, chagrin, déplaisir, souci." Littré, in the 1872–1877 dictionary, exemplifying the use of the word through numerous sources dating to before the eighteenth century, commented: "Dans le style relevé, ennui est un mot d'une grande force et qui s'applique à toutes sortes de souffrances de l'âme : les ennuis du trône ; des ennuis cuisants. Dans le langage ordinaire, il perd beaucoup de sa force et se borne à désigner ce qui fait paraître le temps long." Thus he justified the use made of the term by eighteenth-century Englishmen: by and large, *ennui* meant simply "boredom," but by the end of the eighteenth century it was, clearly, on the verge of meaning something much more serious.

According to J. Ch. Coffin, the eighteenth century witnessed "the return of ennui" to France.[37] It coincided with "the discovery of England" and was directly connected to the attempt of the French public to understand the English malady. The first to connect suicide, spleen, and ennui was that abbé Le Blanc who found English melancholy funny. He spent in England seven years between 1737 and 1744, and in 1745 came out with *Lettres d'un françois,* which were in 1747 translated as *Letters on the English and French Nations.* In it he compared the gay disposition of his nation with the "funereal mold" of the English, noting that "melancholy air" was a part of their "national character," and puzzled why, given this, the English lacked an equivalent of the French word *ennui* "which so well expresses a thing they feel every moment," and why, having borrowed "from the French so many words without any necessity for them," they would not borrow this one. "They better express the *taedium vitae, l'ennui de la vie,* by the desperate resolution they take, when tired of life," he said, "than by any term in their language." "Spleen" and "vapours," thought Le Blanc, were but "feeble substitutes" for *ennui* and, in any case, meant "nothing else but ennui carried to its highest pitch, and become a dangerous and sometimes a mortal disease." This added to *ennui* a new and surprising sense of a potentially mortal disease. When the word "spleen" entered French by the end of the eighteenth century, it was defined as "ennui de toutes choses, maladie hypochondriaque propre aux Anglais."[38]

This identification of ennui and spleen was passed on to the nineteenth and twentieth centuries, as demonstrated by the entry in *Le Grand Robert:* "SPLEEN—1763; spleen, attestation isolée, 1745; var. spline au XVIIIe; angl. Spleen . . . Mélancolie passagere, sans cause apparente, characterisée par le dégout de toute chose.—cafard; 2. chagrin, ennui, hypochondrie, neurasthénie, nostalgie." Remarkably, the fifth edition of the *Dictionnaire de l'Académie française* in 1797–1798 defined spleen without any reference to French experience (and therefore terms that expressed French experience), as "mot emprunté de l'anglois, par lequel on exprime un état de consomption," while "consomption," it explained, was "certaine espèce de phthisie fort ordinaire en Angleterre, qui consume et desséche le poumon, les entrailles; et toute la substance du corps." It was still understood as a purely physical disease, the corrosion of a machine, in which, as already Montesquieu supposed, the spirit did not at all participate. But, before the Revolution, whether or not ennui was associated with spleen, even the most informed Frenchmen had difficulty understanding the English concept. Diderot's letter to Mme Voland in 1760 on the subject made it clear that he considered the experience well nigh inconceivable: "You don't know what *le spline* is, nor English vapours: I also did not know. I asked our Scott [P. Hoop] during our latest promenade, and here is what he said: 'For twenty years I experience a general more or less serious malaise, my head is never free [from it]. Sometimes it is so heavy that it feels like a pulling weight . . . My thoughts are black, I am sad and irritable; I feel comfortable nowhere, don't want anything, have no desires, I try vainly to amuse and occupy myself; joys of others pain me. I suffer hearing them laugh or talk. Are you familiar with the incomprehension and gloom one experiences after sleeping too much? This is my usual state, life disgusts me . . ."[39]

It was nationalism—which caused France to revolt against its *ancien régime* and plunged it into the swirl of anomie and modernity—that made everything clear. The French experienced—and understood—what spleen was. It was, said Chateaubriand, "tristesse physique, véritable maladie," and the most horrible imaginable "souffrance de l'âme." They decided that it was indeed ennui, but not the ennui of the eighteenth century, "non pas cet ennui commun, banal, qui provient de la faineantise," to quote Flaubert, "but that modern ennui which gnaws on one's guts and transforms an intelligent being into a walking shadow, a thinking phantom." One spoke of *la maladie de l'ennui*, one learned what it was to have *le dégoût de la vie*. Baudelaire, who suffered terribly from, and wrote about, ennui and spleen (which, for him, obviously were one and the same, which he equated with "l'Angoisse atroce, despotique," and than which he could find nothing "plus laid, plus méchant, plus immonde") would find the philosophes' naïve disquisitions on them laughable.[40] It was a mortal mental disease, and, even if they did not kill themselves, French people now died of it regularly in mental hospitals. In the twentieth century the eighth edition of the *Academic Dictionary* defined it as "depression" (spleen was long since replaced by this new international concept in the English-speaking countries), explaining: "Il se dit particulièrement de la lassitude morale qui fait qu'on ne prend d'intérêt, qu'on ne trouve de plaisir à rien." It turned out "the English malady" had nothing to do with Easterly wind.

Mental Alienation: Madness in France

The suddenness with which France was hit by madness corresponded to the heaviness of the blow. Virtually unknown before 1789, by 1800 it was considered common. Chateaubriand already in the very first years of the new century found it inexplicable that modern authors had not yet "dreamt about" depicting this singular experience.[41] In France, indeed, he was the first to describe the preclinical and very widespread unipolar depressive variety of it, which was often fatal, even though not leading to hospitalization, writing about this "condition of the soul, which, it seems to us, has not been well observed":

> it is . . . when all the faculties, young, active, whole, but self-contained, are expended on themselves, without aim or object [outside]. The more people advance in civilization, the more widespread becomes this condition of the

[assaulting] wave of passions; because a very sad thing happens then: the great number of examples one has before one's eyes, the vast literature discussing man and his sentiments, make one knowledgeable without experience. One is disappointed before living [through what might disappoint]; there are still desires, but one no longer has any illusions. The imagination is rich, abundant, marvelous—the existence poor, dry, disenchanted. One lives with a full heart in an empty world; and not having taken advantage of anything, one is disabused of everything.

The "bitterness with which this state of the soul colors one's life," he said, "is not to be believed; the mind [*le coeur*] turns around itself and folds itself in hundreds of ways to employ its useless forces." The ancients, he was aware, little knew "this secret anxiety, this pithiness of suffocating passions, all fermenting at once": after all, engagement in public affairs filled their days and left no time to *ennuis du coeur*. In addition, they were not "inclined to exaggerations, hopes, fears without an object, the motility of ideas and sentiments, to perpetual change [of attitude] which is nothing but unchanging disgust." A description of the psychological effects of anomie could not be more exact.

Chateaubriand clearly perceived that anomie was the cause of this "awful misery," even though, obviously, he did not name it thus. He also provided an historical explanation for it—the Revolution: "Never had a people experienced a transformation more shocking and sudden. From the heights of genius, of respect for religion, of the gravity of attitude, everything all of a sudden descended into uncertainty and opportunism,[42] into impiety, into corruption." He knew that the condition he was describing could be fatal. His goal was to fight the particular trend among the young generation, "that leads directly to suicide." He had been close to it himself, confessing in *René*, as he stressed the central experiences of suicidal depression: "I was oppressed by the too much [that] life [had to offer] . . . A secret fear tormented me: I sensed that I was but a traveler . . . Disgusted by life . . . I felt my existence only through a profound sentiment of ennui . . . I decided to take my life . . ."[43] He could be anything, achieve any position, but could decide on nothing and had none; he did not belong anywhere, and, unlike Descartes, whose thought offered him the undeniable proof of his self, Chateaubriand knew himself only through suffering. It appears he was aware that in England the "singular condition of the soul" that he was describing existed earlier, perhaps because monasteries, which offered a refuge to those predisposed to it and prevented it from developing to its full tragic potential, were destroyed in England earlier:

> Once the convents offered retreats to such contemplative souls . . . But since the destruction of the monasteries and the loss of faith one must expect to see in the midst of society (as it happened in England) the increase in the number of loners, overemotional and overrational at the same time, who, unable to renounce the vices of the world around them nor to love this world, interpret hatred of mankind as a sign of genius, renounce every religious and secular duty, delude themselves with vainest hopes, and sink ever deeper in a proud misanthropy that is sure to lead them either to madness [folie] or to death.

Yet, he believed that, in France, this was an independent development, inspired, specifically, by Rousseau's *Rêveries du promeneur solitaire*. There, Chateaubriand argued, "isolating himself from the company of other men, abandoning himself to his dreams, he made masses of young people believe that it is beautiful to thus throw oneself into the wave of life. Later, this poisonous seed was developed by the novel of Werther." Rousseau's *Rêveries* were published posthumously in 1782, while Goethe's *Werther* appeared in 1774; still, it seems, Chateaubriand considered the condition singular to France. It was a "new vice . . . not yet attacked."[44] Neither England nor Germany, apparently, had anything to contribute to its depiction and explanation; France, possibly because of its superior civilization which made it particularly susceptible to it, led the way.

Given the interest in *extravagances angloises* and the repeated attempts to understand "the English malady" throughout the eighteenth century, it is remarkable that Chateaubriand's opinion of the peculiarity of the French *état de l'âme* was widely shared. In fact, several of his compatriots credited Chateaubriand himself with creating it—as part and parcel of French Romanticism! Theophile Gautier advanced this claim in his *Histoire du romantisme*, saying, no less, that he "invented melancholy and modern suffering [*mélancolie et la passion moderne*]," while Baudelaire, even more astoundingly alongside appropriating "spleen" as the proper name for his personal experience, wrote that "the grand school of melancholy [was] created by Chateaubriand." Madness, and specifically depression, like in England, in France hit the educated classes—and, among them, writers (though in this case, prosaics at least as much as poets) first, but, unlike in England, where its literary interpreters were aware that it was a real affliction that came from the objective world outside, in France at least some very important writers believed that it was a product of their literary imagination. This expression of professional megalomania was, in effect, a schizophrenic delusion in reverse, and it contributed not a little to the misunderstanding of psychiatric disease in the West. Their experience was that of a disease which had all the symptoms of "the English malady." A character in *Adolphe* (1816) by Benjamin Constant, for example, complained: "I was experiencing such lack of energy and felt such self-loathing, that . . . quite seriously, I did not think I could go on living." Or consider the description of Étienne de Senancour, another French Romantic, writing in his (autobiographical) epistolary novel of 1804, *Oberman:*

> I sometimes ask myself where will lead me this malaise which chains me to ennui; this apathy which never leaves me; this [sense of] meaninglessness and insipidity of reality from which I can never free myself, [reality] in which everything is unsatisfactory, repugnant, ever-fleeing; in which every probability negates itself; in which efforts are misdirected; in which every [desired] change is aborted; in which expectations are always thwarted, even those of a least bit stirring misfortune; in which one would say that some hostile will is intent to keep me in a state of suspense and inability to act, to lure me with vagueness and evasive hopes, in order to waste my entire existence without ever allowing me to achieve anything, produce anything, have anything.

But they refused to see it as an actual disease. "There is in me," mused Senancour/Oberman, "a derangement, a sort of delusion, which is not one of strong emotions [*passions*], and neither that of mental illness [*folie*]: it is a disorder of ennuis; it is the discordance that they [ennuis] have created between me and the things . . ." When they referred to their experience as a *mal*, which they did, constantly, they used the word as a metaphor, as if it felt like a disease, but was, in fact, something entirely different.

Contemporary literary theorists still put *mal* in quotation marks: it was not really a disease. Christophe Bois writes in his comments on *René:*

> René is the first literary character to feel this "disease" [*ce "mal"*], a mélange of melancholy, disgust with life, and ennui. . . . An entire generation of young adults recognized themselves in the character of René; the rapidity with which this "mal" spread was such that the qualifier "of the century" [*"du siècle"*] was added to it.
>
> This *"mal du siècle"* is caused by the "discordance" between the self and reality: the individual seems not to be made for the reality which he must live; his thirst for the absolute collides with reality. . . . The sentiment of not being understood, like René, comes from this "discordance" with reality, from this maladjustment to one's environment.
>
> The *"mal du siècle,"* it is also the incapacity to act in this world; this incapacity engenders a sense of void to which death is preferable .

A powerful literary device, indeed. The experience, then, is interpreted as a core element of Romantic style. Bois continues: "The individual gripped by this delicious unhappiness is essentially egocentric. . . . He will, therefore, talk above all about himself. . . . The favorite Romantic literary form is that of autobiographical and lyrical confession. . . . One also understands that, among Romantics, poetry is the genre of choice."[45] It takes a theorist par excellence to consider the sort of unhappiness that drives people to suicide "delicious." French Romantic authors were in a grip of depression which, according to their sensitive descriptions, often reached clinical proportions, and *mal du siècle* was no metaphor and no element of style: it was a very real mental disease which was likely what brought literary Romanticism into being. Self-analysis helped the affected authors cope with their disease: the literary form was a form of self-medication, and the fact that the affliction was widespread made these thinly veiled autobiographies popular. Thus an extremely important phase in the development of Western modern literature was, fundamentally, an expression of madness.

French physicians first became aware of madness in the late 1780's, that is, just before the Revolution. They never encountered it before in France.

Having encountered it, they assumed that it has always existed, forgetting that just a few years earlier it was considered a peculiar problem of their neighbors across *La Manche*. They believed that it was their attitude toward mental disease that changed (prompting, among other things, Philippe Pinel to replace chains restraining deranged patients at Bicêtre by strait-jackets—an act which became the symbol of the new approach), because they were much more enlightened now in every respect, not the phenomenon they were observing. Historians of the French psychiatry still believe that, which makes the sudden emergence of this profession in France at the time (and many French scholars believe that it was France at that time that gave birth to psychiatry as such) quite tricky to explain.[46] Psychiatry, however, emerged because madness emerged, and France, like England three centuries earlier, became susceptible to this new disease because of the colossal cultural transformation that was underway in it in the end of the eighteenth century.

The country was aflame with the new sentiment of nationalism; the entire society, as the great Esquirol—"the favorite student" of the father of French psychiatry, Pinel—put it, seemed as if it was suffering from vertigo.[47] Yet, none of the pioneers of French psychiatry associated the curious symptoms of a growing segment of their patients with this. Like in England, insanity in France, inexistent only years before, was spreading rapidly. Esquirol was perplexed and tried to account for the impression of this spread in a memorandum of July 1824, "Existe-t-il de nos jours un plus grand nombre de fous qu'il n'en existait il y a quarante ans?" for the *Académie de médicine*. The assumption that one dealt with the age-old problem of *folie* obscured the nature of the phenomenon and made it impossible to answer the question with any degree of certainty.

Mental illness subsumed under the traditional designation of *folie*, obviously, was as familiar in France as anywhere else. And in France, like elsewhere, the medical profession considered it a part of its province. According to Semelaigne, the author of the 1930 *Les pionniers de la psychiatrie française*, all the medical treatises written before the eighteenth century contained either chapters on mental disorders or observations on them, included in other chapters, "because specialists were unknown," and, in the case of mental problems, the rich clientele (i.e., those who consulted physicians) consulted the very same general practitioners who would be called upon to treat any other disease. Medical treatises focusing on mental diseases were, as elsewhere, rare (as were any specialized medical treatises), but they existed and carried on the Hippocratic and Galenic traditions, which related these, like all the other diseases, to the four bodily humors. The reaction to these treatises might have differed, depending on the circumstances in which they appeared (the time and locale, and specifically the way the church, the ultimate arbiter in every intellectual endeavor, always jealous of its intellectual authority, viewed the medical profession at the moment), but there was no deviation from the tradition and no original ideas in them; what they differed in, if at all, was their literary quality.

Some of these texts contain descriptions of typical cases of *folie* these doctors treated; they present a revealing contrast with the "English malady." In late sixteenth century, for instance, Guillaume de Baillou mentions among particularly interesting cases of his career a case of a delirious man with fever (*frénétique*), kept in bed for nine days. When the doctor came to visit, the patient attacked him, but was persuaded to lie down again. He pretended to be asleep, yet, when the doctor, leaving, found himself in front of the sick chamber, jumped on him from the window. Another of Baillou's mental patients, a nobleman, was subject to epileptic attacks, resistant to every medication. But a sudden "furious delirium" made these attacks disappear. A woman patient suffering of "hypochondriac melancholy" experienced violent pains in the left side of the abdomen each time she drank water mixed with wine, but if she drank pure water, she had no pains. Charles Lepois, who practiced a bit later than Baillou, among others treated hysterical women, one of whom, a lady of good birth, presented with symptoms which struck most experienced physicians with (in the doctor's words) astonishment or horror. During attacks of her malady, the patient would become blind and deaf, and completely lose the senses of smell and touch. Her limbs, sometimes shaking, would be so contracted that it would be easier for a strong man to break her arms than to open them. She would not produce a sound, and there also were abdominal contractions. For a year these attacks, apparently, were quite prolonged; later they became brief, but still happened often and at the drop of a hat.[48]

A number of sixteenth- and seventeenth-century medical authors included in their discussion of mental disorders "insane love" (*l'amour insane*). Only a few, however, met with it in their practice. Jacques Ferrand did encounter a case in the very beginning of his medical career and became so interested in the problem that he wrote in fact two very large books on it—the two considerably different from each other editions (1610 and 1623) of the treatise on the *mal fantastique* of *maladie d'amour ou mélancolie érotique*. The overvaluation of the psychological significance of sex in our day makes some historians consider this treatise an important original contribution to psychiatry. In his work on "lovesickness," writes Michael Stone, Ferrand was a "physician who proved himself able to shuck traditional explanations when they no longer seemed sensible."[49] He did not. Though a doctor of law and medicine, Ferrand, apparently, craved literary fame and would rather be recognized as a scholar and erudite. Much more than a medical tractate, his *Maladie d'amour* was "a speculative courtly essay" on *amor hereos*—erotic desire—which, while a favorite subject of poetry, was, since Plato, defined as a disease of the soul. As sexual desire could in fact, if unsatisfied, make one quite disturbed in body as well as spirit, physicians also treated it as a disease, and, specifically, as a melancholic disease, that is one related to excess or some perturbation of black bile. The commonly recommended treatment for the condition was coitus, whether with the particular object of desire or not. The subject (which is not to be confused with "lovesickness" as defined in England since the sixteenth century) was of interest mostly at Renaissance courts, where people discussed (and, in this case, practiced the principles expressed in) classics of erotic literature. It was one such court—at Toulouse—for which Ferrand wrote, and, though apparently popular with its intended reading public there and elsewhere, his book was not regarded as a medical work. Nobody but Robert Burton, who referred to everything, referred to it (very briefly, in the fourth edition of *Anatomy of Melancholy*) as such in the first two centuries after its appearance, and "[it] is not until 1838, with the publication of Esquirol's *Des maladies mentales* . . . that Ferrand's name reappears in the context of a sustained analysis of erotic monomania."[50] It reappears, however, only to disappear again, for even Esquirol had not sustained this analysis. Whether called "erotic monomania," "erotomania," or "erotic melancholia," the conventional—in the sense of both "familiar" and "literary"—malady, discussed by Ferrand with "encyclopedic inclusiveness," never intrigued psychiatrists, all of a sudden faced with the striking phenomenon of madness, as much as it did courtiers, forced, for lack of a more engaging occupation, to spend their mental energies in and on trivial sexual pursuits. Semelaigne, who devotes to Ferrand a chapter of three pages, dismisses him, saying: "Jacques Ferrand ne s'occupe que de la mélancolie érotique."[51]

Descriptions of what may be recognized as madness or "English malady" (varieties of schizophrenia) begin to appear in French medical literature only in the 1780s. Cases of psychosis before that, mentioned very rarely, are cases of puerperal insanity—i.e., those of women temporarily affected during pregnancy or postpartum.[52] High society physicians focus on *affections vaporeuses*—which appears to be the nervous complaint à la mode, especially among the ladies. The most famous of these, the "celebrated" Dr. Pierre Pomme (whom Semelaigne characterizes as "a capable showman and charlatan of genius") as late as 1769 dedicates to it the fourth edition of his *Traité des Vapeurs* in two volumes, with a new dedication and preface in which he refers to publications such as *Mercure de France* and *Journal de Médecine* of 1767–1769. In it he defines the disease thus: "I call '*affection vaporeuse*' that general or specific illness of a nervous kind which produces [in the nerves] irritability and stiffening. It is referred to as 'hysterical' among women, because the Ancients regarded disorders of the uterus as the sole cause of such illnesses. It is called 'hypochondriac' or 'melancholic' among men, because the same [ancient] authors found its cause in the hypochondrium and the viscera of the lower abdomen."[53] This evidently ancient affliction was apparently remarkably widespread in mid-eighteenth-century France. "One is asked every day why the nervous diseases became so common," wrote Pomme. As an expert he felt duty-bound to respond, listing as the first among the general causes "the growing love of sciences and the expansion of literary culture":

That crowd of presses that roll ceaselessly in Europe, that immense quantity of works which they produce day after day, presuppose the existence of multitudes of people who, perhaps, lack the attributes of scholars, but are more or less exposed to the illnesses characteristic of them. So many authors bring along crowds of readers; and constant reading leads to all the nervous diseases: maybe, of all the causes of ill-health among women the principal one is the infinite multiplication of romances in the past hundred years. From cradle to old age they read these with such ardor that they wouldn't

be distracted for a moment, do not move at all, and often stay awake late
into the night to satisfy this passion—which absolutely ruins their health;
and this is not speaking of those who become authors themselves, a number
which grows daily. A girl who at the age of ten reads instead of running
must at the age of twenty suffer from vapors, and wouldn't be a good
[nursing] mother. [54]

Other general causes included "much increased consumption of hot drinks:
coffee, tea, chocolate, etc."; "the growing prosperity which has made life
cushier for the masters as well as for the servants, and prodigiously multiplied sedentary occupations, the establishment of which, so highly praised,
has at once ruined both agriculture and health"; the proliferation of passions, such as vanity, greed, ambition, jealousy, which are to be expected in
urban centers in times of prosperity and, damaging to health in general,
produce all the nervous problems; love for hot spices; natural degeneration
(ever weaker parents producing increasingly weaker offspring); and overuse
of pharmaceutical remedies.[55]

The symptoms of the characteristic mid-eighteenth century French nervous condition were not those of the "English disease." Its sufferers (especially women) did tend to be sad at times: "Sadness, melancholy and
discouragement poison all their amusements," wrote Pomme, "their imagination is troubled: they laugh, sing, yell, and cry for no reason." But most
of the symptoms were somatic—headaches, ringing in the ears, dizziness,
tremors, uneven or weak heartbeat, coughing, toothaches, leg cramps, and
spasms and seizures of all kinds. There was also nausea, vomiting, and
numerous digestive and elimination problems.[56] Perhaps, indeed, the
patients overused hot spices, or drank too much coffee while reading
romances.

Most of the French late eighteenth-century authors who touched on
mental disease were not high society physicians like Doctor Pomme. Often
starting as army surgeons, they were medical officers in hospitals, i.e., public
facilities for the indigent sick of all kinds, and prisons, and their interest in
mental illness, incidental to such service, was predominantly the interest in
ameliorating the conditions for the mentally ill. When, in 1788, Jacques-
René Tenon, the chief surgeon of the Salpêtrière hospital, addressed to the
Academy of Sciences his *Mémoires sur les hopitaux de Paris* (of which a couple

of pages were devoted to mental patients) the conditions these doctors encountered were appalling. In Hôtel-Dieu in Paris, which was for many the only place of treatment, for example, most mental patients shared beds. There were two rooms for all of them, one for men and one for women. Men's room contained ten beds for four people each and two individual beds; there were forty-two men in it. In the one for women thirty-two patients had the use of six collective beds and eight individual ones. This room was separated by a curtain from the room for women with infectious diseases. "How," asked Tenon, "can one breathe in beds in which three or four madmen [*fous*] lie together, crowding each other, quarrelling, and fighting, each garroted and chained, and in the narrowest of rooms, with four rows of beds?" If the inmates of Hôtel-Dieu after some period showed no signs of improvement, men were moved to Bicêtre and women to Salpêtrière hospitals. According to Pinel's Memoir of 1794, at Bicêtre in 1788, ninety-five out of 151 mental patients admitted died within a year. "Among the causes that exerted such a fatal influence on the lives of the insane at Bicêtre under the old regime," Pinel argued, "one must count the lack of food, since the daily ration of bread was only one and one-half lb, with an ounce or so of a carelessly prepared dish. This ration was distributed in the morning, or rather, it was instantly devoured and the rest of the time was spent in a ravenous delirium." Fortunately, in 1792—after the Revolution, but before Pinel was appointed as "physician for the infirmaries" at Bicêtre— "the hospital administration hurried to do away with this unnatural outrage, and for approximately 2 years the daily ration of bread has been raised to 2 lb, while care was taken to distribute part of it in the morning and part at night. That has stopped all complains about the dearth of food."[57]

Pinel's 1794 memorandum marks the first time a French physician in fact encountered patients who were mad in the English sense of the term— i.e., psychotically depressed or fully schizophrenic—among inmates of the hospital to which he was assigned and understood mental disease (*folie*) as madness. It is significant that the document was based on the experience at Bicêtre—the oldest French hospital with a special ward for the mentally ill, established by the order of Louis XIV, most likely in imitation of London's Bedlam—in Paris. Even at the time other public establishments in, and other parts of, France might not have allowed a similar experience. In 1791, Joseph Daquin published a volume of close to 300 pages, *La philosophie de la folie.* The full title made clear both the practical preoccupation and the theory of the author: it was the book, it announced, "where it is proved that this disease should be treated by moral, not physical, means, and that those who suffer from it are clearly under the influence of the moon." In the vanguard of his enlightened age in the humane attitude towards the mentally ill, Daquin appeared to be somewhat behind it in his belief in the causal role of the night luminary. Though he received his medical degree in 1757, he was a "fervent admirer" of Hippocrates and put his trust in ancient authorities. He became interested in mental disease rather late in life—after serving for 30 years as the general physician in the hospital and the librarian in his native Chambery, and then the natural history teacher at the Central School of the Mont Blanc Department. In 1787 he assumed the directorship of the mental ward of the Chambery hospital. In his book he confessed that he had had little experience with mental disorders (*folie*) before, but the experience he did have convinced him that the problem should be studied with the methods of natural history—through careful observation without prejudice, the only allowable prejudice being the sympathy for the patient. "A person who sees a mental patient [*un fou*] and remains unmoved," Daquin wrote, "or one who is amused by his state, is a moral monster." He was obviously a kind man.

There were about 40 patients in the ward when Daquin took his position. He spent much time in their company, talking to them as well as carrying regular medical examinations. On the basis of such observations he defined the illness of *folie* as "the privation of the recognition of what is true, that is, privation of reason." There were several distinct varieties of persons so deprived: the patients who needed to be tied (*fous à lier*) or the furious, that is, maniacs; the calm; the extravagant; the void of sense (*insensés*); idiots and cretins; and the demented. The furious were agitated and prone to "unnatural" actions; the calm—taciturn, absorbed, sometimes immobile; the extravagant—capricious, garrulous, unfocused, inattentive and incoherent, but almost always inoffensive; the void of sense—limited, incapable of almost any foresight and reflection, with "everything in [them] being reduced to the satisfaction of most ordinary needs of life"; the idiots and cretins were impulsive, unable to reason, "nothing but automata"; and the demented were "completely devoid of reason."

There were no suicidal patients in Daquin's ward. Semelaigne, summarizing Daquin's views as they appeared in the first, 1791, and the second, 1804, editions of *Philosophie de la folie*, writes:

> One is rather astonished to see him affirm that madmen [*les aliénés*] kill themselves very rarely, that they die above all from acute or chronic [physical] diseases, and that those who voluntarily end their own life are simply "unhappy beings, falsely considered *fous*, who kill themselves out of despair." Because loss of reason could not be reconciled with "often most ingeniously premeditated arrangements of the majority of those who think about suicide." The *fous* could not, according to him, resort to such ruses and clever tricks necessary to ward off suspicion. This opinion is hard to reconcile with the experience of a man who had been, by that time [1804], the director of a mental ward for seventeen years.[58]

Semelaigne's astonishment, however, reflects only his inability in 1930 to imagine that the *folie* that Daquin encountered at Chambery was not madness or, as the French would call it, *aliénation,* which in Semelaigne's own day was defined as schizophrenia and manic-depressive illness, but a very different, in some way the opposite, kind of mental dysfunction, in which psychiatrists—faced with the challenge of madness—lost interest in the course of the nineteenth century.

The French government became rather preoccupied with the care of the mentally ill already in the last years of the *ancien régime*. Whether this was because of the change in the nature of mental disorders or because such preoccupation reflected the new enlightened spirit of the age is unclear, but committees were appointed and projects of amelioration designed, the realization of which, according to Semelaigne, was prevented by the Revolution. There were also other changes. In and around Paris, at least, affluent families with mentally disturbed members in the 1770s and 1780s had the option to place these members in private establishments similar to English asylums, where, as we learn from Esquirol, though the proprietors felt their duty was to secure public safety, not to heal the sick, and "never attempted any rational treatment," the sick were nevertheless assured "an existence as tolerable and pleasant as their condition would allow." There were before the Revolution eighteen such establishments; most of their inmates were, likely, still the *fous* of the weak-minded variety (idiots, cretins, demented elderly) observed by Daquin at Chambery. But one of these *Petites Maisons* had the honor of the patronage of Marquis de Sade, for whose care 4.000 livres were paid in 1789 (a considerable sum, given that some of these private homes charged 300 livres per annum), and another had as a patient the revolutionary Saint-Just, who apparently spent his time there, between October 1786 and March 1787, writing "licentious" poetry. However unreasonable, Sade and Saint-Just were no fools.

Pinel was the first to focus on the mentally ill of their kind, pointing out, in Dora Weiner's words, that "gifted and sensitive persons are particularly vulnerable to mental anguish." He called their affliction "mental alienation" and thus implicitly distinguished it from the *folie*. When Pinel assumed his position as "the physician of the infirmaries" at Bicêtre in 1793, there were 200 patients in its seventh ward for the insane. The majority of them, like in the private establishments, probably were weak-minded, but a significant minority was not. Pinel wrote in his 1794 memorandum:

> A large gathering of madmen inspires an undefinable thoughtful tenderness when one realizes that their present state derives only from a vivid sensitivity and from psychologic qualities that we value highly. I find that truth ever more convincing and confirmed by my daily notes. Here is the father of a family whom unexpected losses have thrown into despair; here is a son exhausted by work and vigil to provide for his parents' subsistence; elsewhere a passionate and sensitive young man, victim of unrequited love; there a tender husband, distracted by suspicions and the justified or false umbrage of jealousy; a young warrior thirsting for glory whose vast and ambitious projects failed, his spirit crashed by the harsh experience. Religious zeal claims its victims, as does ardent military fervor, which often expresses all the reveries and excesses of manic fanaticism. Man is most often led from the free use of reason to madness by overstepping the limits of his good qualities and of his generous and magnanimous inclinations.

> The excessive sensitivity that characterizes very talented persons may become a cause for the loss of their reason: I mention this as a well-meant warning without the intention of discouraging them. Groups as diverse as investigators, artists, orators, poets, geometers, engineers, painters, and

sculptors pay an almost annual price to the hospice for the insane. I have on more than one occasion stopped at the cell of a madman speaking about current affairs in the most elaborate terms and with great verve. The exalted imagination of poets also leads sometimes to madness, and I am often importuned by a confabulator who urges me to read his productions, while I see only the urgent need to subject him to treatment for madness. . . . One of the most skillful clockmakers of Paris, infatuated with the fantasy of perpetual motion, spent a long time in the hospice. . . . There are usually some famous painters, at the moment two skilled artists. . . . I also give special care to a man versed in the most profound mathematical meditations who lost his reason because of ever-renewed fears that Vandalism visited upon true Knowledge. How many talents lost to Society and what great efforts are needed to salvage them![59]

There was a new kind of mental disease in France and even among the indigent it hit persons with superior intelligence and education particularly hard. Without explicitly acknowledging its newness, French psychiatrists from the first nevertheless could not regard it as a form of the familiar *folie* and, like the English three hundred years earlier, came up with a special term to designate it. They appropriated the English terms then in use—mania and melancholia, but the French term of preference was *aliénation mentale*—"mental alienation."

In the first years of the nineteenth century, the place of the central publication of the "parti 'philosophique'" in its Enlightenment sense, tell us the authors of *La pratique de l'ésprit humain* Marcel Gauchet and Gladys Swain, was held by the journal *La Décade philosophique*. It was the chief among what today would be considered "intellectual" periodicals for the general cultured public. In 1801 (or year IX of the revolutionary calendar) *La Décade* published a review of Pinel's 1800 *Traité médico-philosophique sur l'aliénation mentale ou la manie*. Pinel's central argument in this work was that mental alienation required and responded to "moral treatment"— not only gentler measures of restraint than chains and better nutrition than the starvation ration of a pound-and-a-half piece of bread a day, but engaging patients in conversation, keeping them occupied in calming activities, physical exercises, etc. The review presented several cases of recovery accomplished with the new method of moral treatment. Several months later *La Décade* informed its readers of another new development touching on the subject of mental alienation. Starting with a declaration that the "*Traité de la manie* has proved that the disease commonly referred to as *folie* is not incurable as believe those not in the know [*le vulgaire*]," it announced the opening of a new private establishment for the treatment of the mentally alienated. "The necessity to isolate the alienated from their families and old relations," the announcement explained,

> has been acutely sensed in London and in Paris. Experience has demon-
> strated that they do not regain their health in their habitual environment
> and that surrounding them with new objects is an essential element of the
> treatment. The expenses involved in private isolation, the danger of treating
> the alienated in homes unequipped for such use; the interest inspired by the
> unhappy victims of over-exalted or over-exhausted nervous susceptibility;
> the desire to offer Frenchmen and foreigners (for whom the change of cli-
> mate alone may be most useful [presumably, the English with their easterly
> wind on top of everything else]) an establishment which will put into prac-
> tice, in every detail, the principles developed in the *Traité de la manie;* these
> are the reasons for the establishment of the *Maison de Traitement des aliénés,*
> established under the authority of C. Pinel, the author of the said *Traité.* . . .
> The patients will be under the care of C. Esquirol, a private student of
> C. Pinel, who has studied mania under the direction of this famous pro-
> fessor, both among the women-patients [*folles*] of the Salpêtrière and among
> some[mentally] ill in the city. This citizen will bring to bear on his work in
> the new establishment the results of his research and the principles he
> derived from public lessons, medical conversations, and the confidence of
> his illustrious teacher.[60]

Some scholars find the interest of *La Décade* in the nascent national psy-chiatry puzzling and in need of an explanation.[61] Since the treatment of mentally alienated clearly was a matter of national honor, the fact that this central cultural periodical of the time followed developments in it so closely could be explained, among other things, by the journal's patrio-tism. But, perhaps, this interest is no more of a puzzle than interest in any other subject profiled in any periodical: papers inform their public about things the public wants to be informed about. This trivial explanation, however, reflects the great transformation in experience, which experts, as so often, do not want to see. The "disease commonly referred to as *folie*" was coming to concern the cultured classes in France. Mental alienation was their problem.

The first task French psychiatrists set for themselves was to describe the symptoms of mental alienation. Unlike both their predecessors and followers, they based this description almost exclusively on their clinical experience, mistrusting the existing (native) literature on the subject, perhaps because it focused on afflictions very different from the ones they encountered in their medical practice. Several features of mental alienation struck them from the outset as characteristic: its periodicity, often coming in attacks separated by intervals of lucidity; the fact that loss of reason (bizarre obsessive ideas) in regard to one particular subject could coexist with perfectly reasonable views in every other regard; the tendency for mistaken self-identification, particularly the prominence of delusions of grandeur, and other regularities which the reader would have no difficulty recognizing as parts of the schizophrenic/manic-depressive profile. For Pinel, Esquirol, and their students, all these were discoveries, phenomena long, maybe forever, in existence, which they believed nobody had noticed before them. They were meticulous in recording their observations, and it is to the efforts of these indefatigable French clinicians in the first sixty years of the nineteenth century that we owe the most accurate characterizations of the disease they were to name *dementia praecox* and to recognize as alternately manic and melancholic, *folie circulaire* or *folie à double forme*. In 1794, of course, none of these names, or detailed descriptions which they captured, existed, but Pinel wrote in his pioneering address:

> Madness may be continuous during a large part of life or show long remissions, increase steadily, without interruption, or occur in regular or irregular attacks. This points to two kinds of madness: one continuous or chronic, the other intermittent or characterized by the most violent recurring symptoms. In continuous insanity, the madman is ceaselessly preoccupied by an exclusive thought or a fixed sequence of thoughts or else led to acts of violence while his reasoning faculties appear intact. He seems dominated by the sinister tendency to harm and to destroy. This derangement of his psychologic faculties stays with him for a large part of his life, with very little change.

One should keep in mind how necessarily and specifically limited Pinel's experience was, being based on observations at Bicêtre, which kept its mentally ill patients of every variety chained and starved, and where, at the time of writing, he worked for one year. Here are some of them:

> In this hospice for the insane there is a melancholic inmate with sinister looks who has been chained for 25 years and who tries to vent his fury on anyone daring to set foot in his cell. He relents only in the presence of women, toward whom he behaves in a gentler manner. Another madman who is just as agitated and violent has been chained for 45 years, and it is only since the harsh winter of 1788 that he is calmer, or rather, advancing age has rendered him harmless. In contrast, neither the change of seasons nor the passage of time has markedly altered the condition of an Irish priest chained for 15 years: he combines a deadly inclination to harm with perfidious cunning, and his polite behavior is designed to detect opportunities for venting his fury.

This leads Pinel to a generalization: "The insanity caused by religious fervor or a zeal for devout thoughts usually persists without interruption until the end of life." And, by association: "Puffed-up ambition or the mad thought of believing oneself a king or prince is just as hopeless, an almost indestructible and seductive illusion. The madman who believes he is Louis XIV and who often hands me Dispatches for the Governments of his provinces is so enchanted with his exalted power that his imagination holds on to it: he would make too great a sacrifice in stepping down from his imaginary throne." There was at Bicêtre also a man "rendered mad by love who, the day before his attack confided to [Pinel] a dream designed to make his lifelong happiness: his love had appeared to him with features of the most ravishing beauty, and he believed that she promised soon to unite her destiny to his." "I have never heard love spoken of with such ardor," recalled Pinel.

Mental alienation, the Doctor insisted in this very first presentation on the subject, "should by no means imply a total abolition of the mental faculties. On the contrary, the disorder usually attacks only one partial faculty such as perception of ideas, judgment, reasoning, imagination, memory, or psychologic sensitivity." Moreover, specifically "errors of reasoning" were much rarer among the alienated than was "commonly thought, for they derive reliable inductions from a particular sequence of ideas that preoccupies them." Pinel, probably, was not aware that he was paraphrasing John Locke's reasons for distinguishing madmen from "natural fools," and adduced an observation from his experience to support this statement: "The white-haired 70-year-old still living at Bicêtre who believes that he is a young woman is in perfect agreement with himself when he obstinately refuses other than feminine clothing, adorns himself with care, is flattered by the polite behavior of the staff and their talk of his prospects of an approaching marriage, or when his modesty seems alarmed at the least indecent gesture." Still, symptoms of mental alienation were remarkably variable and, while "a total upheaval of the rational faculty," expressed in "a bizarre association of the most incongruous and incoherent ideas" was rare, it did occur. Whatever the symptoms, what seemed to follow the attacks was indeed a sense of self-alienation: "they themselves know," wrote Pinel, "that they are not sufficiently in control of themselves to be responsible for their willed behavior."[62]

Pinel's contemporaries called him "the good Monsieur Pinel." Speaking about his contribution to psychiatry in the early twentieth century, Georges Dumas argued that "this affectionate appellation does not seem to indicate that they considered him a genius."[63] Perhaps, they did not. It was not his analysis of mental alienation, but his kindness to those who suffered from it that stayed in the national—and professional—memory. In the present context, however, Pinel's random observations—i.e., observations of what he found at Bicêtre—are of the utmost significance precisely because they are uneducated, unsystematic, and intellectually unambitious, of which he was certainly aware. (He wrote, revealing the state of international psychiatry and much more:

a person who seeks to acquire the right ideas and fixed principles about the psychologic treatment of madness hardly knows where to turn. Medical treatises offer only general views, and in specialized treatises one finds only isolated observations irrelevant for a large group of maniacs. Travelers have not yet brought us specific enlightenment in their reports about various European institutions of this kind. The rights of man are too little respected in Germany to make the study of their ways of handling the insane in public establishments worthwhile. Spain has taken only a few steps toward this great goal. . . . it is mainly England one must envy for the artful wisdom of managing a large group of madmen and effecting the most unexpected cures. Why does that haughty and self-righteous nation spoil such a great gift to humanity by keeping a mysterious silence and guiltily casting a veil over its skill to restore distracted reason? The English proudly display the majestic sight and the internal arrangements of the asylums that Philosophy has dedicated to the unfortunate insane. But they keep the art of managing the insane a deep secret which they apparently want to control and keep from other peoples. I have therefore been restricted this first year to the slim resources of the preliminary studies I had done and to the observations I was making daily; I have carefully examined and compared the several varieties of insanity to deduce firm rules for managing all of them.[64])

He does not attempt to explain what has struck him, just to report it. That what he has observed struck him, in the last years of the eighteenth century, and that he could regard what he observed as a discovery reveals a great deal about the nature of psychiatric mental disease—above all, that this disease is an historical phenomenon.

While French psychiatrists remained, in the first place, clinicians, they rapidly grew intellectually ambitious, among other things, because of the necessity to stay on a par with England. They studied the practices of their English colleagues. Their specialist education improved, they became impressively systematic in their analysis. This analysis swiftly led them to the conclusions reached by English physicians in the sixteenth century (whom, at this point, nobody read any longer), though the French were much more explicit—and lucid—in their formulations. François-Emmanuel Fodéré was, probably, the first, if unlikely, of such analysts, not counting Esquirol, who formed a category of his own. Fodéré is an interesting character. Since 1793 a cousin by marriage of two kings, Bernadotte and Joseph Bonaparte, he finished his medical studies in 1787, and thought of dedicating himself to the study of cretinism. Enthusiasm inspired him to attempt secretly an exhumation of a cretin's body, on the brain of which he wished to perform an autopsy, and this led to some trouble with law-enforcement and medical authorities. This experience moved the young doctor, who barely managed to keep his license, to exchange cemeteries as the theater of his operations for Parisian hospitals, which for three years "he visited assiduously," going to study in London after that. On his return, having served for a while as a doctor in the military and taking part in the Italian campaign, he was appointed to a mental hospice, having been, on his own account, especially interested in the afflictions of the mind.

Fodéré is best known for his pioneering work in legal medicine (specifically, advocating the use of insanity defense in cases of violent crime), but this was spurred by his study of cretinism and a clinical experience with mental alienation, which made him acutely aware of the differences between *folie* and madness. He, therefore, explicitly distinguished between the two. *Folie* was a dysfunction of the intellect, in which the senses remained in good working order, while in madness (which he called *délire*) "the mind cannot correct its judgments, because it is deceived by the images present; it is a state of illness in which there is no freedom."[65] Only acquired idiotism could be considered a loss of mind and thus a variety of madness; cretins, he argued would not have a mind to lose. Chronic madness, in distinction to acute one, is almost never accompanied by fever. It begins with a prodrome, usually depressive and is followed by increasing agitation. Fodéré felt he could not draw clear-cut nosological distinctions: in his practice, he wrote, he did not encounter pure cases and could only report that "the maniacs lost their minds [*étaient en même temps en démence*] during episodes of agitation, while those suffering from melancholia, dementia, and idiotism were very often maniacs." He disagreed with Pinel that mania (as a disease expressed in extreme agitation) could be separated from *délire* and proposed for episodes in which only agitation, but not delirious speech and thinking, was present the term "maniacal rage" *(fureur maniaque)*. Although *délire* in almost every case began with melancholia, he was not certain one could interpret mania as *"mélancholie dégénérée en fureur."* Melancholia, in Fodéré's view was "a child of pride or a product of fear." It could be expressed in several ways: as misanthropy (we would call it "sociopathy" today); as love melancholy—which, significantly, he distinguished sharply from erotic melancholy or erotomania of *amor hereos;* as prophetic melancholy; as superstitious melancholy; and as suicidal tendency. He considered suicide committed for fear of an imaginary misfortune or because one is disgusted with life as a sure sign of mental alienation, which could not be accounted for, as could be cases of suicide cited from ancient history, by values and mores of the epoch. The more frequent were the episodes of maniacal rage the more certainly they abutted a complete loss of mind—dementia, in which both perception and judgment were disordered and of which Fodéré wrote: "in this [state] of eclipse of reason, the patient [*l'insensé*] never engages in any argument and undertakes no action determined by his will."[66]

But it was Esquirol, above all, who should be credited with laying the foundations for the French psychiatry of the nineteenth century—and, since Kraepelin's great classification on which psychiatry everywhere is still based, was in essence a presentation of the accumulated French knowledge, transformed into a "theory" (endowed with great authority by scientifically-sounding Latin names which had meaning only for the experts, and duly obscured under a thick fog of the German *Idee*)—of psychiatry as we know it. In 1817, Esquirol, since 1811 the physician in charge of the mental patients at Salpêtrière—the counterpart of Bicêtre for women—and the most eminent French clinician, established the first clinical course in mental disease. His lectures were attended by students from everywhere in France and, according to Semelaigne, "even from abroad." His "classic book, *Des maladies mentales considerées sous les rapports médical, hygiénique et médico-legal*," say Alexander and Selesnick in their *History of Psychiatry*, "was a basic text for half a century and stimulated his students to contribute new and basic definitions to clinical psychiatry."[67] Indeed, for the next fifty years France would be the undisputed center of psychiatry, and Esquirol's ideas on the nature of mental alienation were very influential.

Esquirol, say Alexander and Selesnick, "did not indulge in philosophical or physiological speculations about mental illness." He believed that madness was an etiologically complex disease, but his main goal (besides alleviating the suffering of the mentally ill) was to describe it and distinguish specific clinical syndromes. Numerous factors participating in its causation could be divided into general and particular causes, which could be physical and cultural (*morales*), with some, in fact, being predisposing conditions and some triggers. He considered it significant, for example, that children were not subject to madness; the disease could develop with puberty, but even this happened in rare cases. Persons who habitually strained their intelligence—intellectuals, we would call them, but the word did not exist in Esquirol's day—were particularly predisposed to it. The question of the affinity between genius and madness having been already raised, Esquirol considered it, ruling: "If one means by this [affinity] that those with very active and unregulated imagination, who are excited by ideas [or, rather, thinking] and whose ideas change rapidly, are quite similar to madmen [*fous*], one is correct, but if one assumes that a great intelligence predisposes one to madness, one is mistaken." The dominant ideas of the time, in his view, directly influenced both the contents of delusions (*délire*) in, and the rates of, madness. Thus, every scientific discovery, every new institution would be reflected in certain cases of madness. Political turmoil, in general, increased the number of the cases. Yet, most madness was caused not by change and instability, as this might imply, but by passions Esquirol considered universal: fear, ambition, emotions caused by vicissitudes of fortune, domestic troubles—and "the struggle," contradictions, between principles of religion (and accepted morality) and these passions. Perhaps, because such struggle would be exacerbated under certain conditions (for instance, those of political turmoil), Esquirol argued that madness could become epidemic and that there were cases of collective madness (*folies collectives*): "As in the atmosphere there exist certain conditions making occurrences of epidemic infectious diseases more or less frequent, there also exist in the minds certain general dispositions conducive to the propagation and spread of mental alienation, its communication to a large number of individuals by a sort of mental contagion." This, he thought, was observed throughout history. The causes and triggers of madness were many. In contrast, Esquirol believed that only one predisposing cause (or condition) deserved the consideration of a clinician: it was heredity, understood, however, as the effect on the offspring of the actual parental disease, and not as the inheritance of a parental predisposition, i.e., quite differently from contemporary genetics.

Esquirol seemed to define specific syndromes as forms of monomania, madness with narrowly focused delusions. Depressive monomania was lypemania, characterized as delusional melancholia (*mélancolie avec délire*), or what we would call a "psychotic depression." Its symptoms were indeed the familiar symptoms of the latter. While lypemaniacs were self-centered, they focused on their inner world; in contrast, active, irritable monomaniacs lived "too much outside"; their dominant emotion was vanity: their characteristic delusions were those of grandeur, and it is among them that one would find enthusiasts of all sorts, the pseudo-prophets and pretenders to thrones; they also believed themselves to be pursued by enemies, using supernatural means. There were three clinical forms of monomania. Monomaniacs, wrote Esquirol, may "start with a false premise and follow it logically without deviation, deriving legitimate conclusions which modify their sentiments and actions of their will; apart from this partial delusion, they feel, reason, and act like every other person; the basis of this mental disorder [ce délire] that I would call 'intellectual' are illusions, hallucinations, wrong associations of ideas, false, bizarre, erroneous convictions." In other cases the emotions were primarily affected and justified by well-reasoned arguments, leading some authors to refer to the condition as *manie raisonnante*. Esquirol, however, preferred to call it "affective monomania." The third kind expressed itself in the impairment of the will, the patient being moved to do things repugnant to him, but "instinctive, irresistible; this [was] monomania without delusions or instinctive monomania." Such was, for example, homicidal monomania, in which "his will injured and subjugated by the violence of the urge, the man is deprived of moral liberty." In all these forms, madness did not consist in the loss of the intellect, but rather in the disassociation between the intellect and emotional and/or volitional faculties of the mind: the mind, in other words, was not lost, but disorganized. One certainly could call this phenomenon "schizophrenia."

Mania, for Esquirol, was generalized monomania. Patients' delusions were unfocused, and all their mental faculties were affected. Esquirol wrote: "The maniacs are recognizable by their false sensations, the illusions and hallucinations, by the wrong association of ideas, which follow one another without any connection and with extreme rapidity; they are recognizable by the errors in their judgment, the perturbation of their affections, and finally by the disappearance of their will." The onset of mania was usually insidious and very often initiated by a state of depression, but this state was only "a sign of mania waiting to explode." Depressive episodes would announce the return of an acute state of intermittent mania. In effect, Esquirol used the term "mania" to designate what we throughout the twentieth century and today would see as acute psychosis of the full-blown schizophrenia, and he saw this disease as explicitly manic-depressive. Kraepelin did not improve much on that—to say the least—when he separated schizophrenia from manic-depressive illness. But, then, Esquirol was just a clinician, and clinicians were regarded as inferior species by German theorists (who happened to regard so many as inferior species).[68]

Esquirol was the premier clinician in France, but it could not have been just a reflection of his renown among fellow-psychiatrists and patients that his name and expertise were expected to be familiar to the entire French reading public. And they were expected to be familiar. It is to the care of M. Esquirol that the mad protagonist's uncle hastens to commit his ailing relative in Balzac's 1832 novel *Louis Lambert*, later included in *Contes philosophiques* of *The Human Comedy*, and the statement is followed by no explanation as to who M. Esquirol is and why Louis should be brought, from the countryside, to him in Paris. For a twenty-first-century historian of mental disease, this is remarkable, as is the novel, in general, describing as it is possibly the first case of classic schizophrenia, "madness in its pure form," in French fiction, and as one of the very first subjects in Balzac's colossal *panneau* of contemporary society. Today's literary specialists say that Balzac became interested in madness because he suffered a minor head injury in a carriage crash (indeed, *Louis Lambert* was written while he was recuperating), and that the question that really preoccupied him was not the nature of madness as such, but the often discussed at the time connection between madness and genius (and, indeed, Louis, before becoming indisputably mad, is portrayed as a person of prodigious analytical powers and imagination, a possible genius). But, then, one must ask why was the question of madness and genius so often discussed in early nineteenth-century France—and discussed by great writers, such as Balzac or Chateaubriand, who were not clinically ill themselves, rather than by persons afflicted by the disease, who have a clear motive to uncover its positive features, as it is today—and why would a minor head injury with no repercussions for all we know make young Balzac interested in madness which in his book he connected to no physical injury of any kind. I believe Balzac was interested in madness because it was all around him, a central experience in the life of his time (which would also explain Esquirol's name recognition among the wide educated public), and the issue of madness and genius was discussed because the disease affected first and foremost people who, at the start, could end either way (as mad or as genius): people who thought too much and lived in their mind.

Balzac was such a man. In *Louis Lambert* before he succumbed to his disease (became acutely psychotic in our words: in the book, on the eve of his wedding to his very ideal, a beautiful, good, sensitive creature, who is also the richest heiress in the province, Louis is suddenly convinced that he is impotent, attempts to castrate himself, and never becomes lucid again) he described himself. His portrayal of Louis's inner world rings so true, because it is based on the careful introspective observation. From childhood, Louis lives in his thoughts and the focus of his thoughts is the mind. He analyses its several faculties, examines its creative powers. As a young teenager he attempts to write "A Treatise on Will"; the will, he concludes, is the central mental faculty:

> New ideas need new words or old words better defined, with enlarged, expanded connotations; Lambert thus chose, to express the essence of his theory, several common words which already vaguely reflected his thought. The word WILL served to name the sphere in which the thought evolved; or, to put this less abstractly, the mass of force by which man can reproduce outside of himself the actions of which his exterior life consists. VOLITION . . . referred to the person's acting on Will. The word THOUGHT, for him the quintessential product of the Will, also designated the sphere in which IDEAS were born . . . He put the Will before Thought. 'To think, one has to will,' he would say . . .

Lambert's material is, again, himself. He is remarkably self-conscious and self-reflective. He is also absolutely fascinated, carried away by language. Language, in Louis' life, is an autonomous force, which Louis follows, as if enchanted, rather than controls. Balzac considers this special relationship as basic to the understanding of his character, focusing on it already on the second page of the novel, just as he begins to introduce Louis Lambert to the reader:

> The analysis of a word, its physiognomy, its history were for Lambert the occasion for a long dreamy reflection [*rêverie*]. . . . Often, he would say to

me, speaking of his reading, I would depart on a delicious voyage, tied to a word in the gulfs of the past, like an insect carried by a current on a blade of grass. Starting in Greece, I arrived in Rome and traversed all the modern ages. What a beautiful book can be written about the life and adventures of a word! Without a doubt it bears the impressions of the circumstances in which it was used; depending on the place, it suggested different ideas; but isn't it even greater to consider it from the triple perspective of the soul, the body, and movement? To look at it, abstracting its functions, its effects, and its acts—isn't there enough in this to fall into an ocean of reflections? Aren't most words shades of ideas which they externally express? To which genius do we owe them? If a great intelligence is required to create one word, how old should human speech be? The assemblage of letters, their forms, the contours they give to a word, draw precisely, following the character of each people, the unknown beings whose memory is in us. . . . Isn't there in the word TRUE some sort of fantastic rectitude? Isn't there in the brief sound it produces a vague image of chaste nudity, of the simplicity of the true in everything? This syllable breathes some sort of freshness. I took as an example the expression of an abstract idea, not wanting to explain the problem by a word that would make it too easy to understand, such as FLIGHT [*vol*] in which everything speaks to the senses. But isn't this so in every word? Each one is full of a living power they derive from the soul, and which they restore to it by the mysteries of a marvelous action and reaction between speech and thought. Isn't this like a lover drawing from the lips of his beloved as much love as he gives? Just by their look, words animate in our mind the creatures which they serve to clothe. . . . [69]

Balzac ended up a great and celebrated writer, not a madman. How did he know that this kind of hyperreflexive cerebration on the mind, this explicit awareness of the autonomy of language, as well as its materiality and sensual qualities, was in fact a characteristic of schizophrenic thinking? A number of persons of similar sensitivity and ideas sufficient to create this impression on him must have ended up mad in his circle. Schizophrenics whom one knew before the outbreak of the disease as brilliant and enthusiastic, if somewhat desultory, intellectuals must have become as familiar a phenomenon in mid-nineteenth-century France as Toms O'Bedlam were in late sixteenth-century England. Delacroix wrote to Balzac upon the publication of *Louis Lambert:* "I have known Lamberts. . . . I myself was somebody like Lambert . . ."[70]

In January 1843, in Paris, the very first specialized (though clearly trans-disciplinary, as we would say today) periodical on mental disease in the world began publication. This was *Annales Médico-Psychologiques.* Its title-page announced very explicitly what it aspired to be: a "journal of anatomy, physiology, and pathology of the nervous system, specifically committed to collect all the materials relative to the science of connections of the body and the mind [*la science des rapports du physique et du moral*], to mental pathology, to legal medicine of the mad [*aliénés*], and to the nature of neuroses." Its editor-in-chief was Jules Baillarger, then the physician attached to the mental ward at Salpêtrière. In the introduction taking the first 27 pages of the first volume, he explained that the idea of the journal belonged to Pinel and his principal students who long wished to realize it "in the name of the French school." However, Pinel was thinking about a periodical focusing solely on pathology, while the sphere of interest of the current editors was broader. "Madness [*la folie*]," wrote Baillarger:

> that cruel disease so long neglected by the majority of physicians, and so often associated with crime by the most civilized governments of Europe, merited such supreme interest on the part of those who, in the beginning of this century, focused on it the meditations of science and the solicitudes of public charity. That was a beautiful day, indeed, when the voice of Pinel woke up the medical mind and called on it to intervene not only in the physical treatment of the unhappy madmen [*aliénés*], but also in the organization and the direction of mental asylums. The general public reacted to this late but energetic awakening, and in the light of this favorable reaction, the idea of a journal exclusively focused on mental pathology would everywhere meet with encouragement.
>
> The situation is different today. The creation of a narrowly specialized journal, which would be an immense contribution in 1800, appears to us insufficient in 1843. Physicians, legislators, representatives of the government, everybody, in the spheres of their responsibilities, cooperate in the study, treatment, and protection of the mad [*aliénés*] and there is no neces-

sity any longer to ceaselessly call for such cooperation. Mental alienation has risen in medicine as well as in public policy to the rank belonging to great disasters [*grandes infortunes;* social problems]. Considerable work has been done . . . it serves as a point of departure for the work that has to be accomplished. The road to reforms and ameliorations is open; one has only to take it. . . . We do not need any longer to concentrate all our forces on a single point, as if the matter was to found a new doctrine or institution. The science of mental alienation exists today uncontested; every day it is enriched by new materials; . . . Our efforts, therefore, may be expended less sparingly . . . and rather than limiting ourselves to the task of focusing the attention of the readers on mental pathology, we could, enlarging the framework of our collection, include in it all the work related to the nervous system . . . the study of mental disease [*folie*], instead of being pursued in isolation, as it was until now, will find itself associated with those [other studies] which must contribute most effectively to its development. . . . The time has come . . . for the diverse elements of the science of man to come together, unite, and mutually support each other. Keeping them separate is . . . to impede the advancement of the science of connections between body and the mind . . .

This explains, on the one hand, the title we have given to this periodical, and, on the other hand, the variety of publications we intend to accept in it. . . . We pursue a general goal: the theoretical and practical advancement of the science of connections between body and mind. . . . In effect, the science of connections between body and mind does not belong exclusively within physiology correctly understood; it enters into the field of pathology, into the study of neuroses, of idiocy, of mental alienation, etc.; it also raises a number of philosophical problems which one can, to some extent, see as foreign to medical sciences. We thus felt it was necessary, taking into the consideration the complex character of the science of connections between body and mind, to assign to that science a special place under the title of medico-psychological generalities. We shall dedicate the second section to anatomy and physiology. The third will be reserved for pathology."[71]

A discussion of the subjects in each of the three planned sections of the journal followed. In regard to "medico-psychological generalities" (general medical psychology, I suppose), in particular, Baillarger made it clear that, while it was impossible to understand mental disease outside this context, the study of mental disease offered a key to the understanding of the mind and was, therefore, the linchpin of the human sciences (*science de l'homme*) in general. Thus the journal was of interest not only to the very many people interested in mental alienation as such, but to a much broader audience, if such could be imagined. Could a physician understand the perversions in human cognition (*l'entendement humain*), he asked, for instance, if he does not examine the influences of education, and of moral and physical environment? "The point is not to accept servilely the teachings, always imperfect, of one or another school of psychologists or social scientists (*idéologues*) whose understanding of moral and intellectual phenomena is very narrow. . . . The point is . . . to examine the laws which rule, in the normal state, the production of our ideas, our sentiments, our sensations, and our actions, in order to discover the pathological laws leading to the disorder in these ideas, these sentiments, these sensations, and these actions in mental alienation and in neuroses." This part of the project, in fact, was rather similar to that of moral philosophers, such as Adam Smith or the contemporary Utilitarians (though the only English philosopher Baillarger mentioned was Locke). The doctor stressed the role of philosophy in it:

> The intervention of philosophy in the scientific research is the more necessary the more the facts under study are complex and related to multiple other facts. Now, such is precisely the nature of the facts under study in the science of man as a moral and intellectual being. . . . [Ill-advised was] the extreme division between different branches of human sciences, which presupposed that they are separated by impenetrable boundaries, in modern education. . . . Man is one, despite the distinct elements of which he is formed. In a marvelous manner combine in him the material forces, the organic forces, and the spiritual forces, which can be conceived in isolation only outside him . . . [72]

At the same time, Baillarger insisted that "the questions of pure philosophy" would be completely excluded from the journal. It would not consider general moral problems, or those of ontology and logic. Metaphysics was a sphere it left to others. The editor was aware that the intention and the central subject of the journal necessarily involved it in the debate on the problem of the duality of man "dominating the science of man as the intellectual and moral being"—the debate between idealism and materialism. He refused to take sides and promised eclecticism in editorial policy. Philosophy was important only in its most obvious connection with the science of human organism:

> Our sights will remain fixed on this organism, and if we'll turn them away for a while, this will be only to explore the spiritual [*morales*] forces which move it and to which it reacts; this will be to explore the mode of action of ideas that impress themselves on and change it. The nervous system is a special instrument of the phenomena of relational life; it is this system which allows the organism to be influenced by the intellectual world, the world of the senses, and the world of the organism itself. Thus our attention will be focused on the . . . operations of the nervous system in order to discover what role it plays in the production of phenomena of man's moral and intellectual life. We must make the whole ensemble of physiological and pathogenic data converge on the understanding of neuroses and mental alienation. . . . Our medico-psychological generalities must have a practical goal, a medical goal, positive and clearly defined.[73]

The emphasis on neuroses (*névroses*), often mentioned alongside mental alienation, in this 1843 editorial introduction to the first issue of *Annales Médico-Psychologiques* is interesting. Baillarger called "neuroses" the subclinical forms of mental alienation, like the latter, disorders of "relational life," expressed in social maladjustment, in a general malaise that affected the so-called "malcontents" in sixteenth-century England—not mad enough to be called mad, but close—and that in contemporary American society seems to be the normal "angst" of young adulthood; in short, what today's experts would regard as "spectrum disorders"—dysthemia, cyclothemia, anxiety disorder, etc. To be considered normal, these conditions must be very widespread. They are, as we know, very widespread among us. Apparently, they were pretty widespread in 1843 Paris as well.

With the founding of *Annales Médico-Psychologiques* the interest of the general reading public in France in mental alienation as a psychiatric disorder treated by alienists, very pronounced and growing since the early years of the nineteenth century, in some way reached its culmination. In Paris, mental alienation must have been the talk of the town in 1843; in intellectual circles it would be very difficult to avoid discussions, and close to impossible to remain unaware, of it. From that point on, it seems, while the interest in mental alienation among the general public continued, judging by the stress on it in fiction, its experience was taken out of the medical context and incorporated into the very fabric of life as yet another (perhaps a central) element of modernity. On their part, the alienists went on with their professional investigations, focused on madness indeed, but including in their scope other, more familiar forms of *folie,* such as idiocy and cretinism.

In November 1843, a young intellectual from Germany, Karl Marx, arrived in Paris to assume the editorship of another new periodical, then in preparation, *Deutsch-Französische Jahrbücher.* The French capital being for him "the new capital of the new world" (as well as "the old university of philosophy") he was excited about moving there, and it is possible that the magazine he planned to edit was really conceived as a collaboration between German and French intellectuals. In general, as Marx stated in a letter to his prospective coeditor, Arnold Ruge, the magazine aimed at "the reform of consciousness" through "self-clarification (critical philosophy) to be gained by the present time of its struggles and desires." Its specific subject was customized. "We want to influence our contemporaries," wrote Marx to Ruge, "particularly our German contemporaries. . . . In the first place religion, and next to it, politics, are the subjects which form the main interest of Germany today. We must take those, in whatever form they exist, as our point of departure." It is nevertheless clear that at this point in his career, human spirit, rather than social institutions, was what preoccupied Marx most—he saw himself as belonging quite naturally within the fold of traditional German philosophy. His authorities were Kant, Fichte, Schelling, and, above all, after 1837, Hegel. It was Hegel's thought he repeated in the famous letter to his father of November 10 that year, when he equated the "activity of history" with "that of the mind." "Life, in general" was for him "the expression of an intellectual activity which develops in all directions, in science, art and private matters"; the world of ideas "a living world"; a real achievement (not to show-off, but "to bring genuine pearls into the light of day") worthy of every effort was to prove "that the nature of the mind is just as necessary, concrete and firmly based as the nature of the body." All this sounds as different as can be from the historical materialism of the later years, from 1846 on, in fact, in which consciousness was reduced to "conscious awareness" of material—mostly economic—reality, and ideas had "no history, no development," but were epiphenomena of their carriers' class positions. It is arguable that Karl Marx of 1843 would find the "medico-psychological generalities" part of the project Dr. Baillarger outlined for *Annales Médico-Psychologiques* congenial.

There were other reasons why the psychiatric concerns of the French reading public might have interested the future father of scientific communism. He was no stranger to mental affliction himself. Though there is no evidence that he ever approached a clinical condition, French alienists would, no doubt, classify him as a neurotic. He also faced in effect insurmountable identity problems (which, in his youthful idealism, he believed to have surmounted): he was a German Romantic nationalist and a Jew—as a German nationalist he was an anti-Semite, and as a Jew he was a target of anti-Semitism and could not feel fully German. Add to this that, as a German nationalist, he suffered from a sense of a national inferiority vis-à-vis, and thus deeply resented, the French, and yet he also admired France, which for him was a model society. In 1837, in Berlin, while studying law and writing Romantic poetry ("marked," as he said, "by attacks on our times" and "complete opposition of what is and what ought to be"), he clearly was socially maladjusted and unhappy, felt isolated, had trouble sleeping, "endured [NB] much internal and external excitement," and turned into "an anemic weakling." His vexation with philosophy, Hegel, in particular, left him for a while "quite incapable of thinking" and he was running "about madly in the garden by the dirty water of the Spree." He was aware that he was ill (attributing this to his "vain, fruitless intellectual labors") and even sought the advice of a doctor, which was to go to the country. There the episode ended. The young man celebrated the regaining of his mental health by burning his poems—and, with them, his earlier self-definition: he was to be a poet no more, from now on he was a philosopher. Karl's father, however, was not certain of the significance of this change, he still talked of "the demon" that possessed his son, suspected that Karl's heart was in disaccord with his head, and doubted that he would ever be capable of "true human, domestic happiness."[74] And timid Jenny von Westphalen, Frau Karl Marx to be, was frightened by her betrothed.

It is suggestive that the two very first essays Marx wrote, "On the Jewish Question," and "Introduction to the Contribution to the Critique of Hegel's Philosophy of Right," both written in 1843 and published in the first (and only) February 1844 issue of *Deutsch-Französische Jahrbücher,* attempted to solve the young man's two disturbing identity problems. The first argued that Jewish "nationality," while fully deserving of the coarsest invectives German nationalists showered on it, was "chimerical," nothing but an illusion, and thus proved that Marx, even were he more predisposed towards the Jews (which he evidently was not), simply could not be Jewish. This thorny obstacle to his chosen (German) identity and participation in the defense of the German cause removed, Marx made his next essay a nationalist manifesto, ingeniously redefining Germany's very inferiority to the model modern nations of England and France as superiority, because Germany alone possessed philosophical ideas that could create a revolution (presumably, in consciousness—that self-clarification of the times he spoke about in a letter to Ruge) allowing for the realization of human potential, which was less of a possibility in self-satisfied England and France, blind to the fact that the existing social arrangements in them prevented it, than in self-critical Germany, and which England and France, therefore, needed more.[75]

Proving, at least to himself, that the widely acknowledged superiority of France was only apparent, but that it was Germany that was the really superior nation, certainly would make Marx feel more comfortable in Paris than he would have been, had he carried with him across the border the sense of national inferiority. What lends further support to this interpretation of the second 1843 essay is the fact that Marx never proceeded beyond the "Introduction" in his contribution to the critique of Hegel's "Philosophy of Right": the task was accomplished. Marx certainly intended to continue. The most significant piece of writing he did in France, the so-called "Economic and Philosophical Manuscripts of 1844," opens with a reference to an announcement of this continuation he placed in *DFY:* "I have already given notice in the *Deutsche-Frazösische Yahrbücher* of the critique of jurisprudence and political science in the form of a critique of the Hegelian Philosophy of Right." But something else caught his attention; while his plans remained the same (he still thought that, in a somewhat roundabout fashion, he would fulfill his promise to the readers), jurisprudence and political science definitely no longer held his interest. Most incongruously for the future theorist of historical materialism, who insisted that being determines consciousness, his focus now was psychology. True, Marx linked it to political economy and nobody can be surprised by the fact that political economy finally, in his twenty-sixth year, attracted the attention of the greatest political economist in history. But Marx talks about constructing the science of man, human science, and insists that it should be one of the natural sciences, focusing on man as an organism with a mind. Indeed, when he gets to a discussion of Hegel in the fifth and last fragment of the manuscripts, it is the *Phenomenology of the Mind* that he discusses, saying, among other things, in his critical comments: "consistent naturalism or humanism distinguishes itself both from idealism and materialism, constituting at the same time the unifying truth of both" and "only naturalism is capable of comprehending the act of world history."[76]

The main contribution of the manuscripts—to be considered of central importance by twentieth-century Marxists—was the development of the concept of *alienation* as related to private property. Marx wrote in German and used the German equivalent of the word—*Entfremdung*—the term also used by Hegel in *Phenomenology of the Mind* in the context of the alienation of the Mind (the Spirit) from itself in the course of history, as it perceived the world of its own creation as something objective and other from itself.[77] It has been a matter of consensus among Marxist scholars that the concept of "alienation" in 1844 manuscripts signaled the beginning of Marx's effort to turn Hegel from his head onto his feet, and thus transform Hegel's idealism into materialism. But it is not at all certain that Hegel's "alienation" of the World Spirit was the phenomenon Marx was trying to understand and explain. Of course, Marx knew his Hegel, and it would be surprising had he not connected his discussion of alienation to Hegel's discussion, but it is significant that the discussion of Hegel is the last fragment of the manuscripts, attempted almost as an afterthought and very probably as something that had to be done, if Marx was to fulfill the promise he gave in print to the readers of his journal.

If it was not the argument with Hegel Marx was engaging in, if Hegel was not the inspiration behind his concept of alienation, who and what was he responding to? Could not this be the alienation of alienists and their patients, alienation as understood in France at the time and that everyone talked about in Paris of 1843—i.e., madness? However marginal was the existence Marx led in Paris and however uninterested he might have been in French intellectual life, it is simply impossible that he would be unaware that this is what "alienation" meant around him when he was writing about it. If at all hoping to remain in Paris for some time and to address the French public as well in his *Deutsch-Französische Jahrbücher,* wouldn't he want to participate in the discussion, and to contribute an original interpretation of the phenomenon, which was of evident interest to this public, even if he did not have personal interest in it? And he did have a personal interest.

The concept of alienation in the 1844 manuscripts bears striking resemblance to symptoms of schizophrenia (and its spectrum disorders) as we see it today. First, there is alienation of man from his product—the denial of authorship, treating one's own creation as objective reality, which is the central characteristic of schizophrenic delusion. Then there is alienation of man from his fellow men, and from his social nature—social maladjustment, the sense of isolation, schizophrenic autism. Most importantly, there is self-alienation, the alienation of man from himself—the schizophrenic "I-problem"—the terrifying and disorienting experience of one's self or parts of one's self as alien forces inserted into one's being and no longer one's own to command. How are we to say that it is not this alienation that Marx is talking about? One could respond that its relationship to private property and division of labor makes this improbable. Let us consider this. Marx writes in the first fragment:

> Every self-estrangement [self-alienation] of man from himself and from nature appears in the relation in which he places himself and nature to men other than and differentiated from himself. . . . Private property . . . results by analysis from the concept of alienated labor—i.e., of alienated man. . . . True, it is as a result of the movement of private property that we have obtained the concept of alienated labor (of alienated life) from political economy. But on analysis of this concept it becomes clear that though private property appears to be the source, the cause of alienated labor, it is really its consequence. . . . How is this estrangement [alienation] rooted in the nature of human development? We have already gone a long way to the solution of this problem by transforming the question as to the origin of

private property into the question as to the relation of alienated labor to the course of humanity's development. . . ."

He adds to these propositions: "First it has to be noticed, that everything which appears in the worker as an activity of alienation, of estrangement, appears in the non-worker as a state of alienation, of estrangement." (Elsewhere in the first fragment, listing the effects of labor on the worker, Marx specifically notes what labor does to the worker's mind: "It is true that labor produces for the rich wonderful things—but for the worker it produces privation. It produces palaces—but for the worker, hovels. It produces beauty—but for the worker, deformity. It replaces labor by machines—but some of the workers it throws back to a barbarous type of labor, and the other workers it turns into machines. It produces intelligence—but for the worker idiocy, cretinism [*sic!*].")

The source of alienation, Marx suggests in the next fragment, is separation of man from man. It is, in fact, the insistence on the self-sufficiency of the individual that alienates the individual from others and leads to one's self-alienation. Communism (even "despotic" communism, Marx stresses) tying individuals into one whole, will "transcend human self-estrangement," because "society is the consummated oneness in substance of man and nature—the true resurrection of nature—the naturalism of man and the humanism of nature both brought to fulfillment." Marx continues:

> What is to be avoided above all is the re-establishing of "society" as an abstraction vis-à-vis the individual. The individual is the social being. His life, even if it may not appear in the direct form of a communal life carried out together with others—is therefore an expression and confirmation of social life. . . . Man, much as he may therefore be a particular individual . . . , is just as much the totality—the ideal totality—the subjective existence of thought and experienced society present for itself. . . . Thinking and being are thus no doubt distinct, but at the same time they are in unity with each other. . . . [In communism, in communal life] man appropriates his total essence in a total manner, that is to say, as a whole man.

Communism, which solves the problem of alienation, is not simply, or even primarily, a form of economic organization; nevertheless, because it reflects the state of alienation (see above), economic organization is the best clue to the understanding of man's psyche. "[T]he history of industry and the established objective existence of industry," writes Marx in the fragment on communism, "are the open book of man's essential powers, the exposure to the senses of human psychology. . . . A psychology for which this, the part of history most contemporary and accessible to sense, remains a closed book, cannot become a genuine, comprehensive and real science."[78]

This sounds like a direct answer to Baillarger's editorial introduction to the first volume of *Annales Médico-Psychologiques:* really, the status of psychology as science could not have been a bone of contention between Marx and Hegel. Thus, the discussion of alienation in 1844 manuscripts could at least as sensibly be interpreted as an attempt to deal with the phenomenon of mental alienation (and neurosis) as putting Hegel onto his feet. The experience of madness, and the desire to account for it, could be at the root of Marx's intellectual project, and the Marxist doctrine. Insanity, the modern mental disease, rather than capitalism, the modern economy, could be the inspiration for the idea and ideal of communism, as well as the foundation of the economic determinism and the analysis of the capitalist economic system which, presumably, made Marxist communism scientific. Shocking as this may be, this is a possibility at least worth exploring. In fact, what a dissertation subject for some ambitious graduate student!

The Fog Thickens: German Madness

It may be asked: if the question Marx focused on in 1844 was essentially psychological and closer to medicine than economics and social engineering, why then did his thought take such a drastic turn just a year later? The answer to this is twofold. Marx was banished from Paris before he could impress French public by his contribution to the mental alienation discourse, and even edit or translate his notes: there was no point in addressing himself to the French audience. And in Germany, the tradition within which this contribution belonged lost relevance precisely at this moment in time. For the 1844 manuscripts clearly belonged to a tradition: they were not only written in German—they were German through and through, obviously informed by German Romantic notions and attitudes. German psychiatry first appeared in the form of Romantic psychiatry, an essentially philosophical and largely academic discourse with a political (or, rather, police, administrative) science bent, and not as a medical specialization. By early 1840s, this tradition, already half a century old, had exhausted itself and, while possibly of interest in France, to which it was foreign, was no longer of interest to those who wished to understand, cope with, treat, or manage mental disease in Germany.

In 1843 and 1844 two articles on mental disease appeared in a medical journal, *Archiv für physiologische Heilkunde*, which signaled the emergence of psychiatry as a medical specialization in Germany. They were written by a young doctor, one year Marx's senior, Wilhelm Griesinger. Griesinger was a son of a hospital administrator killed by a mentally ill piano teacher—thus, personally familiar with dangers of mental disease. While studying medicine at Tuebingen, he focused on physiology and (though philosophy was, likely, a curricular requirement) "refused to attend the psychiatric lectures of the natural philosopher Eschenmayer ... polemicizing against Hegel." In 1838, when Marx was having his "nervous breakdown" in Berlin, Griesinger received his doctorate, for a year studied with alienists in Paris, spent another year as a general practitioner, and between 1840 and 1842 was a resident at an insane asylum. One of the patients there was a physician (a mad doctor, indeed, though not an *Irrenartz*) and naturalist Robert Mayer, who became his friend and had some influence on his psychiatric views. It was this experience that the new-to-Germany ideas Griesinger formulated in his path-breaking articles of 1843 and 1844 reflected.

Griesinger was interested in all sorts of mental disorder—feeble-mindedness as much as "irrationality" of hypertrophied intellect in what his followers in the twentieth century would call functional psychoses of schizophrenia and manic-depressive illness. He was, obviously, unaware of the newness of the latter, although cognizant that in his time the ailment was spreading, and regarded insanity, just like idiocy, as a physical illness—an "irritation in the brain" and the nervous system. His description of symptoms of insanity, based on clinical observation, however, was very sensitive. His experience led him to agree with the view of the French alienist Guislain that insanity in all its forms was one and the same disease, a unitary psychosis, commencing with psychic pain, "the basic depression," and expressing itself in thought and behavior as "sickness of the will." The "essential [mental] change" that the sick brain produced,

Griesinger argued, was the "alienation" of the person's former self, and "simultaneously internalization of, and alienation from, the outer world." The patients, he wrote, "experience their environment as 'having become something quite different,' reject it, replace it with hallucinations, and ultimately dream of or commit destructive or suicidal acts." Apparently, in the Germany of 1844, one could observe this among people "whom one can find more frequently out in the world than in insane asylums, [their disease manifesting] itself in characteristic chronic ill temper and moodiness, suspicion, distrust, envy, and malice." Later, arguing the need for private practice psychiatry, Griesinger spoke about perhaps somewhat different "little known class of mentally ill": "this army of the 'irritable and weak,' the 'sexual perverts,' the psychopaths, compulsives, neurotics." In the 1860s their "weakness" was becoming "conspicuous" not only to astute clinicians such as Griesinger, but—what was at least as important—to themselves as well, and they were turning to privately practicing neurologists and clinical psychiatrists for help.[79]

Why did one find more mad Germans outside than in the asylums in the 1840s and why were German neurotics left without help until 1860s? There were two reasons for that. The first several generations of German psychiatrists—the Romantic psychiatrists—paid no attention to the mentally ill, single-mindedly dedicated as they were to the establishment of psychiatry as a branch of philosophy and an academic discipline. And the first several generations of German madmen and neurotics—the Romantics and their public—defined mental illness as the expression of the human essence, not a disabling disorder to cure, but a precious potential to be cultivated.

The Idee

In sharp contrast to England and France, where the phenomenon of madness provoked the interest in it, and the suffering of those affected and the desire to help them led to what was later called (Germans contributing the term) "psychiatry," in Germany, psychiatry—named at the outset—emerged within the walls of the universities, essentially, if not hermetically, closed to realities of the outside world. Fortunately for me (and preventing accusations of prejudice on my part), some thirty years ago already "it has been proposed that a flourishing philosophical psychiatric literature without a basis in practice was unique to Germany. . . . It becomes a more understandable endeavour when it is seen as an attempt to enhance professorial status and authority at German universities in a rapidly changing society, politically threatened from without and within."[80] In this sense, German psychiatry followed the trajectory of German economics, both creations of a product differentiation strategy on the part of mediocre professoriate in search of an intellectual niche to advance their careers—and both, remarkably—first defined as parts of police (i.e., administrative), or cameralist, sciences.[81] (A comparison between the two would make another excellent dissertation.) A function of the politically disjointed structure of the German lands, there were many more universities in Germany in the eighteenth and nineteenth centuries, than anywhere else in the world. Because of their cultural and specifically linguistic uniformity, these numerous universities constituted a system, and because they were so numerous, the system was autarchic and allowed for the virtual independence of academic careers from their relevance to, or impact on, the outside world (very much the way this is now in the United States). The professors were state employees and therefore attuned to the needs of their princes (thus, the desire to show themselves useful in administration, thus cameralism), but the internal dynamics of the extensive university system made it much more important that they be attuned to the interests, impress, and curry the favor, of their peers—other professors.

There were four overlapping faculties in German universities, with professors frequently appointed to and teaching in more than one: law, medicine, theology, and—the addition of the *Aufklärung*—philosophy, which fulfilled the general education responsibilities. There is no question that the flourishing of German philosophy on the cusp of the eighteenth and nineteenth centuries was made possible by the establishment of this cozy and undemanding environment for people who loved to think and were excited about their own mental life. The mind was the central subject for all the great philosophers of the period, the authorities Marx listed by name in letters to his father (Kant, Fichte, Schelling, and Hegel): it was the central subject for the great German representative of the *Aufklärung* rationalism, Kant, and of the three idealist/Romantic/nationalist opponents of *Aufklärung* and Kant. Therefore, they all were interested in, and occasionally wrote about, insanity—the curious irrational behavior of

thinking men and women, examples of which abounded in their immediate circles and which John Locke, whose essay on human understanding
they, naturally, knew very well, defined as madness. Romantic psychiatrists were the entrepreneurial epigones of these great philosophers. They
were people of completely different motivation and abilities. However
murky and ultimately unhelpful their ideas, the great philosophers were all
men of prodigious originality and seriousness: they were puzzled by the
realities of their experience (including, in the first place, the reality of the
mind); they were driven to resolve these puzzles—nothing forced them to
dedicate themselves to such resolution, yet they felt an inner sense of
urgency, they had, they were called, to accomplish it. They were literally
"inspired" thinkers. In distinction, Romantic psychiatrists were professional men of learning—"professional" in the sense that plying philosophy
or medical theory was for them essentially the way they earned their living and established their place in society. Their chief qualification for
the job was their competence: they diligently read and could quote everything they were expected to read and quote. Their minds, while impressive reservoirs of knowledge, certainly were not fountainheads of ideas.
Competence as the chief characteristic of an intellectual is, by definition,
intellectual mediocrity.[82] To stand out among other mediocre philosophers
or medical theorists our professors had no choice but to appropriate a particular area of competence. Romantic psychiatrists were those who appropriated the great philosophers' discussion of mental disease.[83]

A number of these professors studied with Hegel, some were personal
friends of Fichte, but, of the three idealists, it was Schelling who had the
greatest impact on their views: they all subscribed to his *Naturphilosophie*.
Schelling's philosophy of nature was an outgrowth of Fichte's generalized
(glorified) solipsism, the postulation of the ego (*Ich*) as the creator of its
own "objective" reality and of the "world soul" as the creator of nature.
(However "abstruse" such reasoning may appear to the modern reader,
writes Otto Marx in his review of Romantic psychiatry, it is important to
remember that it led to ego psychology and provided the basis for Freud's
psychoanalysis.[84] This tells us something indeed about Freud's psychoanalysis.) Schelling disagreed with this monistic stand: "Nature should be the
spirit made visible, and the spirit, invisible nature," he wrote in 1797 *Ideen
zu einer Philosopie der Natur*. "Here, in the absolute identity of the spirit

within us and nature outside us, the problem of how a nature outside us is possible must be resolved."[85] He insisted that mind and matter were one, the soul, the spirit being the most developed natural phenomenon, the highest form of nature and thus subject to the same laws. It was also the only self-conscious part of nature, the only one that could uncover these laws. Deductive analysis from the first principles, completely independent of any empirical study, therefore, was the best way to study empirical reality, and carried with it the additional—and most significant—advantage of being home-grown: "a science based on the deductive speculative method came with higher credentials than the empirical science of Newton."[86] All knowledge, what one knew about reality, was instinctual and proceeded from the inner drive. "Man knows only what he has an instinct to know; it is a vain effort to try to make men understand what they have no urge to understand," wrote Schelling.[87] This meant, among other things, that knowledge could not be learned or shared, if it did not already exist within a person and, in the case of insanity, implied that it was "endogenous" and could not be understood from the outside.

As Schelling's thought developed, he came to emphasize that the soul, which was the highest form of nature, was also the divine element in man, the "absolute." The essential sinfulness (the Fall) of man prevented a clear and immediate consciousness of it in most cases, there was "no steady transition from the absolute to the real, the origin of the world of perception is conceivable only as a total break from absoluteness, through a leap . . . a falling away from the absolute." While one's mind and reality were one, there was no true identity between the "world-soul" and nature, which included one's mind, and each individual now stood alone. (One could easily derive from this the conclusion that one's consciousness was likely to be false consciousness and that one was necessarily alienated at once from others, from one's species-being and from one's true self. Indeed, it is hard not to see here the provenance of Hegel's argument in the *Phenomenology of the Mind* or of its reinterpretation by Karl Marx in the terms of historical materialism.) For Schelling, the "most apt simile" for this state of disunity was disease, "the disarray brought into nature by the abuse of freedom," "the true counterpart of evil or sin," and mental disease in particular. Schelling distinguished between the mind as a whole, which he called Spirit (*Geist*) and its constitutive elements: the unconscious emotional element of *Gemuet,* which was natural (and which some translate as "mind"[88]), the conscious volitional element of will and intellect he referred to as spirit in the narrow sense, and the soul (*Seele*), the impersonal divine element. The soul was incorruptible and was supposed to rule the rest of the mind. "The health of the mind and the spirit depends on the constancy of the connection between the soul and the depths of the mind," Schelling argued, while disassociation between them led to mental disease: melancholia in the case when insatiable desire to be what one was not predominated in *Gemuet*, idiocy in the case of the intellect being overpowered by the will of pleasure in the spirit narrowly defined, and insanity, "the most dreadful thing of all," when the intellect was disconnected from the soul. He wrote in 1810:

> [S]ince the human spirit relates as non-being to the soul, it also relates to it as non-understanding. Hence the deepest essence of the human spirit, when contemplated apart from the soul and thus from God, is insanity. Insanity does not originate, it emerges when that which is actually non-being, i.e., not understanding, is actualized, when it wants to be essence, being. Thus the basis of understanding itself is insanity. That is why insanity is a necessary element, that must, however, not emerge, not be actualized. What we call understanding, if it is real, active understanding, is, in fact nothing but regulated insanity. Understanding can manifest itself, show itself only in its opposite, in non-understanding. People who carry no insanity within themselves are people with empty, sterile understanding. Hence the reverse saying: *Nullum ingenium sine quadam dementia.* Hence divine insanity, of which Plato and the poets speak. Namely, when insanity is ruled by the influence of the soul, it is truly divine insanity, the basis of inspiration, of effectiveness.[89]

He concluded just a bit later in the discussion: "Insanity is thus the condition of hell."

The iron logic of German idealist philosophers was rather pliable, clear and consistent definitions were not their strong suit, and blatantly contradictory statements on the same page or pages closely following each other were characteristic of their writings. All this, however, served only to increase their popularity with the public, for which these philosophers performed not an intellectual but an extremely important psychological function. The German public, the educated bourgeoisie—the *Gelehrten* or the *Bildungsbürger*—since the late eighteenth century faced vexatious identity problems, and the three great idealists helped its different sectors to define themselves. The opaque and self-contradictory quality of Fichte's, Schelling's, and Hegel's philosophy made it possible for people of opposing interests and needs to find in it the message promoting their particular interests and pertinent to their special needs.

Schelling helped *Gelehrten* employed in the universities to find a digni-fied professional identity—that of philosophical experts on mental illness—which would allow them to stand out among other professors of philosophy and medicine and increase their value for the princes. To begin with, the name Schelling gave to mental illness, *Geisteskrankheit,* attracted profes-sors' attention to the existence of the phenomenon, for it is not at all certain that they were aware of it before; he also made very explicit its philosoph-ical significance (as well as the significance of philosophy for medicine). And then he offered them plenty of choice as to which of his pronounce-ments on it to take as a guide in their own ruminations. The fact that they were state employees and wanted to be considered of use for the princes made them appropriate the notions that mental illness was at the same time a physical illness, because the mind was a part of nature, that it was (objec-tively) dreadful, and that it had to be regulated and prevented from being actualized. There were, obviously, differences of emphasis, and early in the process it was suggested that there were two warring camps in Romantic psychiatry: the *psychici,* whose leading representative was J. C. A. Heinroth (the first professor of psychotherapy at Leipzig and later the dean of the university's medical faculty), and who claimed that at the root of all mental disease was sin, the cure—or management—thus being a matter of the patient's moral responsibility; and the *somatici,* led by K. W. Maximilian Jacobi (the director of one of the first German asylums, the Siegburg), who insisted that "mental disturbance was invariably a sign or symptom of a physical disruption."[90] The majority of the *psychici* were professors, and many of the *somatici* worked in the newly founded asylums, but it was not necessarily the difference in the experience that explained the differences in their views. The oneness of body and mind Schelling postulated justified both positions to an equal degree, and Otto Marx concludes that it is dif-ficult to draw lines between them: "Their concept of man included faith and religion in addition to reason. Analysis was insufficient. What holds man together was critical for the understanding of man, especially when it came to healing those who were no longer mentally whole. All abhorred a secular view of man, a reality based on external perceptions and a linear concept of the emotions which excluded religious feelings."[91]

The arguably most important figure among the Romantic psychiatrists, if only because he is credited with fathering German psychiatry in particular, and christening the discipline in general, Johann Christian Reil, stood outside both camps. He was older than all the rest, born between the generations of *Sturm und Drang* and the early Romantics. A son of a clergyman, he rebelliously studied medicine and at the age of twenty-nine was appointed professor of medicine at Halle, where he did research in anatomy, pathology, physiology, chemistry, and pharmacology, and saw patients suffering from various physical diseases. He was "an ardent medical politician and fervent German nationalist," a friend of Fichte and the nationalist über-propagandist Arndt, and "an enthusiastic disciple of Schelling."[92] During the Wars of Liberation, "his hatred of the French surpassed even Fichte's. E. M. Arndt described him thus: 'Fichte and Reil were to a certain degree the most tragic people in the capital because of the enormous ardor of their response to contemporary events and their burning hatred of the French, almost more intense in Reil than in Fichte.'"[93] It is remarkable, indeed, how many Romantic psychiatrists were passionate nationalists, and how many passionate nationalists were interested in mental illness.[94]

Reil "had practically no experience with mentally deranged," says Doerner, "when he wrote his basically poetic, literary anthropology," the 1803 *Rhapsodien ueber die Antwendung der psychischen Curmethode auf Geisteszerruetungen* (*Rhapsodies on the Application of the Mental Cure to Mental Disturbances*), "a work generally considered as the start of German psychiatry." Addressing himself to German physicians, governments, and the educated public, and ostensibly writing to ameliorate the condition of the mentally ill, Reil rhapsodized for almost five hundred pages, mostly filled with the discussion of "all the psychological methods the physician may employ in the treatment of mental illness."[95] The introduction, however, was that of a medical politician, astute, if not ardent, and German nationalist: "he started from the primacy of foreign and power politics: Only when the 'body politic' learns to work in harmony like the bodies of nature, can princes, whose loftiest goal is the 'well-being of the people,' also be noble-minded toward the insane and show their 'paternal concern' for the 'socially immature,'" (which, presumably, would allow Germany to take the lead in caring for the mentally ill, and not to lag shamefully behind England and France, as it did in 1803). With supreme self-confidence, personal, professional, and national, Reil proclaimed: "An intrepid breed dares to approach the gigantic idea that makes ordinary man reel, the idea of extirpating one of the most devastating of epidemics from the face of the earth. And it truly seems as if we are approaching and are about to dock."[96]

There are just a few points that are of interest in Reil's book, and all of the Romantic psychiatry literature, in the present context. First, it is absolutely clear that Reil's conception of mental disease was traditional. His typology included four classes: idiocy (*Bloedsinn*), folly (*Narrheit*), mania (*Wuth*), and fixed delusions (*fixer Wahn*). The majority of cases exemplifying these Reil cited from foreign sources, relying heavily on Haslam in England and Pinel and Tissot in France, but he did not perceive that madness and *aliénation mentale* on which they focused was different from all of his categories, that cases that they diagnosed as mania or delusional insanity were not at all like what he defined as such. Indeed, his own cases of *Wuth* and *fixer Wahn* were cases of mental problems obviously related to infectious disease and fever.[97] He was evidently completely unaware of the phenomenon of madness.

Though not directly related to the argument of this book, Reil's curative methods also call for comment. Like some of his Western colleagues, the professor recommended wine with poppy juice under some circumstances. However, treatments he preferred and, in several instances, was the first to suggest were of another kind altogether. They included "hunger, thirst, sneezing powder, blistering plaster, seton, burning moxa, red hot iron, or burning sealing wax dripped into the palm of the hand," whipping with nettles, infecting with scabies, induced vomiting, constant drip, submersion in water, mice under a glass on the skin, and goats to lick salt covered soles. "Reil recognized that he was advocating the use of torture," writes Otto Marx, "but then torture was a venerable European tradition." Reil, the historian continues, "reserved corporal punishment, including the bullwhip, for patients who were aware of their transgressions and who understood the reason for punishment. In any other situation Reil thought it would be 'barbarous.' No attendant was to strike the patients and only the supervisor [the psychiatrist!] was to use the whip." As to patients who could not be brought to their senses by these tactile measures, "Reil proposed grandiose stage settings. A pitch dark cave filled with the strangest live and dead objects, skeletons, 'furmen,' and ice pillars. Cannon shots, drums and firecrackers," and, most impressive for the present author, a cat piano or harpsichord, "composed of live cats whose tails would be hit with nails"!!! "Why does he mention it?" asks Otto Marx, astonished. And: "It is even more difficult to assess what Reil had in mind when we read that all the patients who recovered after [such] music therapy had suffered from fever."[98] Reil, however, is quite clear on this: The duty of the psychiatrist is to "lead the patient from the lowest level of senselessness through a chain of mental stimuli to the full use of reason." This requires that the psychiatrist impress the patient as a terrifying super-man who cannot be resisted and must be obeyed: "Let his speech be terse, brief, and bright. The shape of his body should aid the soul and inspire fear and awe. He should be big, strong, muscular; his gait majestic, his mien stern, his voice stentorian. . . . Mostly he must extemporize the impressions to the patient's imagination and aspirations, depending on the situation and on his gift for forceful and surprising improvisation." (What a gratifying self-image for would-be psychiatrists!) "A few brutal passages through the nervous system" would ensure that the patient has this impression of the therapist. Thus Reil recommends: "Hoist the patient by a tackle block to a high vault so that he . . . may hover between heaven and earth; fire a cannon near him, approach him grimly with white-hot irons, hurl him into raging torrents, throw him in front of ferocious beasts . . . or let him sail through the air on fire-spewing dragons. A subterranean crypt, containing all the horrors ever seen in the realm of the ruler of hell, may be advisable." One may well ask whether our rhapsodist was mad himself. This explanation would certainly be more palatable than ascribing the fertility of Reil's gory imagination and his obvious relish in inflicting suffering on his fellow-beings and defenseless animals to some deep predilection for evil in the German tradition—those with schizophrenic "I-disorders," after all, frequently resort to wanton cruelty as a means of self-assertion. (Just among the examples mentioned in this book, K. P. Moritz and John Nash tortured animals; John Nash enjoyed inflicting pain on small children and those he knew to be vulnerable.) But it is sadly suggestive that sadism, though named after a mad Frenchman, was defined as a special diagnostic category within madness by a German psychiatrist (Krafft-Ebing), while a comparative historian of asylums in 1891 was moved to comment: "the Germans seem to have excelled all other nations in the ingenuity of the torture which they sought to inflict upon their patients."[99] Perhaps, all of the Romantic psychiatrists were, unbeknownst to themselves, madmen.

The foremost *psychicus* among the next (in fact, the first, since Reil stood alone) generation of German psychiatrists, Johann Christian August Heinroth wholeheartedly subscribed to all of Reil's curative methods. He also contributed to the professional vocabulary of psychiatry, coining the term "psychosomatic." He was a remarkably prolific writer, authoring, without much experience, thirty-one "psychiatric" books and numerous articles in German and in Latin—indeed, among his contemporaries, he was famous as an "ink-spiller." Some of these contemporaries, according to Luc Cauwenbergh, our contemporary, who would like to clear Heinroth's name and "do him justice," were also critical of the quality of what this first professor of psychotherapy wrote: "When contemporaneous critics of Heinroth managed to restrain themselves from making fun of him, they hardly said more than that his works were a maze of knots, that his thoughts were absolutely useless or that he left the questions he raised without answer." Cauwenbergh concedes that Heinroth's work is not easy reading, explaining: "The fundamental reason for the difficulty is that each of his volumes gives the impression that there is no consistent line of thought in it, or at least that if there is such, it cannot be detected. What confronts the reader is an abundance of concepts that have no obvious links with one another." But, he insists, this is so only if one confines oneself to Heinroth's thirty-one books and scores of articles. However, "a reading and re-reading of Heinroth's works on the one hand and a familiarity with German Idealistic Philosophy through some writings of its representative proponents on the other, yield[s] promising results." Hegel's *Logic,* in particular, he says, provides the key to the understanding of Heinroth's psychiatry.[100] Indeed, one can see the logic of Hegel (and Karl Marx), as well as the ontology of Fichte and Schelling's natural philosophy, behind Heinroth's theory of mental disease: these were all variations on the same theme, after all.

The central postulate in this theory was that man's purpose in life was to unite in consciousness with God (whose name, of course, could be the "world-soul" or Absolute), this unity being perfect mental health. The opposite of mental health, mental illness was the betrayal by man of his purpose; Heinroth, among other things, referred to it as *menschlich-krankhafte Zustand*—"man sick in his humanity"—Marx could have called it alienation from the species-being. But Heinroth considered mental illness the product of sin. That perfect mental health "happens so seldom," he wrote, "is [man's] guilt, and out of this guilt derive all his troubles, also the disturbances of mental life." As the patient was, therefore, morally responsible for his or her mental illness, it was only proper to punish the mentally ill: treatment (which Heinroth defined as "re-education") by torture was the wages of sin, nothing more, and what recommended it further was that, in addition to restoring the cosmic order, it contributed to "national happiness." The historian of German Romantic psychiatry Otto Marx, who is sympathetic to his subjects, knows how to take the sadistic propensity of Heinroth no more than that of Reil. "Like Reil," he writes, "[Heinroth] too was criticized for listing and not condemning all cruel and unlikely measures from the past." "Some of these abominable measures," he reminds himself despondently, "were not from the past at all [but] were among the newest inventions of German psychiatry. We must accept that [Heinroth] approved them and recommended them in his writings. No one knows what measures Heinroth actually used in his practice, which was certainly limited. He quoted Arnold's cases from the literature because of his own lack of practical experience, and yet he never tired of criticizing others as mere armchair psychiatrists."[101]

The psychiatrists Heinroth criticized were mostly English and French. He did so—remarkably, given the infant state of psychiatry in Germany, whose "actual accoucheur" Heinroth was considered by his professional peers—in his discourse on the *history* of psychiatry, to which some of his voluminous writings were devoted and which, until it arrived in his *Vaterland*, he saw as sorely wanting. German psychiatrists turned historians of psychiatry as soon as they decided on becoming psychiatrists. History of psychiatry helped them in the construction of their professional and national identities and thus was a subject of general interest among them. The first book explicitly focused on it, J. M. Leupoldt's *Ueber den*

Entwicklungsgang der Psychiatrie, was published in 1833; it is in it that Heinroth was credited with bringing the profession into the world. Writing in 1818, Heinroth paid tribute to Reil as the "actual founder" of psychiatry and to Ernst Horn, with whom, he believed, psychiatric practice "has reached its highest development."[102] Ernst Horn, "the disciple of Fichte" and a professor of practical medicine, practiced at the Charite Hospital in Berlin. A firm believer in the principle of *Arbeit macht frei,* Horn forced mental patients at that rather incongruously named institution to dig ditches only to fill them in again, and harnessed them to a wagon to pull other inmates across the grounds. "Military drills were considered an effective method of winning compliance, which was equated with health," writes Doerner. "This therapeutic device, which soon reached other German institutions, was supervised by a military man, a former patient, and was also used with females." But, in addition to useless but exhausting and therefore salubrious labor, Horn "indiscriminately" used other curative methods, including, as might be expected, "sadistic punishment." "If hundreds of pails of cold water were poured down from above or powerful jets of water were aimed at the sexual organ, or the head was packed in ice or subjected to water torture, the explanation was: 'It is conducive to the behavior, obedience, and discipline of the insane; it restores speech to mutes; it stills the drive of those who would take their own lives; it brings the quiet melancholic . . . back to self-consciousness; it . . . serves excellently in some cases to instill fear or as a punishment to maintain order and peace.'" Not only an inspired therapist, Horn was also an inventor, contributing to the extensive arsenal of healing torture devices a contraption bearing his name, "Horn's Bag," "in which maniacal patients were tied from head to foot to restrict their freedom of movement and kept in darkness." In 1818—before Heinroth paid him the compliment of achieving the realization of psychiatry's fullest and most glorious potential—Horn was discharged from the Charite, because one of the irrational patients there died—six years earlier—while being treated by (or, rather, in) the Bag.[103] One could conclude that there was no more justice in Berlin than anywhere else in this world. But this would be an unjust conclusion: Horn's "carreer was not adversely affected," he was appointed professor of therapeutics, continued to teach and publish on "the special therapy of mental diseases," and "was much honoured."[104]

Though he mostly praised his countrymen, it would be wrong to let the reader assume that Heinroth had nothing good to say about the mad-doctors and alienists abroad. In addition to singling out Arnold, on whose clinical cases he relied, as the best among the former, he endorsed the contributions of Pinel and Esquirol among the latter as a "leap forward." (As it happened, this generous sentiment was not returned. Esquirol, we are told, when Heinroth's former student attempted to familiarize the French clinician with his teacher's views, had only this to say: "Ah ça, ce sont de vos obscurités allemandes.") Heinroth did his homework, without a doubt, he studied English and French literature on mental disease and his competence was unassailable. He even adopted from this literature seventeen species of mental illness until then never mentioned in Germany. This, added to the thirty-six varieties at which he arrived by multiplying John Brown's categories of "hypersthenia," "asthenia," and "hyper-asthenia" by the three mental powers of the emotions, the intellect, and the will, and to several subclasses, rendered the impressive total of fifty-seven mental illnesses. For all these Heinroth found names in German and in Latin, though he used them inconsistently. He called mental disease, in general, *Geisteskranke* after Schelling, and also *morbis mentis* and *insanientes*. *Wahnsinn* (the common translation of "madness" or *folie*) was another general term, but also meant "mania," which, in other instances, Heinroth referred to as *Tollheit,* and so on. The evident dislike by the Romantic psychiatrists of clear definitions raises a general problem, writes Otto Marx, bringing "up the difficulties we face in our attempt to understand the psychiatric literature of this period. Some terms, such as melancholia, do not refer to what we mean by it. Others are used by several authors in different ways. Worse still is the problem of translating the German terms. Some turn out to be translations from the English or French literature[!] . . . *Verueckungen* and *Zeruettungen,* as well as *Stoerungen, Narrheit,* and *Wahnsinn* have quite different meanings at times."[105] This unwillingness, on Heinroth's part, specifically, to make his meaning plain, makes it impossible for us to say with any certainty that he understood his English and French colleagues and, given his lack of clinical experience, suggests that he probably had no idea whatsoever of what kind of mental disease they focused on. Knowledge is often quite independent of understanding—

among professors and theorists, perhaps, more often than among others—and it is likely that this was so in the case of Heinroth.

Not to base our conclusions on evidence which may be thought one-sided, we must consider whether it was so in one other case—that of the leading *somaticus,* Maximilian Jacobi. Jacobi was not a professor and differed from Heinroth, whose writings he criticized, and the great majority of Romantic psychiatrists in many other respects. Though close to the early Romantics and, through his father, the philosopher of religion Friedrich Heinrich Jacobi, to the *Sturm und Drang* group in his younger years, he followed his studies in the German universities of Jena (when Schelling was teaching there), Goettingen, and Erfurt, by medical training in Edinburgh and London, translated Tuke's description of the York Retreat, worked as a hospital physician, and directed (first de facto and then as the official director) the 200-bed Siegburg mental asylum, one of the first in Germany, from 1824, when it opened, until his death in 1858. Here is how Jacobi is characterized by an historian of psychiatry:

[He] had extensive clinical experience with thousands of patients. Despite his intensive exposure to Romanticism in Jena, his studies with [the Romantic psychiatrists] . . . in Munich, and . . . Bonn, Jacobi attempted a clear differentiation between his profound religious belief and his medical writing. His father had postulated an intuitive, immediate knowledge in matters of faith. Yet psychiatry like medicine was to be exclusively based on "sober observation of nature and most careful induction." Assured that his philosophical education would guard him from "the labyrinth of uncontrolled speculation" prevailing in psychiatry, he explicitly dissociated himself from philosophy of nature. Of his magnum opus, *The Main Forms of Mental Disturbances In Their Relations to Therapeutics,* only the first volume, *On Mania,*[106] was published after twenty years of extensive practice. Yet throughout his career he stuck to his basic conviction that the immortal soul and its functions were never affected by mental illness. His anthropology differed from that of Heinroth. . . . To Jacobi, anthropology referred to the study of mind in relation to body, with mind limited to that part of it which man shared with animals. The other part, consisting of personal self-conscious mind with "its striving for freedom" and its belief in God, was excluded from psychiatry, since it was never affected by mental illness. . . . Psychiatry was not concerned with moral perversions or "degradations" as Heinroth had claimed. Sin or abuse might lead to degradation of the organism . . . and disturb the functions of its parts, leading to mental disturbances indirectly. But mental disturbance was invariably a sign or symptom of a physical disruption. Hence Jacobi denied a direct role to purely moral or religious agents "in both the genesis and in the fight against mental disturbance."[107]

It is entirely possible that Jacobi's somaticism accurately reflected his clinical experience which simply did not present him with cases of what the English called "madness" and the French *aliénation mentale*. As we know from Griesinger, as late as the 1840s, one rarely encountered such mentally ill in the asylums. Much of Jacobi's 786-page-long volume on mania was devoted to the description of cases he did encounter, and the overwhelming majority of these cases were cases of mental disease clearly associated with physical illness. A typical case was that of patient suffering from a rapidly spreading pulmonary tuberculosis with an intermittent fever and diarrhea. After these symptoms subsided, the mania was cured as well, which prompted Jacobi to comment that, though the patient had been said to suffer from religious mania, he turned to be "incredibly ignorant on the religious subject."[108] Ergo: religious mania did not exist.

Unlike Heinroth, Jacobi distinguished just eight mental disorders. There were two emotional diseases (*Gemuethkrankheiten*) that proceeded from the alienation of desire, heightened desire causing mania (*Tobsucht*) and "depressed" desire melancholia. There were two intellectual diseases, madness (*Wahnsinn*) and fatuous confusion, resulting from the alienation of intellect, the former from its "exaltation," the latter from its reduction. In addition to these there were delirium and folly. These six conditions, though symptomatically distinct, often coexisted or transformed one into another and were caused by the same physical disturbances, the most common of them, according to Jacobi's own statistics, resulting in turn from, in that order, alcohol abuse, puerperal difficulties, sudden loss of blood, typhoid fever, strenuous exertion, hemorrhoidal bleeding and tuberculosis. Finally, two more mental disorders—cretinism and idiocy—were congenital.

As was already pointed out, the views of the *somatici* and the *psychici* on the nature of the mental disease cannot be clearly distinguished, because representatives of both camps of psychiatrists subscribed to Schelling's idea that the mind and the body were one, in sickness and in health. Unlike the French alienists who were willing to consider philosophy only when it was specifically relevant to their clinical work and made no assumptions, German Romantic psychiatrists took philosophy to heart and the fundamental ontological assumption of the body and mind's oneness was necessarily reflected in their views of the sick mind. "Beyond that," says Otto Marx in continuation of an already quoted passage, "we see no easy way to separate those with more extensive clinical expertise from those with less. . . . Jacobi's years at the Siegburg did not modify his basic convictions." Still, two things should be said to Jacobi's credit. First, he was not a sadist, and, though he believed that violent inmates should be restrained, resorting for this purpose to a restraining chair for six to eight hours and cold baths, and did not object to the use of rotating chair, he thought that torture was torture and not a method of therapy, did not invent any new instruments for the "re-education" of his patients, and generally favored treating underlying physical disorders. Almost half of the patients he diagnosed as maniacs (45 of 111 men and 49 of 117 women) recovered. Second, he was intellectually honest enough to recognize that, by the time he was in his fifties, something was changing in the experience of mental disease in Germany and that his interpretation of it, which did not take this change into account, was no longer relevant. That is why he left unpublished most of his comprehensive work on mental disorders—a product of twenty years' labors. *On Mania*, its first volume, appeared in 1844, simultaneously with Griesinger's revelation of madness/mental alienation to the psychiatrists and neurologists of the German nation, and Jacobi, sensitive that he had nothing to contribute to the conceptual advancement of his profession, withdrew from the theoretical fray and dedicated the rest of his life to serving his patients the best he could.

Giving a Higher Note to Their Complaint

Knowing what kind of therapy was practiced in most asylums in Germany, one can easily understand the unwillingness of German madmen and neurotics of higher class to seek psychiatric help and their desire to conceal from the world that they were sick at all. But there was more to their denial than the fear of zealous psychiatrists' intent on saving their souls with methods that made the tortures of Spanish Inquisition look like chiropractic by comparison. For Germans of a particular higher class—the *Bildungsbürger*—began to go mad before the precocious Reil ever conceived his intellectual offspring and gave it its sonorous name. Among continental Europeans, *Bildungbürgertum* was, probably, the first group, i.e., the first population, to experience this new variety of mental disease, being exposed to it by its peculiar—acutely anomic at the time when anomie in continental Europe was not widespread—structural situation. It may be in order to reiterate here that individuals could be placed in such a structural situation, and thus become affected by mental illnesses of schizophrenia spectrum at any time. For instance, acute anomie was obviously the experience of the heirs of the Roman Augustan Imperial family during the first century AD, and, though their psychosis could be due to other reasons, at least Caligula and Nero were, quite likely, schizophrenics. So, closer to our time, arguably might be Luther, because his personal, individual situation could certainly be described as one of acute anomie as well. Such individual cases are interesting and might present an intellectual problem for an exceptionally discerning psychiatrist (i.e., a psychiatrist who understands that these cases are categorically different from any organic mental disease) who nevertheless believes in the organic etiology of all mental diseases. But they do not present an intellectual problem for a sociologist or an historian: such an intellectual problem arises only when the causation can no longer be considered random, i.e., when anomie becomes to some extent systemic and when mental disease, which is its product, affects specific populations. That this is what has been happening since the sixteenth century has been a central claim of the present book and why this happened the question accounted for by its central argument. This argument so far has been that nationalism has been responsible for making anomie systemic and its effects on mental health population-wide, first in England, where in the sixteenth century this completely new view of reality was born, and then, as it spread to Ireland and France, in these newly-defined nations as well. This was different in Germany.

In Germany madness arrived before nationalism. I have already described the situation of *Bildungsbürgertum* in detail elsewhere in this trilogy and, since nothing changed in eighteenth-century Germany in the eighteen years which have elapsed between the time I did so and now, can only repeat here some of what I wrote then.[109] The class, the educated bourgeoisie, was created out of the regular middle class and lower strata by the German universities, and connoted a higher social status than bourgeoisie in general. During the reign of the Enlightenment (*Aufklärung*) in Germany the prestige of the university education was further increased, while a new educational ideal—education (*Bildung*) as the way to the formation (also *Bildung*) of the inner spirit, irrespective of professional utility, specifically increased the prestige of the philosophy faculty. Legally, doctors of law and medicine still stood above the graduates from the far more populous faculties of theology and philosophy: the last sumptuary law in Frankfurt-on-Main grouped Juris Doctors and medical men together with the patricians and the nobility in the highest of the five classes into which it divided the city residents. But, as Mme de Staël was soon to remark, all academic degrees "earned one the entrée" into society. The educated rubbed shoulders with the nobility as if on the basis of equality, because especially humanistic, not occupationally oriented, education, was itself "noble." The universities encouraged the development of elevated self-esteem among its graduates and the expectation of greater deference towards them on the part of the society at large. But those who mattered in this society, i.e., the nobility and the bureaucracy, did not defer to them. Raised above the generally despised common lot, *Bildungsbürger* remained a lower class nevertheless, and were vexed and made unhappy by their position. They were victims of that most pernicious variety of anomie—status-inconsistency.

Toward the end of the eighteenth century, very significant numbers of them also suffered from the condition of trained unemployability. The universities had created a large class: at any point in the second half of the century there probably were somewhat above 100,000 educated commoners in Germany, which, with the addition of their wives and children, would render somewhere between 1.5 and 2 percent of the population of 20 million in 1800—that is, a stratum about equal in size to that of the nobility. The overwhelming majority of these men had no personal means and could not support themselves and their families without gainful employment. Their education thus remained career-oriented despite the ideal of knowledge for its own sake; they hoped to enjoy their *Bildung*, while provided for by sinecures in the legal and administrative branches of the civil service, the church, or university teaching. But the opportunities open to them in civil service dwindled toward the close of the eighteenth century, as the percentage of bureaucrats from the nobility increased, rising to 37.8 percent between 1770 and 1786 and to 45.23 percent between 1786 and 1806. Of course, the best positions were occupied by the well-born. The situation was somewhat better in the legal branch, but not much, and, in 1788, *Berlinische Monattschrift* assessed: "The number of young men applying for posts in the civil service is so great that all the administrative services are overwhelmed. If you compare their number with the number of posts which, even if there were to be an epidemic of deaths, are likely to fall vacant, you can see that there is now no hope whatever of placing all, or even most, of them in any way that bears the slightest relation to the many sacrifices which their training has required of them."

A clerical position was, if anything, even more difficult to obtain, though in this profession *Bildungsbürger* faced no competition from the nobility. Still, the total number of Church appointments between 1786 and 1805 in Prussia was 584, while in 1786 alone the theological faculty at Halle had eight hundred students (out of 1,156 at the university as a whole). Throughout Germany, Doctors of Theology, in anticipation of a living, were becoming tutors to children of the nobility, "hastening from house to house all day," as a reporter reflected in 1785, and barely earning "enough from their lessons to eke out a miserable existence. All of them are withered, pallid, and sickly and reach the age of forty before the consistory takes pity on them." Finally, the universities absorbed another small minority of the vast army of their graduates: all German universities, with the exception of Austria, combined, had 658 professors in 1796. Thousands upon thousands of the educated were employed only sporadically (as tutors) or remained unemployed altogether, forming a large class of "unattached," "free-floating" intellectuals. Many of them turned to freelance writing. There were 3,000 writers recognized as such in Germany in 1771, and 10,650 by 1800.[110] But writing was not, by any means, a moneymaking occupation. "The horde of famished poets is growing daily," wrote in 1776 in *Der teutsche Merkur* Wieland, one of the most successful writers of the time; "the outcome . . . is still starvation. They grow sour and write satires against princes who have not aspired to imitate Augustus and act as wealthy patrons to them or poets who have a regular meal waiting for them on the table at home."[111] Wieland himself ate regular meals thanks to the posts, first, of a town clerk in Biberach, then of a professor at Erfurt, and finally a tutor to Weimar princes. But, it must be said, that he had these posts because of his renown as a man of letters. So, and this was possibly the worst of it, there always was hope.

The promise of higher status did not allow the intellectuals to reconcile with the reality of their situation: they would rather starve than give up the remote possibility of achieving the social position their society told them they deserved. They suffered from the painful discrepancy between their self-esteem, which they had acquired with and because of their education, and which was reinforced by the ideas of the Enlightenment, and the inattention of their essentially static pre-national society, still composed of a given number of social strata, unchanging in their traditional definitions and standing in given, long-established relations to each other. Upward mobility was a new phenomenon in it, which the traditional society could not accommodate, and *Bildungsbürger*, defined by their upward mobility, were psychologically torn. They shared the contempt of the upper classes for the strata from which they came and resented the nobility, the officialdom, and the upper bourgeoisie, which would not accept them. They could not become a part of the society of which they aspired to be a part and did not wish to be a part of the society with which they were in fact associated. "No one lacking wealth and leisure can enter 'good society,'" wrote Christian Garve. "But in the society of peasants, mechanics, journeymen, apprentices, shopkeepers, or students he will find that manners are coarse or loose and that their speech is incomprehensible."[112] They were suspended between two social worlds, out of place in both, and always in agony. Like their representative Anton Reiser, on K. P. Moritz's testimony, they suffered constantly from "the feeling of humanity oppressed by its burgher [middle class] condition."[113] It is no wonder that this experience left so many of the intellectuals gloomy, misanthropic, and bitter—that what French alienists would soon be calling "neurosis" became the bane of the class and that, as early as 1770s, members of this class exhibited unmistakable symptoms of madness.

Because one in ten of the university-educated men was a writer, we can actually base our judgment of their mental health on a plentiful supply of direct and explicit reports, which supplement the suggestive evidence of statistics. The reports that fully justify the claim that madness, in its most impressive as well as subclinical forms, was a common experience among the *Bildungsbürger* begin in the early 1770s, the so-called *Genie* period, or *Sturm und Drang*, and come from the writings of a group of young intellectuals that congregated around Goethe and included among other members always identified with it Herder, Merck, Lenz, and Klinger—and, as a major source of inspiration behind it, Hamann. *Sturm und Drang* was a proto-Romantic (that is, Romantic in everything but name), nationalistic movement of thought, opposing the values and symbols of the Enlightenment (the rational individual, reason in general, learning, conventions, civilization, France as the most enlightened and civilized society, and everything French) and glorifying community, unrestrained emotions, innate—unlearned and unconventional—creativity, bending to no rules (and defined as original genius), nature and anything considered natural, i.e., uneducated and uncivilized—"savages," women, and children, German race and language. The sobriquet *Sturm und Drang*, taken from the title of one of Klinger's plays, the fundamental attitude of the original genius, the man of passion, captured the essence of the young men's worldview, literary style, and conduct. With the exception of Goethe, who came from a patrician family and was a man of independent means, and Klinger, who early discovered that military life offered precisely the kind of excitement he sought among his stormy and pressing friends and went on to have a distinguished career as an officer, all the other members of the core group were caught in the condition of trained unemployability described above in their formative youthful years and suffered wretchedly from anomie to the end of their days. "All the circumstances of life," writes the historian of *Sturm und Drang* Roy Pascal, "seemed to conspire to intensify that temperamental restlessness that is common to *Stürmer und Dränger;* and in these circumstances, this restlessness gained a wider, social, and philosophical significance, it may well be regarded as a typical expression of the malaise of the individual in modern society."[114]

Four of the chief six *Stürmer und Dränger* would be characterized today as mentally ill, two—Hamann and Herder—were manic-depressive or, at the very least, severely cyclothymic, one—Merck—committed suicide, another—Lenz—is confidently diagnosed today on Wikipedia as paranoid schizophrenic. But they were not characterized as mentally ill and did not see themselves as such. Hamann, whose pronouncements were described by his interlocutors as "incomprehensibly queer" (compare to the "bizarre," "unununderstandable" [sic.] schizophrenic thought and language) and who described himself as "more frightened of shadows than the horse of Alexander," also wrote proudly: "I have nothing to do nor any responsibilities . . . and, with the strongest propensity for work and enjoyment, can come to neither, and can only rock to and fro like Noah in his Ark. This anguish in the world is however the only proof of our heterogeneity. . . . This impertinent restlessness, this holy hypochondria is perhaps the fire in which we sacrificial beasts have to be salted and preserved from the corruption of the current century."[115] Their misery thus was holy—divine insanity, the source of inspiration and effectiveness, Schelling and the Romantics would call it later—it was the proof of their originality, i.e., of their innate creativity, and the sign that they remained pure of soul, untouched by the evil of too much civilization. Seen in this complimentary light, mental disorder became a badge of honor, it helped these sick men, who, torn between the ideals and realities of their society, had trouble defining themselves, to construct a lofty identity, one that had the additional advantage (extremely important for people who suffered from a disease of the will and were incapable of sustained effort) that they had to do nothing to claim it: their very condition was the proof of their genius. The lucky Goethe, who undoubtedly contributed much to the development of this wishful idea, commenting on it in *Dichtung und Wahrheit* from the perspective of his mature years, chuckled at his hapless erstwhile friends among thousands of others:

A new world seemed suddenly to come into being. The physician, the general, the statesman, and soon enough anyone who had any pretension to eminence in theory or practice was required to be a genius. . . . The term "genius" became the key to everything, and as it was so frequently employed, people came to believe that what it ought to denote was tolerably common. Since everyone was entitled to demand that his neighbor should be a genius, he came to think that he was one too. It was a far cry from the time when it was believed . . . that "genius" is the power with which man is endowed by the laws and regulations as a consequence of what he does. Quite the contrary: it was displayed only by transgressing the existing laws and over-turning regulations, for it openly claimed that there were no limits to its powers. So it was very easy to be a genius. . . . If someone trotted around the globe with no great notion why he was doing it or where he was going, it was called a voyage of genius. To embark on a thing which had neither sense nor utility was a stroke of genius. Enthusiastic young men, some of them truly gifted, lost themselves in the infinite.[116]

"Herder's unhappy temperament gives us perhaps the deepest insight into the psyche of the *Sturm und Drang*," writes Roy Pascal, "not without justi-fication he has been considered to be the prototype of Goethe's Faust, the supreme imaginative symbol of the movement." He was greatly admired by his friends and acquaintances for his beautiful mind, but was, clearly, a remarkably unpleasant and difficult person to be around: contemporary references to his conduct and character in letters and diaries read very much like personal reminiscences about John Nash. Like Nash, Herder was moody, emotionally unstable (his moods oscillated between "rapturous enthusiasm and melancholy hypochondria"), and very cerebral: "Theory, ideas were much more real to him than things and men." He was extremely ambitious, arrogant and yet, unsure of himself and terrified of criticism which inevitably confirmed his self-doubt. His way of dealing with this was to hurt others. "He attacked his enemies passionately and sharply, often with ostentatious indignation . . . ; to be spiritually or practically indebted to anyone was likely to provoke his resentment, and he taunted his own friends in a personal way that they often found humiliating and unjust." Goethe was so afraid of his "vicious bite" that he concealed his plans for *Goetz von Berlichingen* and *Faust* from him, and Wieland wrote: "The man is like an electric cloud. In the distance the meteor makes a very fine effect; but may the devil have such a neighbor hovering over his head. . . . I can't abide it, when a man is so convinced of his own worth; and worse still, when a strong fellow never stops enjoying making fools and laughing stocks of others, then I'd like to have a dozen pyramids between me and him."[117] One does not have to consider Herder's very influential ideas as delusions to recognize in him the classic features of "schizoid personality"—i.e., in fact, the disease in its embryonic form.

Weimar calmed Herder and he never reached (or skipped) the stage of acute psychosis. But for his younger friend Lenz there was no such reprieve. And yet, nobody around this possibly the first known German schizophrenic considered him sick. His condition looked like sickness—Goethe wrote that in Weimar Lenz had to be treated "like a sick child"—but they saw it as the expression of original genius, and this was not something one would want to cure or even contain. Merck remarked: "One cannot like the lad enough. Such a strange mixture of genius and childishness!" To remain a child into one's adult years was not exactly the same thing as genius, but it was also a good thing: it proved that one had an authentic personality and resisted the dehumanizing effects of civilization. Lenz himself was certain that his suffering was a gift, and that it would be "the greatest misfortune" to be free of it. "My greatest sufferings," he naively confessed, "are caused by my own heart, and yet, in spite of all, the most unbearable state is when I am free of suffering." He suffered from hallucinations, was tortured by a sense of guilt, believed himself capable to raise the dead and, on one occasion, at least, attempted to do so, several times tried to kill himself. In periods of lucidity he was aware that his imagination did damage to him and could observe sadly: "my philosophical reflections must not last more than two or three minutes, otherwise my head aches." His writing was "rhapsodic, broken, often difficult to follow," his essays, in particular, "disjointed, unsystematic." Socially and financially, he had to be taken care of. Goethe supported him—for about five years— inviting him to Weimar as a guest, among other things, but the great man's sense of decorum revolted against what he called "Lenz's asininities," which were downright offensive in these princely surroundings, and, presuming that any individual in his right mind (and Lenz's mind was, by definition, right) should have the responsibility to distinguish where to let his original genius loose and where to rein it in out of simplest politeness, broke with his protégé, had him expelled from Weimar, and the two never spoke again. Lenz died in 1792 in Russia, completely mad, in a country which at the time had no idea whatsoever of madness, and to the last admired by his many friends among the emerging Russian noble intelligentsia. Nikolai Karamzin, Russia's first novelist, wrote of him: "That deep capacity for feeling, without which Klopstock would not have been Klopstock, nor Shakespeare Shakespeare, was his undoing. In other circumstances Lenz would have been an immortal."[118] Like other Russian nobles, Karamzin owned populated estates and thus numerous "souls." He could have been a connoisseur of man's inner life, but it is more likely that he was a connoisseur of German literature, in particular of *Sturm und Drang*, and even more specifically of Goethe, completely taken in (with thousands of European readers, among whom the couple of hundreds Russians who so much wanted to join the European world of letters were the most enthusiastic) by *The Sufferings of Young Werther*. Lenz was, very probably, a model for Werther; for Karamzin, he was certainly the model for Werther, the incarnation of the beautiful ideal: how could such innocence associate the poor man with disease?

Goethe had no problems with his identity as an affluent patrician, and supreme confidence—the confidence of genius, indeed—in his intellectual abilities, which were at any rate generally acclaimed when he was very young. Passionately interested in the world and subject to strong emotions, he was as mentally healthy as one gets—a vigorous and willful personality, in complete control of his inner life. But he was a creative genius and saw more clearly into the temper of his time than his troubled friends who, unhappily for them, represented it. Life provided him with abundant material for observation and he elevated it into art: Goethe, more than anyone else, was responsible for making madness an ideal. *Werther* was much more than a literary event—it was a social phenomenon with remarkably widespread and very grave consequences. The wild popularity of the book was a sign that it fulfilled a tremendous need among the readers: this was the need for an acceptable interpretation of the misery they could not escape, an interpretation, in other words, that would make their suffering sufferable. And Goethe obliged.

There was an epidemic of suicides among young educated men in Germany. To refer to it as the first known case of copycat suicides is not only inadequate (it raises the question: what explains this new phenomenon), but wrong.[119] The epidemic lasted well into the Romantic period—too long to be a case of imitation; and suicide of ratiocinative men is extremely unlikely to be copycat—it is a matter of the individual decision. Henri Brunschwig attempted to account for this strange trend in his brilliant commentary on the Romantic mentality, writing "since *Sturm und Drang*, death is no longer felt to be annihilation but man's liberation. By its means these dreamers aspire to find the solution of the problem of knowledge, to discover what lies behind the external perceived by their senses."

"But," he added, "this philosophy of death, brought into fashion by Werther, will not alone account for suicide; there must be other circumstances to incite these young men to resort to it as a remedy."[120] The reason that all of a sudden so many ratiocinative men decided to end their lives is that they wished to do so for some time, but suicide was considered a sin and, what was perhaps more important for them, shameful. Goethe changed this. He made it, much to his later regret, yet another expression of original genius, thereby sanctioning it, making it morally attractive. Suicide became not only an honorable thing to do, like the Japanese hara-kiri, but a proof of an identity one doubted so long as one's life continued. Thus, killing oneself, one, so to speak, killed two birds with one stone: both putting an end to an intolerable existence and, in this final act, reaching self-realization.

More generally, *Werther* lightened the burden of mental illness for the large numbers of sufferers who thought of but did not commit suicide. Karl Phillip Moritz, as marvelously analytical in his (first to be so called) "psychological romance" *Anton Reiser*, as Goethe was imaginative in his book, wrote of the latter's effect:

[Sixteen-year-old Anton's] self-consciousness, with the sense of being worthless and rejected, was as burdensome to him as his body with its feeling of wet and cold. . . . That he must be unalterably himself and could be no other, that he was shut up in the narrow prison of self—this gradually reduced him to despair. [And then he discovers in succession Shakespeare and *The Sorrows of Young Werther.*] . . . in his spirit he was no longer an ordinary commonplace person, before long his spirit rose above all the outward circumstances that had crushed him and all the ridicule and scorn he had suffered . . . when he felt himself tormented, oppressed, and confined he no longer thought of himself as alone: he began to regard this as the universal lot of mankind. This gave a higher note to his complaints . . . the reading of Werther, like that of Shakespeare, raised him above his circumstances . . . he was no longer the insignificant abject being, that he appeared in other men's eyes.[121]

Shakespeare and *Werther* gave a higher note to Anton's complaints: they provided him with the means to reinterpret and find dignity in his unbearable position, and made it bearable. And for most people like Anton, *Werther* had an additional merit and a great advantage over Shakespeare: it was German. Now hundreds of madmen and thousands of neurotics could take solace in their very suffering, truly enjoy their "joy of grief," as K. P. Moritz called it, because their mental condition offered them a double proof that they were people of a desirable identity, placed above all others— not only were they men of a superior inner life (i.e., more truly human than the rest), but this superiority was the expression of their blood, derived from their bodily constitution—it was German national superiority. Original genius was the most perfect manifestation of the German nation, the universal, the most human nation of all.

Romanticism was called forth by the widespread psychological malaise resulting from the excruciatingly anomic situation in which *Bildungsbürger* were placed in the end of the eighteenth century and an attempt (remarkably successful as it turned out) to assuage it. It was a response, in other words, to mental illness of the madness or mental alienation kind, though, clearly, as elsewhere, the great majority of cases were of subclinical variety. As I have tried to demonstrate already in *Nationalism,* Romanticism provided the mold for German national consciousness, making German nationalism, essentially, a form of Romantic way of thinking and feeling. German nationalism first appeared as an integral part of the Romantic movement of thought in *Sturm und Drang,* with many of its central principles formulated by Goethe and especially Herder. But, while all other elements of Romantic mentality continued to develop, or, at least, to simmer, without interruption, the principles constantly reiterated, the brew constantly stirred and penetrating ever deeper into the souls exposed to its enticing (but, as we were soon to learn, poisonous) vapors, the events in France arrested—and for twenty years kept in abatement—a similar development of German nationalism. All so-called "early" Romantics (people like the Schlegels, Novalis, but also closely associated with them Fichte and Schelling) were cosmopolitans in their young years, expecting the liberators from the West to come and change the social structure of the German societies, as they were doing at home, which would rectify the intellectuals' position vis-à-vis the nobility and the bureaucracy and save them the trouble of changing its image instead. The French did not deliver, but they did something as good: they frightened the nobility and the bureaucracy, who then decided to befriend the *Bildungsbürger* and encouraged them to spell out the nationalistic implications of their grand ethereal

Ideen. Answering the call of the rulers, at the turn of the century the cosmopolitans became ardent nationalists virtually (in some cases literally) overnight. Their nationalism—passionate, savagely xenophobic, and fueled by hatred of the failed liberators—inspired the Wars of Liberation. This time it was in Germany to stay.

The Romantic generation suffered from mental illness in its cosmopolitan and nationalistic days alike. *Bildungsbürger,* in general, were sickly. Tuberculosis was very widespread, syphilis too, though, probably, less so than in the military nobility, but the main complaint was the one with a higher note: they called it "the nerves." Most contemporary chroniclers, according to Henri Brunschwig, stress the prevalence of nervous disorders. Those still unaffected, the employed die-hard representatives of the *Aufklärung,* laugh at this. "illnesses come into fashion and pass out of it . . . like Palais-Royal fashions," writes someone in the periodical *Eumonia* in 1801.

> Instead of seeking the real causes of a disorder, new names are invented for it, and people comfort themselves with the idea that if they are ill, they can at least suffer under the auspices of a fashionable druggist. . . . There was once a happy time when no human being knew that he had nerves. . . . How things have changed! Forty years ago an English doctor . . . was seized with an unfortunate idea of writing a book on the nerves and their disorders. . . . The term gave entire satisfaction and became fashionable; hypochondria, vapors and the like had to yield pride of place. The doctors themselves, compelled to bow to the exigencies of fashion, soon found the term so convenient that nothing on earth could induce them to give it up. Now the entire universe must have nerves. People pique themselves on having strong nerves, irritable nerves, or delicate nerves, as good form requires. A man of nerve was formerly a sturdy and hale son of Adam. Nowadays he is a being whose nerves respond to every impression to the thousandth degree, who swoons at the buzz of a fly, and is thrown into convulsions by the scent of a rose.[122]

But, clearly, whatever was the part of fashion in the widespread "nervous complaint," for very many it was not a laughing matter. "All the Romantics are manic-depressives," Brunschwig declares confidently from the perspective of psychiatrically well-informed post-World War II Paris. Indeed, they constantly complain of their "extreme nervous sensibility." Novalis and his brother exchange epistolary reports of attacks of "hypochondria," "bouts of neurasthenia," and "fits of depression." Caroline Schlegel (later Schelling) suffers "spells" of "nervous fever." According to her daughter, describing one such spell in 1800, the illness was treated with a mustard plaster: "My mother has been really very ill and is still not wholly recovered. She first had a nervous fever, which was very serious for a week; the doctor ordered a mustard plaster on her leg; she kept it on too long, and then they administered the wrong ointment, and that had very serious effects and caused my mother much pain. A relapse ensued, the nervous fever returned, and once it was over, very severe spasms took its place."

"This 'nervous fever,' of which they all speak, is very hard to identify," writes Brunschwig, "It does not seem to worry Caroline unduly; but Wackenroder dies of it at twenty-five." Judging by what the Romantics say of their experiences, it was a form of cyclothymia at best, descending into deep depression. Friedrich Schlegel confesses to his brother: "my feelings have a habit of plunging from heights to lowest depths." A very common description of this latter stage is "anguish" (*Angst*). Jung-Stilling writes of it in his autobiography, calling it "inexplicable." Tieck's literary alias, William Lovell, says: "when I rise to the very peak of enthusiasm, a species of indifference suddenly seizes me, a somber foreboding . . . like the cold dawn breeze that sweeps the mountain peak after a sleepless night. . . . I used to think that this sensation of anguish was a desire for love . . . but it is not that." Tieck's own condition certainly crosses into psychosis. His room was separated from that of his roommate by a glass door. Once the room-mate had a visitor and, seeing the shadows of the two men outlined on the door, Tieck recalled: "I shuddered so strongly that I fell into a species of raging madness, for they suddenly became strangers to me . . . and they too seemed to me to be madmen. That madness is contagious I find more and more evident, and I believe that Hamlet's words are to be understood in this sense, that these fellows will end by making me really mad, for I believe that a man (if he has weak nerves) becomes mad if he passes himself off as mad for any length of time."

It is not clear from this description (which sounds very much like recollections of the schizophrenic girl Renee) what is Tieck's understanding of the "real madness" he speaks about. Hamlet was a model for the Romantics, sharing his condition a sign of mental superiority to be proud of, rather than of a frightening mental disorder. But, whatever the interpretation, his suffering was real enough. Death was preferable. "Ah, if only a beneficent slumber would overtake me," longed the poor poet, "I feel like some wretched phantom wandering, somber and nameless . . . among men; to me they are an alien race."[123]

Nationalism, which was for the Romantics a form of therapy, one way of coping with their affliction, introduced anomie into the wider society, spreading this kind of mental illness beyond the limited circle of the free-floating *Bildungsbürger*. For the majority of these new sufferers, the idea of original genius did not make much sense and, in most cases, they had even less reason to interpret their experience in its terms than the writers. By 1860s, as we know from Griesinger, they wished to be helped. At the same time, the obvious similarity between the condition (the symptoms) of these ordinary mortals and that of the mad genii aroused suspicion that this interpretation did not apply to the latter group as well. The intellectuals would still be affected at a greater rate than other classes, but, from that point on, in Germany too they would be considered just mentally sick, like all the rest. Griesinger considered "neurosis" to be the characteristic disease of the educated class, and claimed that "the poor" were much more likely to become truly insane. If taken literally, however, this claim does not contradict the argument here, which assigns to *Bildungsbürger* the pride of place among German mad. Doerner comments, quoting the first non-Romantic psychiatrist: "The social decline of the educated middle class . . . was symbolized by the fact that the poor were no longer seen as just the lower classes but also as 'the class of the population that, with good education and careful intellectual formation and no other means, is dependent on the steady returns of its sole capital, its intellectual powers, and whose income stops in case of illness, making acceptance in a private asylum generally impossible.'"[124] Intellectuals, now included among the poor, thus constituted a significant, though obviously small numerically, contingent among the "truly" mad of the public asylums. Poor intellectuals!

We Too, We Too! Madness in Russia

The remarkable Russian autocrat Peter I, the Great, had a special liking for the English, and for this reason nationalism was imported to Russia very early, leaving even France behind. Despite this, madness, in fact, reached this vast country only in the second half of the nineteenth century, with the reforms of Alexander II, separated by some century and a half from the Petrine reforms. This was because Russia was in no way ready for nationalism when its determined ruler decided that it should have it, it served no function for—and no interests of—any social group in the population in which the vast majority were slaves, but was the wish of one man. This man being all-powerful, those in his immediate service quickly converted to the new creed, and, because Peter's wish was much more than a command for them, akin rather to a revelation than to an order of an earthly potentate, their conversion was sincere and all-encompassing: they gave to nationalism their souls. But these people were very few—numbering a couple of hundreds as late as 1820s perhaps, they represented a tiny sliver of the nobility, their estate, itself only a tiny sliver of the population. Because these few people, members of the same still fewer families, represented the Russian political and cultural elites in their entirety, and because Russian secular culture was created by nationalism and informed by it to its very core (the religious culture being destroyed by Peter and offering no resistance), both Russian politics and Russian secular culture, in particular literature, were intensely nationalistic and created the impression that nationalism was very widespread. But this was not so. Only with the liberation of the serfs in 1861 and the creation of a large class of *raznochintsy*— "people of different positions" in translation—who flooded the universities did values of nationalism spread among the masses of the urban population and changed their experience. Much more time was needed for these values to penetrate into the rural areas, and it is possible they have not reached this "Russian depth" (*russkaia glubinka*) until today.

The epidemiological history of schizophrenic mental disease and suicide related to it in Russia corresponds precisely to the levels of penetration of values of nationalism in the population and their timing. The only identity problems encountered by the first generations of Russian nationalists were problems of national identity. These noblemen were quite satisfied with their position within the Russian society. The anomie they experienced was by no means severe and whatever there was of it they channeled creatively into the transvaluation of Western values and its end-result—Russian national consciousness. This anomie, and the need for the transvaluation of Western values, was the product of the inconsistency between the assumption that Russia was equal to Western nations which it (following the wishes of Peter the Great) selected as its models—first England, then France, Germany, and the United States, and the deep sense of national inferiority based on the recognition that it was not their equal in any respect, which in its turn led to *ressentiment*.[125] The sense of national inferiority could embitter one's life sufficiently for making voluntary exit from it preferable.

Lenin had a theory (arguably stolen from Disraeli and generalized) that every ethnos contains two nations and two cultures. In Russia, these nations and cultures belong, first, to the intelligentsia, second to "the people." "Sometime around the turn of the 18th century," writes the author of a remarkable book *The Author and Suicide* Grigory Chkhartishvili, "the national body of Russia underwent something like cellular division—and from then on two incommensurable parts of society (their sizes being inversely proportional to their contributions to the common national culture) have existed each according to its own laws." These different laws extended to the suicidal tendencies characteristic of the two parts: the intelligentsia has been far more predisposed to suicide than "the people" and committed it for different reasons: people of "the people" would kill themselves because of alcoholism, constant want, and grinding, inescapable poverty, while members of the intelligentsia (in addition to alcoholism) have been mostly moved to take their own lives by injuries to their sense of dignity.[126] The first wave of suicides among the intelligentsia hit Russia in the 1790s, the dignity of this first generation of suicides being offended by Russia's inferiority to the West. The very first case of intelligentsia suicide, in 1792, should be doubtless attributed to it. It was that of seventeen-year-old nobleman and owner of populated estates M. Sushkov. The young boy was already a published author, and of none other than the novelette *Russian Werther* (*Rossiyskiy Verter*). Sushkov thought that Russia was culturally, politically, morally inferior to Werther's Germany (it was inferior even to Werther's Germany!), so he freed his serfs, wrote a tract justifying the action he was determined to take (it was too long to be called a "suicide note") in Werther's spirit, and shot himself. Thus, in Russia, too, Goethe made suicide a dignified solution to problems of indignity, and this first case in which it was used declared Russian nationalists' dependence on the West when it came to life and death decisions.

Yuri Lotman, the great Russian culturologist, in *Conversations on the Russian Culture,* quotes two letters, the first dated September 29 and the second October 27, of the same year 1792 in which the seventeen-year-old Sushkov concluded that enough is enough, written by one Russian nobleman to another, regarding the suicides of two brothers Vyrubov:

> (9/29) "Have I written to you that yet another young man, a son of Senator Vyrubov, having put a pistol into his mouth, took his own life? This happened in the beginning of this month, apparently: the fruits of becoming acquainted with the English people."

> (10/27) "What an unhappy father Senator Vyrubov is: yesterday another son, an artillery officer, shot himself. In two months two sons so shamefully ended their lives. This English malady threatens to become fashionable among us."[127]

The older generation, insufficiently *au courant,* still thought of this as "the English malady," and well might they be afraid of its spread into their country. But it would be long before it did.

The suicide of Alexandre Radishchev, "the first Russian writer of the new breed" (i.e., preoccupied with questions of dignity) and, indeed, one of the first Russian nationalists, must be mentioned here, precisely because it was rather traditionally motivated.[128] For his *Voyage from St. Petersburg to Moscow* (to which we owe the image of "Potiomkin's villages") Radishchev was tortured and sent by Catherine the Great to a penal settlement in Siberia. Restored in the autocrat's favor under Alexander I and brought into the government service, he was a member of the Legislative Committee headed by Count Zavadovsky. The Committee was entrusted by Alexander to give Russia new, enlightened, laws, similar to those enacted in the "civilized" nations, and Radishchev, taking His Imperial Majesty at his word, suggested the abolition of serfdom, physical punishments, and estate privileges. Count Zavadovsky responded that the famous author must be missing Siberia—perhaps, he was joking. Radishchev, however, panicked. Certain that only Alexander's decision to arrest him again would allow Zavadovsky to say a thing like that, the next morning he took some medicine "against the nerves" and, according to his son, "suddenly grasps a huge glass of very strong vodka . . . and drinks it in one gulp." He knew this would kill him, as it did, after several hours of torment, and wishing to save himself unnecessary suffering, tried to speed up the process by cutting his throat. Unfortunately for him, his son would not let him finish himself off in this efficient manner, and the unhappy man had a miserable death. In the conditions of autocratic Russia, even under the enlightened despot Alexander, and especially for a person with Radishchev's experience, suicide in reaction to a suggestion of another imprisonment was a rational act. It had nothing to do with wounded self-respect, whether national or personal, or the feeling that life as such was intolerable.

On the whole, the 1790s wave of the intelligentsia suicide, while chilly, was quickly spent and did slight damage; Russia was not yet susceptible to the English malady in this or any other form. Madness too, even subclinical, was unknown. Pushkin's Onegin, we are told by the poet, was not happy amid brilliant amorous victories and daily pleasures, although in every respect free and in the flower of his age. No: his emotional excitement waned; high society bored him; he lost interest in beautiful women, grew tired of his own and their betrayals, and even friends and friendship itself lost all their attraction. After all, says Pushkin, he could not always drink champagne and banter witticisms even when bothered by a headache. Onegin became ill: "The malady, whose cause it is long since time to find, similar to English spleen, in a word: Russian *khandra* invaded him gradually; God be praised, he did not attempt to shoot himself, but lost all joy of life. He would appear in society salons like a Child-Harold, somber and languid: neither gossip nor cards nor flirtations—nothing touched him, he paid attention to nothing."[129] Russian *khandra*, however, was not at all like English spleen, which showed that between 1825 and 1832 (when Pushkin's novel in verse appeared in its first, serial form) the nature of the latter was not at all understood in Russia: Onegin was morose, not depressed, haughtily contemptuous of the society around him but self-confident and self-complacent. So was Pechorin, the eccentric antihero of Lermontov's tellingly titled 1840 *Hero of Our Time,* in which the twenty-five-year-old author wished to present "the combined portrait of the vices of our entire generation, in their fullest development." Russian noble *intelligenty* who worshipped Byron, struck the Byronic pose, but did not have a clue as to how tragic the experience of that mad poet truly was. Their malaise was purely imitative and superficial—it was finery they paraded, rather than a pervasive and oppressive condition of the soul. And, while Pushkin, the Russian genius, was clearly aware of this and ridiculed Onegin's posturing, Lermontov took it in all seriousness. He identified with his image of Byron, he was Russian Byron, writing in an 1832 poem (at the age of seventeen):

> "No, I am not Byron, I am another, / Yet unknown chosen one, / Like he, a wanderer, persecuted by the world, / But only with a Russian soul. / I began earlier and will end earlier, / My mind won't accomplish much; / In my soul, as in an ocean, / There is a cargo of ruined hopes. / Who, gloomy ocean, can / Understand your secrets? Who / Will reveal my thoughts to the crowd? / I am either God—or nobody!"[130]

But he had no idea that Byron was mad, no notion what it meant to be mentally ill. Pushkin's poem of 1833, "God Save Me from Becoming Mad," may lead one to doubt this; however, the consideration of his reasons proves that Russian understanding of mental disease at that time did not include the modern variety which we came to call schizophrenia, manic depression, or simply depression. Not that he valued his reason overmuch and was very afraid to lose it, said Pushkin, but here was the trouble with madness: ". . . lose your mind, / And you'll be feared like a plague, / They will lock you up, / Chain the fool / And from behind the bars, like an animal / Will come to taunt you."[131] The horror was in the treatment, not in the condition.

One still has to account for Gogol's 1835 "Diary of a Madman," which is, indisputably, a description—the first in Russian literature and in Russia altogether—of a schizophrenic. The symptoms described in the story include (auditory) hallucinations, delusions of persecution and grandeur, flight of ideas, and bizarre formulations, while the treatment administered to the madman of the title, Ahanty Ivanovich Poprishchin, in the asylum eventually entrusted with his care, is precisely of the sort used in England and France in the early pre-psychiatry days and in Germany well into the nineteenth century. The story may suggest that, by 1835, such asylums housing schizophrenics among other mentally ill already existed in the Russian Empire, at least in the Ukraine, one of its Western parts, and that Gogol, at least, a Ukrainian, was familiar with this novel variety of mental derangement. As with Pushkin's poem quoted above, a closer analysis reveals that this would be a wrong conclusion. The symptoms are taken at their face value: for instance, a hallucination is perceiving something that does not objectively exist, but this something is not what a schizophrenic would perceive. There is no empathy with the protagonist, Gogol does not get into Poprishchin's head and does not take the trouble to imagine what it is like to be mad, but uses his hapless hero's nominal hallucinations and delusions as a vehicle for social commentary and, frankly, for their entertainment value. The story is hilarious—one cannot help laughing out loud throughout.

Poprishchin [132] is a poor, though not by any means destitute, nobleman, employed as a clerk of a low- to middling- rank in some office. He is forty-two and in love with the daughter of His Excellency, the Director. He has a maid who prepares his meals, loves theater, and regularly reads newspapers. We are introduced to him when he has the first strange experience: he sees the object of his tender passion descend from a carriage and enter a fashion shop—and distinctly hears the little dog Maggie, whom she leaves outside by the door, exchange words in Russian with another little dog, passing on a lady's leash, Fidel. Poprishchin is not very surprised and quickly decides to enter into a conversation with Maggie himself, in order to get some information on his beloved and her Papa. The little dog refuses his attentions with a growl, but Poprishchin is not discouraged, because he has overheard Maggie's promise to write to Fidel and decides to lay his hand on the doggy correspondence and get his information from it.

In the meantime, his coworkers at the office have noticed his infatuation with the director's daughter. On November 6, he records in his diary:

—Our chief clerk has gone mad. When I came to the office today he called me to his room and began . . . : "Look here, my friend, what wild ideas have got into your head?"

"How! What? None at all," I answered.

"Consider well. You are already past forty; it is quite time to be reasonable. What do you imagine? Do you think I don't know all your tricks? Are you trying to pay court to the director's daughter? Look at yourself and realise what you are! A nonentity, nothing else. I would not give a kopeck for you. Look well in the glass. How can you have such thoughts with such a caricature of a face?"

May the devil take him! Because his own face has a certain resemblance to a medicine-bottle, because he has a curly bush of hair on his head, and sometimes combs it upwards, and sometimes plasters it down . . . he thinks that he can do everything. . . . I know why he is angry with me. He is envious; perhaps he has noticed the tokens of favour which have been graciously shown me. But why should I bother about him? A councillor! What sort of important animal is that? He wears a gold chain with his watch, buys himself boots at thirty roubles a pair; may the deuce take him! Am I a tailor's son or some other obscure cabbage? I am a nobleman! I can also work my way up. I am just forty-two—an age when a man's real career generally begins. Wait a bit, my friend! I too may get to a superior's rank; or perhaps, if God is gracious, even to a higher one, I shall make a name which will far outstrip yours. You think there are no able men except yourself? I only need to order a fashionable coat and wear a tie like yours, and you would be quite eclipsed.

But I have no money—that is the worst part of it!

There is, obviously nothing mad in this, just an understandable irritation with the unfairness of unfair social arrangements. The next entries, however, remind us that we are reading about a madman. Poprishchin decides to render a visit to the doggy Fidel. He records:

When I had climbed up to the sixth story, and had rung the bell, a rather pretty girl with a freckled face came out. . . . She . . . asked "What do you want?"

"I want to have a little conversation with your dog."

She was a simple-minded girl, as I saw at once. The dog came running and barking loudly. I wanted to take hold of it, but the abominable beast nearly caught hold of my nose with its teeth. But in a corner of the room I saw its sleeping-basket. Ah! that was what I wanted. I went to it, rummaged in the straw, and to my great satisfaction drew out a little packet of small pieces of paper. When the hideous little dog saw this, it first bit me in the calf of the leg, and then, as soon as it had become aware of my theft, it began to whimper and to fawn on me; but I said, "No, you little beast; good-bye!" and hastened away.

I believe the girl thought me mad; at any rate she was thoroughly alarmed.

Poprishchin is very happy with the results of his visit, writing in anticipation: "Dogs are clever fellows; they know all about politics, and I will certainly find in the letters all I want, especially the character of the director and all his relationships." Then he reads the correspondence between Maggie and Fidel, with comments like this: "The letter is quite correctly written. The punctuation and spelling are perfectly right. Even our head clerk does not write so simply and clearly, though he declares he has been at the University."

From the letters he learns details about his superior's and his daughter's household, which seem to be perfectly accurate (it is clear that Gogol wants to communicate to us the information about the Director and his daughter, and not about Poprishchin's thought process) and which Poprishchin, however mad, could not have imagined. In this instance, he appears to be not mad, but oracular: facts of which he cannot be aware are revealed to him. It is certainly peculiar that these facts are revealed by an epistolary correspondence in educated Russian between two dogs, yet, this is also not mad, but rather fantastic. Among other things, Poprishchin learns that the director's daughter is engaged to be married to a Chamberlain (official of a high rank), in reaction to which he writes: "Deuce take it! I can read no more. It is all about chamberlains and generals. I should like myself to be a general—not in order to sue for her hand and all that—no, not at all; I should like to be a general merely in order to see people wriggling, squirming, and hatching plots before me." He is distressed both by the marriage that is to take place and by the social injustice:

December 3rd.—It is not possible that the marriage should take place; it is only idle gossip. What does it signify if he is a chamberlain! That is only a dignity, not a substantial thing which one can see or handle. His chamberlain's office will not procure him a third eye in his forehead. Neither is his nose made of gold; it is just like mine or anyone else's nose. He does not eat and cough, but smells and sneezes with it. I should like to get to the bottom of the mystery—whence do all these distinctions come? Why am I only a titular councillor?

This very sensible commentary, however, leads him to suddenly doubt his own identity:

> Perhaps I am really a count or a general, and only appear to be a titular councillor. Perhaps I don't even know who and what I am. How many cases there are in history of a simple gentleman, or even a burgher or peasant, suddenly turning out to be a great lord or baron? Well, suppose that I appear suddenly in a general's uniform, on the right shoulder an epaulette, on the left an epaulette, and a blue sash across my breast, what sort of a tune would my beloved sing then? What would her papa, our director, say? Oh, he is ambitious! He is a freemason, certainly a freemason; however much he may conceal it, I have found it out. When he gives anyone his hand, he only reaches out two fingers. Well, could not I this minute be nominated a general or a superintendent? I should like to know why I am a titular councillor—why just that, and nothing more?

Yet, though suggestive, even this does not sound like ramblings of a schizophrenic.

From this point on, Poprishchin's condition speedily deteriorates. On December 6 he reads in a newspaper that the Spanish "throne is vacant and the representatives of the people are in difficulties about finding an occupant," the news which very much confuse him. He spends a sleepless night thinking about it. The next entry in his diary reads:

> The year 2000: April 43rd.—To-day is a day of splendid triumph. Spain has a king; he has been found, and I am he. I discovered it today; all of a sudden it came upon me like a flash of lightning.
>
> I do not understand how I could imagine, that I am a titular councillor. How could such a foolish idea enter my head? It was fortunate that it occurred to no one to shut me up in an asylum. Now it is all clear, and as plain as a pikestaff. Formerly—I don't know why—everything seemed veiled in a kind of mist. That is, I believe, because people think that the

human brain is in the head. Nothing of the sort; it is carried by the wind from the Caspian Sea.

For the first time I told Mawra [his servant] who I am. When she learned that the king of Spain stood before her, she struck her hands together over her head, and nearly died of alarm. The stupid thing had never seen the king of Spain before!

The next entry is dated "Marchember 86," the following one "No date. The day had no date." Poprishchin makes himself a "Spanish national costume"—a cloak—out of his new official uniform which he has only worn twice; he uses the scissors himself, since tailors "dabble in speculation, and have become loafers," then records:

I don't remember the date. The devil knows what month it was. The cloak is quite ready. Mawra exclaimed aloud when I put it on. I will, however, not present myself at court yet; the Spanish deputation has not yet arrived. It would not be befitting if I appeared without them. My appearance would be less imposing. From hour to hour I expect them.

The 1st.—The extraordinary long delay of the deputies in coming astonishes me. What can possibly keep them? Perhaps France has a hand in the matter; it is certainly hostilely inclined."

The unfortunate man is committed to an asylum. He is not aware of this: in his mind, he is now in his own kingdom of Spain:

Madrid, February 30th.—So I am in Spain after all! It has happened so quickly that I could hardly take it in. The Spanish deputies came early this morning, and I got with them into the carriage. This unexpected promptness seemed to me strange. We drove so quickly that in half an hour we were at the Spanish frontier. Over all Europe now there are cast-iron roads, and the steamers go very fast. A wonderful country, this Spain!

As we entered the first room, I saw numerous persons with shorn heads. I guessed at once that they must be either grandees or soldiers, at least to judge by their shorn heads.

The Chancellor of the State, who led me by the hand, seemed to me to behave in a very strange way; he pushed me into a little room and said, "Stay here, and if you call yourself "King Ferdinand" again, I will drive the wish to do so out of you."

I knew, however, that that was only a test, and I reasserted my conviction; on which the Chancellor gave me two such severe blows with a stick on the back, that I could have cried out with the pain. But I restrained myself, remembering that this was a usual ceremony of old-time chivalry when one was inducted into a high position, and in Spain the laws of chivalry prevail up to the present day. When I was alone, I determined to study State affairs; I discovered that Spain and China are one and the same country, and it is only through ignorance that people regard them as separate kingdoms. I advise everyone urgently to write down the word "Spain" on a sheet of paper; he will see that it is quite the same as China.

He is subjected to the traditional treatment, his thoughts and writing become increasingly disconnected. Yet, Gogol makes even Poprishchin's description of "hellish torments" he undergoes sound hilarious, and manages to poke fun at Russian views of international relations:

January in the same year, following after February.—I can never understand what kind of a country this Spain really is. The popular customs and rules of court etiquette are quite extraordinary. I do not understand them at all, at all. To-day my head was shorn, although I exclaimed as loudly as I could, that I did not want to be a monk. What happened afterwards, when they began to let cold water trickle on my head, I do not know. I have never experienced such hellish torments. I nearly went mad, and they had difficulty in holding me. The significance of this strange custom is entirely hidden from me. It is a very foolish and unreasonable one.

. . . Judging by all the circumstances, it seems to me as though I had fallen into the hands of the Inquisition, and as though the man whom I took to be the Chancellor was the Grand Inquisitor. But yet I cannot understand how the king could fall into the hands of the Inquisition. The affair may have been arranged by France—especially Polignac—he is a hound, that Polignac! He has sworn to compass my death, and now he is hunting me down. But I know, my friend, that you are only a tool of the English. They are clever fellows, and have a finger in every pie. All the world knows that France sneezes when England takes a pinch of snuff.

The 25th.—To-day the Grand Inquisitor came into my room; when I heard his steps in the distance, I hid myself under a chair. When he did not see me, he began to call. At first he called "Poprishchin!" I made no answer. Then he called "Axanti Ivanovitch! Titular Councillor! Nobleman!" I still kept silence. "Ferdinand the Eighth, King of Spain!" I was on the point of putting out my head, but I thought, "No, brother, you shall not deceive me! You shall not pour water on my head again!"

But he had already seen me and drove me from under the chair with his stick. The cursed stick really hurts one. But the following discovery compensated me for all the pain, i.e. that every cock has his Spain under his feathers. The Grand Inquisitor went angrily away, and threatened me with some punishment or other. I felt only contempt for his powerless spite, for I know that he only works like a machine, like a tool of the English.

The last paragraph of the story is heart wrenching, surprisingly—given all this hilarity. And even here Gogol provides us with comic relief in the phrase with which it ends:

34 March. February, 349.—No, I have no longer power to endure. God! what are they going to do with me? They pour cold water on my head. They take no notice of me, and seem neither to see nor hear. Why do they torture me? What do they want from one so wretched as myself? What can I give them? I possess nothing. I cannot bear all their tortures; my head aches as though everything were turning round in a circle. Save me! Carry me away! Give me three steeds swift as the wind! Mount your seat, coachman, ring bells, gallop horses, and carry me straight out of this world. Farther, ever farther, till nothing more is to be seen!

Ah! the heaven bends over me already; a star glimmers in the distance; the forest with its dark trees in the moonlight rushes past; a bluish mist floats under my feet; music sounds in the cloud; on the one side is the sea, on the other, Italy; beyond I also see Russian peasants' houses. Is not my parents' house there in the distance? Does not my mother sit by the window? mother, mother, save your unhappy son! Let a tear fall on his aching head! See how they torture him! Press the poor orphan to your bosom! He has no rest in this world; they hunt him from place to place.

Mother, mother, have pity on your sick child! And do you know that the
Bey of Algiers has a wart under his nose?[133]

Gogol's lack of sympathy for the hero of his story is absolutely astonishing.
Gogol was a great writer, and what makes a great writer, in the first place,
is the ability to sympathize with his characters, even negative ones, to
identify with them, i.e., experience what they experience in one's imagination. In his other works, comical and not (and much of his work is comical),
Gogol's imagination is unerring. The inability to imagine the suffering of
a mentally sick Poprishchin in the "Diary of a Madman," therefore, cannot
be explained by the fact that the story is a farce. It—and the fact that the
story is a farce—can only be explained by the complete lack of familiarity
with such suffering, by the equation of madness with idiocy or weak-
mindedness, which makes the experience of schizophrenia, in Russia of
1835, unimaginable.

Of course, Russians, like the French before they knew better, and like
the Germans, thought that a madman is a madman is a madman. The
words that they used (*sumasshedshy, besumny*) and with which they translated texts that touched on madness from English, and on alienation from
French, could as well apply to any kind of psychosis, dementia, and even
idiocy. In Russia, as elsewhere, there was plenty of that always. Perhaps, a
certain kind of mental derangement was more common in Russia than
elsewhere—*delirium tremens,* psychosis induced by alcohol withdrawal.
There is, after all, a national disease in Russia too, a "Russian malady," so
to speak, with a long, long history, and it is alcoholism. Another organic
cause of *besumie*—syphilis—was also widespread, especially among all
classes of the military. Men caught it, gave it to their women, who then
transmitted it to children. Throughout the nineteenth century, where
asylum statistics were available (in England, France, and Germany, for
example), patients suffering from general paresis, or general paralysis of
the brain, caused by syphilitic infection, constituted, on average, 8 percent
of the inmate population. They usually died in a state of complete dementia:
it was a degenerative disease showing steady and rather rapid neuropsychi-
atric deterioration. Either of these could have been the "madness" of
Konstantin Batiushkov, the one poet of the early generation, very talented
and greatly admired by Pushkin, who obviously became *sumasshedshy.*

Batiushkov, was twelve years Pushkin's senior, born in 1787, and so old enough to participate in the campaigns of 1807 and 1812 against Napoleon. An officer of the victorious Russian army, he ended the latter in Paris, which, we are told in a Soviet commentary, "enriched him with important knowledge, experience, and many impressions."[134] It is quite possible that one of the gifts he carried with him from the City of Lights was syphilis, though there is also a possibility that his was an inherited disease: Batiushkov's mother became psychotic in 1793, was confined in a private asylum, and died there in two years. However this may be, in 1822 he already was severely mentally ill. He became depressed and paranoid, burnt his latest manuscripts and library, and several times tried to kill himself. His family and friends consulted physicians, hiring one to travel with him, and sent him to recuperate in Crimea. This did not help; in 1824 Batiushkov wrote an incoherent letter to Alexander I, requesting leave to enter a monastery. The Emperor, advised by another good poet and friend of Batiushkov, the royal tutor Zhukovsky, instead sent the ailing man to *maison de santé* in Sonnenstein at the government expense. It is not surprising that, after spending there four years, Batiushkov showed no sign of improvement. Clearly incurable, apparently rarely lucid and continuously deteriorating, he was eventually moved to a family estate in Vologda, where he died of typhus in 1855. Very little is known of the nature of Batiushkov's disease; his symptoms are consistent with general paresis, but, though this is most unlikely, he could have been a schizophrenic.

For the generation of Russians born the year Batiushkov died, schizophrenia among educated Russians, poets in particular, was unlikely no longer: in 1861 Alexander II, with a stroke of a pen, placed a rather large class of his people in an excruciatingly anomic situation and Russia lost its immunity to mental illness of this new kind. The abolition of serfdom, which allowed peasants who did not wish to stay on the land to move to towns, significantly increased the small Russian middle class—that is, the class that was in Russia, insofar as its rights and style of life was concerned, literally in the middle, between the nobility and the peasantry—the so called *raznochintsy*, people of all sorts of, or of mixed, ranks. The majority of these people were artisans and merchants, but smaller categories were also included, such as the lower clergy, petty clerks, "soldiers' sons," and "scullery maid's sons"—which, presumably, was a general reference to free domestic workers and their children. The overwhelming majority were uneducated and, probably, illiterate. Nevertheless, "people of mixed ranks" from the outset were a major source of recruits for the newly established secular educational institutions of the secondary and tertiary levels (gymnasia, technical and professional schools, and universities) and thus an important sector in the intelligentsia, the cultural elite, the majority of which came from the nobility. Until the Reforms of Alexander II, the Russian educated middle class was pitifully small. Secular education in the great empire dated only to the eighteenth century, the first medical school being founded in 1706, the first secondary school with general educational purposes in 1725, and the first (Moscow) university in 1755. It was estimated that, by the end of the eighteenth century, all the secular educational institutions together had produced around 8,000 graduates, about 4,000 with a university, or a university-level degree, and possibly a somewhat larger number of those with advanced secondary education. A large proportion of the university graduates (the majority, if we except medical schools) were nobles, which leaves us, by 1800, with the Russian *Bildungsbürgertum* of 6,000 to 6,500 people.

Hundreds of new gymnasia and many new universities were established in the course of the nineteenth century, and by 1900 the educated middle class, recruited from "people of mixed ranks," grew to several hundreds of thousands. Most of the growth had occurred after 1861, as a result of the liberation of the serfs. This one stratum was about 23 million strong.[135] Now free to move, a minority in it, nevertheless counting in the millions, flooded into the cities, providing grist, among others, for the educational mills. This large educated class proved most fertile breeding ground for schizophrenia in all its forms—it was a mentally ill class from the beginning, and much of the Russian history in the fateful half a century between 1861 and 1917 was a direct result of its mental disease.

The situation of the educated middle class was doubly, perhaps triply, anomic. To begin with, its very name, *raznochintsy,* "people of mixed ranks (or positions)," which in the singular, *raznochinetz,* meant "a person of mixed ranks (or positions)," made the formation of an individual identity problematic for its members: they belonged between positions, they were not of any rank fully, they were, by definition, a little bit of this and a little bit of that, and, of course, they fell between the chairs. Given the profoundly nationalist character of the Russian cultural elite since the days of its noble infancy, and of the culture this elite created, secular education of any level in Russia could not but promote the nationalist image of reality and make those whose consciousness became national, as elsewhere, worshippers of equality. But Russian reality negated equality, and no one felt this more acutely and was more insulted by this than educated *raznochintsy*, for it was their personal equality to people of the high rank and position that was negated. They felt eternally humiliated, denied respect they knew they deserved, and wounded in their dignity. For what it did to them they profoundly disliked their society. The sense of national inferiority added to their discomfort (it wounded them in their dignity as Russians), but at the same time allowed them to attribute their personal unhappiness to a shared, national problem, in regard to which they could claim every patriot's sympathy. Many of them thus found solace in nationalism as a cultural and political movement, Westernist—if they believed that Russia was actually inferior to the West socially, politically, culturally, and, most important, morally, Slavophil—if they thought that it was the West that was blind to Russia's superiority, but usually a mixture of the two. Nationalism was to inspire and bring about the revolutions of the twentieth century, but it definitely alleviated the psychological effects of the anomic situation, created in part by national consciousness, which each of the *intelligenty* from *raznochintsy* had to face alone. Participation in the revolutionary movement could not help those who were affected to the point of clinical mental illness, but was a serviceable therapy for those who experienced a milder form of the malaise, the "malcontents" as the sixteenth century English would call them, or the "neurotics" of French alienists. There, obviously, were many more of such than of those who could not cope at all. The great majority became revolutionaries, a small minority went mad or committed suicide.

According to Chkhartishvili, the second wave of suicides among the intelligentsia hit Russia in the end of the 1870s, as the first post-Reform generation was coming of age. Indeed, Dostoyevsky devoted most of his *Writer's Diary* for 1876 to the "epidemic of suicides" among young educated people. "Self-destruction is a serious thing, however stylish it may be considered" he wrote, "while epidemic self-destruction, which is on the increase among the intelligent classes, is serious in the highest degree and should be constantly watched and studied." In another entry he noted: "Really, numbers of suicides have increased so much among us recently, that nobody even discusses them any longer," and, horrified, asked: "Dear, kind, honest [young people], why are you leaving, why has the dark, silent grave come to attract you so? Look, there is bright spring sun in the sky, the trees are blooming, and you have tired yourselves, not having lived at all."[136] The great writer thought "disenchantment" (or, as he called it, "realism") was to blame: young educated people lost their faith in God and meaningful life. But most of the intelligentsia suicides were in fact idealists, with such an intense sense of pervasive meaningfulness of reality and such fervent belief in and commitment to transcendental forces that were the source of it (often identified with Lord Jesus), that these very fervor and intensity made their lives unlivable. They were mad and their beliefs were delusions.

This second suicidal wave drove its victims to the fatal act for the thirty remaining years before the revolution of 1917, and in ever-greater numbers. While suicides of the 1870s puzzled acute observers such as Dostoyevsky, those of the late 1880s and following pre-revolutionary decades were almost invariably (among poets and writers invariably) attributed to mental disease.[137] The specific mental disease believed responsible was denoted by the translation of Schelling's *Geisteskrankheit*, "the disease of the soul" (*dushevnaya bolezn'*), i.e., it was madness, and, after Bleuler's invention of the term, referred to as "schizophrenia." The most famous case of such suicide was that of Vsevolod Garshin, a writer of short stories, credited with introducing the genre into Russian literature. Garshin was a son of an "eccentric" retired army officer; his wife left him for a house tutor when the boy was five. One of Garshin's elder brothers shot himself, and so it is not surprising that Garshin experienced the first episode of illness while still in high school. He went on to study in a Geological Institute (college) and participated in the Balkan campaign, where he was wounded. In 1880, when he was twenty-five, he experienced a second, much more violent, episode, was put into a straitjacket and committed to an asylum. The illness was interrupted by periods of lucidity, during which he worked as a geologist and wrote his stories. Writing, however, was a torment to him; he said it drove him mad. Annually returning episodes were becoming worse and worse after 1884. Garshin committed suicide at the age of thirty-three, in 1888, throwing himself into the stairwell of his apartment building.

When Garshin's condition is discussed today, it is said, "he was, probably, manic-depressive." According to Chkhartishvili, his disease "expressed itself in depression, apathy, physical and spiritual fatigue, terrible sleeplessness."[138] Judging by Garshin's own description of it, it was classical schizophrenia. The experience of madness is the subject of Garshin's best-known story, "The Red Flower," written in 1883. The events of the story take place in an asylum; its hero is a violent madman, who is brought in, in a straitjacket, in the first paragraph. Though he had struggled with the officers committing him, he believes himself to be the inspector, sent by the special order of Peter the Great:

> He was frightful to see. His gray suit, torn to shreds during the attack, was partially concealed by the coarse canvas jacket, whose long sleeves clasped his arms crosswise on his breast and were tied behind. His bloodshot, distended eyes (he had not slept for ten days) sparkled with a motionless, fiery luster; the lower lip twitched convulsively; tangled, curly hair fell with a crest over his forehead; with quick and heavy footsteps he walked back and forth from one corner of the office to the other, searchingly examining the old cabinets containing documents, the oilcloth-covered chairs, and occasionally giving a glance at his fellow-travelers.

This is, unmistakably, the author's self-portrait.

The new patient is familiar with the place; he had already been there. Nevertheless, when brought into the bathroom to be washed, in accordance with the doctor's orders, he is terror-stricken.

> Thoughts distressing and absurd, one more monstrous than the other, flew about in his head. What was this? An Inquisition? Some secret torture chamber where his enemies had resolved to end his life? Perhaps it was hell itself? Finally he came to the conclusion that it was a test of some kind. Despite his desperate struggles he was undressed. His strength doubled by his disease, he easily threw several of the attendants who tried to hold him on the floor; but in the end four of them mastered him, and, holding him

by the hands and feet, lowered him into the water. Boiling it seemed to him, and in his crazed mind there flashed an incoherent and fragmentary thought about having to undergo a test with boiling water and red-hot iron. Almost smothered in his speech by the water which filled his mouth, he continued to struggle convulsively with arms and legs, which were held fast by the attendants. He gave utterance to both prayers and curses. He shouted till his strength was gone, and finally, with hot tears in his eyes, he ejaculated a phrase which had not the least connection with his other utterances: "Great martyr St. George! I give my body into thy hands. But the soul no; oh, no!"

After he is bathed and bled, the patient falls asleep, and, on awakening, at first does not know where he is, but then recalls the events of the last month and understands that he has been ill and the nature of his illness. The head physician comes to talk to him. Garshin records the dialogue:

"Why do you look at me so intently? You will not read that which is in my soul," said the patient, "but I can read yours clearly! Why do you do evil? Why did you gather this crowd of unfortunates, and why do you hold them here? To me it is all the same; I understand all, and am calm; but they? Why this torture? When man has attained that state when his soul harbors a great thought a universal thought to him 'tis immaterial where he lives or what he feels. Even to live, or not to live. . . . Is it not so?"

"Perhaps so," replied the doctor, sitting down on the stool in the corner of the room, that he might more easily observe the patient, who walked rapidly from one corner of the room to the other, dragging noisily his enormous horseskin slippers . . .

"But I possess it!" exclaimed the patient.

"And when I found it, I felt myself born over again. My senses have become more acute; my brain works better than ever. What once required a long path of reasoning and conjecture I can do now intuitively. I have attained that degree in fact which has been projected in philosophy. I am experiencing those ideas in which time and space are essentials. I am living through all ages. I am living without space; everywhere or nowhere, as you wish. And that is why it is immaterial to me whether you hold me here or give me liberty, whether I am free or bound. I have noticed that there are several here such as I. But for the bulk of the inmates here the situation is terrible. Why don't you free them? Who needs . . ."

"You remarked," the physician interrupted, "that you live without space or time. However, you cannot but agree with me that we are within this room, and that now . . . is half-past ten A.M., on the sixth of May, of the 18 . . . th year. What say you to that?"

"Nothing; it's all the same to me where I am and when I live. If it's all the same to me, does it not mean that I'm everywhere and always?"

The physician smiled. "Rare logic," said he, rising. "I think you're right. Good-by. Will you have a cigar?"

"Thank you." He stopped, took the cigar and nervously bit of it the end. "This helps one to think," said he. "This world is a microcosm. On one end is alkali, and on the other acids. . . . The same equilibrium has the world, in which the opposing ends become neutralized."

The patient is emaciated. He weighs 110 pounds on admission and, despite good appetite, a pound less every following day. He is constantly in motion and he does not sleep at all. When he looks through the window on his first day at the asylum, his attention is riveted by a large red poppy on the lawn. Garshin describes his state of mind:

He was conscious that he was in an insane asylum, and was also aware that he was sick. Sometimes, as on the first night, he would awaken amidst the stillness, after a whole day of turbulent motion, feeling rheumatic pains in all his organs and a terrible heaviness in the head, but nevertheless in full consciousness. Perhaps this effect was produced by the absence of sensations in nocturnal stillness and dusk; or perhaps it was due to the weak efforts of a suddenly awakened brain, enabling him to catch, during these few moments, a glimpse of reason, and to understand his condition as if he were in a normal state. With the approach of day, however, with the reappearance of light and the reawakening of life in the hospital, the other mood would seize him again; the sick brain could not cope with it, and he would become mad once more. He was in a strange state of sound reason mixed with absurdity. He understood that all around him were unwell; at the same time he saw in each one of them some secretly concealed face which he had known, read or heard of before. The asylum was inhabited by people of all ages and all lands. Here were both the living and the dead. Here were celebrities and heroes and the soldiers killed in the recent war. He saw himself in some enchanted sphere, which concentrated in itself the entire power of the earth; in proud enthusiasm he regarded himself as the centre of this sphere. They all, his comrades in the asylum, had gathered there to accomplish a deed, which appeared in his fancy as some giant undertaking toward the extinction of evil on earth . . . He could read the thoughts of other people; . . . the hospital building, indeed an old one, he regarded as a structure of Peter the Great's time, and he was confident that the Czar occupied it at the time of the battle of Poltava. He read this on the walls, on the crumbling wall plaster, on broken bricks and tiles found by him in the garden; the entire history of the house and garden was inscribed upon them. . . .

(One observes here features common to schizophrenic thinking everywhere, but also some national coloring. In Russia, as elsewhere, madmen are extremely attuned to the national culture.)

Allowed into the garden on a sunny day, the patient again sees the poppy and is convinced that it concentrates within itself all the evil in the world and that it is his mission to destroy it and liberate mankind. He wants to break the flower off the stem but this is forbidden and he is frustrated in his efforts by a watchman. In the end, he succeeds, but at that point there are already two poppies and he has to destroy the other one too.

He had not slept a wink through the night. He had broken off this flower because he saw in his action a duty. At his first glance through the glass door the red petals had attracted his attention, and it now seemed to him that he had fulfilled that which he was to accomplish on earth. In this bright red flower was concentrated all evil. He knew that opium was made out of poppy; perhaps it was this thought which, growing and assuming various monstrous forms, had created in his mind the fearful fantastic idea. The flower, as he saw it, ruled over evil; it absorbed in itself all innocently-shed blood (that is why it was so red), all tears and all the gall of humanity. It was an awful and mysterious being, the antithesis of God, an Ahriman presenting a most unassuming and innocent appearance. It was necessary to break it off and kill it. But this was not all; it was also necessary not to permit it at its death to discharge its evil upon the world. And that is why he put it in his bosom. He hoped that by morning the flower would lose its strength. Its evil would transplant itself to his breast, to his soul, and there it would be vanquished, or else it would vanquish; then he would perish, die, but die like an honest combatant, as the first champion of humanity, because until now no one had yet dared to wrestle at one onset with all the evil of the universe.

"They did not see it. I saw it. Can I permit it to live? Better death."

And he lay there, succumbing to a visionary, non-existing struggle. In the morning the assistant physician found him barely alive. Nothwithstanding this, however, in a short while he seemed to regain his vigor; he jumped out of bed, and as formerly he traversed the hospital, conversing with the inmates and with himself in a louder tone and more incoherently than before. He was not allowed in the garden. The doctor, noticing that his weight was growing less, that he did not sleep and that he walked and walked all the time, prescribed morphine. He did not struggle; fortunately at this moment his insane thoughts seemed agreeable to the operation. He soon fell asleep . . . He slumbered and ceased to think of everything, even of the second flower, which it was necessary to sever from its stem.

He succeeds in destroying the second flower and sees the bud of a third one. In his struggle with evil he exhausts himself physically. His weight goes down, he stumbles when he walks but walks constantly; the doctors decide to tie him. In an astonishing fit of strength he breaks his bounds, unbends iron bars on the window, climbs down the wall, and kills the last poppy. The next morning he is found dead with the red flower clutched in his hand.[139]

It is hard to see this as dealing with the same subject as Gogol's "Diary of a Madman." In the half a century separating the two stories everything changed in the experience and understanding of madness in Russia. To laugh at madmen, to write a comic story with a mad person as a protagonist in the 1880s, would be impossible. The awful mental disease was, obviously, no more understood in the great empire which it reached by the end of the nineteenth century than elsewhere where it has been known, and, as Chekhov's tragic "Ward No. 6" demonstrates, most people were not at all certain where the dividing line lay between being mad and thinking unconventionally—which is quite in line with today's definition of delusion, as we know. But it was clear as day that there was hardly any suffering worse than that of the mad, and that the mad were not idiots. The disease was starkly visible in Russia now and decimated the rows of the intelligentsia.

Russian psychiatrists, whose pioneers, born in the 1850s, belonged to the generation of the first Russian madmen, while being statistically astute and aware of the steady increase in the rates of *sumashestvie,* which they blamed on the pressures of the time, tended to regard madness as an organic disease. These first psychiatrists were, without exception, patriots, very concerned with the national dignity, and, remarkably, Russia's dignity and international prestige required that they subscribe to these two contradictory positions. Much (if not most) of the documents pertaining to the early history of psychiatry in Russia, dating to the three eventful decades before the Revolution, from the 1880s on, has been lost. No library in the world has the complete set of the first Russian psychiatric periodical, *Arkhiv psychiatrii, neirologii i sudebnoi psychopatologii* (Archives of Psychiatry, Neurology, and Legal Psychopathology), which began publication in 1882 and existed until 1913, or of other psychiatric journals which proliferated at a great rate since the late 1880s. Collections containing separate volumes in provincial Russian cities are, in effect, inaccessible. The richest holdings in this area, however much they leave to be desired, fortunately, happen to be in the United States—in the National Library of Medicine in Bethesda, MD, and the Library of the New York Academy of Medicine. On the basis of the materials there it is possible to conclude that, by the end of the 1880s, the psychiatric establishment in Russia, then at most ten years old, was robust, that having such an establishment was a matter of national honor, because all the "civilized" nations had one, and that the view prevailed that the degree of a nation's civilization was reflected in the rates of mental disease in it; the extent to which mental derangement was spread, in other words, measured how far it was advanced on the road to human perfection. This, of course, was a view quite common in the farthest advanced nations, such as Great Britain, France, Germany, and the United States, in relation to which Russia measured its own worth.

One of the oldest psychiatrists writing in Russian (among other languages), who practiced in Warsaw since 1867, belonging to the first generation of Polish psychiatrists, Dr. A. I. Rote, contributed to *Arkhiv psychiatrii* a lengthy and very informative "Survey of the History of Psychiatry in Russia and Poland." He was inspired to write it, he said, by the recent publication of histories of psychiatry in Spain and Germany, and had to divide his history into two unequal parts, because, while Poland followed, however belatedly, the trajectory of development common to most European countries, "Russian psychiatry developed in its separate ways and at every step has been different from the history of this development in Western Europe." This was so, in the first place, because "culture and civilization penetrated into the East so late, took root so feebly, and so little spread there." As before the introduction of Christianity in 988, so after it until the end of the sixteenth century, the Russian "people was almost at the first stage of its mental development"; its "vital needs could be easily fulfilled [and] there were no moments which could create traumas conducive to the development of mental diseases." Indeed, Dr. Rote wrote, no document from that period suggests that there were any deranged persons (*pomeshanye*) in the society. The people "was not subjected to the deleterious influence of alcohol," nor did "psychological and moral exhaustion exist, because the entire people considered significant and valued only brute force."

From the eleventh century on, indigent sick were cared for at monastery hospitals; they probably included "demoniacs" and fools, which were called *yurodivye* (the name in the nineteenth century applied to idiots and epileptics), who were also referred to as "blessed" *(blazhennye)*. Like court jesters in the West (or King Lear's fool), they had certain privileges, not only as persons not responsible for their actions and words, but also because they were believed, in their innocence, to speak the Truth, and were treated kindly. These weak-minded individuals, however, were not considered mentally deranged or mad. The first reference to such, according to Dr. Rote, we find only in the laws of Ivan the Terrible in the late sixteenth century, where those "possessed or deprived of reason" are listed among those who must be the object of public charity. Mentions of any mental disease remain very few with the ascendance of the Romanov dynasty in the seventeenth century. But in the end of the seventeenth century there is a change, "the main reason for it [being] the mentally ill from the free privileged classes." Traditionally, epileptics and idiots (or "demoniacs" and fools) from these classes were sent by their families to the same monasteries, which cared for the indigent population; the families remained in control of the property of their sick, presumably, paying the monasteries in some way for them. In 1677, a law was issued which formally sanctioned such removal of control over property from the hands of the weak-minded, stipulating that persons who were deaf, blind, or mute could manage their property, but "if they are drunkards or stupid (weak-minded)," they should not be allowed to do so. Five years after this, in Dr. Rote's view, groundbreaking law, Peter the Great took over the reins of power, imposed nationalism on his nobility, and the period of change par excellence, which encompassed all spheres of social life, began in Russia. But even in the course of this memorable reign only one law, in 1722, addressed the problem of the mentally ill and that without in the least changing the way in which mental illness was understood. The point of it was that people of all service ranks (i.e., of privileged estates to begin with) had to inform the Senate of their idiot relatives so that it could examine whether indeed they were incapable of any service to the state and, in that case, deprive them of their rights of inheritance and marriage.

It is an axiom in Russia that Petrine reforms dramatically advanced civilization in Russia, and, according to Dr. Rote, in the upper classes, which bore the brunt of the great Tzar's brutal tactics, created "the most fertile soil in which derangement (*pomeshatel'stvo*) could perfectly develop." Under Peter's (by all accounts, borderline idiot) grandson and namesake, Peter III—whom his wife, the clever Catherine, was to quickly depose and murder—the case of two "mentally ill" (*dushevno-bol'nykh*) brothers Princes Kozlovsky inspired the Tzar to write a special instruction: "not to send the demented (*bezumnykh*) to monasteries, but to build a special house for them, as tollhouses [Russification of German for Fool's Houses] are usually established in foreign states." A week later, in the end of April 1762, the Senate formally requested the Academy of Sciences for information on madhouses and care of the demented abroad. "None of the professors," writes Rote, "could provide a satisfactory answer," even though the majority were Germans. The best they could do is to point to travel guides, such as "*Les délices de la France, de l'Angleterre et de Pays Bas,*" "*État de la France,*" and "Description of London." In 1765, already under Catherine, the German historian A. L. Schleutzer, who was a Russian academician, was asked by the Academy to visit some of the foreign establishments for the mentally ill. He visited a couple and was particularly impressed by the house for the "demented" in Lueneburg. There he found "11 deranged [persons], all of them weak-minded, 'stupid,' among them I did not find any 'furiosus' who would be chained." The mayor of the town, Schleutzer explained, was in charge of the establishment and appointed its personnel. "The same," he suggested, "should be done in Russia as well, but the big difference between a German and a Russian magistrate increases the difficulty of such an arrangement." The historian ended his report with the following consider-ation: "It is hard to believe what glory and amazement would accrue to Catherine II, if, because of her desire, similar establishments will be founded in Russia. Such a rich people as Russian must very soon surpass all the others the moment it would not lack charitable establishments. What is important is not to make mistakes now in the beginning, for that reason one must follow the example of Peter the Great and thoroughly learn abroad how such establishments are constructed."

In the memorable year 1776 the first Russian madhouse was built in Novgorod. In 1779, it was decided to construct one in St. Petersburg. In 1810, there were fourteen such establishments in all of Russia, in 1814— twenty-four, in 1860—forty-three, with the total of 2,038 inmates. All these, Rote says, were houses of containment, rather than care or even less so treatment. But, he adds, "this should not surprise us, because our first establishments date to the last years of the [eighteenth] century, when in all of Europe such establishments were not much better." As late as 1828, such houses for the mentally ill, including the ones in St. Petersburg, operated not only without participation of a psychiatrist, for the reason that there "was no psychiatrist" in Russia at the time, but without any medical involve-ment; they were welfare, rather than medical establishments. Of all Russian cities, St. Petersburg was best provided with them, and in 1847 even had a private asylum, founded by M. Leidersdorf; it had twenty-five inmates. And then, "with the ascension to the throne of the Emperor Alexander II, a new epoch began for psychiatry" in Russia. In 1888, the year with which Rote ends his survey, there was one bed for mentally ill for 434 residents in St. Petersburg. The madhouses were (very slowly, as we know from Chekhov) turning into places of medical treatment and they were constantly and increasingly overcrowded.[140] Civilization was not coming to Russia cheap.

The most active Russian psychiatrist in this early period was, probably, P. I. Kovalevsky. Born in 1850, he was a Professor of Psychiatry and Nervous Diseases at Kharkov University. In Kharkov, in 1882, he founded and served as editor-in-chief of and main contributor to *Arkhiv psychiatrii, neirologii i sudebnoy psychopatologii*. He had, according to all evidence, an extensive clinical practice, both in Kharkov and at the balneological spa in Piatigorsk, and was centrally involved in the organization and subsequent work of the Russian Psychiatric Association, founded in 1887. The first issue of the *Arkhiv* is lost, but we have Kovalevsky's introduction, dated December 25, 1892. This is what he wrote there:

> Beginning the publication of the first issue of this journal I had one goal in mind—to offer my fellow-specialists the opportunity to publish their work in one place and thereby make it convenient for them to get acquainted with original works and foreign literature in psychiatry, which has grown by now to a rather considerable size. Soon after the foundation of our *Arkhiv* another periodical in psychiatry and neurology appeared in St. Petersburg, which showed that the Russian Empire has enough scientific power to support two specialist publications in the same field, and the ten-year-long existence of these journals fully justified this supposition.[141]

Kovalevsky then expressed his thanks to his colleagues for their support and confidence in their work "for the science, as well as the practice of our Motherland," and ended the editorial with the promise: "Foreign literature is annually growing—also growing is the interest in it among our comrades, while reading it in the original is possible to too few by far. That's why I consider it my duty to satisfy this interest of the comrades by broadening the section of reports [on the foreign literature]. In everything else we'll be following the previous direction [of the journal] in our profound desire to serve science and Motherland."

While in the first few years of publication, many of the articles published in the *Arkhiv* were translations and most literature reports summed up foreign works, by the mid nineties the contents of the journal were in the great majority of cases of native origin. Indeed, in 1898, Kovalevsky wrote in one of these reports, a review of *Lectures on General Psychopathology* by Professor N. M. Popov: "Russian medical literature already contains

enough original treatises in every field of medical knowledge—isn't it time
to cut down on translations of foreign works, which even today are often
produced without any need or reason?"[142] Moved by the patriotic spirit of
the practitioners, within at most a dozen years of its emergence, Russian
psychiatry was recognized as a leading national tradition in the field; a
number of Russian psychiatrists, such as Bekhterev and Korsakov, who
lent their names to previously disregarded disorders, were considered
authorities all over Europe and North America. The editorial board of the
Arkhiv in 1892 was sixty-two psychiatrists strong, including twelve from
the provincial city of Kharkov only; and four of its members, in addition to
Kovalevsky, were professors of psychiatry in the universities of Derpt,
Kazan' (two), and Warsaw. St. Petersburg, as was mentioned, was home to
another psychiatric periodical for almost a decade at the time, provided
care for the greatest number of mentally ill in its hospitals and private
clinics, and, most probably, had the largest community of psychiatrists
among Russian cities. (This was just as well, for, according to Kovalevsky,
the capital had "for each 10 people necessarily 9 afflicted with nerves."[143])
Moscow was not much behind it. In 1893, Bekhterev started his own
journal, *Nevrologichesky Vestnik,* in Kazan', and similar publications proliferated in the following years.

Remarkably, as the number of translations of psychiatric literature,
especially from English and French, diminished relative to Russian works
and Russian psychiatry, for all intents and purposes, came onto its own,
the attention paid by the psychiatrists specifically to madness, i.e., to the
mental disease of unknown organic origin which would be soon divided
into schizophrenia and manic-depressive illness, markedly diminished as
well. Russian psychiatry was inseparable from neurology; it was emphatically biological from the first and defined mental disease as an organic
disease. This is also explained by the psychiatrists' concern for national
dignity; nationalism lies at the root of the Russian psychiatric tradition.

The tireless toiler Kovalevsky was skeptical about the commonplace
proposition that the rate of mental diseases in a society is directly proportional to its level of intellectual development or "civilization." Nevertheless,
he mentioned it in his opening address on "The Condition of the Mentally-
Ill in the Russian Empire" to the second Congress of the Society of Russian
Doctors. Even though the rate of mental disease might be lower in Russia

than in Europe ("assuming that in the Russian Empire, instead of 4.5 mentally-ill per 1000 of healthy persons [as in Europe], there is only 1 per 1000"), he argued, "even then in our Fatherland there would be more than 100,000 mentally-ill," i.e., more, in absolute numbers, than anywhere else. Moreover, this colossal number was increasing year after year. "To prove this," Dr. Kovalevsky said,

> I'll cite the evidence pertaining to a small group of people, with which I am closely acquainted, namely, the students of Kharkov University in the last 10 years. We say that in Western Europe, on average, there are 4.5 mentally-ill individuals per 1000 who are well. At Kharkov University, per 1000 students 10 years ago there were 10, but this year are 24, individuals suffering from mental and severe nervous diseases per 1000 [of students who are well]! And this is the flower and ornament of the society, the future hope of the state![144]

On the basis of this example the speaker concluded that Russia was in the throes of "a pandemic of mental diseases. Madness (*sumashestvie*) does not spare anyone," he said. "Poor and rich, educated and uneducated—all are equally prone to become sick with psychoses. And there is no family, which does not have a near or a distant relative who is mentally ill."

But Kovalevsky's evidence warranted no such conclusion. A very large percentage of the presumed 100,000 mentally dysfunctional individuals, especially among the peasantry, which constituted 80 percent of the general population and, as such supplied the great majority of the population of the sick, according to his own testimony elsewhere in the address, were congenital idiots. Kharkov students certainly did not belong to these, and there is no indication that the rates of idiocy were increasing. Nor was there any increase in the rates of alcoholism and syphilis, to which Russian psychiatrists believed *sumashestvie*, i.e., psychotic mental disease (which idiocy was not) was mainly attributable. In an 1894 tract, *Nervous Diseases of Our Society*, Kovalevsky wrote:

> the life of a civilized man each year brings more and more upsetting, burdening and simply morbid influences on the nervous system, so the increase of mental [*dushevnykh*—of the soul] and nervous diseases in our time should

not seem surprising; this in turn represents a natural social, causal moment for the even greater increase and spread both of nervous diseases, and the degeneration of the Russian society. . . . [Among the causes] pathological heredity (the nervousness of the parents) is of incomparably lesser influence [than] two other horrible morbid factors. These deadly factors, relentlessly driving the human race to degeneration in the broadest sense of the word are alcoholism and syphilis.[145]

(Kovalevsky also wrote: "the reforms of Alexander II, which had many bright aspects, gave birth to an unstable generation, which, in turn, produced another one, still more morbid . . . —hence dissatisfaction with life even among children, apathy, suicides without cause, hopelessness, drastic nervousness. . . . These are the causes which gave birth to the American illness (neurasthenia) in Russia, and possibly in a greater measure than in America itself." Syphilis, by the way, he referred to as "the French disease.") Psychoses were defined by delusions and hallucinations, in their own turn seen as persistent false beliefs and false sense perceptions. (As we know, this view of what constitutes a delusion still persists.) Neither alcoholism-induced psychosis, *delirium tremens,* nor the mental derangement resulting from syphilis, paresis or general paralysis of the brain, presented with the peculiarities of thought and language characteristic of schizophrenia. They also differed from the latter in course and outcome, both having an acute onset which implied a drastic change in personality and behavior, rather than, as in schizophrenia, only exacerbating the existing personality traits and peculiarities of conduct (schizoid personality and negative symptoms) and starting with a lengthy prodrome; and while schizophrenia is a chronic condition, *delirium tremens* could very well end after one episode, and paresis would in most cases, after degenerating into a total dementia (which is not a tendency in schizophrenia) end in death within three to five years of being diagnosed. In addition, the three diseases could be distinguished by the nature of their hallucinations: those characteristic of *delirium tremens,* tactile, communicating the feeling of insects or reptiles crawling inside and on the body, are specific to this particular psychosis, as much as hearing voices is specific to schizophrenia, while syphilitic hallucinations, though non-specific, appear to be usually visual. However, Russian psychiatrists could not distinguish between the three diseases, because they did not suspect that they were different diseases and thus could not compare them; they considered them one and the same disease: psychosis, madness, *sumashestvie*. Moreover, unlike their counterparts in Western European countries and North America, who (long before the name) concentrated their attention on schizophrenia, because, while the rates of other psychoses remained stationary, rates of this disease were rapidly increasing, Russian psychiatrists focused on the far more widespread in actual numbers organic psychoses which affected all classes of society indiscriminately (nevertheless basing their claim that their rates were increasing on the observation that rates of severe mental disease were growing among the tiny educated elite in cultural centers). The reason they did so was that, despite its rapid spread in certain circles which it devastated, there was too little actual madness in Russia: even those Russian psychiatrists who, like Kovalevsky, considered the notion "absurd," felt that, to justify their nation's claim to a place among "civilized" societies, they needed to show that there were very large numbers of mentally ill, psychotic, deranged people in it. Russia's international standing demanded this.

It was, therefore, from a certain point of view fortunate that the rates of alcoholism in Russia were indeed staggering and, as a result, disorders associated with it, whether physical (such as cirrhosis of the liver) or mental could be expected to be very high as well. Alcoholism was also comorbid with any other disease in Russia, because it was the commonest national affliction; the statement the lore credits to Prince Vladimir, *veselie russkoye est' pitie* ("Russia's joy is drinking") is cited as the reason for that great monarch's choice of Christianity, which was tolerant of drunkenness, rather than Judaism or Islam, which he considered alongside it but rejected because they looked at inebriating spirits askew, as his realm's monotheistic religion. Cases of *delirium tremens*, individual and collective, assailing entire villages, were quite often described in the psychiatric journals, but were not necessarily recognized as such, instead being presented as examples of delusional psychosis in general.[146] Similarly, syphilis, the cursed "French disease," which was very widespread everywhere in Europe, was very widespread in Russia, and supplied its share of sufferers from the effects of the havoc it wrought on the brain. In the West, syphilisology in the second half of the nineteenth century was a legitimate academic discipline (somewhat as Sovietology in the second half of the twentieth century, and as long—or short—lived); medical libraries contain sets upon sets of impressive-looking periodicals in all the European languages whose speakers aspired to a place in the universe of science, bearing its name. Russia was too young (too "uncivilized," so to speak) to have its own syphilisology establishment, but its doctors, psychiatrists in particular, were passionately interested in the morbid subject. As much as half of the contents of the early psychiatric journals, sometimes almost entire issues, dealt with syphilis; all Russian psychiatrists of importance wrote about it. Kovalevsky believed that it was the main reason for the spread of mental disease in Russia and the world, because, he argued, increasing numbers of people were contracting it in his day of greater self-indulgence than before. (Sexual abstinence was the only means of avoiding new infection, but, he thought, there was so much of it in the blood already that most of those developing the disease—and its most horrible psychiatric form—would be its innocent victims, exposed to "the poison of syphilis" indirectly.) In his clinic in Piatigorsk, at least, he treated predominantly syphilitics, whether or not they were mentally ill, and not, as could be expected, mentally ill, whether or not they were syphilitics.[147]

It was the definition of psychosis as an organic disease, a result of the necessity to focus on organic psychoses, in turn explained by the desire of the Russian psychiatrists to defend the dignity of their nation, which, in the twentieth century allowed Soviet authorities to diagnose political dissenters as schizophrenics, confine them in psychiatric hospitals, and there ply them with chemicals which were certain to destroy the minds of the sanest people. Combined with the definition of delusion as a persistent false belief (i.e., a belief which most of the society considers false), the committing officers could do this in all sincerity and with the full support of science behind them. This is yet another example how serious, in sciences that may affect people in any way, the business of definitions is.

7

Madder Than Them All

From the Records of American Insanity

No tongue can declare
The torment I bear,
It my heart-strings doth tear,
So keen are the pangs of the Hypo.

I start 'cross the floor,
Then pitch out the door,
As if ne'er to enter more,
In order to fly from the Hypo.

I then dodge and run
Which often makes fun,
Till my race is quite done,
I am so bother'd by the Hypo.

I pick up a chip,
A stone or a whip,
And along hop and skip,
And this is to fool the Hypo.

And 'tis not in vain,
For my object I gain,
And I will not complain,
For hereby I muster the Hypo.

I see people laugh,
Though they'd better cry by half,
But I then seize my staff
And rush to the combat with Hypo.

I could sit down and cry,
And pour floods from my eye,
And weep till I die,
I am so afflicted with Hypo.

But this will not do
I plainly do know,
For it adds to my woe,
And only increases the Hypo.

No, I must resist,
As if fighting with fist,
And sometimes must twist,
Or soon I shall die with the Hypo.

This poem appeared in the first issue of the *American Journal of Insanity* (hereafter referred to as *AJI*).[1] The quarterly periodical began publication in July 1844, in Utica, New York, and despite its suggestive title, was not an early precursor of *MAD* magazine, but a serious professional journal that some eighty years thence would become *The American Journal of Psychiatry*. Its "principal Editor" was Dr. Amariah Brigham, the physician and superintendent of the New York State Asylum for the Insane, founded in Utica several months earlier. The poem was called "Hypo"—"hypo," as was mentioned in the previous chapter, was a synonym of "spleen," i.e., all the varieties and the entire range (from subclinical to acutely psychotic) of madness, since the eighteenth century. It was included as clinical information on one of the eight patients from the Asylum, the description of whose cases the first issue of *AJI* presented as "Article V."

In the third issue of the journal, the editor published a notice:

We are pleased to be able to state, that we think the Journal of Insanity is established on a permanent basis, though the list of subscribers is small. We hope those who now receive it, who are friendly to such a periodical, will call the attention of others, especially Physicians, Lawyers, and Clergymen to the work, and induce them to subscribe for it. We venture to make this request, being convinced from numerous communications, that the work is thought to be valuable and worthy of being sustained and the price is very low. . . . The object of this Journal is to popularize the study of insanity,—to acquaint the general reader with the nature and varieties of this disease, methods of prevention and cure. We also hope to make it useful and interesting to members of the medical and legal profession, and to all those engaged in the study of the phenomena of the mind.

Mental philosophy, or metaphysics, is but a portion of the physiology of the brain; and the small amount of good accomplished by psychological writers, may perhaps be attributed to the neglect of studying the mind, in connection with that material medium which influences, by its varying states of health and disease, all mental operations.

We regard the human brain as the chef d'oeuvre, or master-piece of creation. There is nothing that should be so carefully guarded through all the periods of life. Upon its proper development, exercise, and cultivation, depend the happiness and highest interests of man. Insanity is but a disease of this organ, and when so regarded, it will often be prevented, and generally cured, by the early adoption of proper methods of treatment.[2]

In these few lines Dr. Brigham summed up the position of his journal, which was more or less the same that Jules Baillarger presented in as many pages in the first issue of *Annales Médico-Psychologiques*. The Americans received the news that the French beat them to the establishment of the first psychiatric periodical in the world, if only by some months, when the first issue of Brigham's journal was ready to go to print, and, by the time the third issue of the *American Journal of Insanity* came out, its principal editor was, probably, familiar with Baillarger's lengthy statement. Perhaps it was that statement—reflecting the scientific consensus, which in the 1840s was formed under the aegis of the French psychiatric establishment—that he summarized. The only characteristically American contribution to Brigham's brief note was the assertion that his journal was a very good bargain.

It is clear that in the first decade of the journal's existence American psychiatrists (superintendents of the asylums for the insane) deferred to the French alienists: almost every issue included translations from the works of the French luminaries, many of them from the *Annales*. They were also very respectful of the British mad-doctors, and reprinted many of their publications. Nevertheless, at least another half a century had to elapse before knowledge and understanding of the subject would be measured by the number of references to professional authorities. In the beginning, the judgment of whether or not an "expert" deserved to be quoted depended on the correspondence between the expert's views and the American author's clinical experience: empirical knowledge was the final arbiter. Thus the second issue of *AJI*, of October 1844, contained, as article I, an essay "Definition of Insanity—Nature of the Disease." Also penned by Dr. Brigham, it laid out the view prevailing among the superintendents of asylums for the insane in the new world. Dr. Brigham began explicitly:

> By Insanity is generally understood some disorder of the faculties of the mind. This is a correct statement, so far as it goes; but it does not define the disease with sufficient accuracy, as it is applicable to the delirium of fever, inflammation of the brain, and other diseases which are distinct from insanity.
>
> Insanity, says Webster's Dictionary, is "derangement of the intellect." This is not merely too limited a definition, but an incorrect one, for in some varieties of insanity, as Prichard remarks, "the intellectual faculties appear to have sustained little or no injury, while the disorder is manifested principally or alone, in the state of the feelings, temper or habits."
>
> We consider insanity, a chronic disease of the brain, producing either derangement of the intellectual faculties, or prolonged change of the feelings, affections, and habits of an individual. In all cases it is a disease of the brain, though the disease of this organ may be secondary, and the consequence of a primary disease of the stomach, liver, or some other part of the body; or it may arise from too great exertion and excitement of the mental powers or feelings; but still insanity never results unless the brain itself becomes affected.[3]

With the parsimony which the readers would soon recognize as characteristic of him, Dr. Brigham distinguished insanity from mental disorders of known organic origin; separated it from idiocy, on the one hand, and temporary psychosis, on the other; stressed its etiological uncertainty and the possibility that its cause may lie within as well as outside the body; and at the same time pointed to its necessary reflection in the brain. His view was not inferior to that of psychiatry of our day in respect to what is actually known about the disease to which he referred with deplorable nineteenth-century directness and which we call schizophrenia or manic-depression, and in agreement with it regarding the importance of the brain, being arguably more open-minded in respect to what was (and is still) not known about this disease.

Brigham then expanded on his brief introduction, getting somewhat confused regarding the relationship between the mind and the brain: indeed, the dualist mind-body ontology within which he necessarily thought could not allow him to escape conceptual entanglement. In the 1840s, "intelligent persons who have paid much attention to insanity," he argued, regard it

> as a disease of the body, and few at the present time, suppose the mind itself is ever diseased. The immaterial and immortal mind is, of itself, incapable of disease and decay. To say otherwise, is to advocate the doctrine of the materialists, that the mind, like our bodily powers, is material, and can change, decay, and die. On this subject, the truth appears to be, that the brain is the instrument which the mind uses in this life, to manifest itself, and like all other parts of our bodies, is liable to disease, and when diseased, is often incapable of manifesting harmoniously and perfectly the powers of the mind.
>
> Insanity then, is the result of diseased brain; just as dyspepsia or indigestion is the result of disordered stomach; but it is only one of the results or consequences of a disease of this organ. The brain may be diseased without causing insanity; for although we say, and say truly, that the brain is the organ of the mind, yet certain portions of the brain are not directly concerned in the manifestations of the mental powers, but have other duties to perform. Certain parts of the brain confer on us the power of voluntary motion, but these portions are distinct from those connected with the mental faculties.
>
> We may say . . . that insanity is an effect of a disease of only a part of the brain—the outer or grey part. In most cases, insanity is the consequence of very slight disease, of a small part of the brain. If it was not so, the disease would soon terminate in death—for severe and extensive disease of the

brain soon terminates in death. We see, however, numerous instances of insane persons, living many years, and apparently enjoying good health. We have seen several persons who have been deranged 40 and even 50 years, during which they enjoyed in other respects, good health. On examining the brain after death, in such old cases of insanity, but little disease of this organ is often found, though a little, we believe may always be found. . . . It is as if, in some very complicated and delicate instrument, as a watch for instance, some slight alteration of its machinery should disturb, but not stop its action. Thus we occasionally find that violent mental emotions—a great trial of the affections—suddenly to derange the action of the brain, and cause insanity for life, without materially affecting the system in other respects.

[Brigham cited several examples from Esquirol's practice, in which insanity is connected to disappointment in love, as well as some literary English sources, tying madness to other emotional traumas, and continued:] A little injury of the brain—a slight blow on the head, has often caused insanity, and changed the whole moral character. . . . We have known a most exemplary and pious lady—a most excellent wife and mother, whose mind had been highly cultivated—transformed by a little injury of the head, into one of the most violent and vulgar beings we ever saw, and yet the intellectual powers were not very much disturbed. . . . Such cases teach us to be cautious and tolerant in cases where change of character and misconduct are connected as to time, with injury or disease of the head, or even with general ill health. . . . Most experienced physicians must have noticed striking and permanent changes of character produced by disease. The insanity of some persons consists merely in a little exaltation of some one or more of the mental faculties—of self-esteem, love of approbation, cautiousness, benevolence, &c. A man received a severe wound on . . . his head, after which his mind became . . . affected, especially as related to his benevolent feelings, which were perpetually active towards man and beast. He was disposed to give away all that he had, and finally was placed in a Lunatic Asylum in consequence of the trouble which he made in his endeavors to benefit others and relieve suffering. Whenever he saw any cattle in a poor pasture, he would invariably remove them to a better; and whenever he heard of a destructive fire or shipwreck, he would hasten even to a great distance to endeavor to afford relief.

Among the insane in Lunatic Asylums, we sometimes see not only exhibitions of strength, mechanical and musical skill, powers of language, &c., far superior to what the same individuals ever exhibited when sane, but also a remarkable increase and energy of some of the best feelings and impulses of our nature, prompting them to deeds of self-sacrifice and benevolence . . .

We very rarely find the whole mind destroyed or disordered in insanity, except in cases of long continuance, or of unusual severity. A majority of patients in Lunatic Asylums have considerable mind left undisturbed, and some of them conduct with propriety, and converse rationally most of the time, and on all but a few subjects. We have seen an individual who believed that he directed the planets and caused the sun to shine and the rain to descend when he chose, yet he was a man of much intelligence and conversed rationally on other subjects, and was remarkable for gentleness of manner and amiability of disposition. We could cite very many cases nearly similar, and to those who have frequently visited this Asylum, we can appeal for the verification of the statement—that patients decidedly insane on one or more subjects, still manifest acute and vigorous minds, and appear to be sane on others.[4]

From these various examples, most of them taken from his own clinical experience, Brigham derived the following conclusions regarding the mind, which he prefaced by a statement of conscious agnosticism:

Having seen that insanity consists in the derangement of one or more of the faculties of the mind produced by disease of only a part of the brain, we conclude that there is no one faculty of the human mind but may become disordered. If, therefore, we actually knew what mental faculties mankind possess, we might then know all the various forms of insanity, all the varieties of mental aberration to which these faculties are liable. But we don't know. Philosophers have ever disagreed as to the number of the faculties of the mind, and even as to what constitutes a faculty.[5]

The doctor had no interest in getting into a discussion with philosophers, rather "appealing to common observation for the correctness of what" he thought on the subject. "In contemplating the phenomena of mind," he said, we can not fail to perceive the variety of its faculties, and that there is an obvious general division of them into intellectual and moral, the latter comprehending the propensities and impulses. These faculties, both the intellectual and moral, are originally possessed by all, and are alike dependent upon a healthy state of the brain for their proper manifestation. . . . The intellectual faculties are but a part of our mental powers, and contribute but little in fact towards forming what we call the character of an individual. . . . The character is determined by the moral faculties or propensities, by the affections, benevolence, love, selfishness, avarice, &c. The difference in the activity and energy of these, create the differences we see in the characters of men; these constitute the man himself, or the soul of man, while the intellectual faculties are but instruments to administer to the wants and demands of the propensities. Without these propensities or moral faculties, the intellectual powers would not be exerted at all, or but feebly. The stimulus or urgency of the impulses of our moral nature, of benevolence, love, avarice, & c., impel men to action—to gratify these the human race have forever toiled.[6]

We see here that the American psychiatrists' view of the mind (which, or a part of which, Brigham did not hesitate to equate with "the soul") in the 1840s was quite complex. Based on "common observation," instead of inherited beliefs—in established theories taught in graduate schools—it distinguished between various "faculties" of the mind: intellectual, emotional, and what, given the phrasing ("propensities," "wants and demands," "impulses," "impel to action"), appears to be what in this book was called "the will." The three "faculties" were seen as closely integrated, with the emotions and will acting as one, "moral" faculty—the word "moral" standing at the time for both "social" and "mental"—and the intellect, though more independent, being in a way subservient to the "moral" faculty.

This view of the mind naturally led to a complex and open understanding of mental disease, in particular insanity, and precluded both the separation of affective illness from thought disturbances, and the definition of what we shall regard as "madness in its pure form"—schizophrenia—as a degenerative disease culminating in dementia. In this Dr. Brigham already had to argue with the contemporary lay, and, specifically, legal opinion. "It is to these important faculties, the propensities of our moral nature," he wrote, that we wish to call particular attention . . . to the fact that they as often become deranged as the intellectual. They as truly use the brain for manifesting themselves; consequently when certain parts of the brain become diseased, they become deranged, and not unfrequently without the intellectual powers being noticeably disturbed. A man's natural benevolence or propensity to acquire, or to love, may become deranged from disease of the brain as truly as his powers of comparing, reasoning, &c.

Yet evident as this is from Physiology and Pathology, and from daily observation in Lunatic Hospitals, it is a fact, and an alarming fact, that when disease causes derangement of the moral faculties, and changes the character and conduct of an individual, he is not deemed insane, provided the intellectual powers are not obviously disordered. It may be said that such a person has reason still left to guide him, as is evidenced by his ability to converse rationally on many subjects, and even to reason well against the very crime that he commits. All this may be true, and yet the person may not be accountable, for although reason is given to prevent us from doing evil, it cannot be expected to resist a diseased and excited impulse. . . . Numerous cases have fallen under our observation, where a great change in the moral character occurred and lasted a year or two, and then the intellect became affected. This change of character was noticed and lamented, but those thus affected were not considered insane until the intellect itself became involved; while in fact they were insane from the first. We wish all to be assured that a sudden and great change of character, of temper and disposition, . . . although the intellect is not disturbed, is an alarming symptom; it is often the precursor of intellectual derangement, and if not early attended to, is apt to terminate in incurable madness.[7]

Here, clearly, Brigham is talking about the progression from the schizophrenic prodrome (manifesting itself in negative symptoms or as schizoid personality) to the delusional stage of psychosis, i.e., what we observed, for instance, in the case of John Nash. Would the nineteenth-century superintendent's view still prevail a hundred years later, Nash's illness could be recognized much earlier than it was in fact and his fateful deterioration might have been prevented. Perhaps, he would not then get the Nobel Prize in Economics, but the tragic consequences of his disorder for himself and the people around him (his two sons named "John," and their unhappy mothers above all) might have been averted and the overall degree of suffering experienced and caused by him lessened drastically. Would such exchange be worthwhile for the society? Has the benefit of recognizing the brilliance of Nash's equilibrium justified the costs of little John Stier's pining in foster homes or Alicia's agony? Only those who bore these costs have the right to decide.

We entertain no similar doubts regarding Jared Loughner of the "Tucson Massacre" fame, or the two dead teenagers, responsible for the Columbine school shooting: we would recoil from thinking that these miserable youngsters, too, perhaps, had their fate turned differently, might receive Nobel Prizes in their sixties in one field or another. Whose fault it is that they will not? Dr. Brigham offers us something to ponder on in this regard, writing:

Most persons have seen individuals who are crazy, and consider themselves qualified to judge whether a person is deranged or not, yet on inquiry we find that nearly all expect irrational and incoherent talk from those that are deranged, or wild and unnatural looks, or raving and violent conduct. Their opinions respecting insanity are derived from having seen raving maniacs, and not from observation in Lunatic Asylums. . . . Owing to such limited and erroneous views respecting insanity, many persons are not disposed to believe in a kind of mental disorder that may impel men to commit crimes, unless such individuals exhibit derangement of the intellect, or conduct in a manner that they have been accustomed to see deranged persons conduct. But notwithstanding this common opinion regarding insanity, it is a well established truth, that there is a form of insanity, now called by many moral insanity, . . . which may impel men to commit great crimes, while the intellect is not deranged, but overwhelmed and silenced by the domination of a disordered impulse.[8]

"In some cases of insanity," he adds, "the faculties of the mind are so acute, that it is exceedingly difficult for a stranger to detect the mental aberration."[9]

This, then, was the starting point of American psychiatry. Insanity was the disease of the will (disordered impulse); it expressed itself in abnormal affect as well as intellectual derangement, which, in their turn affected the diseased person's actions, which he or she could not control. Affective insanity was far more common than intellectual insanity, and often went hand in hand not only with the ability to think and talk rationally and coherently, but with an intellect of exceptional acuity. It could not be confused with idiocy or dementia. It was a very common disease (Dr. Brigham presumed as a matter of course that "most persons" of his day encountered raving maniacs, i.e., individuals in the state of acute psychosis; this is understandable, because acute psychosis was, probably, the necessary condition for commitment, and so would occur outside of the hospital walls, but is nevertheless remarkable even today).

What were the views of our early psychiatrists based on? They did not acquire them at the lectures in medical schools, although such existed in the new country as early as 1765, and the majority of the superintendents of the asylums for the insane were medical school graduates. A major source of their understanding was English literature—above all Shakespeare, as we saw in an earlier chapter, but also the numerous descriptions of madness in the eighteenth- and early nineteenth-century poetry and fiction; these physicians, clearly, were broadly educated, well-read men. During the first decade of its existence, almost every issue of *AJI* carried detailed analyses of fictional or autobiographical accounts of insanity by English authors. American psychiatrists also followed closely the English and French specialized, psychiatric, literature. However, all this second-hand information was meticulously checked against the superintendents' clinical experience—their own observations in the asylums for the insane they superintended. Clinical case descriptions appeared in issue after issue, beginning, as was seen above, with the first one.

The author of the jarring poem that opens this chapter was one of the eight cases from the Public Asylum in Utica reviewed there. He was, we are told, a man of about fifty, "slightly deranged" for twenty years. His father was "hypochondriacal" and brother "insane." "He is a man of education, intelligence, and piety," wrote of him the attending physician,

> of kind and amiable feelings and manners, and converses rationally on most subjects; yet he is unable to walk, or to attend to any business requiring bodily exertion without much mental agitation and reflection, and not then without the most ludicrous movements. If he attempts to walk from one room to another, or out of doors, he hesitates a long time, appears much

agitated, his countenance exhibiting great terror and excitement, and then he seizes a chair, or whatever is near him, and rushes with the utmost speed. But he rarely moves without much urging, and would remain in his room all day, if not compelled to move—while at the same time, his inclination to leave his room would be strong. He can give no distinct account of the feelings, or reasons, that induce him thus to act—the most common explanation he gives, is, that if he did not act thus, he should commit some awful crime, that would subject him to the vengeance of the Almighty forever. [10]

Perhaps, the poem "Hypo" was written to provide such an account. The attendants recognized that "hypo" was what the patient suffered from. His specific diagnosis was "long-continued mental derangement, with singular peculiarities."

The doctor had somewhat more to say about inmates whose reason was gone together with rhyme. The loss of the former seemed to become more transparent in prose. Thus, he commented on another man in his fifties, whose current (third) "attack of insanity [was] caused apparently by too great and constant mental exertion and political excitement." He observed that, "He is usually very quiet, harmless, and sociable, imagines himself the Prince of Wales and Emperor of the world. . . . In this state he continued with but little variation nearly three years, busily engaged in reading, writing, and conversing, and mostly for the purpose of establishing or asserting and making known throughout the world his right to govern it. For this purpose he addressed numerous letters to the rulers of different countries." (One is immediately reminded of Matthews and John Nash, and also of Saul Bellow's *Herzog*.)[11] In this case, too, the *AJI* presents us with a specimen of the patient's writing:

Mahomet Ali, Governor of Egypt.

Dear Sir:

I was born in the city of Philadelphia, July 26, 1789. On the father's side I am descended from the Roman Emperor Constantine who built Constantinople in the fourth century. On the mother's side I am descended from Mary Stuart, daughter of James V., King of Scotland. It is my intention to dethrone the Sultan if I live long enough—none of the crowned heads in Europe have any right to reign, and will be one and all dethroned either by me or my successors. A son of Joseph Bonaparte, ex-King of Spain, who is my nephew, is the intended King of Italy. The Pope and all other divines will be taught to mind their appropriate business, the cure of souls. I can and will get along without them. I regret the destruction which was made among my subjects at Acre. We shall have a war with England which will end in the overthrow of the tyrannical House of Hanover. I can in one campaign take every inch of territory which that House possesses on this Continent. I have been confined myself for nearly two years and prevented from supporting you in your contest with the Allied Powers. The downfall of the Thiers ministry in France prevented the French from aiding you. Thiers is my friend, so is Mr. O'Connell, and so is every Republican in Europe, and some of the Nobility. I care very little for the Nobility. William the Conqueror was a bastard and never conquered the Britons. My ancestors sought an asylum in these western wilds, and have not yet been conquered. I have some of the native Indian blood in me of the Mohawk Tribe, and mean to teach our white oppressors that we owned this country before the discovery of Columbus. The race of men are bound to obey me as their lawful head. I intend to conquer my inheritance, and then see if I can't govern it better than it has been. I was placed under the protection of General Washington, and have married his grand-daughter. It is my intention to tread in the footsteps of that great man. His limits were the United States. My government embraces the world, and of course must be a military one. The world always has, after a fashion, been governed by the sword, but there has been too many commanders-in-chief. The world will be at peace only so fast as it obeys me.

I am, very respectfully, Yours, & c.,, Prince of Wales, and Emperor of the world.

P.S. The Emperor Napoleon was my uncle, having married a sister of my mother for his first wife.

This megalomaniac patient, we are told, "was always gentlemanly in his conduct, and in his conversation not relating to himself, interesting and instructive."[12] The personnel of the asylum tried by various means to distract his mind "from his particular delusions, but without effect" that was more than temporary. "At one time political and historical works were withheld from him, and he was furnished with works on natural history.

For awhile he talked less about his supreme command of men, but formed projects for improving the races of other animals, and was for sending agents and directions throughout the world for the purpose."

The delusion that one was the emperor of the world was, apparently, rather common in the young republic: among eight clinical cases reviewed in the first issue of the *AJI* there were two such claimants. The second patient was a younger man, aged thirty-three. He, the journal reports, had "a strong hereditary predisposition to insanity, his father and one or more brothers, being insane." The description of his case is illuminating in several respects in addition to the stress laid on the characteristic delusion of grandeur and pre-psychotic focus on status:

> He possessed a mind of much natural activity, with great love of distinction, and strong hopes of obtaining it, by literary and scientific pursuits. At the age of twenty-one, he commenced a systematic course of study, which he successfully pursued for two years; gaining much credit for his acquirements, and enjoying a high standing among his associates and friends, for his mental and moral worth. At this time, his health became somewhat impaired by sedentary habits, and too constant application to study. At the same period, also, he became somewhat involved in political excitements, which, operating on a system already highly predisposed, developed the phenomenon of insanity. His course of study being thus interrupted, has not since been resumed.
>
> Since the time of his first attack, which is now more than ten years, he has, at different periods, been nearly or quite well, and able to pursue some kind of business, but has relapsed again, when placed in circumstances calculated to excite his feelings. When he came to this institution, he had been in a state of high excitement for a number of months; wandering from place to place, attired in gaudy military trappings, claiming to be President of the United States, and Emperor of the world. While in this state of mind, he was capable of making speeches on various subjects, executing vocal and instrumental music with much effect.
>
> He had been much deceived and flattered by those with whom he had associated, in regard to his character and standing, which had doubtless contributed very much to strengthen and establish his delusions. For about two months, he continued to believe himself Emperor of the world, and to

value his own person in proportion. He passed much of his time in making speeches, and promenading the halls, as a General, with his associates as soldiers. He was at all times good humored and polite, if kindly and respectably treated; but excitable, and occasionally violent, if his statements were doubted, or his supposed prerogatives encroached upon. . . .

As his excitement passed off, he became much depressed in his feelings, lost his fluency of speech, and his facility for musical performance. From a character possessing great hope, decision, and conscious importance, he became timid, apprehensive, and gloomy; ready to do the bidding, or submit to the requirements of all who approached him. In this state of depression, he remained for a number of weeks. . . . [13]

While in two of the cases above the proximate, or "immediate exciting," cause for the psychotic episode that brought the patient to the asylum was of a political nature; in three other cases it was religious excitement. For example, the insanity of a twenty-year-old farmer, of industrious habits, and good character, "was believed to be the result of unusual interest, and attention to the subject of religion." As in other cases, the description included a patient's letter, characterized as "a fair specimen of his mental exercises after his high excitement [acute psychosis] had passed off, but while his mind was yet perplexed and confused":

Dear B——; It is now some time since I have heard from home, and it being near harvest time, all must be life and animation there. I enjoy good health, though not my usual degree of strength. When you receive this, I hope you and yours will be happy and well. As for myself, I ask nothing; I know the Great Redeemer lives. . . . God has declared that heaven and earth shall pass away, though not one jot or tittle of his word should pass away. Who is God, and how many Gods are there? For here are a number of persons who say, by God, and my God, not your God. What means this? How long will this be? "In the beginning was the word, and the word was with God, and the word was God." Then who is God now?

Now there are many going about saying, Lo, here is Christ. I say the Spirit of Christ should dwell in every heart, then we shall be sure to have him here, there, and everywhere; because he is a spirit which we cannot see. Time passes like a dream, for it seems but as yesterday that I parted with you. I hope you will write to me as soon as possible, and state the particulars concerning the people at home. I do not know when I shall be able to meet you there. It has been said that the time will come when we shall all be laid in the dust. What are we but dust? How are we laid? Do we not rise? How do the dead rise? Our spirits are continually rising, while our flesh is consuming. If all are to be laid in the dust, how will it be done, or who will do it? The angels of heaven will come and bury the dead bodies. We are all dead, what is it that keeps our frames together? If we are dust, we are going through the air continually; the wind carries the dust, but the rain falling lays it low.

What is the soul of man? Where can be anything to say? My soul! It must be the feeling of this heart, when the mind is absent from the body. I will praise my Maker while I have breath, and when that is lost, it is found with him in his heavenly kingdom.

Let me receive an answer from you as soon as possible; let me know how father's health is, and mother's also, and all the rest. Think if you please, that I am foolish and crazy, but do not think, as some tell me, that I am a devil, or have one, although I hope to see devilish spirit cast from every heart, before I am accused again of any such thing. Who thinks himself wise? God is an all-wise being who exists eternally in the heavens. If any would be wise, let him search the wisdom and glory of God. But that is past finding out— His wisdom is unsearchable. I have seen so much of the wickedness of man, that I have chosen death, that I might dwell with spirits in heaven. But there is no such thing as choosing, for life and death. At this my heart trembles. What is the world, or the foundation thereof? I think it cannot be anything more than rocks, mountains, air, and water; some of which move themselves, but God, who made the earth and all the things therein, is able to make a new heaven and a new earth. He wills not that any should be lost, but that all should be saved; therefore, we should all know the saving knowledge of the truth. We cannot all think and see alike, therefore, cannot all be alike. Some delight in tormenting, some in doing evil, some are liars, some go about busying themselves about they know not what, thinking themselves able to turn the world round, and keep it moving: so let it be.[14]

There are several remarkable features in these clinical descriptions. All the psychotic patients are seen by the clinician as highly intelligent people and, moreover, people with a very active intellect—they are neither demented nor idiots. (One of the eight cases is, in fact, a case of sudden and brief idiocy, apparently induced by a physical ailment; this condition is clearly distinguished from the psychotic disease.) The doctor constantly emphasizes that the psychotic episodes are brought about by too much thinking or study. The exciting factors are of an intellectual kind: politics and religion; at least four out of six (psychotic episodes) are obviously associated with ambition and preoccupation with status, which the clinician emphasizes. (In the case of one woman among the eight patients described, a psychotic thirty-one-year-old old maid, "much disposed to engage in religious exercises by exhorting, praying, &c.," this concern with status in addition to some mildly excessive self-complacency—"I am a wonderful child"—expresses itself in her self-pity for being homely and a decision to apply to a magistrate to change her title to "Mrs.,"—a wife of a reverend doctor.) In the case of a religiously excited young farmer, the confusion in his mind is intellectual itself: he is unable to come to grips with the contradictions between various claims of religion and between these claims and his own experience and rather realistic, natural-scientific, views. The only other causal factor in such intellectual psychosis suggested (but suggested consistently) is heredity, and it is important to remember that 1844 is long before the very existence of genetics is suspected. It would be interesting, indeed, to know, what did the American protopsychiatrists mean, when they spoke of "heredity." When mental disease is associated with an organic problem (in the case of brief idiocy and another one of psychosis connected to alcoholism), heredity is not mentioned. Alcoholic psychosis, which ends in the death of the patient, is clearly recognized as *delirium tremens*. The description reveals extraordinary sensitivity to the language and thought process of non-organic psychotic patients as a clue to their disease, as well as to its recurrent and bipolar nature, with episodes interrupted by periods of near-functionality. Delusion as a persistent false belief has not yet become the marker of insanity, and non-organic psychosis is not seen as two distinct diseases, one affecting emotions and the other intellect. Finally, the term "depression" is already used in its sense current today.[15]

In January 1849, the *AJI* published an account of "Mental Depression," furnished by the patient, E. B., then seventy-one-years-old. The account was mostly of the last and recent episode, of a seven-months duration (February–August, 1848), which occurred after E. B.'s "unfortunate precipitation down a long flight of stairs." But it was supplemented by samples of his cogitations dating to previous episodes. He "experienced but little local pain at the time [of his fall]," E. B. remembered,

> but . . . great distress of the mind, and confusion of the intellect; settling, as it soon did, into the deepest and most uncontrollable state of nervous depression and agitation, such as can hardly be at all conceived of, except by its unhappy subject. Having experienced some years since . . . much of these sort of infirmities, I felt at once to what my peculiar condition was evidently tending; the contemplation of which was as that of a deep and awful gulf yawning with its dark caverns before me, increased much undoubtedly by my fearful agitations and anticipations of what seemed to be before me. And I can truly say that from the first moment of my fall, "a change (a most fearful change) came o'er the spirit of life's dream." The aspect and contemplation of every object of nature and of art, and in the moral and intellectual world, experienced to my views and comprehension a most dark, fearful and disastrous change; not such, I suppose, as the poet tells us, sometimes "perplexes monarchs," but certainly most deeply perplexing to poor human nature, whoever may be its unhappy subject. One of the immediate and constant incidents of my condition was that—"tired nature's sweet restorer balmy sleep," became a stranger to my restless and gloomy couch . . . and between restless and uncontrollable agitation of body and mind at one time, and torpid indifference to everything around me at others, by day and by night, I, for those seven long months, lingered out those most dark and wearisome hours of what seemed to my beclouded reason, an objectless and purposeless life. Such was the utter derangement of my entire nervous system that it appeared as though every one of my natural senses was but the avenue and conductor of pain and distress to my exquisitely sensitive system, and every incident of my past or present life, but a theme for melancholy and forbidding reflection. . . . Or as is Byron's version of that dark scene—"It was not night, it was not day, / For all was blank, and bleak, and gray, / 'Twas but vacancy absorbing space, / And fixedness without a place."

Despite the wealth of literary allusions, reflecting E. B.'s general education, his description of an experience of what is clearly manic (i.e., bipolar)
depression is barely distinguishable from Kay Jamison's or others we have
encountered before. Just like our depressed contemporaries, this unhappy
American living in the first half of the nineteenth century recognized that
he was no longer in control of himself, that he had lost his mind, and that
what was happening to him was madness:

> perfectly conscious that both the natural and the spiritual world around me
> had suffered no change, and were the same as in other days, "when the
> candle of the Lord shone upon me," I could not by any exertion of my dis-
> torted reason make it so to me; . . . my mind moved in a world of its own
> creating, but no less real to me than once had been the actual existing one.
> These and other like considerations go to confirm me in the opinion which
> I have long entertained, that many of the wretched insane are fully con-
> scious of their own insanity, and yet are wholly unable to resist the feelings
> and impulses under the influence of which their thoughts and actions are
> dictated.

He enclosed "various sketchings" of his thoughts and emotions, including
"two or three printed articles, thrown into *measure* and *rhyme*" (he would
not call this "poetry," he said), written during this and previous episodes of
his illness:

> Oh! that it were in the power of any language which I can command,
> to give to my friends an adequate idea of that awful prostration of body
> and of mind which seem wholly to incapacitate me from making even an
> effort for breaking out of that dark prison of suffering despair, which con-
> fine me within its dreary walls,—under the influence of which I can look
> upon no earthly object, person or scene, however once dear and inviting to
> me, with the least complacency, or satisfaction,—while on the other hand
> every one of those persons and objects present themselves to me as a melan-
> choly contrast to the inviting forms in which I once delighted to view and
> enjoy them . . . existence is to me a dark and painful blank, from which I
> can relieve myself only by retiring from it within the gloomy recesses of my
> own solitary cell, there, if possible, to forget myself, or to commune only

with my own melancholy thoughts, and my own dark spirit . . . oh! that I may be enabled to submit to [all these misfortunes] with Christian resignation and composure, and not be left to the horrors of confirmed insanity or idiocy, on the very borders of which I seem to be a wandering and lost traveler!

My life is very desolate,
My heart is very sad;
Dark phantoms flit across my brain,
And visions wild and mad. . . .

At another time, he wrote a poem, entitled "My Mind's a Tablet of Unutterable Thoughts"; it ran:

Oh! could this bursting, bleeding heart,
Its bitterness disclose;
Its maddening tale of grief impart,
And speak its hidden woes.

But this dark dream of life to tell,
Nor tongue nor pen is found;
No charm can break the lucid spell
Which wraps the soul around.

From morning's early dawning light,
'Till evening's shades arise,
No welcome sun's glad cheering ray
Breaks on my wistful eyes.

And when night shadows, dark and drear,
Thick gather round my bed,
No guardian spirit hovers round
To sooth my fevered head.

God of my life!—thy light impart
To cheer my darksome way;
And on this sinking, sorrowing heart
Pour out celestial day.

And when at length in death's dark gloom
This throbbing pulse shall cease,
In mercy close the parting strife
And let the end be PEACE!

"It may seem a strange, if not impossible phenomenon," E. B. continued,

that one in the full exercise of consciousness, and whose actions and general conduct are as yet apparently under the control of his reason, should feel sensibly that his mind is approaching to a state of insanity, or a deprivation of the full exercise of his rational powers. But that this is the case at times, (how often I know not,) I am fully convinced of in my own unhappy present condition; knowing, as I do, that there has never been a moment since my fatal fall seven months since, when the world in all its relations, natural, social and moral, has presented itself to my senses and feelings in the same aspect that it had done before; either in the hours of sleep or of wakefulness. These aspects are either those of extreme agitation, anxiety and anguish of feeling, impelling both body and mind into a state of desperation of purpose, or of torpid despair and indifference to every worldly object . . . I have endeavored all in my power to escape from this fearful thralldom, and to brace and tranquilize my mind against its approaches, but alas, all in vain. It continues to advance upon me like an armed man in his strength, and will not let me go . . . And under that dreary and dark cloud it is that every thing in and about me ever admonishes me that my wandering and beclouded sun is, e'er long, to sit in the forlorn region of dread insanity, madness or idiocy.

"Almighty Father!" he begged,

stay that chastening hand,
Thus stretched in judgment o'er a writhing worm;
Rebuke those frowning storms—those clouds disperse,
And with the lamp of life, at truth's own altar lit,
That twilight path illumine! Ere it leads
The way-lost pilgrim down its gloomy shades,
Where light, and life, and joy can never break

The three-fold bars of madness' cloistered cell.

This did not differ much from "Edward Allwills"'s pleas of poor mad Lenz in late eighteenth-century Germany or from the free-form lamentations, considered literally prize worthy by serious literary critics, of our nearer contemporaries. Madness remained what it was from the beginning, easily recognizable to its victims and observers alike. That so many of the observers among us stopped recognizing it can be explained only by the fact that its victims have become so numerous that we consider their horrible condition normal.

E. B. had added a postscriptum to his case history. "It may be well," he wrote,

> as better elucidating the entire case, to state that I have twice before, although apparently from different exciting causes, been for a long time the victim and subject of similar bodily and mental distemperaments, with those which I have attempted very imperfectly to be sure, to portray, during the past year. In both of the former instances, I was inclined to attribute them to a too free course of living, connected with too little bodily exercise, great reverses of fortune in my wordly affairs, and consequent intense anxiety of mind growing out of this state of things. These came on somewhat gradually, and ceased as gradually; that of the present year came on at once, and simultaneously almost with my bodily precipitation, and vanished almost as rapidly.

The editors of *AJI* thought his case "an encouraging one, for all those who have long suffered from extreme mental depression and despair, accompanied by bodily infirmities; for although his last attack was of but short continuance [seven months was "short continuance" for an extreme depression in their opinion], the previous ones were of several years duration." In their "Note" to E. B.'s account they also wrote: "It may not be improper to add, that the distinguished gentleman has ever been remarkable, when in health, for activity of body and mind, and having heretofore been much engaged in public life, and among the leading members of Congress during the war of 1812, and always fond of reading, his mind is well stored with information which he is ever ready to impart for the gratification and improvement of others. His health and spirits are now very good; long may they thus continue."[16]

The subject of the *American Journal of Insanity* was mental disease but its focus madness properly defined. Indeed, madness was a very old problem in the new nation. It was transplanted into America with the first English settlers, for whom it was a familiar experience—a part of reality—in the mother country. Americans recognized it before they recognized themselves as Americans. This early acquaintance did not deepen their understanding of the phenomenon (it did not do so in England either), but their knowledge of it was empirical, rather than derived from theories, and, for this reason, their attitude to madmen was one of profound sympathy born of the consciousness that the mad were one's afflicted brethren, people just like oneself, only hit by a terrible misfortune, that "there, but for the grace of God, go I." The psychiatric views of the Pilgrim Fathers, especially those of clerical calling among them, were different from those of the nineteenth-century physicians and not unexpectedly reflected the confusion that reigned on the subject in seventeenth- century England. Dr. Brigham, who evidently considered the study of his predecessors' views relevant, wrote:

> In former times, insanity was attributed to the agency of the devil, and the insane were supposed to be *possessed* by demons. Something of this opinion is still prevalent, and it appears to have been embraced by our Pilgrim Fathers. Cotton Mather, in his life of William Thompson, thus remarks: "*Satan,* who had been after an extraordinary manner irritated by the evangelic labors of this holy man, obtained the liberty to *sift* him; and hence, after this worthy man had served the Lord Jesus Christ, in the church of our New English *Braintree,* he fell into that *Balneum diaboli,* a black *melancholy,* which for divers years almost wholly disabled him for the exercise of his ministry."

And yet, even in the judgment of Cotton Mather we find sympathy for those thus victimized, the acceptance that madness was the possibility constantly facing righteous, godly men, and—remarkably—the recognition that it was visited on the chosen people of this American, New England with especial frequency. One bore no responsibility for one's insanity. Satan himself, thought the worthy divine, was but an instrument in God's hands and used bodily weakness, not sin, to insinuate himself into the soul and wreak havoc there. Mather wrote:

> There is no experienced minister of the gospel, who hath not in the cases of *tempted souls,* often had this experience, that the ill cases of their distempered *bodies* are the frequent occasion and original of their *temptations.* There are many men, who in the very constitution of their *bodies,* do afford a *bed,* wherein busy and bloody *devils,* have a sort of lodging provided for them. The *mass of blood* in them, is disordered with some fiery *acid,* and their *brains* or *bowels* have some juices or ferments, or vapors about them, which are most unhappy engines for *devils* to work upon their souls withal. The vitiated humors, in many persons, yield to *steams,* whereunto *Satan* does insinuate himself, till he has gained a sort of *possession* in them, or at least, an opportunity to shoot into the mind, as many *fiery darts,* as may cause a sad life unto them; yea, 'tis well if *self-murder* be not the sad end, into which these hurried people are thus precipitated. *New England,* a country where *splenetic* maladies are prevailing and pernicious perhaps above any other, hath afforded numberless instances of even *pious people,* who have contracted those *melancholy indispositions,* which have unhinged them from all service or comfort; yea, not a few persons have been hurried thereby to lay *violent hands* upon themselves at the last. These are among the *unsearchable judgments* of God![17]

Schizophrenia and manic-depressive illness have been a problem in this country long before they were so named. It is not widely known, but the United States was one of the very first societies to institute arrangements for the care of the "insane," of which a few existed before the Revolution. In the pre-independence period there was no significant pauper population in the new society, the sick were cared for at home, and the first general hospital was founded only in 1751. The main purpose of this Philadelphia establishment, which, unlike early hospitals in Europe, was, from the outset, a medical institution in which inmates were attended by physicians, was to treat indigent patients. But its declaration of intent, penned by Benjamin Franklin, also made provisions for taking in other than charity cases, if place was available. For several decades the Pennsylvania Hospital was the only hospital in the colonies, and already in 1752 it was taking in mentally ill—specifically "insane," according to the *AJI*—patients. ("Pennsylvania Hospital for the Insane" the *AJI* referred to it, commenting: "This is a branch of the Pennsylvania Hospital—the oldest institution in the country in which regular provision was made for the treatment of insanity." In 1781, Dr. Benjamin Rush, declared by tradition to be America's first psychiatrist, joined the medical staff of the hospital.) In 1773, the Eastern Lunatic Asylum was established in Williamsburg, Virginia.[18] Such institutions proliferated in the first decades of the nineteenth century. Pennsylvania Hospital proving insufficient for the accommodation of the Quaker state's afflicted, the "Asylum for the Relief of Persons Deprived of the Use of their Reason," or the "Friends Asylum," was established near Philadelphia in 1817. Massachusetts acted on the need to provide a refuge for the native mad a year later, opening the McLean Asylum for the Insane in Somerville in 1818.[19] Within fifteen years one asylum in a suburb of Boston proved not enough: thus, the State Lunatic Asylum was established in Worcester in 1833, and Boston Lunatic Asylum followed in 1839. Several asylums were added in the 1820s: in 1822 a state institution in Columbia, South Carolina; in 1824 another state institution in Lexington, Kentucky, and Connecticut Retreat for the Insane at Hartford; and in 1828 Western Lunatic Asylum in Staunton, Virginia. Madness was apparently blind to the Mason-Dixon Line. Remarkably, New York did not feel the pressure until 1830, when the first of its asylums, Hudson Private Lunatic Asylum, was founded. It caught up with the leading states quickly, however: there followed the establishment of the City of New York Private Lunatic Asylum and the New York City Lunatic Asylum on Blackwell Island in 1839, New York State Lunatic Asylum in Utica in 1843, and Bloomingdale Asylum—the Lunatic Department of the New York City Hospital. The list of "Lunatic Asylums in the United States," published in the first issue of *AJI* in July 1844, included twenty-four institutions, which existed in fifteen states: Connecticut, Georgia, Kentucky, Maine, Maryland, Massachusetts, New Hampshire, New York, North Carolina, Ohio, Pennsylvania, South Carolina, Tennessee, Vermont, and Virginia. Several other states and territories, it was reported, were about to open establishments for the insane. The number of inmates in the institutions already in existence, by July 1844, was 2,561.[20] The estimated number of "insane and idiotic" in the nation as a whole, for the population of 17,069,453, was 17,457, producing the ratio of 1 to 977.[21] "Insanity" (the polite American term for "madness") was a much narrower category than "mental disease" today, sharply separated from congenital idiocy, and applying to mental disorders with a relatively late onset (not before adolescence) and chiefly of uncertain organic basis. Throughout the nineteenth century it included psychoses associated with pregnancy and childbirth (so-called "puerperal insanity"); paresis, or general paralysis of the brain, whose connection to syphilis was but poorly understood; and even epilepsy. But the vast majority of the patients in the various asylums and hospitals were "manic" and "melancholic," which not always distinguished and rather inconsistent diagnostic groupings answered to the description of today's schizophrenia and/or manic-depressive illness.

The early institutionalization of the psychiatric profession (*avant le nom*) in the United States—the establishment of the Association of Medical Superintendents of American Institutions for the Insane, which was to become the American Psychiatric Association, and of its official organ, the *American Journal of Insanity*, in 1844—was also indicative of the precocious familiarity of the young American society with the problem of madness. In their pioneering efforts the thirteen founding fathers of the national psychiatry had no organizational example to follow. If similar professionalizing efforts were made simultaneously in Britain and France, this was unbeknownst to the American superintendents: the decision to form the association and to found the journal was reached before the news of the French *Annales* arrived, and it is certain that the Americans believed they led the world in an attempt to confront insanity in this characteristic, "grassroots," concerted way. As demonstrated by the appearance in 1812 of the first internationally acclaimed original American contribution to its understanding, *Medical Inquiries and Observations upon the Diseases of the Mind* by Benjamin Rush, the premier general physician in the country, the interest of American physicians in the disease dated to a much earlier date.[22] This interest—itself a reflection of the frequency with which insanity was encountered in this country—prompted a growing number of general physicians to specialize in it, making psychiatry the very first American medical specialization (just as it was in Britain and France). The "original thirteen" of the Association—Drs. Luther V. Bell, Amariah Brigham, John S. Butler, Nehemiah Cutter, Pliny Earle, John Minson Gait, William McClay, Thomas Story Kirkbride, Isaac Ray, Charles

Harrison Stedman, Francis T. Stribling, Samuel White, and Samuel Bayard Woodward—were among the first specialists, but the fast growing list of the organization's members attests that there were dozens more. In October 1847, the first "Professorship of Insanity" was announced. The *AJI* celebrated the event: "We are gratified to learn that a Professorship of Insanity has been established at one Medical School," the journal stated. "The Willoughby University, Columbus, Ohio, has appointed Samuel M. Smith, M.D., Professor of Medical Jurisprudence and Insanity. We think there should be a distinct course of Lectures on Mental Maladies, at every Medical School."[23] Thus the United States, a very young nation, was one of the very first nations to have a psychiatric "establishment."

Given the early presence of madness in the United States, the focus of our inquiry, the main question addressed in this chapter to test the central historical argument of the book, must be different from the focus of the chapter dealing with the spread of madness in Europe. While the question regarding Europe was "when had madness reached particular European countries?" the one in respect to the United States is "has there been an increase in the rates of insanity?" In both instances we are testing the same argument, namely, that madness (insanity, the psychotic disease of unknown organic origins that came to be diagnosed as schizophrenia and manic-depressive illness) is a product of the inherently and pervasively anomic nature of nationalism, the form of consciousness (i.e., culture) implied in the secular, egalitarian, and based upon popular sovereignty image of reality, which forms the cultural foundation of modern existential experience. Thus, this mental disease emerged in England—the birthplace of nationalism and the first society redefined as a nation, and spread to other societies only when they were redefined as nations as well, when nationalism became the form of consciousness of a considerable minority, if not the majority, of the population, and anomie reached this (part of the) population. In the cases examined (Ireland, France, Germany, and Russia), as I hope the reader has seen, all the available evidence supports these propositions. Having established that, indeed, madness reached various European societies with the penetration of nationalism into certain masses of population, our inquiry into the history of schizophrenia and manic-depressive illness in them could end. But this is not so with regard to this country which was born with national consciousness (though not defined at first as a separate nation) and madness already present. The fact that madness exists in, and has existed since the inception, of the United States, supports, but adds nothing to the already existing support of, the argument. However, the American experience would add significantly to this support, if the rates of this disease have increased in proportion to the growing freedom and prosperity, in general, and, in particular, to the exposure of new large groups in the population (women, descendants of slaves, second-generation immigrants, social strata previously satisfied with basic education, whose children are now expected to go to college, etc.) to the choices in self-definition implied in nationalism, and the increase in the number of such choices (for example, multiculturalism and redefinition of "alternative lifestyles" as biological predispositions and their legitimization, which made non-orthodox sexual orientations a matter of choice; or, more recently, the possibility of changing one's sex, which, combined with the reinterpretation of this biological marker in terms of socially constructed gender ("gender reassignment"), made sexual identity a matter of choice as well, and a rather varied choice at that). Thus, we must ask: has insanity (schizophrenia and manic-depressive illness) been on the increase throughout the history of the United States?

So Has It Been on the Increase?

All the available evidence suggests that it has. An unprejudiced discussion of this evidence seems timely today. According to the latest and most authoritative statistics, the rates of schizophrenia and manic-depressive illness have approached proportions that without much exaggeration may be characterized as catastrophic. The lifetime prevalence of major depression alone—and only among Americans between the ages of eighteen and fifty-four—is estimated by the 2002–2003 Replication of the National Comorbidity Survey (NCS-R) of the National Institute of Mental Health at over 16 percent, which translates into about 35 million people. Schizophrenia, estimated at 1.7 percent, adds to this impressive number another 4 million, and, presumably, at least as many are added by bipolar disorder (which is not always specifically distinguished and often estimated for life prevalence at as high as 5 percent).[24]

Ronald Kessler, the head of the NCS team and a recipient of many awards for his work on the statistics of mental disease, noted in 2006: "Mental disorders are really the most important chronic conditions of youth in America," and, in 2007, insisted again that "mental illness is the chronic disorder of young people in our nation."[25] But NCS-R leaves out a large part of this most vulnerable group—teenagers under 18. How many millions of American manic-depressives and schizophrenics would one find by the end of the first decade of our brand new century if thirteen- to seventeen-year-olds were included in the national survey? Not to exaggerate, let us say that between one in ten (according to NIMH statistics, obviously an underestimate) and one in five Americans are likely to become severely mentally ill in their lifetime, which means, because these diseases are chronic and often have an early onset, to suffer from them for most of their lives.[26] Between one in ten and one in five Americans (one in ten to one in five senators and congressmen, corporate executives and employees, college professors, lawyers, physicians and psychiatrists, scientists, school teachers, soldiers and military officers, etc.) are likely to become and be, as another age—less inclined to euphemisms but more sensitive to human suffering—would put it, *mad*. The statistics may be, as is often claimed, confusing and unreliable.[27] But these *are* the most relied upon statistics, they are the findings of the world's best statisticians, and we have none better. If they are to be believed, schizophrenia and manic-depressive illness not only constitute the greatest public health problem faced by this society but pose a real danger to its very survival, if only for the reason that even one gravely mentally disturbed person in ten policymakers or generals would make its existence precarious by definition.

Whatever is the attitude one adopts towards the NCS-R estimates, they are consistent with the relevant economic data. Already in the early 1990s schizophrenia and manic-depressive illness constituted "the single largest disease category for federal payments under the Supplemental Security Income (SSI) and Social Security Disability Insurance (SSDI) programs"— that is to say that they cost the United States taxpayers, in living assistance to disabled persons, more than the two top natural killers, heart disease and cancer. When costs of hospitalization are taken into account, in 1991 alone, writes E. Fuller Torrey, "it was estimated that [schizophrenia and manic-depressive illness] together . . . cost the United States $110 billion" in direct and indirect costs.[28] Translated into 2012 dollars, this makes $185.6

billion—quite a sum even compared to the $787 billion of the American Recovery and Reinvestment Act (of 2008), especially given that this was a one-year expenditure for one disease category and not a five-year budget for the saving of the entire U.S. economy. The latest study of the costs of schizophrenia, in 2002, found that this relatively rare disease alone cost the United States eighty billion in 2012 dollars.[29] Schizophrenia and manic-depressive illness thus constitute a major, in fact an enormous, burden on the American economy, and this burden is growing heavier. Were this a purely economic problem, we could not be overly concerned about solving it. But, obviously, the economic costs are but its minor aspect.

What do all these numbers really mean? According to the Director of NIMH, Tom Insel, about 90 percent of suicides in the United States are caused by mental disease.[30] This includes anorexia and substance abuse-related disorders (often co-morbid with manic-depressive illness and schizophrenia), but manic-depressive illness and schizophrenia on their own contribute the largest number. Already for several years in the new century suicide represents the eleventh leading cause of death in the country. Deaths by suicide are increasing by about 0.7 percent a year (among some groups, in particular white women between the ages of forty and fifty, they have increased by a much larger percentage in the last decade). In 2007, 32,000 Americans ended their lives by their own hand. This number was far above the number of deaths from AIDS (20,000), considered an epidemic and often compared to the plague that devastated medieval populations, and only three forms of cancer, those of colon, breast, and lung, have mortality rates surpassing the annual rate of suicide. About 20 percent of people with major depression (manic or not) and perhaps 13 percent of schizophrenics commit suicide, but, of course, only a tiny proportion of these do so in any given year. Given the prevalence of these diseases in our society, we are facing a somber prospect. Currently, suicide is the second leading cause of death among twenty-five- to thirty-four-year-olds and the third leading cause of death among fifteen- to twenty-four-year-olds.[31]

To a certain extent, suicide is hereditary (whatever is the nature of this very complex concept): the risk of taking one's own life increases dramatically among people who have had suicide in their household before. This means, among other things, that suicide due to mental disease in one year is likely in the years that follow to contribute more suicides to the 10 per-cent percent of this grim statistic that are attributed to other causes. Death by suicide is unlike any other death and its effects on survivors in the circle of one's family and friends tend to last longer and be more profound than those of death due to old age, heart disease or stroke, and even the more frightening, because more mysterious and indiscriminate as to age, death from cancer, or AIDS. It is not only that suicide is quite common among young people for whom it is uncommon to die at all; more important is that it is chosen, unnatural, and preventable. Of course, the death of any loved person is very difficult, in the beginning impossible, to come to grips with in our modern secular society, which offers no argument against its finality. But, at the very least, the surviving child, sibling, spouse, parent, and friend has, as a rule, little to reproach oneself for—it is not in one's power to prevent death from natural causes or, in the vast majority of cases, even accident. And then there is the consolation that the life that ended was, nevertheless, worth living, that the dear departed had enjoyed it, per-haps had been happy. There is no such consolation in the case of suicide. And the survivor always doubts: was it my fault? What have I done wrong? What should have I done differently to prevent it? The life of a child whose parent had committed suicide would be forever under a dark cloud of such doubts. A survivor of the death by one's hand of a sibling, a spouse, or a close friend would never live again completely at peace with oneself. And the life of a parent whose child took his or her own life can only be imag-ined as hell on earth—year after year after year. Taking the circle of sur-vivors of a suicide to be just three people on average, this means that 32,000 suicides leave about 100,000 Americans grieving forever, unsure that life is worth living and unable to live full lives. In ten years there are a million such Americans. These people are not depressed in the clinical sense, not mentally ill—just deeply and irreparably unhappy. And suicide, insofar as the effects of mental disease are concerned, is just the tip of the iceberg.

"The greatest cost of manic-depressive illness," write the authors of a 2005 manual on this particular disease, "is the personal toll it takes on affected individuals and their families. It is . . . incalculable."[32] The same, obviously, can be said of schizophrenia. It may be argued that any serious disease affects a family's life. Cancer disrupts the family routine for long months, interferes with settled plans, hangs a cloud over every interaction;

diabetes requires a routine of its own, rules out certain foods and activities, etc. There is fear and worry and regret. But the effect of manic-depression and schizophrenia are more profound and all-encompassing. These diseases estrange family members from each other, changing the very nature of the family relationship, corroding the connections that make it a family, suffocating affection and destroying trust. They leave members who are healthy helpless and hopeless, exhausted by constant and necessary watchfulness, guilty of letting their minds wander to other concerns, of having interests and desires which the sick no longer share, deeply, sickeningly unhappy. If, again, like with suicide, we take the immediate circle of a person with either of these diseases to consist just of three people, for one in ten to one in five such people there would be three in ten to three in five family members and friends affected by their illness—30 to 60 percent of the American population, 100 million to 200 million people not mentally ill themselves, but nevertheless suffering because of manic-depressive illness and schizophrenia. Which of these two estimates is closer to the actual number at this point becomes already immaterial. Even the low figure of 100 million (*sic!*) is unimaginable; it is impossible to believe that it can be true. But two plus two makes four, do what you will. This is a colossal social problem, quite possibly the greatest social problem faced by American society today, and one can well get emotional about it, though this would be out of place here and won't help us resolve it.

Instead of dwelling on today's disputed statistics, I'll endeavor to show my reader how things stood in the good old days. When insanity was already a problem serious enough in the United States to inspire the formation of the association of asylum superintendents, the first issue of *The American Journal of Insanity* assessed, it affected the U.S. population at the rate of 1 in 977 persons, lagging behind Britain (where Scotland led with 1 in 648, followed by Ireland at 1 in 774, and England at 1 in 807) though already slightly ahead of France (1 in 1000), and far ahead of other nations included in the comparison (such as Spain, which trailed far behind its eastern neighbor with the pathetically miniscule 1 in 7180). The *London Medical Gazette* from which the *AJI* statistics were copied also reported numbers (ratios of insane and idiotic to the population) for several cities, which, unfortunately, did not include any American ones. They were 1 in 200 in London, 1 in 222 in Paris, 1 in 361 in Brunswick, 1 in 3142 in St. Petersburg,

1 in 3400 in Madrid, and 1 in 23,572 in Cairo. Thus in London the ratio was four times that of England in general and even in Madrid it was about double the one that characterized the obviously backward (in so far as madness was concerned) Spain. Civilization, clearly, was taking its toll.[33] Throughout the nineteenth century, the *AJI* (similarly to its counterparts in other countries) stressed how rare insanity was in the "uncivilized"—or what we today would call "developing" part of the world.

The third issue of *AJI* carried a letter from a reader, E. K. Hunt, MD, of Hartford, CT, with some statistics on suicide. It was based on "the careful examination of one newspaper, the *New York Mercury*, or *Weekly Journal of Commerce*, for a period of twelve months." Dr. Hunt "noticed, First; the number of persons committing this act. Second; the age of each person, at the time of committing it. Third; the time when it was committed. Fourth; residence. Fifth; the remote cause. Sixth; the proximate or immediate cause. Seventh; the civil condition of each." Altogether, the *New York Mercury* reported 184 suicides, thirty committed by women, 154 by men. The ages ranged between sixteen (of whom there were three) and eighty-one, but were not always given. The month in which the suicide happened was reported in 172 cases; the largest number of these (two) occurred in July, the smallest (eight) in March. This, Dr. Hunt observed, confirmed the pattern already described in France on the basis of "a very extended and minute investigation of this subject." In the State of New York there were forty-four suicides, in Pennsylvania twenty-five, in Massachusetts twenty, and in Louisiana thirteen, the rest of the country contributing in single digits (from nine in Maine to one each in Indiana, Rhode Island, Tennessee, Alabama, Delaware, Long Island, and Florida.) For 101 suicides no cause was stated, but for the remaining eighty-three cases, the causes assigned were: "mental derangement" in twenty-nine cases; "habitual intemperance" in nine; "depression of mind" in eight; domestic trouble and "intoxication and the temporary use of intoxicating drinks" in four cases each; *Millerism* (which will be discussed later) and "dissipation" in three cases each; "weariness of life," jealousy, and remorse in two cases each; the following being the causes of one case each: dyspepsia, ill-health, seduction, infidelity of wife, murder of neighbor, *delirium tremens,* apprehended insanity, fever, dread of death, want of enjoyment, poverty, violent passion, love, disappointed love, unlawful love, desertion of lover (which makes five cases of love-related suicide), gambling, and being a homeless orphan.

The favorite method of doing away with oneself, according to Dr. Hunt's statistics was hanging: of the total of 142 men and twenty-nine women of whom this detail was reported, fifty-four men and ten women used the rope. Guns were widely available, but only twenty-six suicides, all men, availed themselves of them. Advanced technology, clearly, was not the decisive factor. The majority followed the long tradition of cutting one's throat or arteries, drowning, and taking poison, one man actually stabbing himself with a poisoned stiletto. There were fourteen immigrants in the group: "8 Germans, 2 Irishmen, and one from each of the following countries: England, France, Austria, Spain, and Poland," making for 7.6 percent of the total number. Finally, out of the ninety-three cases of known civil condition, fifty-nine were married, thirty-two single, and two widowed. Dr. Hunt concluded:

> I am far from claiming that an accurate estimate can be made from the data before us, as to the number of suicides committed throughout the country, or in any particular portion of it. We certainly have no right to infer that because one weekly newspaper has furnished a record of 184 suicides, that every other contains an equal number. Indeed the inference is legitimate that a weekly published in the largest city of the country, and containing—as does that from which my list of cases was taken—all the reading matter, excepting advertisements, of the daily for the previous six days, will contain a much larger number than those of a similar character, but published elsewhere. Moreover, were it the fact that the above furnished an average of the number of suicides committed, as found in the weekly newspapers throughout the country, it would still be impossible to make up a correct estimate until we had ascertained the number copied from one into the other. Notwithstanding this, however, the list before us is large enough to satisfy all, that the annual number of those who commit suicide is fearfully large.[34]

Admittedly primitive, though with sophisticated reasoning behind them (which is, generally, better than the other way round), Dr. Hunt's statistics were supplemented, in a response immediately following, by a compilation from the tireless pen of Dr. Brigham. Brigham began by saying that Dr. Hunt's list of 184 suicides is, beyond all doubt, an underestimation of the actual number of suicides committed that year in the United States. As evidence, he said, he would "adduce the fact that as many have been committed in the city of New York alone, as are assigned to the whole State in the foregoing account." He relied in this on the Reports of the City Inspectors for the preceding thirty-eight years (1805–1843), and quoted the annual numbers, which I summarize here by decade. The decade averages of suicides committed annually in the city of New York were: 1805–1814: twelve; 1815–1824: seventeen; 1825–1834: 24.5; 1835–1843: 34.5 (in 1837, 1838, and 1839, the years of economic trouble, however the numbers were forty-two, forty-three, and forty-five, respectively). The population of the city grew rapidly during these years, being 75,770 in 1805; 100,619 in 1815; 166,086 in 1825; 270,089 in 1835; and 312,852 in 1840. The rate of suicides, therefore, basically reflecting the rate of population growth, and even lagging behind it somewhat. Brigham then compared these statistics to the reported numbers from France for the four years 1836, 1837, 1838, 1839 (they grew steadily from 2,310 to 2,717, the population of France being 33,500,000—about twice as large as that of the United States—in 1840); from England and Wales (where it was estimated that, with the population of 15,900,000 in 1840, 1,000 persons annually were "ascertained to commit suicide, and nearly as many [were] returned as drowned"), and from "chief capitals of Europe" for whatever years statistics were available. This latter comparison is particularly illuminating. For example, the ratio of suicides to the total population increased in Berlin from 1 to 4,500 between 1788 and 1797 to 1 to 2,300 between 1799 and 1808 to 1 to 750 between 1813 and 1822; in Paris in 1836 it was 1 to 2,700, in St. Petersburg in 1831, 1 to 21,000, in Naples in 1826, 1 to 173,000.

From all these comparisons, Dr. Brigham concluded: "That suicides are alarmingly frequent in this country, is evident to all," adding: "as a means of prevention, we respectfully suggest the propriety of not publishing the details of such occurrences. 'No fact,' says a late writer, 'is better established in science, than that suicide is often committed from imitation. A single paragraph may suggest suicide to twenty persons. Some particulars of the act, or expressions, seize the imagination, and the disposition to repeat it, in a moment of morbid excitement, proves irresistible.' In the justness of these remarks we concur, and commend them to the consideration of the conductors of the periodical press."[35] This determined the policy of *AJI* regarding the distressing subject in the years to come: well-established facts in science, as we know, are not to be argued with. Suicide statistics, however, continued to appear. In January 1848, Dr. C. H. Nichols, Assistant physician to the Utica Asylum, compiled the numbers of suicides in the State of New York between December 1846 and December 1847. Based on "about fifty principal newspapers published in different sections of the State," Nichols found a total of 106 cases of suicide, forty-two more than in 1846 and thirty-two more than 1845 (which means that in 1846 there were ten cases less than in 1845). In New York City, suicide was "more than four times as frequent" as in the State as a whole. Since similar results were obtained in France, it was possible to conclude that

> in *great cities* when compared with the country, all the human passions are exercised with more than fourfold constancy and intensity, and that reverses of fortune and disappointments of desire, are more frequent by fourfold, and are accompanied by a shock of the intellect or affections, more than four times as severe, and by more than four times the liability to that temporary or continued overthrow of reason, which induces self-destruction;— reflections which should go far to teach country-man longing for the town, contentment, and should warn the dwellers in cities, of the vast importance of the most rigid discipline both of body and mind.

In thirty-eight cases, it was unknown what drove the unfortunate to the fatal action. For the rest, among the "assigned causes, given mainly in the words of respective authorities," the commonest was "insanity," which carried away the lives of thirty-one individuals (though only twenty-four of them men and six women). It was followed by a distant second, responsible for six deaths (three for each of the sexes)—"melancholy." Other causes listed included "pecuniary embarrassment" and "disappointment in love," with two victims each (but there were also "destitution," responsible for two suicides, and "loss of property," responsible for one, which, one assumes, complemented the former of these causal categories, and "seduction and desertion," driving to suicide two women, and "receiving a disagreeable valentine," deciding the fate of another one, which likely added to the latter.) A plurality of suicides occurred among people under the age of thirty. These data, aided by some preexisting knowledge, led Dr. Nichols to conclude thus:

> Recollecting, moreover, that a disposition to suicide is common among the insane who never commit the act; that unwarned suicide has occurred in one and insanity in another member of the same family hereditarily predisposed to mental derangement, and that it is most frequent at the time of life when the conservative instincts are strongest, we are led to the belief to which our feelings strongly incline us, that the awful deed of self-murder is rarely committed in well-regulated Christian communities by persons of sane mind,—that *suicide is generally one of the accidents of insanity.*[36]

In 1848, the number of suicides in the New York State dropped. This was reported by another Assistant Physician to N. Y. S. Lunatic Asylum at Utica, Dr. George Cook, who examined the relevant sources for the period of December 1847–December 1848, and published his statistics in April 1849. There were a total of only ninety-one cases. Dr. Cook commented:

> the number of reported suicides, in proportion to the population, has considerably diminished since last year; . . . the reduction, according to our account, has taken place chiefly in the city of New York. . . . It is an interesting fact, that suicides in New York have been gradually diminishing for several years, while in many other large cities they have increased in frequency. A comparison of recent with former reports would seem to exhibit this fact very clearly. Thus, for the five years from January, 1805, to January, 1810, there was an average annual proportion of one case in five thousand three hundred and thirteen and a fraction of the inhabitants; for five years, from January, 1835, to January, 1840, there was a yearly average of one suicide to every seven thousand six hundred and twenty-eight; and last year, there has been one to about every twelve thousand six hundred and ninety-seven of the population. From this, it appears that they have diminished in frequency more than one-half since 1810, though the relative number is still considerably greater than in the country.

It appeared that, at least in New York, in the late 1840s, like in the Soviet Union under Stalin in the late 1930s, according to the well-known statement oft-repeated by children in schools and kindergartens, "life [was becoming] better, full of jollity." The approximate numbers per 100,000 of New York population thus were twenty suicides between 1805 and 1810; thirteen suicides between 1835 and 1840; and eight suicides in 1848. These numbers were "still considerably greater than" in the State of New York and, presumably, in the United States as a whole. (According to Dr. Hunt's statistics of several years earlier—which Dr. Brigham, we will remember, considered an underestimate of the actual number—in the country as a whole there were somewhat more than ten suicides per 100,000. But Dr. Hunt did not pretend his statistics to be accurate.) Similarly glad tidings, strongly suggesting that the numbers of suicides proportionally to population were steadily declining, were reported for the United States, as the readers of the *New York Times* are undoubtedly aware, for the decades between 1920 and today.[37] Nevertheless, in 2007, 32,000 Americans took their own lives, which still renders the ratio of about 10 per 100,000. Did the rate of suicide decline? Increase? Remain stable? Who knows. One thing Dr. Cook was certain about, namely, "that insanity is the most frequent cause of suicide."[38] This implied that, if the rates of insanity increased, rates of suicide were likely to increase also.

The Ever-Unreliable Statistics

Insofar as statistics of insanity were concerned, nothing was certain: these statistics were disputed from the very first. In the United States, the trend was set by Dr. Edward Jarvis of Dorchester, MA, who discovered a glaring error—a blunder, actually—in the 1840 census. According to the census, as was mentioned, the ratio of "insane and idiotic" to the population in all of the United States was 1 to 977, but it differed from state to state, with New England states leading and leaving the rest of the country far behind. The leading state in 1840 was Rhode Island, where the ratio was 1 to 503; it was closely followed by New Hampshire (1 to 563), Connecticut (1 to 572), and Massachusetts (1 to 580), which was the most populous state among the leaders and thus contained the largest number of such mentally

ill. On the other extreme, there was the Iowa Territory with the ratio of 1
to 3,919, and the states of Louisiana (1 to 3,524) and Michigan (1 to 3,265).
So far, so good. The "insane and idiotic," however, were divided into
"whites" and "colored," and herein lay the trouble. In numerous instances,
the census reported numbers of "colored pauper lunatics" (i.e., patients
supported at public charge) in Northern towns that had "*no colored inhabitants*"; and in Worcester, Massachusetts, it apparently placed all 133 of the
white pauper lunatics in its Hospital "under the head for the colored." In
January 1844, Dr. Jarvis published an article, "Insanity Among the Colored
Population of the Free States," reprinted in a number of medical journals,
with a detailed discussion of this misleading reporting. This is what he
wrote about the incident in his *Autobiography*, which in 1873 he dictated to
his wife.

> He wrote an article for the *Philadelphia Medical Journal* on the gross errors
> of the census of 1840, in misrepresenting the number and proportion of the
> insane among the free colored population. For this purpose he examined
> the census of each town in the whole country and compared the number of
> the free colored living with the members stated to be insane. In the tables
> of population there were columns for ages, sexes, insane, idiots, blind, &c.
> The columns of the white insane were next to those of the colored insane.
> These columns were long and many towns on a page, and it required a very
> accurate eye and careful discipline to select the proper column for a fact,
> and to follow it down from the heading. But, for want of this care, the fig-
> ures representing the white lunatics of many towns were placed in the
> column of the colored. Consequently towns which had no colored popula-
> tion on one page, were represented on the other as having colored lunatics;
> and in many others the number of colored lunatics was more than that of
> the colored living; others were stated to have a large part of their colored
> people insane. The result of these statements made every fourteenth colored
> person in Maine insane, every twenty-seventh in Michigan, and every
> forty-fourth in Massachusetts; and through all the northern states, every
> one hundred and forty-fifth.
>
> He was deeply interested in this discovery for the enormous proportion
> of insanity among the free negroes had staggered him from the moment he
> saw the report. It had astonished and grieved most people, certainly in the

North, but it had delighted the slaveholders, for herein they found a strong argument for the support of the system. Mr. Calhoun said, "Here is the proof of the necessity of slavery. The African is incapable of self care, and sinks into lunacy under the burden of freedom. It is a mercy to him to give this guardianship and protection from mental death."

... In 1845, it was brought up before a meeting of the Statistical Association. It was voted to ask Congress to amend the census in this respect. Mr. William Brigham, Mr. John W. Thornton and Dr. Jarvis were directed to prepare a memorial which Dr. J. wrote, pointing out these inconsistencies and many others in reference to education, manufacture, trade, &c.

Mr. John Quincy Adams took the charge of the matter in the House of Representatives, and Mr.__ of Connecticut in the Senate. The memorial was printed by Congress, and also by the *Merchants' Magazine* of New York. It was referred to a committee who, Mr. Adams said, made no report; and Dr. J. thought that they never met.

Mr. Bencan of Georgia told Dr. Jarvis that the census was in an error in this respect, "but," he added, "it is too good a thing for our politicians to give up, and many of them have prepared speeches based on this, which they cannot afford to lose." ... the error went abroad, and was published and believed by some in Europe. Dr. Boudin in his admirable work, *Traité de Geographie et de Statistique Médicales,* says that cold is destructive to the mental health of the African, as shown in the United States where only one in 2,117 is insane in Georgia the warmest state, and one in fourteen in Maine, the coldest.

[In 1860, visiting Paris, Jarvis pointed out the mistake to Boudin.] Dr. B. was very thankful; he said it was not in accordance with all his notions in anthropology, yet as he found the fact stated in so reliable a document as the census of the United States, he could not deny it, but admitted it into his book.[39]

French scholars of our day, it seems, remain faithful to the admirable tradition, long since abandoned by their American counterparts, of blaming the theory, rather than the facts, in cases of disagreement between the two. Given that this tradition was common to the scholars of both countries in the nineteenth century, one is inclined to forgive Boudin for taking the statements of the U.S. census on their face value. Dr. Jarvis, however, had numerous other facts to juxtapose to these statements. His discovery of the glaring mistakes in the census regarding the insanity among the free colored population in the United States, tied as this was to the most sensitive issue of the time, slavery—and the obnoxious glee these mistakes inspired among the gentlemen of the South—colored the attitude of the liberal northern public towards insanity statistics in general and generated the tendency to regard them as unreliable, unless proven otherwise. Ironically, this very public, as we saw in a previous chapter, has remained convinced, despite all the evidence to the contrary, that schizophrenia and manic-depressive illness affect African Americans at a greater rate than the general population, disagreeing with slave-owners of the 1840s only in respect to the causes of their special vulnerability: while Mr. Calhoun believed freedom to be the culprit, today's epidemiologists predominantly blame poverty.

In July 1849, Dr. Isaac Ray, the Superintendent of the Butler Hospital for the Insane in Providence, RI, published a critique of the statistics of "Insane Hospitals." This paper deserves an extended discussion for several reasons—among them its reflection of the contemporary view of madness: its distinguishing characteristics, types, and causes, but also the perfect applicability of Dr. Ray's criticisms to today's epidemiology despite the almost completely changed view of this disease (as well as to social science, more broadly). Very few persons, Dr. Ray postulated, were satisfied with the statistics published by managers of the asylums, for, in general, "thus far, statistics, with all its show of accuracy, has been, comparatively speaking, singularly barren of results." "It would be difficult," he wrote, "to mention any great principle of physical and moral science, as having been established chiefly by statistical inquiries. A volume would not hold the instances in which they have failed of success, though undertaken with every promise thereof, but I will mention only one, of recent origin, and well known to us all." The instance Dr. Ray had chosen was, unsurprisingly, the census of 1840, which, he insisted, "with all its pretension . . . can be received as reliable authority for no single fact whatever." The most egregious proof of that was in the census's reporting on insanity among the free colored population in the United States. "On the faith of the Census of 1840, it was proclaimed to the world with no ordinary emphasis, that the free colored population is more liable to insanity than the white, and the fact thus inferred was exultingly held up by one of our most distinguished statesmen, as a signal blessing of slavery. The Census has gone to every great library in Europe, but without the exposure of its errors, and in many a future work, no doubt, will be found the record of this stupendous lie."

Statistics, in fact, were only as reliable as the thinking of people who produced them, and this thinking, to be reliable, needed to focus on numerous so to speak "pre-statistical issues" before ever it turned to quantitative methods. It was the inattention to these "pre-statistical issues"—of proper definition and categorization—that defeated the purpose of the statistics issued by superintendents of asylums for the insane. For example, in regard to the question of the curability of insanity, it was a universal practice among asylums to report the number of their recoveries, but what constitutes a recovery was never agreed upon or even consistently discussed. Dr. Ray argued:

Statistics can be properly applied only to incidents and events that have an objective existence, for such only are cognizable to all men and admit of neither doubt nor mistake. Just so far as they have a subjective relation to the mind—are merely matters of opinion—to that degree they are incapable of being statistically expressed. Thus the event of recovery, limited solely to its objective character, only amounts to a certain degree of improvement. Whether the change is a real cure of disease, or a state where diseased manifestations are absent merely from want of a suitable opportunity for displaying them, or a temporary intermission of disease governed by that law of periodicity to which nervous affections are closely subjected,—these are questions which every individual will answer by the aid of his own experience and judgment, and consequently with all the diversity which is utterly incompatible with statistical accuracy. I presume I am uttering no scandal when I say, that the cases are not few which one man would pronounce to be *recoveries*, while another of less sanguine temper, or more knowledge of insanity, would regard them as merely *improvements*. . . .

It is obvious therefore that the question must first be answered, what degree of restoration can be rightfully called *recovery*. . . . It is one of the laws of nervous disease, that it may be suspended or checked for a period indefinitely varying in length, and then, after intervals measured by weeks, or months, or years, renewed in all its original severity. The intervals may or may not recur with the utmost regularity. They may continue for many months, or appear to be merely a transition-state marking the passage of the mind from one paroxysm to another. The restoration may be apparently perfect, or marked by many a trace of disease. . . . it is clear that some conventional rule is necessary for determining among the various intermediate forms and degrees of restoration, what should be reported as recoveries. Now admitting that such a rule might be made, for I would not prescribe limits to human ingenuity and acuteness, there is a more serious difficulty remaining, that of recognizing the condition or event to which the rule is to be applied. . . . For instance, we might agree to call a lucid interval which continues six months or upward, a recovery, but upon the main point, whether a lucid interval has really occurred, how are we to prevent conflicting opinions?

It was a common practice, pointed Dr. Ray, to divide cases of insanity in asylums into old and recent, based on the belief that curability was the function of the duration of the disease before admission. But often it was impossible to decide "whether the disease has or has not commenced within the period allotted to recent cases." After all, he argued, "the earliest aberrations of the disordered mind differ so little from its ordinary movements, that they are readily confounded by the careless or unskillful observer," and madness was, admittedly, a recurrent, chronic condition. He wrote:

The large class of periodical and paroxysmal cases presents insuperable difficulties to every attempt to bring them under any general rule. The question of their origin is complicated with that of their recovery, and we are under the same kind of embarrassment in deciding upon the former, that we experience with regard to the latter. If we are to regard every fresh attack that has been preceded by a distinctly marked lucid interval of considerable duration, as a recent case, can we adopt any rule that will prevent us from bringing within the same category those cases in which the interval is scarcely more than a brief remission of the disease? A single instance will be sufficient to illustrate the difficulty. A person is subject to paroxysms of high excitement when he is destitute of all self-control, and for the sake of decency and safety, must be kept in close confinement. In this condition he is placed in a hospital where the excitement passes off, and he is discharged. He returns home, engages in his customary pursuits, and for all practical purposes certainly, appears as sound as ever. In the course of a few weeks or months, the excitement returns. . . . [Is] every discharge a recovery? . . . During the alleged interval, is the mind really clear and unclouded by disease, or are its obscurations less dark only because the absence of excitement leads the patient to withdraw himself from the common notice, and refrain from obtruding his fancies upon others?

Similar objections could be raised, Dr. Ray argued, against the division of cases into curable and incurable, a question which also could not be decided by statistics, because statistics were only as good as the definitions on which they were based. These definitions being in dispute, he could not see "how any candid mind can help drawing from [the existing statistics] the conclusion, that the curability of insanity is as far from being settled as that of many other diseases that have been scarcely subjected to statistical inquiries." Confusion and inconsistency reigned in everything pertaining to insanity, in fact, making meaningful statistics altogether impossible (as, it must be reiterated, they do today). For instance, some patients died while hospitalized, and it was the prevailing practice in American asylums to state the causes of death when it occurred. "I am aware that in our hospital reports," wrote Dr. Ray,

we always find some deaths attributed to "*disease of the brain,*" some to "*inflammation of the brain,*" and others to "*acute cerebral disease,*" by all which terms it is probably meant, that the patients sunk under the violence of the maniacal attack. Then, why not say so? As these terms are often used to designate affections unaccompanied by insanity, I see no propriety in applying them to a form of disease which is characterized by mental derangement, especially as the term *acute mania* and its congeners have long been sanctioned by nosologists, and convey an exact, well understood idea. If there were any pretension to consistency in the matter, it might be asked why, in the same table, some deaths are attributed to *general paralysis* which is a specific form of mental disease, and not to *disease of the brain,* &c., which may be as properly applied to it as to mania.

These tables indicate great confusion of ideas, evidently arising from the want of well settled, well understood views of pathology.

Then as now causes of insanity excited much speculation, becoming a central subject of hospital statistics. And Dr. Ray's judgment, in this context, is indeed as applicable now as then. "It would not be the first time," he wrote (nor, unfortunately, the last),

> if the very importance of the subject has raised a determination to arrive at results of some kind, but not a corresponding anxiety for their soundness. It would not be the first time, if an imposing array of names and phrases, were mistaken by their authors for substantial contribution to knowledge, nor would it be strange if others were led to participate in the pleasing delusion. I fear that the careful inquirer will seldom rise from the examination of these tables, with the conviction that they have thrown much light on the origin of insanity. Perhaps no point within the range of our professional studies, demands a clearer insight into the laws both of psychology and pathology, than the successful elucidation of the causes that lead the mind astray from the line of healthy action. Here if anywhere, it will appear, whether our studies have led us to a higher philosophy than that which consists in repeating catch-words . . .

As regards the hospital statistics of causes of insanity, the chief defect was "their total want of precision and uniformity in the use of language which are now justly deemed essential in any scientific inquiry really worthy of the name." "The most remarkable step ever made in the pursuit of natural science," Ray insisted (and we may insist with him today, for the point has not really sunk into the collective consciousness), "one which marks the transition from idle and anile speculation on the one hand, to sure and valuable acquisitions on the other was the adoption of a language the terms of which are so precise and well-defined as to convey the same idea to every mind, in every time, and every land." Logical formulation of hypotheses was not possible without precise and consistent definitions of terms; logically faulty hypotheses could not be tested against evidence; and the lack of the possibility to test hypotheses inevitably led to the perpetuation of errors and misunderstanding.

The examples Dr. Ray adduced in support of his argument, nevertheless, were revealing not only of the logical problems, which precluded any
advancement of the psychiatric knowledge, but also of the experiences,
and circumstances that appeared to his contemporaries as particularly conducive to the loss of mind—and this has a separate claim to our attention.
The following contains the list of causes of insanity American psychiatrists
emphasized, with Ray's accompanying commentary:

> In one and the same table, are cases charged to "domestic trouble," "bad
> conduct of children," "jealousy," "infidelity of wife," "ill-treatment of par-
> ents" and "abuse of husband." Surely, it would not be easy to find stronger
> manifestations of "domestic trouble," than are indicated by all these events,
> and we are therefore obliged to conclude that the term "domestic trouble"
> which appears to have given rise to so much insanity, is used in a sense very
> different from the ordinary, but one to which we possess no clew [*sic*]. In
> another table a number of cases are charged to the account of "disappoint-
> ment," but whether they were disappointed in love, or politics; in the
> struggle for honor or wealth, does not appear. Another gentleman is more
> precise, and subdivides the general affection into "disappointed love," and
> "disappointed ambition." Another uses all three terms, and cases are referred
> by him respectively to "disappointment," "disappointed affection," and
> "disappointed ambition;" and another extends the list of disappointments
> by adding "disappointed expectation." What idea are we to attach also, to
> such vague phrases, as "mental excitement," "anxiety," "exposure," "fright,"
> and a host of others too numerous to mention?

The centrality of love and ambition in this list is too obvious to stress.

Finally, Dr. Ray addressed the issue of the classification of the different
forms of insanity. Unlike today, there was not much agreement on how
many, or what, these forms were, though we, of course, always find among
them the usual suspects: mania (mono- or plain), melancholia, and
dementia (to which in a few years would be added the adjective *praecox*).
"No one, I apprehend," claimed Ray, "can be sure that by monomania,
melancholia, moral insanity, and many other terms that are used to designate different forms of mental derangement, he understands precisely what
his neighbor does . . . these terms have never been clearly defined." But

this was not the main problem. It was the fact, like today, "that in a large proportion of cases, the form of the disease changes in the course of its progress [, that] the same case, at different periods, may present the aspects of melancholia, monomania, and dementia" that was, in his words, "fatal to such attempts at classification." Insanity was one disease—often emotionally bipolar, which could disorder thought and emotions in equal measure, mostly emotions, or most obviously thought—and statistics which purported to establish which of these transient forms was more prevalent, curable, or deadly were, by definition, unreliable.[40]

An example of the well-intentioned and punctilious, but not sufficiently thought-through, work to which Dr. Ray was reacting was provided by the statistical analysis of the records of the Bloomingdale Asylum by Dr. Pliny Earle, who was the physician there, which was published in the *AJI* in January 1848 under the title "On the Causes of Insanity." Dr. Earle had analyzed the records of his hospital from June 16, 1821, to December 31, 1844. "In many of the cases of Insanity," Dr. Earle began, "it is extremely difficult to fix upon any particular influence which we are satisfied was the origin of the disorder. Sometimes two causes are found, and it is impossible to tell which is the predisposing and which is the exciting." He nevertheless decided "to enter upon the subject of hereditary predisposition before proceeding to other causes," so privileging this supposed but entirely unexplored factor, of which nothing was known in his time, because he believed that "that constitutional condition of the system, transmitted from one generation to another, a condition, which although recondite in its nature, facilitates to a greater or lesser extent the invasion of mental derangement, . . . is invariably a remote or predisposing cause. According to our belief, wherever this natural condition exists, the person will retain the healthy action of his mind until he is subject to some other influence, more immediate, more active, more potent, and the tendency of which is to derange the physical functions of the system, so as to impair the manifestation of the mental powers." Of the 1,841 patients whose records were available for the twenty-three-year period reviewed, 323 (or 17.5 percent) had at least one relative insane. Dr. Earle himself was dubious of these statistics. "It is not to be presumed, however," he wrote, "that this is even a near approximation to the number actually having relatives of disordered mental powers. During the first years of the existence of the Asylum, there appears to have been but little attention paid to this particular subject, and hence the records thereupon are imperfect." His conclusion was measured:

> Insanity being a disordered manifestation of the mind, dependent upon some disease of the body, either functional or organic, is subject to the same laws as many or most other maladies to which the human race is subject. Like consumption, gout, diseases of the liver and of the heart, it may attack any person whatever, but is certainly somewhat more likely to prevail among those whose ancestors have suffered from it. . . . It is obvious that the foregoing statistics are not sufficiently full or definite to be adopted as accurate data from which to estimate the proportion of the insane in whom an inherent predisposition exists, the comparative number in whom it is transmitted from the father's or the mother's side, or any of the other important questions involved in the subject. In some persons, although none of their family either in a direct line or an immediately collateral branch may have ever suffered from mental disease, there is a natural idiosyncrasy or peculiarity of constitution which facilitates the invasion of insanity. This peculiarity probably exists in the intimate structure of the nervous system, although Dr. Rush appears to have thought it to be in the blood. In which system of organs soever it may be, it is probably very similar in its nature to that which constitutes the hereditary predisposition, and in this way the latter springs up in families among whose members it has never before appeared."

Like today, whether the evidence supported the presupposition of hereditary predisposition (or vulnerability, as we prefer to call it) or did not, it was presupposed all the same; the statistics, after all, were unreliable, and one was free to interpret them whichever way one was inclined.

From this conclusion regarding the importance of hereditary predisposition, Dr. Earle proceeded to enumerate and comment upon the supposed (apparently exciting) causes of insanity. These were divided "according to the general method, into physical causes or those which act immediately upon the body, and mental causes or those whose influence is primarily exerted upon the mind." There were 1,186 patients for whom relevant data were available. For 664 of them, the cause of insanity was believed to be physical. Women's reproductive problems led the way with 142 cases (including ninety-four cases of puerperal insanity, associated with pregnancy leading to labor and its immediate aftermath; five cases of abortion, 30 cases of irregular menstruation, 10 of menopause, 14 of unspecified uterine disorder, and 2 of hysteria). This was followed by intemperance (i.e., alcoholism) in 117 cases (ninety-seven of these men, alcoholism being the male equivalent of child-bearing—a fearful joy, indeed); undefined "ill health" and masturbation (the former responsible for the derangement of twenty men and seventeen women, the latter affecting men exclusively) with thirty-seven cases each; cerebral disease with thirty-four (thirty men and four women; a separate category of "cerebral congestion" added to these one man and one woman). Injury from falls (twenty-eight men and three women) and assorted fevers (twenty men and eleven women) accounted for the insanity of thirty-one patients each; dyspepsia was responsible in twenty-six cases (sixteen men and ten women); and epilepsy for twenty-three (nineteen men and four women). A multitude of physical causes explained the remainder: tuberculosis accounted for the loss of mind of eight patients, for example; sedentary life for that of three; drinking cold water and "kick on stomach from horse" for the derangement of one each.

The list of "moral" (earlier in the article referred to as "mental") causes, responsible for the mental disease of 522 Bloomingdale Asylum patients, 310 males and 212 females, deserves to be reproduced in full (see table). If the rest of the records Dr. Ray considered in his critique were of the same nature, he certainly had a good reason to be annoyed.

Dr. Earle commented on his compilation: "Almost all the older authors upon insanity entertained the opinion, that mental causes were more prolific of insanity than physical. Within a few years however, the opposite opinion has been gaining ground,—an opinion which is sustained by these statistics." Substance abuse, Dr. Earle thought, was clearly the major cause of madness. Not only did intemperance occupy "the highest rank in point of numbers, among the physical causes" (though not if we united the many categories related to female reproductive cycle into one), but an additional thirteen cases (five men and eight women) resulted from the use of narcotics—"too abundant indulgence in opium, snuff and tobacco." Anticipating the recent anti-smoking focus among sociologists of mental health by more than a century and a half, he considered tobacco as particularly pernicious and argued:

> The action of these narcotic substances upon the nervous system is very similar to that of alcoholic liquors, and a recent French writer not only maintains that this action is precisely the same, but asserts that he has proved it to be so. If, therefore, one of the necessary effects of alcohol is to establish in the system a condition which will prevent the healthy action of the mind,—and we are but too well aware that this is the fact,—it follows that the narcotics in question would produce an identical effect, and cause insanity. . . . In reference to tobacco . . . several modern authors . . . concur in the belief that, when excessively used, it may be the principal cause of mental derangement, and cases thus produced have been reported at a

"Moral" causes of the mental disease of Bloomingdale Asylum patients, according to Dr. Earle

	Males	Females	Total
Pecuniary difficulties	118	15	133
Want of employment	11		11
Religious excitement, &c.	51	42	93
Remorse	5	6	11
Death of relatives	16	27	43
Disappointed affection	12	26	38
Home-sickness	2	1	3
Application to study	30		30
Mental excitement	6		6
Fright, fear	4	15	19
Mental shock	2		2
Domestic trouble	22	43	65
Anxiety	12	10	22
Mortified pride	8	6	14
Disappointed ambition	3	1	4
Disappointment	1	2	3
Faulty education	4	4	8
Ungoverned passions	1	3	4
Avarice	1		1
Jealousy	1	4	5
Seduction		3	3
Novel reading		3	3
Dealing in lottery tickets		1	1

Pliny Earle, "On the Causes of Insanity," *American Journal of Insanity* 4 (January 1848): 195–196.

number of institutions. The immediate action of this substance upon the
nervous system, in persons of a highly excitable temperament, is so powerful, that when smoking, they feel a peculiar sensation of thrill even to the
remotest extremities of the limbs. A constant stimulus of this kind upon a
nervous temperament can hardly be otherwise than deleterious. Tobacco,
particularly when used by smoking, tends to disturb the function of the
liver; and disordered action of this organ is not an unfrequent cause of
mental disease. . . . tobacco is likely to produce dyspepsia, a disease which,
more than almost any other, by acting sympathetically upon the brain,
affects the manifestations of the mind. Who has not experienced or observed
this deleterious influence, producing depression of spirits, dejection, taci-
turnity, and inability to contend with the cares of life; gloom, despondency,
and perhaps a disposition to self-destruction, or actual insanity in the form
of melancholia?

Masturbation was another practice to be avoided. Attention to it could
be counted among the advances of the young psychiatric science. For a
long time, Dr. Earle remarked, it "has been known as one of the many
agents tending to destroy the balance of the mind, but it is not until within
a few years that its influence was supposed to be so great as it is at present
by most physicians to institutions for the insane." Dr. Earle, however, did
not follow the prevailing opinion blindly. "Although [masturbation] is
acknowledged to be a very prolific cause, yet there is danger of misappre-
hension upon this point," he cautioned. "The habit is, undoubtedly, in
many cases, the *effect* of the disease."

The comments on "moral," or "mental," causes also deserve quoting.
Wrote the doctor:

Connected as this Asylum is with a city almost purely commercial—a city,
the majority of whose active adults are subject to the cares, the perplexities,
and the fluctuation of trade, it is not remarkable that among moral causes,
pecuniary difficulties should occupy the most prominent position. . . . There
is, perhaps, no mental influence which, if examined in all its bearings and
relations, exercises so extensive and controlling a power upon men in civilized countries, and more particularly in the United States, as that arising
from his pecuniary condition. Connected with this are many if not all his

hopes, and schemes of ambition, preferment and aggrandizement—all his prospects of present and future temporal comfort, and all his affections that are enlisted in the welfare of the persons constituting his domestic circle.

A constant business, moderate in extent and sufficiently lucrative to afford a liberal subsistence, can never, in a mind well regulated, operate as an exciting cause of mental disorder. The sources of the evil are, on the one hand, the ambitious views and the endeavors rapidly to accumulate wealth, and, on the other, the extremes of excessive business, of bankruptcy and of poverty, the fluctuations and the unwholesome disposition to specula-tion. . . . The moral cause which ranks next in point of numbers among both the men, and women, is the anxiety and other mental influences in reference to religion. . . . In a country of universal toleration upon religious subjects, and sheltering under this broad banner congregations of almost every sect that has ever appeared in Christendom, it is to be supposed that the religious sentiment would act under its greatest possible variety of phases, and in every diversity of gradation between the extremes of apathy and fanaticism. The accurate observer of the events of the last twenty years, to say nothing of a period more remote, cannot fail to perceive that this is actually the fact. Under these circumstances, and when we consider the whole scope and bearing of this sentiment, and the eternal interests which are its subject, we can not but perceive how important an influence it may exert.

It was America, and not religion as such, which made religion a cause of mental illness. "It is difficult to believe that 'pure religion and undefiled' should overthrow the powers of the mind to which it was intended to yield the composure of a humble hope and the stability of a confiding faith," wrote Dr. Earle. But the idea of universal toleration (however limited the toleration was in fact), apparently, was antithetical to pure and undefiled religion, for it was difficult to decide which of the equally legitimate vari-eties of it was the one; one's faith was no longer confiding, and, clearly, the hopes one entertained were anything but humble. Thus the doctor believed that "a great majority of the cases of insanity attributed to religious influ-ence, can be traced to the ardor of a zeal untempered with prudence, or a fanaticism as unlike the true religion which it professes, as a grotesque mask is to the face which it conceals." In other words, one had to be already quite insane to make religion contribute to one's insanity. He singled out

Millerism as the example: "The exciting doctrines of Miller, the self-styled prophet of the immediate destruction of the world, gained but little hold of the public mind in this vicinity, but in those sections of the country where they obtained the most extensive credence, the institutions for the insane became peopled with large numbers, the faculties of whose minds have been overthrown thereby."

Of love as a mental cause Dr. Earle had to say just that: "Forty cases, twelve males and twenty-six females, are recorded as having originated from disappointed affection . . . ," leaving the subject in mid-sentence, perhaps as too perplexing for a lengthier consideration and, definitely, disturbing enough to interfere with one's arithmetic. Like his sixteenth-century predecessors in England, the superintendent of the Bloomingdale Asylum, however, stressed the dangers of over-much study, offering this advice:

> In students, whether young or of middle age, if a proper equilibrium be maintained between the physical powers and the intellectual faculties, the development and energies of other portions of the body being so promoted and sustained by exercise, that they may preserve their due relations with an enlarging brain, there need be no fear that mental alienation will result from application to study, but unless this precaution be taken, the midnight oil consumed by the student as a beacon light to guide him towards the temple of fame, may become an *ignis fatuus* leading the mind into the labyrinth of insanity. Even in persons of strong constitution, and of great physical strength, severe and prolonged study exhausts the nervous energy and impairs the functions of the brain. How much greater must be these effects in a frame naturally delicate, and how much more alarming still if the body be debilitated by the want of exercise![41]

It is worth noting that, in Dr. Earle's view, the student consumed the midnight oil not in a disinterested search of enlightenment for its own sake, but to reach the temple of fame, study being, in less highfaluting prose, an instrument of social ambition. But many of his contemporaries prescribed "forgetful dullness" as an antidote to the "pain of thinking" and considered study, even if pursued as an end in itself, mentally dangerous. Under the heading of "Miscellany," the *AJI* for July 1847 published the following excerpt:

Particular professions and modes of living exercise a considerable influence in the development of insanity. Deep study and intense application, with the want of rest both of mind and body, which ardent pursuits bring on, are as prone to derange the mind as the fervor of the enthusiastic imagination. Calculating speculations are as influential on the mind as versatility in ardent and passionate pursuits. While we recognize these predisposing causes, we must also take into account the habits of many enthusiasts, too frequently irregular, and which add materially to their morbid sensibility; and genius is too apt to let the passions flow a headlong course. In the ratio of the social qualities and agreeable converse of men of talent, are they exposed to the temptation of fascinating enjoyment. In deep, sordid speculation, or in ardent scientific disquisitions, disappointments are bitterly felt, and the mind not unfrequently becomes blunted by exclusive pursuits which admit of no repose. In both these conditions, although most opposite, the physical functions become disturbed. In the one case, the circulation of the blood is hurried, and the vital fluid is unequally distributed, occasioning fever, congestion, and excitement. In the plodding man of business, careworn by anticipations rarely realized, the digestive functions are disturbed, and their energies destroyed, the epigastric region becomes the seat of tumultuous action, with all its fearful train of sympathies, and under their baneful influence insanity ensues.[42]

Abstinence was the recipe for preventing insanity among many other ailments: to avoid mental disease one was to abstain from using the mind. One has the feeling on occasion that in some of the "particular professions" mentioned above this medical advice was taken very seriously. But, according to the statistics, rates of insanity continued to rise nevertheless.

The discovery of the blunder regarding the numbers of "colored insane" in the 1840 census by Dr. Jarvis planted a seed of doubt in the reliability of statistics of insanity in general in the mind of the public interested in such matters, and this seed bore a splendiferous fruit: these statistics, pursued ever more frequently and diligently, and with ever greater expenditures of money and effort, would never and in no respect be considered reliable. Among the people in the know—psychiatrists and psychiatric epidemiologists—this skepticism most often expressed itself in the belief that the statistics *under*estimated the actual number of the insane, even though in certain sectors there were factors that encouraged overestimation. Thus Amariah Brigham wrote in his comment on the 1840 census in the first issue of the *American Journal of Insanity:*

> We presume these estimates of the number of the insane and idiotic in the United States are considerably below the actual number, though we believe them as accurate as the statistics of other countries on this subject. It will ever be difficult to ascertain the precise number of insane and idiotic. While many monomaniacs and those but little deranged will not be enumerated because not considered actually insane,—the insanity of others will be concealed by their friends. On the other hand some who are not deranged, but whose mental faculties have become impaired by old age or by defect of vision or hearing, and some who are merely eccentric, hypochondriacal, and intemperate, will be included. The number of the insane reported by Committees of Inquiry who are anxious to establish Lunatic Asylums, is, we apprehend, often too large;—certainly much larger than requires removal to a Lunatic Asylum. Many thus included, if deranged at all, are but partially so, and are living quietly and pleasantly with their friends, and capable of supporting themselves by their labor, and would in no respect be improved by being removed."[43]

Their experience suggested to the experts that they should take the reported figures with a grain of salt. But this grain of salt flavored the attitude of non-experts undiluted in the stock of experience, and, with respect to the question of the possible increase of insanity in the nation, paradoxically, the statistics—which consistently reported increasing rates[44]—were accused of exaggerating the extent of the problem.

Nobody was better aware of the shortcomings of existing statistics than Edward Jarvis. In 1851 he weighed in on the debate, delivering a speech before the Association of Medical Superintendents of American Institutions for the Insane during the annual meeting held in May of that year in Philadelphia. He began by recouping the expert position: in both Britain and France the opinion prevailed that "'Insanity has increased in prevalence of late years, to an alarming extent, and that the number of lunatics, when compared with the population, is continually on the increase.' A very similar apprehension exists in America, and the known facts and the public records seem to confirm it. There are certainly more lunatics in public and private establishments; they attract more of popular sympathy; they receive more of the care and protection of the government; more and more hospitals are built; and the numbers of the insane seem to increase in a still more rapid ratio." This conclusion, however, Dr. Jarvis asserted, was not statistically demonstrable at the moment. The existing statistics were plainly insufficient to be the basis for a judgment, pro or contra, on this question. The premier statistician explained:

> it is impossible to demonstrate, whether lunacy is increasing, stationary, or diminishing, in proportion to the advancement of the population, for want of definite and reliable facts, to show, how many lunatics there are now, and still less to show, how many there have been at any previous period. Wanting these two facts, we cannot mathematically compare the numbers of the insane or their proportions to the whole people at any two distinct periods of time, and thus determine, whether lunacy increases or retrogrades. It is but a recent thing, that any *nation* has enumerated its insane. And I cannot discover, that any nation has ascertained and reported this twice, and thus offered us data for comparison.

The existing statistics would support the claim that insanity was on the increase, were it kept in mind that the disease was of recent historical origin, unknown before the sixteenth century in England and much later elsewhere, because the current numbers they reported were consistent with this. But in 1850 nobody in the United States remembered (if anyone ever knew) that this was so. It was already assumed that, at some level, this devastating illness has always existed. At most, it was recognized that the interest in insanity was of recent origin. Several governments, argued Jarvis, had ordered an investigation into the numbers of the mentally ill within their borders, but none, he claimed, "have done it thoroughly and completely. Most have been contented with estimates, or with such general enquiries as were answered entirely or in part by estimates and conjectures. They have not gone from house to house, making diligent and minute enquiry in every family, to know, whether there were any insane, and how many of these there might be, and what were their form and degree of disease." Of course, the government of the United States had done that, in the census of 1840, and again that of 1850. But then it was common knowledge (though never repeated often enough) that the census of 1840 was not to be trusted: "There was such a manifest carelessness and inaccuracy in some of the officers or clerks, who had the management of, or who performed the work of that enumeration and its presentation to the public, as to throw doubt over the statements of the whole of that document." And the results of the census of 1850 had not yet been published.

Jarvis examined the insanity statistics in Belgium, France, and Great Britain, and found them all wanting, chiefly because, like in the United States (apart from the census), they were based on the numbers of inmates in the asylums. He commented on these calculations, summarizing them while doing so:

> The number of patients in the hospitals must bear some relation to the numbers of the insane in the countries to which they respectively belong: that is, they cannot have inmates unless there are insane among the people, and the inmates cannot exceed the whole number of the lunatics in the country or district unless they come from abroad. But there are so many other elements to be taken into the calculation, that as yet the hospital population is no indication of the prevalence of mental disease in any community. It is rather an indication of the degree of civilization, and of general intelligence, especially in respect to mental disorder, of public generosity, and of popular interest, in behalf of the afflicted. Thus we find, that whenever the seeds of this interest are once sown, and allowed to germinate, and grow, it spreads continually thereafter. Whenever the attention of the people of any country is called to this subject, and a hospital is built, there follows a remarkable increase of the cases of insanity revealed to the public eye, and seeking for admission.

These, as we have seen, remain popular arguments in defense of the claims that (a) the rates of schizophrenia and manic depression do not increase in the West, and (b) that these diseases are spread uniformly, at a "normal rate" in all human societies. As today, in Dr. Jarvis's time, they did not hold water, either logically or empirically. Logically, they depended on the faulty definition of civilization: on what grounds, it could be asked, could China or India (in which insanity was not observed) be considered as less civilized than the much younger societies of the Western "Old" and New worlds? And, empirically, the observations outside of the core Western societies (core in the sense of their commitment to the Western values of individual liberty and equality), as we saw in the cases of Germany and Russia, did not support the assertion that calling the attention of the public to mental illness and even building hospitals in itself increased the numbers of patients. Before the insane population actually appeared (which might happen several generations after the attention of the public was attracted to the phenomenon and in 1851 had not yet happened in Russia, for instance), the hospitals stood half-empty or were filled with idiots and alcoholics.

The American data Dr. Jarvis presented following these disclaimers were, nevertheless, impressive. One needed, indeed, all the arguments one could muster to insist, in their face, that insanity was not on the increase in this land of the free. Dr. Jarvis summarized:

In the year 1832, when the McLean Asylum at Somerville, Massachusetts, contained 64 patients, the State Lunatic Hospital was established at Worcester, for 120 patients. This was as large a number as was then supposed would need its accommodation. In 1836 one new wing, and in 1837 another new wing, and rooms for 100 more patients were added to the Worcester Hospital, and at the same time the McLean Asylum contained 93 lunatic inmates. In 1842, the Worcester Hospital was again enlarged by the addition of two new wings, and now these are filled to the over flowing, having 450 patients in May 1851, while, at the same time, there were 200 at the McLean Asylum, 204 at the City Lunatic Hospital, at Boston, and 115 in the country receptacles for the insane at Cambridge and Ipswich, beside 36 in the jails, making 1,015 lunatics in the public establishments of Massachusetts in 1851, instead of the 184 which were there in 1832. . . .

The State Hospital at Augusta, Maine, was opened in December 1840, with only 30 patients. In 1845, it was so crowded that the trustees asked for more rooms. In 1847, the building was enlarged, and 128 patients were admitted. In 1848, the house was all filled, and more were offered than could be accommodated, and the superintendent asked the Legislature to build still another wing to enable him to meet the increased demand.

The New Hampshire Hospital was opened in 1842, and received 22 patients: these were all that were offered. In 1843, these were increased to 41; in another year, 1844, there were 70; in 1845, there were 76; in 1846, there were 98; and in 1850, they reached the number of 120. In the meantime additions have been made to meet this growing demand for more and more accommodations.

The number of patients in the Eastern Virginia Asylum, at Williamsburg, has increased more than 200 per cent in 15 years,—from 60 in 1836 to 193 in 1850. Those in the Western Virginia Asylum, at Staunton, have increased more than 800 per cent in twenty-three years,—from 38 in 1828 to 348 in 1850.

The average number of patients in the Ohio State Lunatic Asylum, at Columbus, was 64 in 1839, and 328 in 1850, being an increase of more than 400 per cent in eleven years.

"It will readily be supposed," argued Dr. Jarvis, "that the opening of these establishments for the cure and protection of lunatics, the spread of their reports, the extension of the knowledge of their character, power, and usefulness, by the means of the patients that they protect and cure, have created, and continue to create, more and more interest in the subject of insanity, and more confidence in its curability. Consequently, more and more persons and families, who, or such as who, formerly kept their insane friends and relations at home, or allowed them to stroll abroad about the streets or country, now believe, that they can be restored, or improved, or, at least made more comfortable in these public institutions, and, therefore, they send their patients to these asylums, and thus swell the lists of their inmates." The numbers of mentally ill in the asylums could reflect much more than the rate of the illness in the population, therefore, and it was not clear whether they reflected the rate of the illness in the population at all. "We see also," Jarvis continued,

> from the very great difference of hospital accommodations, and of the use made of them by the people of different nations, and at different periods by the same nation, that we have no means of knowing what number of lunatics abroad those in these establishments represent. The statistics,—the ascertained and enumerated facts—then, are not sufficient to enable us to determine this question satisfactorily. . . . To infer the number of lunatics in the community from the number in the hospitals, is about as unsafe as to infer the number of births from the number of children in the schools. The

first element here is wanting; that is, the proportion of all the children that are sent to school. Now as this is very different in Massachusetts, and England, and Spain, and Egypt, and Siam, no reasonable man would venture to compare the number of births in these several countries by the population of their schoolhouses. The provision for the cure and the custody of the insane in these countries differs as widely as their provision for the education of children; and yet, writers have given us the comparative numbers on this ground, as, in London one in 200, because there were 7,000 in the metropolitan Hospitals, and in Cairo one in 30,714, because there were 14 in the hospital of that city.

This was a persuasive argument—assuming that we were not comparing societies with clear evidence of a juvenile population in and out of schools with societies in which the only evidence that children were born there at all was the presence of some native specimens in classrooms. It was silly, of course, to imagine societies with so few children. But was it as unreasonable to suppose in 1850—given that there was no evidence to the contrary— that Cairo, indeed, had no schizophrenics or sufferers from manic depression among its residents?

But Dr. Jarvis, while an excellent statistician, keenly aware of the pitfalls and shortcomings of the mental illness epidemiology of his age, was also a very intelligent man. Therefore, after a lengthy explanation why the existing statistics did not allow for an answer to the question whether insanity was—or was not—on the increase, he declared:

> Nevertheless, as all the enumerations, estimates, and computations, from whatever source, give larger numbers of the insane at each succeeding period, and as none of them give less, except the enquiry in Massachusetts, by the State Commissioners in 1847, and as, in almost all states and countries, the history of whose hospitals through several years has come to us, there are more and more that ask for hospital accommodations, and they increase as fast as rooms in the hospitals increase, and in some places faster, there is plausible ground at least for the supposition that insanity has been increasing for the last half century, and is now on the increase; and there is certainly a manifestation of more and more lunatics in these communities, if not a development of more and more insanity, among their individual members.

It was not any particular set of statistics, but the *remarkable degree of consistency* among them all that made the supposition that insanity was on the increase plausible (and the counter-supposition that it was not implausible). And this plausibility was made stronger by considerations which—though considerations of an eminent statistician—were not of statistical nature altogether.

"Not finding the facts of history and statistics," argued Dr. Jarvis,

> sufficient to determine, whether insanity is an increasing, or diminishing, or stationary disease, we may derive some additional light from an examination of the origin and sources of this class of diseases, and see whether the causes are more or less abundant, and act with more or less efficiency now than formerly, and are likely to produce more or less lunacy.
>
> Esquirol says, that "insanity is a disease of civilization and the number of the insane is in direct proportion to its progress." "The progress of civilization multiplies madmen (*fous*)." So certain is he, that this progress of society causes this disorder, that he asserts, that the insane have a right to demand that civilized society should remedy the evil which it causes. "It is not pity, nor benevolence, but justice that should restore madness." "If it is true, that madness has a direct relation with civilization, it is the duty of society not only to ameliorate the lot of the insane, but it is right even to compel it to diminish their number."
>
> Nothing can be more positive than this opinion of one of the ablest and most learned writers on diseases of the mind; and he sustains it at length by various observations on the proportion of lunatics in countries of different degrees of civilization. "There is less insanity in Spain than in countries where civilization is more advanced." "There are fewer insane in the northern parts of Norway where civilization is the lowest, than in the southern provinces where civilization is the highest."
>
> Humboldt made diligent enquiry and found none among the Indians of America. Travelers find none in Africa, and the general opinion of writers, travelers, and physicians is, that this disease is seldom found in the savage state, while it is known to be frequent in the civilized state.

The combined authority of Esquirol and Humboldt was, apparently, blinding enough to prevent the usually careful logician Jarvis from seeing that he was now making an argument which contradicted his assertions a few pages (or minutes, given that they were parts of a speech) ago, to the effect that the advancement of civilization only attracted the attention of the public to the problem of insanity, rather than caused—and increased—it. Moreover, he forgot that Esquirol's "observations on the proportion of lunatics in countries of different degrees of civilization" were based on the very statistics which, according to Jarvis, could not in themselves provide such a basis. But so it was in the United States of the 1850s: statistics were insufficient and unreliable, but evidence of one's senses could not be denied. All around one, insanity was increasing. "Civilization" being implicitly defined, especially in the innocent New World, in quantitative terms and chiefly as advancement in science and technology, it was natural to connect the two and was constantly done, *AJI*, writing several years previously (anticipating Nietzsche by some forty years and Freud by sixty, as it happened):

> Insanity is of rare occurrence in barbarous nations. Civilization appears to favor the development of madness. This circumstance may be attributed to the restraints imposed upon the indulgence of the passions, the diversity of interests, and a thirst of power; long-continued excitement of the mental energies, and disappointment in affections and anticipations. The wants of the savage are circumscribed: he gives vent to the burst of passions without control, and their violence subsides when they are gratified. In a more polished state of society, man dwells upon his injuries real or supposed, acts silently, and cherishes hopes of enjoyment, amongst which the sweets of revenge are not the least seductive. Such a condition, when followed by humiliating disappointment, must naturally tend to develop mental diseases. It is probable that the diseases of civilization, which act chiefly on the nervous system, may have led to the original foundation of hereditary predisposition, transmitted by a shattered constitution, and disturbed functions.

The advancement of civilization was, therefore, the culprit. American civilization was advancing at a neck-breaking pace; the young nation was poised to outrun its old-world rivals. Technological innovations also necessarily occasioned frequent reversals of fortune, and as the author or editor of the above-quoted remarks (they were published under the heading of "Miscellany") noted: "Both sudden prosperity and adversity madden."

And so Dr. Jarvis was "led to examine the causes of lunacy, and see how far they are necessarily connected with, or grow out of, the improving condition of civilized society." Systematic as usual, he divided these causes into "the Physical" and "the Moral," defining the former as "those which primarily act upon the body and disturb the brain, and then its functions, deranging thus the mind or the moral affections," and the latter as those which "affect the mind and the moral affections primarily, and through them they reach the brain." There were eighty-nine of such. As with the physical causes, Jarvis began by asking the question "whether these disturbing causes are increasing, stationary or diminishing," and answering provisionally "that some of them are increasing in frequency and in force, some are probably stationary, and a few are diminishing with the advancement of civilization. Some of them are essentially inherent in man, in every condition, the savage and the refined nearly alike, and are to be found throughout the world and in all ages." The following were the moral causes that were increasing in frequency and in force:

In a higher state of refinement, the sensibilities become more keen, and the tender passions more powerful and more relied upon as sources of happiness. Then the affections between the sexes are more ardent and abiding, and have a more controlling influence over them, than in a ruder state, and a rupture of the proposed union, a disappointment in love, the failure in tenderness, of respect, or of fidelity in a partner after marriage, would produce a keener anguish, a more effective shock, and wear upon the spirits more in a refined, than in a less cultivated state of society, where less was hoped, and less suffering would follow failure or disappointment. Therefore, we may look for more insanity from disappointed love or domestic trouble now than in former ages . . .

The causes connected with mental labor, in its manifold applications have increased and are increasing continually. In the progress of the age, education has made rapid advances, both in reaching a wider circle of persons and in multiplying the subjects of study. The improvements in the education of children and youth have increased their mental labors, and imposed more burdens upon their brains, in the present than in the preceding ages. The proportion of children who are taught in schools increases every year in the United States, and in most civilized nations. There are more and more of

those whose love of knowledge, whose sense of duty, whose desire of gratifying friends, and whose ambition, impel them to make their utmost exertions, to become good scholars. Thus they task their minds unduly, and
sometimes exhaust their cerebral energies and leave their brains a prey to
other causes which may derange them afterwards. The new sciences which
have been lately discovered, or the old sciences that were formerly confined
to the learned, but are now simplified and popularized, and are offered to
the young as a part of their education, multiply the subjects of study and
increase the mental labor of almost all in schools. Men and classes of men,
such as in the last century would have thought of nothing but how they
should obtain their bread, are now induced to study subjects and pursue
sciences, and burden their brains with great and sometimes excessive labor.
New fields of investigation have been laid open within the last hundred,
and especially within the last fifty years. New inducements are offered, so
that a greater variety of tastes is invited to their peculiar feasts of knowledge. Many persons now study phrenology, metaphysics, mathematics,
physiology, chemistry, botany, and other branches of natural history, to say
nothing of mesmerism, biology, & c., and thus they compel their brains to
labor with more energy and exhausting zeal than those of any former generation. In this multiplication of students, there are some who attempt to
grapple with subjects, that they cannot master, and sink under the burden
of perplexity which they cannot unravel.

In the nineteenth century, Americans, a new people, were discovering that
thinking is a difficult job. Being from the outset oriented towards raising
their standard of living, bettering themselves in the sense of increasing
material benefits (i.e., comfort) and decreasing material costs (or effort),
and exceptionally good at inventing labor-saving devices, they would soon
deal with this problem. But there was more in what Dr. Jarvis saw than the
dangers of natural history, mesmerism, and biology. "In this general
increase of mental activity," he wrote, "some men become interested in and
give their minds intensely to the study of public topics, politics, State or
National affairs and the subjects of legislation, the banking system, tariff,
anti-rent, anti-masonry, the license question, &c., or to public moral questions, anti-slavery, temperance, and general or special reforms, any or all of
which impose upon them great anxiety and mental labor."

All these political preoccupations, he knew, were new and widespread, and as the interest in them grew, insanity in the country increased in prevalence. Jarvis was a religious man, early in life choosing Unitarianism as his faith of preference and remaining a conscientious participant in the church affairs to the end, but he stressed in his remarks that, as politics emerged as a significant contributing cause to the deterioration of the national mental health, so religion receded in its importance as such. "The causes connected with religion," he said, "have doubtless diminished within the last thirty years." Still, it was not the obvious ascendancy in the public mind of the new political interests that drove the rates of insanity upward. Far more important was the increasing number of choices the American society offered its members and the growing extent of social mobility in it.

"In this country," Jarvis asserted,

> where no son is necessarily confined to the work or employment of his father, but all the fields of labor, of profit, or of honor, are open to whomsoever will put on the harness and enter therein, and all are invited to join the strife for that which may be gained in each, many are in a transition state, from the lower and less desirable to the higher and more desirable conditions. They are struggling for that which costs them mental labor, anxiety, and pain. The mistake, or the ambition, of some, leads them to aim at that which they cannot reach,—to strive for more than they can grasp,—and their mental powers are strained to their utmost tension; they labor in agitation, and they end in frequent disappointment. Their minds stagger under the disproportional burden; they are perplexed with the variety of insurmountable obstacles, and they are exhausted with the ineffectual labor.
>
> There are many whose education is partially wrong, and some whose education is decidedly bad. These persons have wrong notions of life. They are neither taught to understand the responsibilities that they must meet, nor are they prepared to sustain them. They are filled with false hopes. They are flattered in childhood and youth, but they are not accustomed to mental labor, nor disciplined and strengthened to bear burdens. They are led to expect circumstances that will not belong to them. They look for success, honor, or advantages, which their talents, or education, or habits of business, or station in the world, will not obtain for them. Consequently, when they

enter responsible life, they are laying plans which cannot be fulfilled, they are looking for events which will not happen. They are struggling perpetually and unsuccessfully against the tide of fortune. They are always hoping, but they are frequently disappointed. Their ineffectual labor exhausts them, and their disappointments distress and disturb them. They are thus apt to become nervous, querulous and despondent, and, sometimes, insane.

How much better for one's mental health was it to live in a closed society which limited one's freedom! In a less "advanced," not as civilized society, in other words. "In an uneducated community," Jarvis pointed out,

or where the people are overborne by despotic government or inflexible customs, where men are born in castes, and die without over-stepping their native condition, where the child is content with the pursuit and the fortune of his father, and has no hope or expectation of any other, there these undue mental excitements and struggles do not happen, and men's brains are not confused with new plans, nor exhausted with the struggles for a higher life, nor overborne with the disappointment in failure. Of course, in such a state of society, these causes of insanity cannot operate. But in proportion as education prevails, and emancipates the new generations from the trammels and condition of the old, and the manifold ways of life are open to all, the danger of misapplication of the cerebral forces and the mental powers increases, and men may think and act indiscreetly, and become insane.

One could see these forces plainly at work in the economy, where choices augmented with particular rapidity. "There are many new trades and new employments," argued the observant doctor,

there are new schemes of increasing wealth, new articles of merchandise, and speculations in many things of new and multiplying kinds. All these increase the activity of the commercial world. The energy of men of new enterprises gives a hope of actual value, and a momentary market value to some new kinds of property. The consequent inflation or expansion of prices, to a greater or lesser degree, makes many kinds of business more uncertain, and many men's fortunes more precarious. This increases the doubts and perplexities of business, the necessity of more labor and watchfulness, greater fear and anxiety, and the end is more frequently in loss, and failure of plans, and mental disturbance.

These universal pressures of the open society were especially strong among those whose choices included the top social positions. "Besides these uncertainties which may happen to any, there are more that enter the free and open avenues to occupations which hold out high and flattering promises, and for which they are unprepared, in which they must struggle with greater labor and anxiety than others, and in which they must be more frequently disappointed." Social mobility—an implication of the unquestioned values of liberty and equality, of the promise that in this free nation one could rise as high as any other—was not an unmitigated good, in the eyes of our first great epidemiologist, in other words, even though he had never said so explicitly. What he said, instead, was:

Besides these causes of mental disturbance in the new and untried fields of study, business, and commerce, there are other causes in the social position which is subject to like changes. Many are passing, or have passed, from a comparatively retired, simple and unpretending, to the showy, the fashionable or the cultivated, style of life. In this transition state there must be more mental labor for those who are passing from one condition to the other; there must be much thought and toil, much hope and fear, and much anxiety and vexation, to effect the passage, and to sustain one's self in the new position . . . and then nervousness, frequently, and insanity, sometimes, follows.

Thus we see, that with advancing civilization, and especially in the present age and in our own country, there is a great development of activity of mind, and this is manifested in most of the employments, in the conduct of the mechanic arts, agriculture, trade and commerce, in the attention to the professions, and to other subjects of study, and to politics. This increase of mental activity, and of cerebral action comes without a corresponding increase of discretion to guide it, and of prudence to restrain it.

And so Dr. Jarvis concluded his speech "On the Supposed Increase of Insanity":

In review of this history of the causes of insanity, we find that very few of them diminish with the progress of the world. Some are stationary, remaining about the same in the savage, the barbarous and the civilized state, while many of them increase, and create more and more mental disorder. Insanity is then a part of the price which we pay for civilization. The causes of the one increase with the developments and results of the other. This is not necessarily the case, but it is so now. The increase of knowledge, the improvements in the arts, the multiplication of comforts, the amelioration of manners, the growth of refinement, and the elevation of morals, do not of themselves disturb men's cerebral organs and create mental disorder. But with them come more opportunities and rewards for great and excessive mental action, more uncertain and hazardous employments, and consequently more disappointments ... more groundless hopes, and more painful struggle to obtain that which is beyond reach, or to effect that which is impossible.

The deductions, then, drawn from the prevalence and effects of causes, corroborate the opinion of nearly all writers, whether founded on positive and known facts, on analogy, on computation or on conjecture, that insanity is an increasing disease. In this opinion all agree.[45]

Well, "nearly all," and perhaps even not that nearly.[46] But Dr. Jarvis was, before everything else, an empiricist, and the evidence of his own experience weighed more with him, than the opinions of others—and even statistics.

The Travails of a Pioneer Psychiatrist: Dr. Edward Jarvis

Dr. Edward Jarvis for thirty years practiced whatever was psychiatry in his time and may well be regarded the first American epidemiologist of mental disease, conducting and publishing numerous statistical studies on the subject. His contribution to the understanding of the problem in the United States, however, extends beyond such professional publications and practice. He left two invaluable documents—his already quoted *Autobiography* and his diaries—which allow us a glimpse into the motivations and character of a mental disease specialist in those early days, as well as into the special nature of American society which made this ailment so common in it.

In however mild a form, Dr. Jarvis, throughout his life, was clearly afflicted by the illness he found he was best equipped to treat. It is possible that what kept him from succumbing to it and becoming a patient, rather than a healer and observer, was that he grew up in a community with a stable and unquestioned set of values, that he early acquired a circle of life-long friends who shared these values, and, above all, that he enjoyed a long and happy marriage to a woman from this community, whom he knew and loved since the school bench and to whom he got engaged at the young age of twenty-three. He entered life, in other words, in a psychological cocoon and was lucky to keep this insulating spiritual garment as long as he lived. Its padding afforded him protection from the ever-repeated challenges of the wider society to his identity and prevented them from profoundly disrupting his sense of self.

Edward Jarvis was born in 1803, in Concord, Massachusetts, into what by all accounts may be called a (middling) New England gentry family. His father, Francis Jarvis, was a respected, educated farmer. Edward early developed a taste for reading. "His father had a small library which was composed principally of histories, travels, sermons, philosophical treatises and a few novels. There was a good public library of which his father was one of proprietors and officials." Edward first read the "tales," such as *Robinson Crusoe*, but soon found "the heavier works of history . . . even more interesting than the lighter works of romance." When he was sixteen, "casting about for a profession for life, he would have selected a literary profession and followed his brother to Cambridge, but it seemed that the burden of educating Charles [Edward's elder brother] was as great as his father could bear"; thus Edward, who was fond of mechanics, was apprenticed to the owner and manager of a small woolen factory in Stow. However, the boy "longed for a different and more intellectual employment." He remembered his eighteen months there as "the absolute misery," recording in his diary:

> My hostess was a virago. My master a tyrant of a conceited squire, thinking all must be done as submissively as his workmen did. I despised him, refused . . . I lived here miserably, my only comfort was reading, which I summoned indefatigably having nothing else to take my attention . . . he often attempt to disturb me in this only enjoyment. I read Shakespeare,

Chesterfield, Scott Novels . . . during the spring-summer 1820 Cranston [the owner] and I became tired of each other. I wanted none of his littleness . . . haughty tyranny. . . . He charged me with laziness with being more fond of books than work. I did not deny this: but I did what was to be done, my reading did not interfere with his business. The truth was he kept much help, he had not work for all at all times. So often I had not an hours work a day to do. I kept a book in this factory to read while the others lay still though they invited me to join with them, felt envious or jealous of me. They were ignorant/bigoted like their master.[47]

Supported by some elder friends, Edward begged his father to allow him to continue his schooling and prepare for college, to which the latter immediately agreed, as a result of which in the fall of 1822, he entered Harvard.

There, the environment was all that the young man desired. But he fell short of his expectations from himself. The Diary reports in March 1823: "Soon after [the second] term began I went & learned my rank in the class and found it to be the 56th. I was much mortified . . ."[48] He endeavored to study better and succeeded in raising himself to the twenty-first rank, but in June 1824, wrote despondently again: "so my route continued falling, in the spring it was the 27th and now it fell to the 29th. . . . I began to despair of doing any thing as a scholar." He was dissatisfied with himself and also worried about money and lack of opportunities (for which its lack was responsible) to cultivate contacts with prominent Boston families. These worries and dissatisfaction, according to the *Autobiography* led to dyspepsia. He was to graduate in the class of 1826. Shortly before Commencement he made a trip to New York. He went from Salem, in a coaster, around Cape Cod, through Long Island Sound. Jarvis recorded in his *Autobiography:*

In the morning they were in the sound, and there they met the New York steamer going to Providence apparently filled with passengers on the decks—ladies, gentlemen—all seemingly enjoying the luxury of the most comfortable means of travelling. This was a new experience to Jarvis. He had never been on board or even seen a steamer, except the ferry boats in Boston Harbor. Comparing that mode of travelling with the coaster in which he was sailing, the steamer's ample dimensions and the show of cabins and staterooms, with the narrow and stench cabin where he had slept below, it seemed to him that there was a luxury much beyond his present power to enjoy.[49]

Almost fifty years later, the memory, clearly, retained the power to rankle.

Medicine was not Edward's calling. In the *Autobiography*, we read:

> Jarvis's predilection was to be a minister. To him there was something indescribably attractive in the profession. The nature of the employment, as teacher of holiness and as messenger from God to men, the opportunity to put forth those exact and elevated notions of right and wrong, of leading people, by love, to the paths of wisdom; there seemed to him a beauty and a grace in this position and relation more than any other, and he wanted to devote his life and power to it. But his friends—especially his brother Charles—thought that this was not his field of service. His speech was indistinct, his enunciation was imperfect, and he could not succeed as a minister. People would be unwilling to hear him, and perhaps his severe notions of life and duty, and, probably, unfeeling way of presenting them, would rather repel than draw hearers to his preaching. As none advised him to study this profession and some positively dissuaded him, he gave up the cherished hope and took that which alone seemed not to be closed to him, and studied medicine. But his first affections were not so easily given up, and afterward, while studying anatomy, medicine and healing, his thoughts too often wandered to his friends at the divinity hall, their delightful studies and their lovely prospects of usefulness in the field of humanity. His sympathies with the profession remained through life. His best and most intimate friends of college became ministers . . . [50]

The young man thus longed for authority and status—these were the "indescribable" attractions of the clerical profession at the time—but was denied them through ministry because of the lack of natural aptitude for it. It is no wonder that he could not work up much enthusiasm for the profession he chose as a default option—medicine—for it, apparently, required no aptitude.

But there was more to that. The *Autobiography* states:

As soon as J. began to read on practical medicine, and the statement of the remedies prescribed for disease, he began to inquire farther as to the precise relation of the agent to the evil that it proposed to influence . . . the question remained as to the effect of these agencies and interferences on the disordered state of the body. Did these remove fever, cool the skin, allay the thirst . . . or in pneumonia did they remove the fullness of the lungs and difficulty of breathing? He saw people thus diseased and medicated, and yet the disorder continued, but gradually left the patient . . . the doubt arose in his mind whether, in many cases the action of the medicine and the cause of the disease were not two independent series of facts, or events, co-existing in the same body, perhaps with or without an active influence upon each other. From reading, conversation and observation, it was seen that for the same diseases, or same series of marked events, as fever, pleurisy, dysentery, &c. at different times, in different places, by different persons, various and different medicines had been and were given; the physical form had been and was very differently acted upon by these agencies, and yet one event of death happened to a few, and the other event of recovery to many, about in like proportion under these manifold kinds of treatment. The remedies that were supposed to be effective in removing disease in one age, were forgotten in the next; and others used with the same apparent effect in their stead, and these, in turn, yielded to a new means of treatment, and these again to the later inventions. Means believed to have power to annihilate disease in one place, and in one physician's hands, were rejected by others for the same kind of malady.

In short, medicine, which Edward Jarvis studied and was expected to practice, he discovered, was far from an exact—or any kind of—science. It was a matter of belief and convention, and these happened to be a belief Jarvis did not share and a convention he did not care for. He was a skeptical medical student, doubting the worth of the profession for which he was preparing. "These doubts and inquiries," he wrote in the *Autobiography*, "began with his earliest studies of the theory and practice of medicine, and in various degrees have followed him ever afterward, and although he studied this branch of the profession with earnestness, yet he felt that, thus far, it had partaken very much of the nature and result of the search for the philosopher's stone, and offered less hope of practical reward."[51]

What made matters much worse was the fact that the profession Jarvis chose for lack of a better option and which he quickly found unworthy of his own respect, in the early nineteenth-century United States was not quite as prestigious and certainly not as well-paying as he would like.[52] During the first six years after he graduated from medical school in 1830, Jarvis first practiced in Northfield, MA, then a town of 1,757 inhabitants, "almost exclusively farmers," where "there was no sound to be heard save the lowing of cattle." He had sufficient practice to afford room and board, but not enough to begin paying the debts he accumulated during his studies. Moreover, he "felt a great loneliness there. He was ambitious of a larger field of service, of association with a wider circle of people of high and broad culture, especially in medical and other science. . . . he longed to be nearer the active world, to live among men who had a larger share in its great responsibilities, and took a larger part in its movements."[53] In his *Diary*, which was in these years interrupted by much "anxiety," Jarvis wrote in January 1832: "I confess, I have a secret bending for notoriety. I like to keep myself before the eyes of others." And then:

> My mind is in undisciplined state. I have accustomed myself from early youth to day-dreaming. I delight to revel in reveries, in imagining myself in certain conditions, with certain means of doing good and in power, in afflu-ence, in respectability. This has unhinged my mind. I find my eyes on any book, my thoughts far from it. . . . In these reveries my thoughts in their creation have always created for me a pure character one with industry, energy, talent virtue means. . . . Some good has arisen from this, for this has been my conception of a perfect character, which has tended to fix my moral principles, to choose my notions of right and wrong in certain condi-tions. Nevertheless . . . it has lessened the power of their conceptions, their influence over me. I confess this day-dreaming is wrong. I confess that I have indulged it against conscience. It has had a power like a charm over me, with its siren influences has very often drawn me very far from my duty. I know my failing. I was conscious of being astray, but my enchanter threw

such a veil over the sin, such a beauty over the temptations that it dulled my moral perceptions for the moment and I was happy . . . in sin![54]

In September 1832, Jarvis went to visit his family in Concord and learned that one of the physicians there left for a different town that very morning. On the spot, Jarvis decided to stay. "No place was more desirable than Concord," states the *Autobiography*. Concord offered greater scope for the young man's intellectual activity, but did not much improve his income, which "did not justify house-keeping." Until 1835, Jarvis, already married, still "took rooms" (though now parlor and chamber, rather than chamber alone) and board, and, when the health of the landlord failed, rented an old house "which was the only one that could be obtained in that neighborhood, for $90 a year" the doctor could afford. There, the young couple (which remained childless) took boarders, "and, from these and the profession had sufficient income to pay the expenses." They had no servant. Again the *Autobiography* strikes a sad note:

> he had not succeeded in his profession as he supposed he had reason to expect. He still owed the debt with which he began his profession. Although he was satisfied with his first and second years of practice, he had made little or no advance beyond those years. He had barely sustained himself in all his Concord life. His income from both profession and boarders had only supported his family living with the most rigid economy. He took care of his horse himself. He rode horseback always except when he was sleighing. . . . His earnings had all been consumed in his living; none devoted to the payment of his debt which was not diminished since he began his professional practice. He began to despair of farther increase of reputation, business, or income. . . . It was apparent . . . that in Concord Dr. J. must . . . receive a meager support. . . . This conviction wore upon his spirit and made him feel that his present position was not the best that he ought or, at least, hoped to enjoy. Possibly it was in himself, his want of fitness for his profession . . . or it might be that Concord was not his true professional field. . . . Nevertheless he began to cherish the willingness, at least, to change either his profession or his abode for another, in the probability that any other would profit him more.

And at this time, something wonderful happened to Jarvis.

A new and unexpected experience was thrown open to him in 1836. A young man in Cambridge was taken insane. . . . The physician in charge advised the friend to send him to the care of some young physician who would watch over him, and take such care of him as should be necessary. He suggested Dr. Jarvis of Concord. . . . Then one was sent from Cape Cod who had been long insane and past recovery. . . . A third, a lady of Boston, was sent by Dr. James Jackson of Boston, and was three months in Dr. J.'s family, and was then taken to the McLean Asylum.

This turned Dr. J.'s active attention to the subject of insanity, and changed his whole professional course of thought and life. He had not paid attention to mental disorders before, but when the matter was brought to him, he found it more consonant to his mental habits and taste, than the care of physical disease. This seemed to be the opinion of others, besides those who had sent patients to him and who advised him to open a house for the special care of the insane.

"The offer of the insane patients," Jarvis also writes, "came as a relief" in the midst of his self-doubts and mild depression associated with them, "and their continuance showed that there was a talent in him, and a field in the world for its exercise, whereby he might work with more success. This gave him comfort and hope, and removed much of the cloud that hung over him."[55] The insanity of others thus was balsam for the soul of the unhappy Dr. Jarvis; he found in their misfortune a therapy for his own mental troubles and, at the age of thirty-nine, in his mind, at least, turned psychiatrist.

He would be forty, however, before this ideal self-definition aligned itself with objective reality and even then not to the extent Dr. Jarvis wished them to be aligned. For several months the possibility of being appointed the superintendent of McLean was dangled before him. "At no time in his life was such a prize so desirable both to his mind and taste, and to his fortune, ever held out to the eye of Dr. J. It seemed to offer to him a field for the highest exercise of his mind where he could develop his talents more than in any other. Here was opportunity for the employment of all his philosophical training. It seemed to open a way for his broadest culture and the best refinement. His heart was strongly fixed upon it, and he waited with anxious hope." But, in January 1837, Luther Bell was selected for the position instead. Jarvis's interest in insanity survived the bitter disappointment, but when the Association of the Medical Superintendents was formed, he was not among the founding thirteen, though well known to all of them through his statistical publications, in fact he was never to become a superintendent of a mental asylum. Unable to achieve any of his goals in his native New England, he left in 1837 for Kentucky and practiced for five years in Louisville as a general physician. His bad luck pursued him there: in that land of opportunity, he happened to spend precisely "the time of the great commercial and financial depression, 1837 to 1842," when there were no opportunities. He was able to pay all his debts, published quite a lot, and became involved in numerous cultural activities. Still, in five years "he had become weary of Kentucky. . . . He went there with the hope of earning a large income and acquiring a competence and independence in a few years. His eyes were very early opened to this error." Kentucky too turned out not to be the place for him; he was still unable to find his place. He determined to look for it again back at home.

The main reason for Jarvis's dissatisfaction with his situation in the wide West was that new and attractive choices seemed to emerge in the East. "The interest in mental disorder still remained in his mind, and the desire of a position in a [mental] hospital still burned within him. It seemed to him that his field of usefulness was there, and that he could in that way do a greater good for humanity and accomplish a higher purpose for himself." A visiting friend told him that there was expected a vacancy in the superintendency of the Boston Lunatic Hospital, for which he could be an excellent candidate. At the same time he heard that both S. B. Woodward of the Worcester Hospital and Bell of the McLean intended to leave. His desire for a position in a lunatic asylum, inflamed by these rumors that in the end turned to be false, "took leading hold of Dr. Jarvis's heart and made him discontent with his position of general physician."

Accordingly, on the 14th of July, 1842 . . . Dr. and Mrs. J. left Louisville never to return to live there. . . . In Philadelphia Dr. J. visited the Insane Hospitals under care of Drs. Kirkbride and Earle, and in New York, the Bloomingdale Asylum. In these he was received so cordially by the superintendents, they spoke so kindly about his writings and his interest in the matter of insanity, they expressed so much hope that he would be called to join their corps, and co-operate with them, that he felt encouraged in his hope, and went to Massachusetts with a more ardent desire than ever, of entering this new field of employment, and a determination to leave no stone unturned that should lie in his way of being made superintendent of an insane hospital.[56]

Self-realization seemed to be so near! Jarvis in quick succession proposed his candidacy for the superintendencies of Boston Lunatic Hospital and Hartford Retreat, and was in both cases not elected. He wrote in the *Autobiography:*

> Here was the third defeat in his candidacy for the superintendency of an insane hospital. He had supposed that therein was his best field of development of his complete professional character, where he could bring his talents and taste more effectively into use and where he could enjoy scientific and professional life better than in any other. Yet the results of these three attempts seemed to show that the world thought differently, and that they could find men who would work in this sphere more satisfactory to them. He must therefore be content to take his chance, and find what fortune the world had to offer him in the field of general practice.[57]

On the advice of friends, however, he opened a private mental clinic in Dorchester, taking patients and caring for them in his home. It was immediately successful and profitable. He continued it until his retirement, three decades later. He was an active participant in the work of the Statistical Association and the Association of Medical Superintendents of the Asylums for the Insane, a respected member of several culturally-important communities, some of them country-wide, and a dear friend of many famous people, much better known than he. He never realized his ambition for status and, as we know from the *Autobiography*, at least until his sixties, remained somewhat dissatisfied with his position. He was not happy, but not deeply unhappy either. His life was one of relative success.

Jarvis never suffered from want, he always lived in what the overwhelming majority of his contemporaries and countrymen would consider as comfort. He belonged to the upper classes, the affluent (moderately or immoderately), the educated, the gentry. Objectively speaking, his life was devoid of problems: it was the relativity of his success and prosperity that made it problematic. His friends were more successful than he, some of them were more prosperous. There were too many possibilities, which seemed to offer him greater success (i.e., status) and wealth than the ones he enjoyed at any particular moment, too many choices, in other words. American society offered too great a scope for the imagination, encouraged the imaginative to strive, and exposed them to constant disappointments. So much was possible, so little could actually be attained. Thus Dr. Jarvis, who was perfectly well off from the objective point of view, all his life suffered from the anomic malaise which made his insane patients truly and grievously ill. He did not see the connection. The bent of his intellect was statistical, not philosophical. In his case, at least, the interest in psychiatry was not a result of the interest in the nature of psychiatric disease (as it was not a result of the sympathy with the suffering of the mentally ill and desire to alleviate it), but, rather, a product of "role-hybridization," connecting the skills of one, less prestigious social role (in Jarvis's case, that of general physician) to the authority of another, more prestigious one (that of an intellectual, minister to the souls),—incidentally, very much like in the case of Freud.[58]

The situation of Dr. Jarvis was rather common, as, judging by numerous memoirs, diaries, and autobiographies, was his malaise. It is quite possible, therefore, that his route to psychiatry was not entirely exceptional among the practitioners of that pioneer generation.

Throughout the nineteenth century, the issue of possibly increasing rates of insanity was a matter of a passionate and continuous debate in all the countries where the disease was observed. In Britain, the United States, France, and other countries large-scale statistical surveys in the second half of the nineteenth century were conducted repeatedly. Their findings suggested that insanity was on the increase. But the statistics everywhere, like today, lent themselves to numerous criticisms and were not considered reliable. This left the question "Is Insanity on the Increase?"[59] open, and a large part of the public committed itself to the view that it could not be. The main reason for such commitment, however, was not the unreliability of statistics but the fact that the possibility of increasing insanity was very frightening. In the United States, in the end of the nineteenth century many well-informed people were still alive in large cities who remembered when no need was felt for a mental institution in their community and insanity was not considered a pressing problem. Sixty years later every major American city had a mental hospital bursting with patients and it was absolutely "safe to say throughout the United States generally . . . that in urban districts the ratio [of insane to healthy population was] 1 to 350, and in rural sections 1 to 500." The same, it was claimed, applied "to all civilized countries,"[60] which meant that the United States stood now breast to breast with the frontrunners in this sad race. "Civilized countries," at the time, were limited to countries of Western Europe and North America, all the reports (obviously impressionistic) continuing to suggest that the rest of the world was still blissfully unaware of insanity. What, could an American ask, would happen if the ratio of insane to mentally healthy Americans doubled to tripled again, or, banish the thought, quadrupled, reaching, for an outlandish example, the full 1 percent of the population?!

This nightmare vision was all too quickly becoming a reality. On October 5, 1906, the front page of the *New York Times,* carried the following piece of news: "London, Oct. 4.—The delightful forecast of the world gone mad is held up to us by Dr. Forbes Winslow. 'According to the statistical figures on insanity,' says the doctor in an interview, 'it can be shown that before long there will be actually more lunatics in the world than sane people. The burning problem of the day is how to prevent this increase of insanity. What is the use of wasting time and energy on an education bill when we have before us this absorbing problem, the contemplation of an insane world, to deal with?'"[61] The message was phrased jokingly but considered important enough to be specially cabled to the paper. No, this sort of prospect was not to be entertained.

Despite the fervent belief of the general public that this could not be so, insanity (i.e., schizophrenia and manic-depressive illness to be) in the United States was on the increase. This was reflected not only, and not even mostly, in the statistics doomed to be forever regarded as unreliable. Perhaps, a better indicator was provided by the luxuriously ramifying American psychiatric establishment. In the fifty-six years of the nineteenth century remaining after the foundation of the *American Journal of Insanity* and the Association of Medical Superintendents of American Institutions for the Insane in 1844, this establishment—the numbers of psychiatric asylums, clinics, and hospitals, of the superintendents and doctors working in them, of public officials and lawyers from the first involved with these institutions and their potential patients, of members of the association and contributors to its journal, etc.—grew by leaps and bounds. This trend is exhibited by the Reports of the Proceedings from the Annual Meeting of the American Association of the Superintendents of Mental Asylums published annually in the *American Journal of Insanity*. There were thirteen members in attendance at the second annual meeting of the Association in 1845, twenty-six during the fifth annual meeting in 1850, although three of the previously attending members (two of them the founders, S. B. Woodward, the first president, and Amariah Brigham, the vice-president) died. Thereafter, the attendance (presumably reflecting the membership) doubled every ten years, increasing tenfold by the turn of the century. The only ten-year period in which the attendance at the association's convention was not increased by a factor of two occurred between 1855 and 1865. By 1895 it was deemed necessary to create a second association for the Assistant Physicians of Hospitals for the Insane.[62] But the supply always lagged behind the demand. The numbers of persons in need of the care the establishment sought to provide seemed to increase faster. Annual reports of the existing institutions consistently showed increasing inpatient population; new institutions within months of opening would fill to capacity; shortage of asylum space and hospital beds was a constant complaint.[63]

The United States, as the reader saw, was not the only country to bend so under the apparently increasing burden of chronic mental illness with uncertain causation. The situation in both Britain and France was very similar.[64] This also supports the conjecture that it was increasing in America. In the course of the century, institutions for the mentally ill began to appear in many other countries of Western Europe. With their numerous universities and large professorial class ever in need of new specializations, German principalities led the way in establishing psychiatry as an academic discipline.[65] Eastern Europe followed. In 1883 the first Russian psychiatric periodical began publication, adding a contingent of Russian specialists, soon to be considered among the leaders of the new profession, to the growing international community of practitioners and researchers, the clinics for mentally ill began to crop up around the vast territory of the Russian Empire, and the premier Russian psychiatrist, P. I. Kovalevski, claimed, on however impressionistic basis, that Russians suffered from "the American disease"—neurasthenia—at a greater rate than Americans themselves. The question of increasing insanity was discussed everywhere.

It was eclipsed early in the new century. There was no longer any thrill in contemplating an insane world in the future, as the condition of its mental health became quite absorbing in the present. The hospitalized insane population in the United States numbered 74,028 persons in 1890 but 187,791 in 1910, while the general population of the country increased only 46 percent. In 1955 there were over half-a-million hospitalized psychiatric patients—in fact 558,922, i.e., about the same number over half a million as there were in total in 1890.[66] By the 1950s coping with insanity at its current rates became one of the top national priorities. Sloan Wilson, in the iconic *Man in the Gray Flannel Suit*, the probing portrait of the post-World War II decade, considered a very good likeness, tellingly makes the establishment of improved mental health services the target of the broadcasting campaign, the success of which it is the job of the novel's hero to ensure and in which the hero's aging boss sees a justification of his own otherwise meaningless workaholic life and family breakdown. The clue to the success of the said campaign? Government involvement. Clearly, mental disease was no longer a problem that associations of health professionals, or even municipal and state authorities could be expected to solve—no one but the Federal Government had sufficient resources to cope with it. This was no fiction: by the end of the 1940s, insanity in the United States had reached the levels which required the existence of a special federal agency; this agency, the National Institute of Mental Health, was formed in 1947.

The question "Is Insanity on the Increase?" would still, from time to time, be raised in specialist publications, but it no longer occupied the public mind. It was decided that the point was moot. One of the most eminent American psychiatrists today, Edwin Fuller Torrey, has long argued that "insanity" specifically defined as schizophrenia and manic-depressive illness had increased in prevalence throughout the nineteenth century and continued to grow steadily in the twentieth century as well. According to his figures, between 1880 and 1980 these severe psychiatric disorders became nine times more common.[67] Several studies done since 1980s have suggested that the prevalence of these disorders has been "much higher" in the cohorts born since 1940.[68] Summarizing these findings in 2005, Torrey wrote in regard to manic-depressive illness: "The possibility that manic-depressive illness may be increasing in prevalence should be considered an open question, since definitive data are lacking. Of major concern, however, is the fact that the National Institute of Mental Health collects virtually no data with which to answer such a question. . . . Even more remarkable is the fact that there appears to be no interest in studying this question."[69]

In the end of the nineteenth century, the existence of insanity in their society at the rate of 1 percent (i.e., one insane person in every one hundred individuals) was a terrifying prospect to Americans; today, it is estimated in 2004, it exists at the rate of 20 percent. This is the number combining major depression and schizophrenia, major depression alone being responsible for 17.2 percent. As I am writing these lines, on April 26, 2011, I receive the news from my campus newspaper, *BU Today,* its front-page news: "Depression and anxiety on college campuses have risen to epidemic proportions . . . 20% of BU students surveyed fit the criteria for major depression."[70] It can be claimed, of course—I am sure, it will be claimed—that Boston University is just one of many universities and cannot be considered representative of the American college population, and that college population is not representative of the population in general. Indeed. No statistical study is reliable. Nevertheless, *taken together, and with other supporting evidence,* the accumulated statistics of the last 170 years chart an undeniable trend.

Whatever one thinks of the skills of our statisticians, it appears to me, this lays the question of whether insanity has been on the increase in this mighty nation of ours to rest. To hide, ostrich-like, from this evidence will not do. The answer to this question, without a shadow of a shadow of a doubt is "yes." The American case, our case, lends a resounding support to the argument of this book. How sad! How very, very sad.

American Insanity as a Mass Phenomenon

As everywhere, in the United States, the subclinical forms of madness, first called "neuroses" by French alienists, have been far more common than the clearly psychotic, clinical forms, which required containment. It was E. H. Van Deusen, the Superintendent of the Michigan Asylum for the Insane, in a supplement to the annual report for 1867–1868, who subsumed the French neuroses under the general caption of "neurasthenia." Dr. Van Deusen's "Observations on a Form of Nervous Prostration, (Neurasthenia,) Culminating in Insanity" was published in *AJI* in April 1869. He explained his choice of the name: "As to the term *neurasthenia*, it is an old term, taken from the medical vocabulary, and used simply because it seemed more nearly than any other to express the character of the disorder, and more definite, perhaps, than the usual term 'nervous prostration.'" "Our observations have led us to think," wrote Van Deusen,

> that there is a disorder of the nervous system, the essential character of which is, well expressed by the terms given above [in the title], and so uniform in development and progress, that it may with propriety be regarded as a distinct form of disease. . . . Among the causes, excessive mental labor, especially when conjoined with anxiety and deficient nourishment, ranks first. It is also traceable to depressing emotions, grief, domestic trouble, prolonged anxiety and pecuniary embarrassment. . . . Its leading symptoms are general malaise, impaired nutrition and assimilation; muscular atonicity, changing the expression of the countenance; uterine displacements, with consequent results, and neuralgias of debility, cerebral anaemia, with accompanying tendency to hyperaesthesia, irritability, mental depression, impaired intellection, melancholia and mania.

Despite the medicalese verbiage, which was speedily replacing the vernacular used in the *American Journal of Insanity* in its early years and becoming de rigueur after the publication of Darwin's *Origin of the Species,* which dramatically elevated the authority of science in the United States, and the concomitant turn of American superintendents to the more "scientific" (at least in vocabulary) German psychiatry at the expense of its previous, English and French, models, "neurasthenia" is easily recognizable. "Neuroses" would survive it as the diagnosis by many years; on many occasions it would be called "hysteria"; today we refer to it as "bipolar spectrum diseases"—dysthymia, cyclothymia, generalized anxiety disorder, and so on. According to Dr. Van Deusen, it "occurred . . . in the persons of those occupying positions of great responsibility, the duties of which were of a nature to make heavy demands upon the nervous energies of the individual, and at the same time deprive him of the large amount of sleep rendered requisite by the exhausting labors of the position." In Michigan, it in particular affected women, especially educated lower-middle-class women. Wrote Van Deusen:

> The early married life of the wives of some of our smaller farmers seems especially calculated to predispose to this condition. Transferred to an isolated farm-house, very frequently from a home in which she had enjoyed a requisite measure of social and intellectual recreation, she is subjected to a daily routine of very monotonous household labor. Her new home, if it deserves the name, is, by a strict utilitarianism, deprived of everything which can suggest a pleasant thought: not a flower blooms in the garden; books she has, perhaps, but no time to read them . . . The urgency of farm work necessitates hurried, unsocial meals, and as night closes in, wearied with his exertions, the farmer is often accustomed to seek his bed at an early hour, leaving his wife to pass the long and lonely evening with her needle. Whilst the disposal of his crops, and the constant changes in the character of farm labor afford her husband sufficient variety and recreation, her daily life, and especially if she have also the unaided care of one or two ailing little children, is exhausting and depressing to a degree of which but few are likely to form any correct conception. From this class come many applications for the admission of female patients.

This description could not be faulted for insufficient sympathy. Its logic, however, was faulty. Why would the daily life of a farmer's wife become more depressing if she had to care for little children, for instance? Should not have such cares provided her with at least some variety and recreation that his exertions, the disposal of his crops, and the constant changes in the character of farm labor afforded her husband? No, it was not the hardship of the life on a farm that was the source of the neurasthenia among farmers' wives. It was, rather, that they could imagine a different, more genteel, life, and made a bad choice. It was the problem of Carol Kennicott of Sinclair Lewis's *Main Street* which won him the Nobel—the book called "a remarkable diary of the middle-class mind in America"—half a century after Van Deusen's "Observations" appeared in *AJI*. Carol did not fit in

Gopher Prairie, the small-town Minnesota community into which she moved after marrying its doctor, who, like the majority of the citizens, was quite content there. And what was Carol's way to deal with her maladjustment? She decided that Gopher Prairie was not good for its inhabitants and needed to be reformed. This would continue to be the problem "of the middle-class mind in America" (and Carol's "solution," would continue to be its solution). Indeed, Van Deusen recognized that farmers' wives were not the only ones susceptible to "nervous prostration." "The hot-house educational system of the present day," he wrote, "and the rash, restless, speculative character of many of our business enterprises, as well as professional engagements, are also strongly predisposing in their influence to debilitating forms of nervous disorder."[71]

Later in 1869, George Miller Beard also referred to the apparently widespread condition of "nervous prostration" or "nervous exhaustion" (for which "asthenia" was a common term in particular in Germany, though originating in Scotland) as "neurasthenia." Beard's article was published in the *Boston Medical and Surgical Journal*, which, perhaps, was more popular than the *AJI*, at least with some of the Brahmins.[72] William James, who was diagnosed as a "neurasthenic," helped to popularize the concept, referring to neurasthenia as "Americanitis." The term was borrowed from an author named Annie Payson Call whose 1891 book *Power Through Repose* James reviewed favorably, finding in it apparently helpful guidance for reducing the nervous tension which was cause of this national disease. Payson Call wrote: "Extreme nervous tension seems to be so peculiarly American, that a German physician coming to this country to practise . . . finally announced his discovery of a new disease which he chose to call 'Americanitis'. . . . we suffer from 'Americanitis' in all its unlimited varieties."[73] In James' case, the condition appeared to be more serious than usual, for his depression involved ideas of suicide. The eminent psychologist considered it quite normal, though; "I take it that no man is educated," he opined, "who has never dallied with the thought of suicide"—even unusually complicated neurasthenia, he thought, apparently, just as we think of "teenage angst" today, was only a stage in one's usual development. However bad it was, his neurasthenia never progressed to a level of clinical mental disease, but not everyone in his immediate family was as lucky.

George Miller Beard felt the scope of this particularly American problem warranted writing a several-hundred-page long "supplement" to his earlier work, titled *American Nervousness: Its Causes and Consequences* (1881), in the preface telling the reader:

> A new crop of diseases has sprung up in America, of which Great Britain until lately knew nothing, or but little. A class of functional diseases of the nervous system, now beginning to be known everywhere in civilization, seem to have first taken root under an American sky, whence their seed is being distributed.
>
> All this is modern, and originally American; and no age, no country, and no form of civilization, not Greece, nor Rome, nor Spain, nor the Netherlands, in the days of their glory, possessed such maladies. Of all the facts of modern sociology, this rise and growth of functional nervous disease in the northern part of America is one of the most stupendous, complex, and suggestive; to solve it in all its interlacings, to unfold its marvellous [sic] phenomena and trace them back to their sources and forward to their future developments, is to solve the problem of sociology itself. . . . [74]

Every one of the New World's contributions was a contribution on a truly mass scale, forever bigger, if not necessarily better, than anything that came from the puny storehouses of Western European countries. Moreover, the United States was a true democracy. And so, when at last this young colossus had a disease of its own, this was not just the "American disease"—it was the all-American disease.

In his "Observations," Dr. Van Deusen noted: "It is a well recognized fact in mental pathology, that in the asthenic the earliest marked morbid psychical symptom is distrust. It is true that this is usually preceded by irritability and other modifications of temper and disposition—grave symptoms always . . . but, as before remarked, the first clearly marked morbid sentiment is distrust. If the sufferer be an individual of deep religious feelings, to whom there is but the only, great and vital interest, there is distrust of God's promises, morbid views of personal relations to the church, and to society—in fine, what is improperly termed 'religious melancholy'. If the acquisition of gain and the possession of broad acres have been the great object of life, there are torturing apprehensions of poverty; the poor-house stares the patient in the face, and pauperism is his inevitable fate. Title deeds are filled with flaws, his notes are forgeries, and even gold and silver to him are worthless. If the conjugal relations have been peculiarly close and tender, there are the tortures of jealousy. In a few exceptional cases the morbid feeling has been general in its application." In sixteenth-century England, the English having a knack for calling a spade a spade, people suffering from such *disaffection* (or social maladjustment) were named "malcontents." American neurasthenics were uncomfortable in their society; they could not find a proper place for themselves in it; everything was suspect, because they were not sure of their own identity. If not relieved "from previous cares and anxieties" by a change of scene and occupation, and preserved by special "hygienic and medical agencies," Dr. Van Deusen believed, these neurotics were certain to develop "confirmed melancholia or mania," i.e., become clinically insane. In the open, pluralistic, and tolerant United States, the great majority of the sufferers, however, were able to successfully self-medicate. This self-medication consistently took the form of passionate if not fanatic dedication to causes that lacked the remotest connection to the personal interests of the people so dedicated, but had the attraction of presenting the American society in a critical light and thus justified their sense of disaffection and discomfort in it.

In the 1840s, a popular movement spread over the northern states, which was deemed by the psychiatric community to be a species of collective insanity. It was of a religious nature and called "Millerism" after the author of its central doctrine, Mr. Miller, who predicted the imminent destruction of the world. *AJI* devoted an article to this movement in January 1845. "We do not intend to give a history of [the doctrine]," it stated, "or to show that it is but a revival of a delusion which has often prevailed before, to the great injury of the community. The evil results from its recent promulgation are known to all, for we have scarcely seen a newspaper for some months past but contains accounts of suicides and insanity produced by it." A paper in upstate New York, for example, wrote: "Our exchange papers are filled with the most appalling accounts of the Miller delusion. We hear of suicides, insanity, and every species of folly." Another one, in Boston, reported "one lady and one gentleman, belonging to this city, were committed to the Insane Hospital last week from the influence of this horrible delusion. The man cut his throat but was stopped before he severed the large blood vessels. Another man cut his throat from the same cause, producing instant death." Similar accounts came from Connecticut, Philadelphia, and Baltimore. The Utica Asylum had an influx of patients "who became deranged from attending upon the preaching of this doctrine," most of them recovered, but some were considered incurable and remained. According to the reports of mental hospitals in the northern states for 1844, just three of them admitted 32 patients whose insanity was attributed to Millerism. In the opinion of the *AJI* author, "the prevalence of the yellow fever or of the cholera has never proved so great a calamity to this country as will the doctrine alluded to." This was so, because the suicides and commitments to asylums reported were but the tip of the iceberg: "Thousands who have not yet become deranged, have had their health impaired to such a degree as to unfit them for the duties of life forever; and especially in this case with females. The nervous system of many of those who have been kept in a state of excitement and alarm for months, has received a shock that will predispose them to all the various and distressing forms of nervous disease and to insanity, and will also render their offspring born hereafter, liable to the same." It was common of the unaffected to think that such delusions properly belonged "only to the dark ages of the world, or spread only among the illiterate and ignorant." But this was not so, because Millerism was embraced by "many intelligent and well-disposed persons." In fact, declared the *American Journal of Insanity,* "we believe for the most part, the promulgators and believers of this doctrine were sincere and pious people. We entirely acquit them of any bad intentions. In fact, such moral epidemics appear always to spread . . . 'without aid from any of the vices that degrade our social nature, and independent of any ideas of temporal interest.'"

Clearly, early American psychiatrists were more charitable towards those espousing beliefs they considered erroneous and even dangerous—they had more respect for the American people—than the vocal judges of those with opposing opinions today. In the opinion of the *AJI,* Millerism was an illness, an *epidemic* or *contagious monomania,* and it was as silly to place the responsibility for subscribing to the doctrine on its victims, as it would be to blame a tuberculosis patient for contracting the disease.

In 1845, apparently, Millerism was already on the wane, *AJI* stating, "This doctrine for the present, we presume is dead, and probably will not soon be revived," but, it predicted, there surely would be other such epidemics. "Let us inquire if there is no *improvement* to be made of it," the journal suggested, and if there can not be some measures adopted to prevent the spread of equally injurious though dissimilar delusions thereafter. The prevalence of one such delusion prepares the way for others. We must therefore expect them, and those who wish well to the community ought to strive to prevent their being extensively injurious.

Talking to the already injured did no good, the authors of the article argued,

> Reasoning with those thus affected is of no use. In fact, we were assured by one of the believers in the late delusions, that according to his observation, it but tended to confirm them. They are monomaniacs, and the more their attention is directed to the subject of their delusions by reasoning with them, the more is their *diseased faith* increased. We do not believe that much, if any, good has resulted from the numerous sermons and tracts that have been published exhibiting most clearly the calculations and predictions of Mr. Miller to be erroneous.

Instead, they issued the following recommendation, addressed particularly to heads of families:

> Do not go to *hear* any new, absurd and exciting doctrine taught, and keep away all those over whom you have influence. This need not and should not hinder you from obtaining a knowledge of all new truths and new doctrines; for such are in this country immediately published. Read about them if you wish, but do not go to *see* and *hear—to swell the throng of gazers and listeners,* for as has been said, such things spread chiefly by *contagion* and *imitation.*[75]

The wisdom of the preference for reading (as encouraging rational consideration of issues, over other ways of delivering information, which might wrap these issues in emotions clouding one's perception and discourage such consideration) aside, this advice was, most probably, wrong in its essence. It is unlikely that the popularity of Millerism was due to contagion. Rather, it reflected the pre-existing condition of neurasthenia among the doctrine's subscribers. This condition was already very widespread in the 1840s in the advanced European nations, such as Britain and France; it must have been widespread in the explicitly freedom-oriented and rapidly articulating the implications of its nationalism United States. Indeed, as we saw, within just a few decades it would emerge as "the American disease."[76] In the 1840s, apparently, Millerism provided relief from it for many, helping them to make sense of their uncomfortable experience (explaining why they felt the way they did and legitimating their feelings) and thus orienting them and providing some form of a structure that they lacked in their lives. This very general need for therapy would persist and increase in the course of American history.

However accurate or mistaken in regard to the contagious nature of collective insanity, the early writer for *AJI* was right in predicting that the country won't see the last of it with the waning of Millerism. Similar movements would convulse sectors of American population. The message or doctrine at their center would often be as delusionary (i.e., a product of pure fantasy without any connection to objective reality), but in the later cases, such "diseased faith" would be of a political, rather than religious, nature. Of course, in the United States, politics and religion have interpenetrated each other: politics, from very early on, became the American religion, while traditional religions were essentially reinterpreted in the light of, and as, American nationalism, which made the two very easy to combine and extremely difficult to distinguish. As schizophrenics are exceptionally attuned to their cultural environment, this interpenetration has been clearly evident in the writings of that portion of the asylums' insane whom we would today diagnose as such from the first moment such data were collected. And yet, even these intricately confused ruminations demonstrated the ascendancy of the political realm over the religious.[77] In their mysterious way, such schizophrenic maunderings reflected the transformation of the culture around them as a whole. Those suffering from the mild, run-of-the-mill, all-American form of mental disease, or neurasthenia, *represented* the culture as a whole.

As we saw in Jarvis's discussion of increasing causes of insanity, early American psychiatrists noticed the rise of politics vis-à-vis religion as a disturbing factor in the consciousness of the community. *AJI* referred to it in a matter-of-fact fashion, as if self-evident and requiring no explanation. Dr. Brigham, for instance, wrote in April 1849 in his capacity as the editor:

"All great excitements are represented by their victims in Mad Houses. The French Revolution, the American Revolution, the Reformation of Luther, all produced an increase in insanity. Dr. Macdonald, late Physician of the Bloomingdale Asylum, near New York, says, 'within the writer's own experience, the Anti-Masonic excitement, the Jackson excitement, and the Anti-Jackson excitement, the Bank excitement, the Abolition excitement, and the Speculation excitement, have each furnished the Asylum with inmates.'" Brigham did not see much difference between all these "excitements," and his editorial was a preface to a survey of episodes of "money-making mania," but most of the "excitements" he mentioned were of obviously political nature.[78]

Then there was the announcement of a new form of clearly political insanity from Germany. This was the "democratic disease," whose "virus," according to the author of the doctoral thesis in medicine, "De morbo democratic, nova insaniae forma," a certain M. Groddeck, "has of late circulated throughout the Continental Nations with a rapidity contrasting strongly with the solemn and stately march of cholera." An editor of *AJI* commented in 1851, "Its development, indeed, has been all but simultaneous in the great European Capitals, but we know not that it has before occurred to any one to treat it medically."[79] It appears from this reaction that, while he did not consider the diagnosis of the democratic insanity surprising, he was not sure that the disease was serious enough to justify psychiatric intervention. In the early period on which I decided to focus, the *American Journal of Insanity* drew most of its examples of "moral epidemics" or "collective monomanias" of political nature from Europe. Europe was far away, and in the United States, by 1851, no political "excitement" reached the level of "contagious monomania." This might have been the lull before the storm, for this truly democratic society, worshiping equality above any interpretation of God, of so many of which it has been so tolerant, would certainly have its share of strictly political—and clearly democratic—"moral epidemics."

In June 2005, the *Washington Post* announced that, according to the latest numbers, "the United States is poised to rank No. 1 globally for mental illness." The study on which this cheery announcement was based was the famous National Comorbidity Survey—Replication, headed by Ronald Kessler of Harvard and NIMH, and already referred to in this book on several occasions. According to the *Washington Post* correspondent, "The survey focused on four major categories of mental illness: anxiety disorders (such as panic and post-traumatic stress disorders); mood disorders (such as major depression and bipolar disease); impulse control disorders (such as attention-deficit/hyperactivity disorder); and substance abuse. Almost half of Americans meet the criteria for such an illness at some point in their lives, the survey found." The correspondent quoted Kessler as saying that, "because schizophrenia, autism, and some other severe and relatively common disorders were not included, actual prevalence rates are somewhat higher."[80] We can conclude from this that one in every two Americans is at the very least a "neurasthenic." Of course, we no longer call the national disease by this completely outdated name. Though "neurasthenia" remains a diagnostic category in the World Health Organization's *International Classification of Diseases* (*ICD*), the *Diagnostic and Statistical Manual of Mental Disorders* (*DSM*) of our own American Psychiatric Association— the descendant of the Association of the Medical Superintendents of American Institutions for the Insane—no longer uses the term. We now refer to this widespread illness in a more scientific manner—sometimes, indeed, as anxiety disorders, impulse-control disorders, and also as mild depression. What William James considered "Americanitis" is mild by comparison with schizophrenia and manic-depressive illness. It is a mild form of the insanity on which the asylums focused—the persistent malaise of the sort that affected Edward Jarvis, the inability to find one's place in an open, fluid, competitive society with ever increasing amount of choices. Today so many young Americans suffer from it (the *Washington Post* report says "mental illness is very much a disease of youth. Half of those who will ever be diagnosed with a mental disorder show signs of the disease by age 14, and three-quarters by age 24") that it is considered normal, dismissed as a troublesome but inevitable developmental stage, like menstruation or menopause in women. It is not a severe mental disease that would lead to the confusion of subjective and objective realities, just a mental discomfort, however profoundly felt. Does the term "Americanitis" fit it?—after all, only half of the American population, according to the latest statistics, not more that 160 million people, suffer from it. Perhaps to call it the "American disease" (as some Russian psychiatrists were wont to do) is an exaggeration? And statistics are unreliable anyhow.

Afterword

Madness was not brought about by the progress of civilization. It was brought about by nationalism, the cultural framework of modernity, by the best this secular, egalitarian, essentially humanistic and democratic image of reality has to offer: its insistence on the dignity and creativity of man, and on the value of the human life, on equality and liberty of members in the political community, on their right and capacity to construct their own destinies, to love, and to be happy. It is the other side of the coin, a proof that, as with most things in life, benefits are usually associated with costs. But, having been brought about by its best features, madness has continuously fueled nationalism's most destructive passions, caused an appalling amount of harm, and may well end by destroying the Western civilization. We must understand it well, become aware of its implications, and stop it. And this presupposes the development of a reliable way to acquire objective knowledge about human affairs—the development of *human science,* capable of progress.

In this sense, the approach I took has already proven to be remarkably (and unpredictably) productive. It seems to have uncovered a spring veritably gushing with research questions and possibilities, which could not be asked or considered within the conventional paradigms embedded within the old mind-body ontological framework. The reason for this is that, in distinction to the conventional paradigms, this approach, connecting as it does the mind and its symbolic environment, and treating the mental process on the individual and the collective level (mind and culture) as one, allows for discerning the very mechanisms of the causal chains that lead from the cause to the effect in every case of human affairs. Whichever aspect of specifically human reality one attempts to understand (be it the economy, international relations, religious institutions and movements, family relations, or what not), the causes and effects are always symbolic, i.e., cultural, but the mechanisms through which the former translate into the latter are psychological—they occur on another level. This, in turn, makes readily imaginable links between human phenomena that appeared obviously independent before: new hypotheses simply pop up all around.

Given the ways we used to think about most important human phenomena, however, many of these new questions and possibilities may appear truly disconcerting, so that at times one wishes to replace the metaphor of a fertile spring of ideas with that of Pandora's box. As I was writing this book, I was constantly surprised by evidence of connections of madness, in its clinical and subclinical forms, to numerous aspects of modern life. This evidence was "unintentional" in Bloch's sense, its sources were "witnesses despite themselves," and I neither expected to find it nor planned to interrogate them on the particular subjects they were illuminating. This testimony, unsought for and unwittingly offered, however, was not to be denied. It was no idle prattle: madness has been at the root of a wide range of phenomena one would never think of as its effects. To me, in fact, the consistent suggestion of the documents that so it was, in every case, came as a shock. Yet, in every case, upon consideration, this possibility turned out to make perfect sense logically. And, just as with the contents of Pandora's box, once out in the open, it could not be disregarded.

The first such connection to strike me was the role schizophrenic mental disease played in shaping modern literature. (I hope it goes without saying that I had not set out to prove any such thing.) English language modern poetry, it now appears to me undeniable, has been a creation of madness. From eighteenth century on it was not simply the work of people admittedly suffering from manic depression or full-blown schizophrenia, but has been both saturated with peculiar-to-schizophrenics abnormalities of thought and language, that is, uncontrolled linguistic creativity characteristic of schizophrenia, and represented a characteristic of such sufferers turn to language for help, a desperate, though unconscious attempt to name, and thus make sense of, their horrifying experience. The undesigned (and often formless) form to which the vain efforts of these very sick people gave rise, was perceived by their audience, much of which shared their plight, though at a lower degree of severity, and thus was naturally drawn to and appreciative of what they wrote, as *art,* i.e., as *intentional aesthetic construction,* and, as a result, acquired its authority. This, in turn, allowed succeeding generations of literary aspirants to study this form and craft it consciously. Today one does not have to be a madman to write poetry, but madmen continue to turn to language for help as before and very often it is the poetry of madmen that strikes one as the most poignant.[1]

For a lover of poetry and an occasional poet in English, this discovery is troubling enough. However, the role of madness in shaping modern literature has not been limited to the English-speaking world, and neither has it been confined to one particular genre. It has been at the root of arguably the most important, formative literary style of the modern period—Romanticism—leading to it, and molding it, both in Germany and in France. Romanticism, in the creation of which the Romantics whom we know by name in fact participated unselfconsciously, that is, only passively, too, was taken by innocent critics to be an intentional artistic device: Chateaubriand, said already Gautier, invented melancholy and modern suffering. So now students of literature study it as a stage in a secular aesthetic trend. But Romanticism is far more than just an extremely important literary style: it is a pervasive variant of modern consciousness or "mentality,"[2] often dominant and, if not, vying for dominance with the other major variant, that of Enlightenment rationalism. As such, it colors attitudes to reality and thus our existential experience, and informs much of our conduct in life and specific actions, including political actions. This turns into a vicious circle: madness generates Romanticism which generates more madness which generates Romanticism which . . . , and so on and so forth.

The shock of these literary discoveries had hardly worn off when I had to cope with a worse one. A specter from my past, which haunted my earlier decades, was confronting me—the specter of Karl Marx. I firmly believed to have already said everything I could ever want to say about him;[3] there was certainly no place for him in a book about schizophrenia and manic-depressive illness. But no, here he was—in Paris precisely at the time when the first psychiatric periodical in the world began publication and all the lights of the City of Lights blazed upon *aliénation mentale*—again taunting me and demanding attention. Madness as the inspiration for Marxism? For the most influential social doctrine and political ideology of our time? In my life, it has been such: I grew up in the Soviet Union; my parents' lives were consumed, broken by the Marxist state; my grandparents were Bolshevik revolutionaries, if not of the first, certainly of the second rank— and paid for this with the same coin of separation from their young children, effectively orphaned, of long years of imprisonment and convict labor in the worst camps of the GULAG, in the case of my mother's father, of death under NKVD torture—never giving up their Marxist beliefs. I would not want to think that the problem underneath it all was mental disease, that the mighty historical force we thought ruled our destinies was madness. But I had to reexamine "The Economic and Philosophical Manuscripts of 1844": Marx's focus on alienation in Paris in 1843–1844 was too startling to be dismissed as a mere coincidence. To me, this reexamination provided sufficient proof that it is indeed the alienation of the French alienists that lies at the basis of the Marxist doctrine that still guides the lives of so many. I shall resist the temptation to develop this proof and make it sufficient for others: I am done with Marx (I hope). But it is clear that those who are not done with him, whether as social theorists or as political actors, will now have to take the connection between madness and his doctrine into account, because it might radically change this doctrine's very nature.

And yet, however shocking is the discovery of madness at the root of modern English poetry, Romantic mentality, and Marxist doctrine, it is much less important than the possibility, very strongly suggested by "unintentional" and thus eminently credible evidence, that madness lies underneath modern violent crime and—still more distressing, because we want political actors to be rational actors who know the difference between right and wrong—politics. On the whole, violence before the age of nationalism (or outside it, since every historical time is geo-politically located) was *rational* and, in its own way, as natural—nature being inescapably red of tooth and claw—as that in the wild. It was, of course, very common. Rape was in a day's work and considered a crime only insofar as it concerned property of someone whose property was a matter of social concern, while murder, or mutilation which one would accidentally survive, which usually was considered a crime on the individual level, was committed whenever it would most efficiently lead to the achievement of any desired goal, be it robbery or political victory. This instrumental rationality applied on the collective level as well. Genghis Khan wiped out entire populations of settlements which resisted his conquest, leaving no man, woman, or child alive, but he did so neither because he enjoyed depriving sentient creatures of life nor because he felt called to do so by some power on high, and he was not, so historians tell us, a cruel man. One's heart bleeds for the wide-eyed helpless cubs whose sire can no longer protect them, but can a lion that devours the young of another in an attempt to claim the females of the tribe for his own be called cruel? Murder could also be committed as a duty because it was, traditionally, the right thing to do, as in family vendettas of the early feudal period. It was not one's decision that this was the right thing to do, but a dictate of a tradition which one perceived as inviolable universal law and thus had no choice but to obey. The rationality in such cases was value rationality. Already to sixteenth-century Englishmen it was apparent that acts of violence committed by madmen did not answer to either of these descriptions. The legal preoccupations of the early psychiatric establishments (it is remarkable that most of the first psychiatric periodicals, in France, the United States, Britain, Russia, and even Germany were medicolegal publications and showed a strong interest in criminology[4]) reflected this awareness. Indeed, it is obvious that madness has changed the very nature of violent crime, dramatically increasing the irrational element in it, making the action in many instances expressive, rather than instrumental, and undertaken for the sheer pleasure in inflicting suffering, and making individual responsibility—the pivot of modern law—a consideration largely irrelevant to its understanding and prevention. Even when seemingly politically or ideologically motivated (one can as well think about Lee Harvey Oswald as Jack the Ripper) acts of violence by *individuals,* on examination, more often than not turn to be brought about by the "nawghtye mallenchollye," similar to that of the Elizabethan Peter Berchet—which throws a formidable wrench into the innermost workings of the legal machine and undermines the legitimacy of the penal system. (Remarkably, just as the part of mentally ill people among violent criminals skyrocketed, detective fiction—the fiction of super-rationality par excellence—made its appearance, and the battle of masterminds, the criminal's and the detective's, became one of the most engrossing forms of modern entertainment. Here is a subject for another dissertation—in English, comparative literature, or sociology of literature.) But it is precisely in the ideological motivation that the larger problem lies. The majority of the famous cases of murder, which provoke an outcry of, and terrify, the community, such as campus shootings, serial killings, and political assassinations, are indeed "ideological," involving the identification of a specific individual (e.g., President Lincoln, Congresswoman Giffords, Berchet's intended victim Sir Christopher Hatton) or group (for instance, prostitutes in the case of Jack the Ripper or athletes in school shootings) as the incarnation of evil, which the killer is called on to exterminate. Such ideological motivation is no less delusional than the implacable reasoning of Garshin's hero in "Red Flower," and the delusionally inspired murderers are as desperate and as careless of their own lives in pursuit of their goal. I would venture a hypothesis that all such murders are committed by people who are severely mentally ill and suggest that early diagnosis is what the efforts of those who wish to prevent them should be focused on.

Madness Writ Large

Nineteenth-century psychiatrists, as the reader saw, were also aware that politics increasingly supplied exciting causes for mental illness. Among other publications on the subject in the *American Journal of Insanity* there was, reproduced via London *Lancet*, Brièrre de Boismont's letter to *L'Union Médicale* on the "Influence of Revolution [of 1848] in Developing Insanity in Paris." The eminent alienist wrote there, among other things, about "patients, whose derangement might be fairly attributed to the working of the new political ideas":

> These were not dejected and sad; on the contrary, they had proud, gay, and enthusiastic looks, and were very loquacious; they were constantly writing memorials, constitutions, &c., proclaimed themselves great men, the deliverers, and took the rank of generals, members of the government, &c. It has long been maintained, that madness often bears the imprint of pride. I declare that I never saw this fact so forcibly borne out as with the patients whom the Revolution of February drove mad; particularly those, who, imbued with socialist, communist, and regenerating ideas, believed themselves destined to play a conspicuous part in the world. Going through the wards, a few days ago, with one of my professional brethren, we stopped with one of those patients whose disposition was originally of a kind and

peaceful description, but who had grown restless and enthusiastic, by being torn from his usual and regular occupations by the excitement of the times, and flung into the street, the clubs, and amidst the working classes. He spoke as follows . . . : "I perceive that people want to make it appear that I am mad, but I am proud of the glory which will be shed on my name when posterity will do justice to me, and ask, with painful astonishment, how the author of such useful and philanthropic views could ever have been thought mad! Why should I grieve at this injustice, however; was not Tasso locked up under the same suspicion?"[5]

It was always encouraging to be in a good company. In accordance with the belief then prevailing in the psychiatric community that such events were "moral epidemics," which spread by contagion, articles of this nature concentrated on the contribution of political "excitement" to the increase of inmate population in mental asylums, but the descriptions contained in them suggested, rather, that certain kinds of politics were a magnet for already sick people. The cases of the Russian Revolutions of 1905 and 1917, in which more evidence on this subject presented itself, support this suggestion.

As the discoveries of the connections between madness and all these central aspects of modern life were completely unpremeditated, I have not planned to include an extensive discussion of madness in politics in this book. It would deserve, at the very least, a separate chapter. The subject is extremely provocative and, for a political scientist, tantalizing, but its improvised examination in an afterword would be out of place. I shall, therefore, limit myself to the formulation of a series of hypotheses, organized in the form of twelve points containing premises and conclusions, which place the connection between mental disease and political action within the general argument of the present study and make clear the logic behind it. To test these hypotheses would be the task of other scholars and books.

1. Nationalism implies an open society, which makes anomie pervasive and the formation of individual identity one's own responsibility, and therefore problematic.

2. This general problematization of individual identity and specific problems with the formation of identity lead to degrees (clinical and subclinical) of mental impairment, derangement, and dysfunction, today recognized as

schizophrenia and manic-depressive illness, the common symptoms of which are social maladjustment (chronic discomfort in one's environment) and chronic discomfort (dis-ease) with one's self, the sense of self oscillating between self-loathing and delusions of grandeur, megalomania, most frequently (in cases of unipolar depression) fixing on self-loathing, and in rare cases deteriorating into the terrifying sense of a complete loss of self (in the acute psychosis of full-fledged schizophrenia).

3. This mental disease—madness—reaches its clinical level in a minority of cases (even if it is a very large minority, as in the United States). But the pervasive anomie of modern national societies affects very large numbers of people—statistics claim, close to 50 percent of Americans today, for example—and therefore, makes very large numbers of people socially maladjusted and deeply dissatisfied with themselves—i.e., as the English were the first to recognize, "malcontent," dis-eased, uncomfortable in their existential experience.

4. In itself, even before it leads to, and irrespective of, such general malaise among the carriers of the national consciousness, nationalism radically changes their social and political experience. Because of its secularism, egalitarianism, and insistence on popular sovereignty, as I have argued in the first two books of this trilogy and various essays, it makes people activist. It follows logically from the explicit or implicit recognition that man has only one life, that social reality, at least, is a thing of his making, and that all men are equal—that nothing can justify this one life falling short of giving full satisfaction, that men are responsible for all its disappointments, and that everyone has the right to change reality that disappoints. It becomes relatively easy to mobilize national populations in causes of social reform and civil society comes into being.

5. But it is very often mental disease that shapes the causes for which the population is mobilized, thus profoundly affecting the nature of social and political action in nations. Specifically, madness makes for "ideological" activism—which is, in effect, delusionally inspired. On the individual level, as already noted, unless spent in the pursuit of red flowers, this leads to the characteristic modern murder. On the collective level it takes the far more problematic form of ideological politics.

6. Ideological politics is a specific form of politics brought about by nationalism. They are irrational in the sense of being motivated by a dedi-

cation (passionate, if not fanatic) to causes which in the large majority of cases lack the remotest connection to the personal experience—and therefore objective interests—of the participants, but are characterized by their capacity to justify and explain the discomfort these participants feel with their self and social environment. At their core invariably lie visions that bear the most distinctive mark of a schizophrenic delusion: the loss of the understanding of the symbolic nature of human social reality and the confusion between symbols and their referents, when the symbols themselves become objective reality.

7. All *revolutions*—a modern form of political action, in contrast to spontaneous rebellions and uprisings, which happen everywhere throughout history—are of this kind. It is significant that, in distinction to the majority of participants in rebellions and uprisings, who come from the lower classes, revolutionaries are mostly recruited from the privileged, and specifically from the educated, strata particularly affected by mental disease. The majority of them, especially in the leadership ranks, are activated not by specific, pragmatic interests, but by a desire to change the society radically on the basis of some vaguely defined ideal. The change is predicated on the destruction of what the ideal is to replace. Thus, while the ideal is vague, the destructive, violent impulse is clearly focused and, with symbols and their referents confused, actual people are killed because of what they represent, rather than because of what they do.

8. The core ideal and the enemy which the revolutionary movement targets are delusions and are very likely to emerge in the disordered minds of, and offered by, actual schizophrenics. However, the overwhelming majority of those who accept and carry on the message, i.e., of the revolutionaries, participants in the revolution, must be of necessity recruited from among the mildly mentally ill, those suffering from the general anomic malaise, neuroses or neurasthenia, from what we refer to today as spectrum disorders. In effect, they use the schizophrenic's delusions as therapy for their minor ills. Their presentation of these minor personal ills under the cover of a general cause serves to conceal their mental illness from themselves and from others. Their recognition of a schizophrenic's delusion as a general cause conceals his/her major mental disease, presents him/her (and allows him/her to self-represent) as a prophet, a genius, etc., and may elevate him/her to the position of the revolutionary leader, if he (or she) is

available for this. (I asked the reader earlier to ponder what might have happened to John Nash, if he were a German rather than an American, and born in the previous decade rather than in 1928. Let me ask now, in a similar vein, might not Hitler have ended up in a mental hospital, rather than becoming the adored Führer of his people, were he an American?)

9. Schizophrenics are singularly attuned to the surrounding culture. I have characterized the schizophrenic mental process as free-ranging culture in the individual brain; their mind being completely deindividualized, and their will completely incapacitated, it is culture in general that processes itself in their healthy brain and language itself that speaks through them. Schizophrenic delusions consist of familiar and suggestive tropes, which make their claims persuasive and even self-evident. This explains the centrality of two themes in violent ideological politics of the last two centuries in the West: the evil rich (capitalism) versus the good poor; and Jews (now Israel) against the world. To demonstrate that this is indeed a trope, I will share with you an old Soviet joke. A certain innocent (perhaps a college student) asks: "Who is responsible for the silting of the Lake Baikal?" and receives the answer: "Jews and bikers." Surprised, he asks: "Why bikers?" Somehow it appears self-evident that Jews would be responsible for every disaster.

10. Different types of nationalism favor different types of self-medication through social/political activism. Thus individualistic nationalisms, naturally, encourage individual activism, and this, in cases of activism prompted by madness, translates into the delusionally inspired violent crime. It is in England that we have Jack the Ripper as well as first political assassinations of this sort, and it is the United States that today supplies us with most examples of serial killings and school/university shootings. Obversely, individualistic nationalisms discourage violent collective activism. Individualistic nations are no strangers to ideologically or delusionally inspired collective action. Such action in them, however, is usually nonviolent (though activists may approve of violence by others) and has a number of other characteristics which distinguish it from what is likely to happen in collectivistic nations. Even as participants in collective actions members of individualistic nations retain a strong sense of their individuality, separateness from the collective. They do not meld with it; the pervasive individualism of their national consciousness makes them believe that they act

as individuals. When suffering from the anomic malaise, each one of them turns against the society that makes them, each individually, uncomfortable, their own society, their own nation, that is. Thus American political activism has been very often anti-American, whatever specific problem happens to be at the core of the activist ideology in any particular case. Another outlet delusional activism finds in the United States is hard to characterize as "ideological" at all—early American psychiatrists, I am sure, would see in it episodes of temporary collective monomania. This outlet is offered to the sufferers from "Americanitis" by presidential elections. One year out of four such ardor seizes a sector of the American public (small but vocal), that a naturalized American such as myself can only helplessly shrug shoulders. It appears as if the election of a particular candidate is a matter of life or death for millions, while it is obvious that it cannot possibly have anything even remotely approximating such an effect, and is likely not to have much effect at all, the United States being a true democracy, which runs itself.

11. Collectivistic nationalisms encourage violent collective action. Thus all the great revolutions—the French Revolution, the Russian Revolution, the German, that is, National Socialist, revolution—happened in collectivistic nations. Such political activism is more likely to have anti-Semitic motivation in the framework of ethnic nationalisms, and anticapitalist motivation in the framework of civic nationalisms. But, of course, the revolutionary ideology in most cases would combine these two "pure" motives. In addition, in collectivistic and especially in ethnic nationalisms delusional politics often take the commonly recognizable form of nationalistic xenophobic politics—that is, the form of hostility to the other: we have numerous examples of this in the past twenty-five years, in the former Soviet Union, Eastern Europe (especially Yugoslavia), Africa, and so on.

12. The sense of national inferiority—which is a common characteristic of ethnic nationalisms—in addition to encouraging delusionally motivated violent xenophobic collective activism as therapy for the psychological, mental ravages of anomie, contributes to mental disease on its own. It adds to the problems with one's individual identity the dissatisfaction with one's national identity, in which one tends to seek comfort from personal dissatisfactions. This might explain certain kinds of political activism in the Middle East today. It clearly appears that there we are dealing with the

phenomenon of existential envy on the collective level: one is so ashamed of
one's national self—i.e., of one's national identity, of being a member of
one's nation (which, in ethnic nationalism, if one sees oneself as such, one
cannot abandon), that the only way of coping with this is the destruction of
those other nations vis-à-vis which one feels one's nation to be particularly
inferior. One's self-loathing (personal and national) is reoriented onto such
others, and the anger and violence, which would, under different circumstances, lead to suicide, are diverted into terrorism (which for those who
still have the secret desire to do away with themselves has the additional
advantage of being easily combined with suicide). Paradoxically, in general,
the rates of severe (clinical) mental disturbance should be inversely proportional to the possibilities of engaging in ideologically motivated collective
activism, that is, necessarily the highest in individualistic nations, and
higher in collectivistic civic nations, than in ethnic ones. Thus most aggressive and xenophobic nationalisms—the worst for the world around—would
be, in fact, of all nationalisms, the best for the mental health of their individual members. Yet another reminder, sadly, that there is no free lunch.

The above remarks, it should be emphasized, are not empirically proven
claims, but only possible directions for further study. They are, however,
logically plausible and strongly suggested by preliminary and—what is
more—unintentionally gleaned evidence, and so deserve serious consideration.

A Note on Education

But whether or not political activism offers therapy to some sufferers from
schizophrenia and manic-depression in their clinical and subclinical forms,
clearly, very many continue to suffer from these awful, debilitating conditions. Therefore, whatever the additional and unforeseen effects of madness and whether they exist at all, the primary task is to stop it—to arrest
the increase in its rates and to prevent its development in individuals. Can
this be done? Yes. But there is no easy way to do it and one cannot expect
results by tomorrow. There are no magic pills and individual psychotherapy
will not do. The disease is essentially cultural, it is society itself that must

be cured, and what is required, therefore, in this society, at least, is nothing less than revamping of the entire system of education, from kindergarten through college, beginning with the education of educators. From very early age, children should be taught about the nature of modern society, its positive features and its negative features, not in a moralistic and judgmental, "good guys versus bad guys," but in a clear-sighted realistic, "this is what there is" way. The national values of freedom, equality, choice should be cultivated, because we cherish them and will not give them up, but children should be taught the psychological price they come with. If one must meet the costs, it is best to be prepared for them. They should be taught that they are expected, by the nature of society they inhabit, to be in control of their social self-construction (and thus destiny), that, ultimately, they are in control, but that the indispensable condition for being in control is knowing themselves. They should be taught to analyze their likes and dislikes, to separate interests imposed from the outside from those that spring from within. The message should be reinforced at every stage of continuing education and remedial resources should be made available at every next stage for cases in which it fails to sink in at the preceding one. Preparing young people to cope with the systemic demands of modern society, and most specifically with the responsibility for the formation of one's identity, should be the focus of general education, and general education should be the focus of the educational system. The teaching of history, philosophy, literature, and civics at every level should be geared to that. Every existing component of, and every addition to, the school and college curricula should be most carefully examined for present and possible consequences for identity formation, and everything that might interfere with it or make it problematic should be eliminated, unless provided with an antidote.

This would obviously involve a dramatic change in educational philosophy and, in higher education, specifically, a turn away from the prevailing emphasis on technical subjects and professional training, a result of badly misunderstood priorities, in turn reflecting the complete lack of understanding of the colossal cultural problem, unprecedented in the history of the human mind, we are faced with. Let us keep in sight the probability (approximating the certainty of a fact) that, even if we produce ten times as many engineers and computer specialists as today, this would not keep

China from taking our place as the most powerful economy in the world within a decade, but if we keep increasing the rates of schizophrenia and manic depression among us, our position in the world and—far more important—our quality of life will continue to deteriorate. Revamping the educational system, admittedly, is an arduous task, it would be very difficult to do it well and dangerous to do it badly. But it would be suicidal not to do it at all. This, unfortunately, is what there is. Modern society is exceedingly complex, and our inability to cope with this complexity makes us mad—surely avoiding madness is worth the most strenuous effort.

The inexorable rise of China, which is very much on the American mind today, brings to mind that persistent "anomaly" in the findings of Western epidemiologists, puzzling them since the early days of their profession: the remarkably low rates of the very kind of mental disease that ravages the West in Asia. Fear not: it is not the relative absence of madness that makes China rise (though it will certainly help it not to fall). But this still leaves the question: what makes these, in some cases definitely modern, in all others modernizing with astonishing rapidity, societies, all embracing nationalism and implementing its principles of secularism, egalitarianism, and popular sovereignty at least as successfully as Europe did in the nineteenth century, immune to the modern mental disease? Why don't the orienting principles of nationalism disorient the Orient? Would monotheism and logic have anything to do with this? Could the root of the problem (not its cause, perhaps, but a necessary condition) lie deeper than nationalism, reaching to the very foundation of our civilization? Even a most tentative answer to this question would be premature at present. But it is clear where I am led by the great forces that form our projects: to a comparative study of civilizations.

Notes

Introduction

1. The phrase is Luhrmann's; T. M. Luhrmann, *Of Two Minds: The Growing Disorder in American Psychiatry* (New York: Vintage, 2000), 13.
2. Liah Greenfeld, *Nationalism: Five Roads to Modernity* (Cambridge: Harvard University Press, 1992) and *The Spirit of Capitalism: Nationalism and Economic Growth* (Cambridge: Harvard University Press, 2001).
3. I first developed this idea in the 2004 Gellner Lecture at the London School of Economics, "Nationalism and the Mind," *Nations and Nationalism* 11, no. 3 (2005): 325–341.
4. Marcia Angell, "The Epidemic of Mental Illness: Why?," *review* of *The Emperor's New Drugs: Exploding the Antidepressant Myth*, by Irving Kirsch; *Anatomy of an Epidemic: Magic Bullets, Psychiatric Drugs and the Astonishing Rise of Mental Illness in America*, by Robert Whitaker; *Unhinged: The Trouble with Psychiatry—A Doctor's Revelations About a Profession in Crisis*, by Daniel Carlat, *New York Review of Books*, June 23, 2011.
5. Jules Baillarger, "Introduction," *Annales Medico-Psychologiques* 1 (1843): vii.
6. Karl Popper, "Conjectures and Refutations," *Objective Knowledge: An Evolutionary Approach* (New York: Oxford University Press, 1972).
7. Émile Durkheim, *The Rules of Sociological Method* (New York: Free Press, 1982); Max Weber, *Economy and Society* (Berkeley: University of California Press, 1978).
8. Marc Bloch, *The Historian's Craft* (New York: Putnam, 1953), 60–65.
9. Ibid., 151.
10. I first used this term in "Communing with the Spirit of Max Weber," *Nationalism and the Mind: Essays on Modern Culture* (Oxford: OneWorld, 2006), 176–202.
11. See Marc Bloch, *Feudal Society* (University of Chicago Press, 1964).
12. Angell, *Epidemic.*
13. Susan Seligson, "Students in Crisis," *BU Today,* April 26, 2011.

14. See chapters 3, 4, and 8.

15. Kim Hopper et al. eds., *Recovery from Schizophrenia: An International Perspective* (New York: Oxford University Press, 2007).

16. Luhrmann, *Two Minds*.

17. "Bolsheviks"—"those of the majority"; "Mensheviks"—"those of the minority."

18. As the example of Freud, indeed, demonstrates. See Joseph Ben-David and R. Collins, "Social Factors in the Origins of a New Science: The Case of Psychology," *American Sociological Review* 31 (1966): 451–465.

19. See chapters 3 and 4.

20. Louis Sass, *Madness and Modernism: Insanity in the Light of Modern Art, Literature, and Thought* (New York: Basic Books, 1992), 381. Regarding the accidental discovery of drugs; see also Denis S. Charney and E. J. Nestler, *Neurobiology of Mental Illness,* 2nd ed. (New York: Oxford University Press, 2004), 491.; Arvid Carlsson, "A Paradigm Shift in Brain Research," *Science* 294, no. 5544 (2001): 1021–1024; Arvid Carlsson and D. T. Wong, "A Note on the Discovery of Selective Serotonin Reuptake Inhibitors," *Life Sciences* 61, no. 12 (1997): 1203; and David Healey, *Let Them Eat Prozac: The Pharmaceutical Industry and Depression* (New York: NYU Press, 2004), 18–19. Regarding neuroleptics, specifically, see David Healy, *The Creation of Psychopharmacology* (Cambridge: Harvard University Press, 2004).

21. See, in particular, Sass, "Appendix: Neurobiological Considerations," *Madness*.

22. William Cromie, "Half of us suffer from mental illness, survey finds," Harvard Gazette, June 16, 2005 http://www.news.harvard.edu/ gazette/2005/06.16/05-suicide.html (accessed June 26, 2012).

23. See Paul Linde, *Of Spirits and Madness: An American Psychiatrist in Africa* (New York: McGraw-Hill, 2002).

24. E. Fuller Torrey, *The Invisible Plague: The Rise of Mental Illness from 1750 to the Present* (Piscataway, NJ: Rutgers University Press, 2001), 315.

25. See George Cheyne, *The English Malady* (London: Strahan, 1733); Cecil A. Moore's "The English Malady," in his *Backgrounds of English Literature, 1700–1760* (Minneapolis: University of Minnesota Press, 1953); Vieda Skultans, *English Madness: Ideas on Insanity, 1580–1890* (Piscataway, NJ: Routledge and Kegan Paul, 1979).

26. Marcel Gauchet and Gladys Swain, *La pratique de l'esprit humain* (Paris: Gallimard, 2007); also Roy Porter and Mark S. Micale, eds., *Discovering the History of Psychiatry* (New York: Oxford, 1994).

27. Michel Foucault, *Folie et déraison: Histoire de la folie à l'âge classique.* Paris: Union Générale d'Éditions, 1961. Translated by Richard Howard as *Madness and Civilization: History of Insanity in the Age of Reason* (New York: Pantheon Books, 1965) see also H. C. Erik Midelfort, "Madness and Civilization in Early Modern Europe: A Reappraisal of Michel Foucault," in Barry Smart, ed., *Michel Foucault: Critical Assessments* (New York: Routeledge, 1995), 117–133.

28. I am using this concept in the sense in which it was used by Michael Polanyi in "Life's Irreducible Structure" *Science* 160, no. 3838 (1968): 1308–1312; i.e., in the sense of the "strong form of emergence." A more extensive discussion is to be found in chapter 1.

29. The way it was envisioned by Durkheim; see, in particular, *The Elementary Forms of Religious Life* trans. Karen Elise Fields (New York: Free Press, 1995).

30. See appendices to chapters 3 and 4.

31. See Durkheim, *The Division of Labor in Society*, trans. W.D. Halls (New York: Free Press, 1997) and *Suicide* ed. George Simpson, trans. John Spaulding and George Simpson (New York: Free Press, 1997).

32. Rick Weiss, "Study: US Leads in Mental Illness, Lags in Treatment," *Washington Post*, June 7, 2005.

33. Kant quoting Horace.

1. Premises

1. The term "empirical" was first used to refer to ancient Greek doctors who replaced dogma with observation of their patients; see Carlo Sini, "Empirismo," in *Enciclopedia Garzanti della Filosofia,* eds. Gianni Vattimo et al. (Milan: Garzanti Editori, 2004). In philosophy, it commonly refers to the view that only experience of the senses provides us with knowledge (view attributed to David Hume). Here, empirical is used in the broader sense of anything actually experienced.

2. Questions that would now be referred to as "philosophy of mind" were, in ancient Greece, tied to discussions about the immortality of the soul. See Plato, *Phaedo,* 78b–84b.

3. Popper, *Objective Knowledge.*

4. Solipsism, in one form or another, has been a constant preoccupation in Western philosophy—no philosopher has been able to prove it wrong. Consider Gorgias in ancient Greece; Descartes in *Discourse on Method;* Husserl in *Cartesian Meditations;* Wittgenstein.

5. Even Plato had to appeal to a God–demiurge to explain the existence of order in the universe (Plato, *Timaeus* 29a–31b). See also Paul Eidelberg, *A Jewish Philosophy of History* (Lincoln: iUniverse Inc, 2004), 134–137.

6. G. E. R. Lloyd, *Early Greek Science: Thales to Aristotle* (New York: Norton, 1974).

7. Aristotle, *Metaphysics* IV, 3. Before its formulation by Aristotle, however, the principle of non-contradiction was used as a method of attaining truth in almost all Platonic dialogues. See Plato, *Meno,* 71a–80b. Also see Dmitri Panchenko, "Thales and the Origin of Theoretical Reasoning," *Configurations* 1, vol. 3 (1993): 387–398 and *Thales and the Origins of Theoretical Reasoning* [in Greek] (Athens, 2005).

8. Their "realism" is very different from the "naïve realism" of everyday life. In our everyday life, we believe that the world that we see exists as we see it and

are often ready to admit that it can be chaotic, mysterious, or just incomprehensible. But science believes in the reality of the world as constructed by scientific theories, i.e., in an ordered universe ruled by universal laws. Its realism is therefore a belief not in the reality of the external world but in that of its own theories. See Stathis Psillos, *Scientific Realism: How Science Tracks Truth* (London: Routledge, 1999).

9. See Kant, *Critique of Pure Reason,* trans. J. M. D. Meiklejohn (Amherst, NY: Prometheus Books, 1990) for the argument that causality is not something that exists in the world out there but a category of our understanding, which we impose upon phenomena.

10. See Descartes, *Discourse on Method,* IV; and discussion by Nietzsche, *Beyond Good and Evil,* 17, 54.

11. Thomas Kuhn, *The Structure of Scientific Revolutions* (Chicago: University of Chicago Press, 1962).

12. Greenfeld, *Nationalism,* 78–86; R. K. Merton, *Science, Technology and Society in Seventeenth-Century England* (Atlantic Highlands, NJ: Humanities Press, 1970).

13. The immediate reason why science was institutionalized in England so early in the age of nationalism, while reflecting the growth of the national consciousness, was not directly related to the epistemological revolution it brought about. It was, rather the inherent competitiveness of the national consciousness and the fact that the English felt their literature not competitive with those of Latin countries, which made them opt for a new area of cultural creativity—science, which did not really exist anywhere else—in which to challenge its chosen rivals. But we need not concern ourselves with this part of the story here.

14. See Plato, *Phaedo.*

15. Most solutions to this problem in Western thought were formulated between the sixteenth and eighteenth centuries, George Berkeley and Julien de la Mettrie representing the two extremes, and Descartes, Leibniz, and Spinoza in between.

16. See Dennett, *Darwin's Dangerous Idea: Evolution and the Meanings of Life* (New York: Simon and Schuster, 1996).

17. Ibid.

18. George H. Lewes (*Problems of Life and Mind: first series: the Foundations of a Creed,* vol. 2 (London: Kegan Paul, Trench, Turbner, and Co., 1875) is credited with the first use of the term. The uses of the terms "emergence" and "emergent phenomenon" can be divided into two categories: "weak" or "epistemological" emergence and "strong" or "ontological" emergence. See Peter Corning, "The Re-Emergence of 'Emergence': A Venerable Concept in Search of a Theory," *Complexity* 7, no. 6 (2002): 18–30; Philip Clayton, "Conceptual Foundations of Emergence Theory," in *The Re-Emergence of Emergence: The Emergentist Hypothesis from Science to Religion,* eds. Philip Clayton and Paul Davies (New York: Oxford University Press, 2006), 1–31; David Chalmers, "Strong and Weak Emergence," in ibid., 244–254.

2. The Mind as an Emergent Phenomenon

1. Ernst Mayr, *This is Biology: The Science of the Living World* (Cambridge: Harvard University Press, 1997), 231–233.
2. For the difference between my and Terrence W. Deacon's view of the transformation from signs to symbols, see in particular Chapters 2 and 3 in his *The Symbolic Species: The Co-Evolution of Language and the Brain* (New York: Norton, 1997).
3. Irene Pepperberg, *Alex & Me: How a Scientist and a Parrot Discovered a Hidden World of Animal Intelligence—and Formed a Deeper Bond in the Process* (New York: HarperCollins, 2008).
4. Arthur Schopenhauer "Parerga and Paralipomena" trans. T. Bailey Saunders in *The German Classics of the Nineteenth and Twentieth Centuries* eds. Kuno Francke et al. (New York: J. B. Lyon, 1914), 74.
5. Among others, see Jennifer Arnold, *Through a Dog's Eyes: Understanding Our Dogs by Understanding How They See the World* (Spiegel and Grau / Random House, 2010); Alexandra Horowitz, *Inside of a Dog: What Dogs See, Smell, and Know* (New York: Scribner, 2009); Stanley Coren, *The Intelligence of Dogs: A Guide to the Thoughts, Emotions, and Inner Lives of Our Canine Companions* (New York: Free Press, 2005); Robert H. Busch, *The Wolf Almanac* (Guilford, CT: The Lyons Press, 1995); L. David Mech *Wolf: The Ecology and Behavior of an Endangered Species* (University of Minnesota Press, 1981).
6. Jean Marc Gaspard Itard and François Dagognet, *Victor de l'Aveyron* (Paris: Allia, 2009); also see, Susan Curtiss et al., "The Linguistic Development of Genie," *Language* 50, no. 3, (1974): 528–554.
7. Bloch, *Craft*, 27–29.
8. See Larry R. Squire and Eric R. Kandel, *Memory: From Mind to Molecules* (New York: Henry Holt, 2000).
9. Jeffery A. Dusek and Howard Eichenbaum, "The Hippocampus and Memory for Orderly Stimulus Relations," in *PNAS* 94, no. 13 (1997): 7109–7114.
10. Albert Einstein, *Albert Einstein: Autobiographical Notes,* trans. and ed. Paul Arthur Schilpp (La Salle, IL: Open Court, 1979), 7.
11. Ernest Thompson Seton, "Lobo, the King of Corrumpaw," *Wild Animals I Have Known* (New York: Charles Scribner's Sons, 1898); *Heart of a Lioness* (Animal Planet) http://animal.discovery.com/fansites/wildkingdom/lioness/lioness.html (accessed June 6, 2012).
12. See Daniel Goleman, "Finding Happiness: Cajole Your Brain to Lean to the Left," *New York Times,* February 4, 2003.
13. See Chapter 5.
14. See, for example, Michael S. Gazzaniga, "Are Human Brains Unique?" in *Human: The Science Behind What Makes Us Unique,* (New York: HarperCollins, 2008).
15. I borrow this analogy from Mark Simes.

16. Marian C. Diamond et al., "The Effects of an Enriched Environment on the Histology of the Rat Cerebral Cortex" in *The Journal of Comparative Neurology* 123, no. 1 (1964): 111–119.

17. See Chapters 5 and 6; for the example of mathematics I am indebted to a Strathclyde mathematician, Michael Grinfeld, and specifically to his convincing argument against the cognitive science-inspired *Where Mathematics Comes From: How the Embodied Mind Brings Mathematics into Being* by George Lakoff and Rafael Núñez.

18. Einstein, "Geometry and Experience" in *Sidelights on Relativity* trans. G. B. Jefferey and W. Perrett (New York: Dover, 1983).

19. Edith Wharton provides a marvelous example of an unerring fashion imagination in the person of Lawrence Lefferts, "the foremost authority on 'form' in New York," in *The Age of Innocence* (New York: Modern Library Edition, Random House, 1999).

20. See O'Keefe and Nadel, *The Hippocampus as a Cognitive Map* (New York: Oxford University Press, 1978).

21. Kandel, *Memory: From Mind to Molecules*.

22. See Chapter 1.

23. Ibid.

24. See Richard G. Niemi and M. Kent Jennings, "Issues and Inheritance in the Formation of Party Identification," *American Journal of Political Science*, 35, no. 4 (1991): 970–988.

25. Czesław Miłosz, *The Captive Mind*, (New York: Vintage, 1990).

26. In this context, it is useful to consider Harold Bloom, *Genius: A Mosaic of One Hundred Exemplary Creative Minds* (New York: Warner Books, 2002), which, unfortunately, deals only with literature.

3. Madness in Its Pure Form

1. Irving I. Gottesman (with D. L. Wolfgram), *Schizophrenia Genesis: The Origins of Madness* (New York: Freeman, 1990), 15–16, emphasis mine; Daniel Nettle, *Strong Imagination: Madness, Creativity and Human Nature* (New York: Oxford University Press, 2001), 19; Louis A. Sass, *Madness and Modernism: Insanity in the Light of Modern Art, Literature, and Thought* (Cambridge: Harvard University Press, 1994), 13.

2. T. M. Luhrmann, *Of Two Minds: An Anthropologist Looks at American Psychiatry* (New York: Vintage, 2001).

3. Here the definition becomes circular and, therefore, a tautology.

4. There is no definition of "delusion" anywhere in the *Diagnostic and Statistical Manual of Mental Disorders*, 4th ed., (hereafter cited as *DSM-IV*).

5. *DSM-IV*, 273–274; Sass, *Madness*, 155.

6. For a discussion of economics as academic discipline see Greenfeld, *Spirit of Capitalism*, 162–171.

7. The term "definitive categorizer" is Gottesman's, *Schizophrenia Genesis,* 7; Bénédict Augustin Morel, *Traité des maladies mentales* (Paris: Masson, 1860).

8. Jean Christophe Coffin, *La transmission de la folie: 1850–1914* (Paris: Editions L'Harmattan, 2003).

9. Jaspers quoted in Sass, *Madness,* 17.

10. Ibid., 4, 7–8.

11. Kim Hopper et al., eds., *Recovery from Schizophrenia: An International Perspective; A Report from the WHO Collaborative Project, The International Study of Schizophrenia* (New York: Oxford University Press, 2007), xi, 277, fn.1. But see for example, Alex Cohen et al., "Questioning an Axiom: Better Prognosis for Schizophrenia in the Developing World," *Schizophrenia Bulletin* (2008): 229–244.

12. Paolo Fusar-Poli and Pierluigi Politi, "Paul Eugen Bleuler and the Birth of Schizophrenia (1908)," *American Journal of Psychiatry,* 165 (2008): 1407.

13. Michael Lyons, Lecture on Schizophrenia "Schizophrenia: An Overview" (lecture, The Seminar on Modernity, Boston University, Boston, MA, January, 2007); also see Gottesman, *Genesis,* 15.

14. Sass, *Madness,* 402 n. 28.

15. Gottesman, *Genesis,* 23; Remarkably, though the presentation of several or even one of the first-rank symptoms of schizophrenia immediately raises a red flag, they are neither sufficient nor necessary to *diagnose* the disease! Only 58 percent of patients with a schizophrenia diagnosis show any of these symptoms; 20 percent of patients never show them (Carpenter and Strauss, "Cross Cultural Evaluation of Schneider's First Rank Symptoms of Schizophrenia: A Report from the IPSS," *American Journal of Psychiatry* (1974): 682–687); and approximately 10 percent of patients with different diagnoses present them as well (Mellor, "The Present Status of First-Rank Symptoms," *Br J Psychiatry* (1982): 423–424).

16. J. E. Cooper, *Psychiatric Diagnosis in New York and London: A Comparative Study of Mental Hospital Admissions* (London: Oxford University Press, 1972).

17. J. M. Davis et al., "A Meta-Analysis of the Efficacy of Second-Generation Antipsychotics," *Archives of General Psychiatry,* 60 (2003): 553–564.

18. See Fenton and McGlashan, "Natural History of Schizophrenia Subtypes," *Archives of General Psychiatry* 48 (1991): 978–986.

19. Lyons, Lecture "Schizophrenia: An Overview"; according to Gottesman "at least 10 percent," *Genesis,* 37.

20. Hopper et al., *Recovery,* 23–38.

21. Louis Sass represents an exception, devoting to it several very illuminating chapters.

22. Gottesman, *Genesis,* 18–19; *DSM-IV,* 280.

23. A. Pulver, "Risk Factors in Schizophrenia: Season of Birth, Gender, and Familial Risk," *British Journal of Psychiatry* 160 (1992): 71.

24. Fuller Torrey et al., "Seasonality of Schizophrenia and Stillbirths," *Schizophrenia Bulletin* 19 (1993): 557–562.

25. Jarl Flensmark, "Is There an Association Between the Use of Heeled Footwear and Schizophrenia?" *Medical Hypotheses* 63 (2004): 740–747.

26. For a short summary, see E. Fuller Torrey, "The End of Psychiatric Illnesses," in *The Way We Will Be 50 Years From Now: 60 of the World's Greatest Minds Share Their Visions of the Next Half Century,* ed. Mike Wallace (Dallas: Thomas Nelson, 2008), 22–23.

27. Nettle, *Strong Imagination,* 48; see also G. E. Schafft, *From Racism to Genocide: Anthropology in the Third Reich* (Chicago: University of Illinois Press, 2004).

28. See M. Avila et al., "Genetic Epidemiology and Schizophrenia: A Study of Reproductive Fitness," *Schizophrenia Research* 47 (2001): 233–241; and J. Haukka et al., "Fertility of Patients with Schizophrenia, their Siblings, and the General Population: A Cohort Study from 1950 to 1959 in Finland," *American Journal of Psychiatry* 160 (2003): 460–463; Gottesman, *Genesis,* 102–103.

29. Nettle, *Strong Imagination,* 56.

30. Hopper et al., *Recovery,* 280, xiv, 278–9.

31. M. J. Owen, M. C. O'Donovan, and I. I. Gottesman, "Schizophrenia," in *Psychiatric Genetics and Genomics,* eds. McGuffin, Owen, and Gottesman (New York: Oxford University Press, 2002), 247–266.

32. Gottesman, *Genesis,* 88.

33. Lyons, Lecture "Schizophrenia: An Overview."

34. Nettle, *Strong Imagination,* 82–83. (No specific connection to schizophrenia was found.)

35. Sartorius in *Recovery,* Hopper et al., 3.

36. Ibid.

37. Gottesman, *Genesis,* 1.

38. P. Carlson, "Thinking Outside the Box," *The Washington Post,* April 9, 2001.

39. Gottesman, *Genesis,* 4, 75.

40. Gottesman, *Genesis,* 73–75.

41. J. McGrath, "A Systematic Review of the Incidence of Schizophrenia: The Distribution of Rates and the Influence of Sex, Urbanicity, Migrant status and Methodology," *BMC Medicine* 2 (2004): 13.

42. About one-fourth of the membership in the United Nations; S. Saha et al., "A Systematic Review of the Prevalence of Schizophrenia," *PLoS Medicine* 2 (2005): 0413–0433.

43. World Health Organization World Mental Health Survey Consortium, R. C. Kessler et al., "Prevalence, Severity, and Unmet Need for Treatment of Mental Disorders in the World Health Organization World Mental Health Surveys," *JAMA* 291 (2004): 2581–2590.

44. Assen Jablensky, "The 100-Year Epidemiology of Schizophrenia," *Schizophrenia Research* 28 (1997): 111–125.

45. Saha, "Review."

46. Hopper et al., *Recovery,* 277–282.

47. T. J. Craig et al., "Outcome in Schizophrenia and Related Disorders Compared Between Developing and Developed Countries. A Recursive Partitioning Reanalysis of the WHO DOSMD Data," *The British Journal of Psychiatry* 170(1997): 229–233; also see Kim Hopper and J. Wanderling, "Revisiting the Developed Versus Developing Country Distinction in Course and Outcome in Schizophrenia: Results from ISoS, the WHO Collaborative Followup Project," *Schizophrenia Bulletin* 26 (2000): 835–846.

48. A. Blomqvist et al., "The cost of Schizophrenia: Lessons from an International Comparison, *Journal of Mental Health Policy* 9 (2006): 177–83; Ronald Kessler writes that NCS and NCS-R results are conservative prevalence estimates and underrepresentative of "several important population segments," Kessler et al., "Prevalence, Severity, and Comorbidity of 12-Month DSM-IV Disorders in the National Comorbidity Survey Replication," *Archives of General Psychiatry,* 62 (2005): 617–627.

49. World Heath Organization World Mental Health Survey Consortium in *JAMA* 291(2004).

50. See Linde, *Spirits and Madness.*

51. J. J. McGrath, "Myths and Plain Truths about Schizophrenia Epidemiology—the NAPE lecture 2004," *Acta Psychiatrica Scandinavica* 111 (2005): 9.

52. Jablensky, *Schizophrenia Research,* 117.

53. Gottesman, *Genesis,* 4.

54. Sartorius in *Recovery,* Hopper et al., 3.

55. Carole Siegel et al., "Predictors of Long-Term Course and Outcome for the DOSMed Cohort," *Recovery,* 39–49. Stability was rated on a scale from one (high) to three (low). This is all we are told of its definition.

56. In these remarks, no criticism of the epidemiologists involved is implied: it is the duty of the social sciences to provide them with the concepts for the analysis of culture. The failing, therefore, is ours, not theirs.

57. With the exception of the second-year follow-up, when Agra was the second best, Ibadan in Nigeria, which was not included in later studies, showing the best results. Sartorius in *Recovery,* Hopper et al., 5.

58. K. C. Dube and Narendar Kumar, "IPSS: Agra, India," in *Recovery,* Hopper et al., 77.

59. Kim Hopper et al., "An Overview of Course and Outcome in ISoS," in *Recovery,* 23–38

60. Siegel, ". . . DOSMed Cohort" in *Recovery,* 48–49.

61. Assen Jablensky, Norman Sartorius, et al., "Schizophrenia: Manifestations, Incidence and Course in Different Cultures: A World Health Organization Ten-Country Study," *Psychological Medicine Monograph Supplement* 20 (1992): 1–97; cited as the most influential study by M. Lyons.

62. McGrath, "Myths," 4–11.

63. Norman Sartorius, "Early Manifestations and First-Contact Incidence of Schizophrenia in Different Cultures: A Preliminary Report on the Initial Evaluation

Phase of the WHO Collaborative Study on Determinants of Outcome of Severe Mental Disorders," *Psychological Medicine* 16 (1986): 909–928.

64. R. Faris and H. Dunham, H. W., *Mental Disorders in Urban Areas: An Ecological Study of Schizophrenia and Other Psychoses* (Chicago: University Chicago Press, 1939).

65. W. Eaton, "Social class and chronicity of schizophrenia," *Journal of Chronic Diseases* 28 (1975): 191–198.

66. Gottesman, *Genesis;* Goodwin and Jamison, *Manic Depressive Illness* (Oxford University Press, 2007), 182.

67. Sass, *Madness,* 13.

68. S. S. Reich and J. Cutting, "Picture Perception and Abstract Thought in Schizophrenia," *Psychological Medicine* 12 (1982): 96; quoted in Ibid., 133; see also G. E. Berios, "Positive and Negative Symptoms and Jackson: A Conceptual History," *Arch Gen Psychiatry* 42 (1995): 95–97; T. R. Insel, "Rethinking Schizophrenia," *Nature* 468 (2010): 187–193.

69. Declaring that the word "schizophrenia" is a polymorph, as does Jeff Coulter obviously does not solve the problem. Coulter, "The Grammar of Schizophrenia" in *What is Schizophrenia?* eds. W. Flack, D. Miller and M. Wiener (New York: Springer-Verlag, 1991).

70. Irving B. Weiner, *Psychodiagnosis in Schizophrenia* (Mahwah, NJ: Lawrence Erlbaum, 1996), 85–86.

71. Sass, *Madness,* 122–125, 164.

72. Ibid., 124.

73. Nettle, *Strong Imagination,* 3.

74. John Haslam, *Illustrations of Madness,* ed. Roy Porter (New York: Routledge, 1988).

75. Matthews in *Illustrations of Madness,* ed. Haslam, 53–4.

76. Ibid., 48–49.

77. Ibid., 38–40.

78. The "famous empty smile"—a characteristic of the negative symptom of abnormal (or flat) affect—term originally employed by Rümke, in 1941 and quoted in Sass, *Madness,* 112.

79. Haslam, *Illustrations of Madness,* 30–38.

80. Ibid., 59–67.

81. Ibid., 72, 74.

82. Chemistry was just born, in fact. More: we do not suspect Ian Flemming, with all his fantastic but plausible gadgets, or the makers of high-grossing movies, such as *Eternal Sunshine of the Spotless Mind* or *The Matrix,* of being mentally disturbed.

83. Tausk is credited with developing the loss of ego boundaries in a article published posthumously in the *Internationale Zeitschrift für Psychoanalyse* in 1919 titled, "On the Origin of the Influencing Machine in Schizophrenia"; Sass, *Madness,* 217.

84. Ibid., 241, 216–218; Anna Freud quoted on page 218.
85. "To work events"—in Matthews' terminology to bring about desired actions by the victims.
86. Haslam, *Illustrations of Madness,* 80; italics mine.
87. Ibid., 2.
88. Roy Porter, introduction to *Illustrations of Madness,* by Haslam app 3, lvii–lxiv.
89. Sass, *Madness,* 215. In what follows I rely on the documentation assembled by Sass in *Madness*—without a doubt, the best "thick description" of schizophrenia in the literature.
90. Ibid., 229, 232, 233.
91. Ibid., 234–237.
92. Ibid., 121.
93. *DSM-IIIR* defines the "illogical thinking" of schizophrenics as "thinking that contains obvious internal contradictions or in which conclusions are reached that are clearly erroneous, given the initial premises." (152) The manual does not elaborate to whom the internal contradictions are obvious, though this is an important question.
94. This is the way Soviet scientists Polyakov and Feigenberg, refer to it (Sass, *Madness,* p. 127.). Instead of responding to cultural stimuli the expected way characteristic of other people in their environment, schizophrenics respond in ways that would be most unlikely for others. This does not mean that their responses are wrong—their distinguishing characteristic is that they are highly unlikely for their environment. In different circumstances, responses of this nature may be the preferred type of response. For instance, the ability to perceive possibilities unlikely for the members of a certain scientific discipline makes scientific outsiders, i.e., people coming from a different field, so prominent among innovators in science; Sass, *Madness,* 127.
95. Richard Noll, "Ambivalence," *Encyclopedia of Schizophrenia and other Psychotic Disorders,* 3rd ed. (New York: InfoBase Publishing, 2007), 15.
96. Quotations from Sass, *Madness,* 130, 144, 139.
97. Indeed, some experts consider such loss of "seriatim functions" (Silvano Arieti)—i.e., the loss of an ability to organize experiences into a time, and therefore, causal, sequences—as another fundamental feature of schizophrenia. They lack an explanation for it, however. Jaspers' patient quoted in Sass, *Madness,* 148.
98. Quoted in ibid., 158.
99. Sass, *Madness,* 155.
100. Ibid., 160. Sass is, therefore, wrong in attributing to schizophrenics the "perspectivist" attitude characteristic of modernist art and literature. The numerous perspectives that are suggested to schizophrenics are for them aspects of reality; they have no control over them, they are unaware that it is their minds that produce these perspectives—their disintegrated minds, in fact, have no such power.
101. Sass, *Madness,* 125–126; (italics mine).

102. Ibid.,175–176.

103. Ibid., 178, 206.

104. Ibid.,179.

105. Ibid., 43–44.

106. Ibid., 45.

107. Quoted in ibid., 47.

108. Ibid., 49.

109. Ibid., 68.

110. Ibid., 60–61 (Jaspers quoted in ibid.).

111. Sylvia Nasar, *A Beautiful Mind: The Life of Mathematical Genius and Nobel Laureate John Nash* (New York: Simon & Schuster, 2001), 16.

112. Per Nasar, 353.

113. Ibid., 13, 14.

114. Ibid., 26–30.

115. Ibid., 32–33.

116. Karl P. Morritz, *Anton Reiser: A Psychological Novel* (Oxford: Penguin Books, 1997).

117. Nasar, *Beautiful Mind,* 37, 36.

118. Albert Einstein, *Autobiographical Notes,* trans. P. A. Schilpp (La Salle: Open Court, 1979), 9.

119. Nasar, *Beautiful Mind,* 34–35, 38–39.

120. Ibid., 49, 50, 40–48, 67–68, 68–71, 83–85.

121. Significantly, Nasar writes: "the economist who first posed the problem of the bargain was . . . Francis Ysidro Edgeworth, in 1881. Edgeworth and several of his Victorian contemporaries were the first to abandon the historical and philosophical tradition of Smith, Ricardo, and Marx and to attempt to replace it with the mathematical tradition of physics." Ibid., 88.

122. Ibid., 92–94, 99, 102, 118–119; Nasar's italics.

123. Ibid., 184–187.

124. Ibid., 233, 235, 242–244,246.

125. Ibid., 299, 324.

126. Ibid., 326–327. NB the tenses Nash uses in this conversation with his biographer after getting the Nobel Prize and when, presumably, in remission.

127. Ibid., 255–256, 258, 318.

128. On March 19, 2010 Sylvia Nasar delivered a lecture in the Intellectual Biography Series of the Philosophy Department at Boston University. I asked her on that occasion about the state of John Nash at the time. She responded that he was well. (I expected this: the plot of her story, which made it a story, was that Nash had recovered.) From other sources (fate, one may say, placed my home in the closest possible vicinity of McLean Hospital, and gossip among neighbors does not abide by professional ethics standards), however, I learned that Nash still had psychotic episodes. Are my sources trustworthy? I don't know. But their information is more consistent with the course and outcome of the overwhelming majority of schizophrenia cases, than Nasar's, and I am willing to leave it at that.

4. Madness Muddled

1. F. K. Goodwin and K. R. Jamison, *Manic-Depressive Illness, Bipolar Disorders and Recurrent Depression,* 2nd ed., vols. 1 and 2 (New York: Oxford University Press, 2007).
2. Ibid., 19–20
3. According to Kessler et al. "Lifetime Prevalance and Age-of-Onset Distributions of DSM-IV Disorders in the National Comorbidity Survey Replication," in *Archives of General Psychiatry* 62 (2005), the lifetime prevalence of Major Depressive Disorder and Bipolar Disorder among American adults is 16.6 percent and 3.9 percent respectively. The NCS-R also indicates a 20.4 percent lifetime prevalence rate of "Any Mood Disorder."
4. Goodwin and Jamison, *MDI,* xix.
5. Ibid., xix–xx.
6. See Goodwin and Jamison, *MDI,* 178–180 for global burden of disease studies, and the WHO The Global Burden of Disease: 2004 update, part 4. http://www.who.int/healthinfo/global_burden_disease/2004_report_update/en/index.html (accessed July 9, 2012).
7. Goodwin and Jamison, *MDI,* 8
8. *DSM-IV,* 317.
9. Ibid., 320
10. Goodwin and Jamison, *MDI,* 66.
11. Campbell quoted in ibid., 66 (emphasis mine).
12. Mayer-Groll et al., in ibid., 66.
13. Jaspers (1913), Campbell (1953), quoted in ibid., 67.
14. Kraepelin (1921) quoted in ibid.
15. Ibid., 66.
16. Bleuler (1924), Kraepelin (1921) cited by Goodwin and Jamison *MDI.*
17. K. R. Jamison, *An Unquiet Mind* (New York: Vintage, 1996), 66–70.
18. Goodwin and Jamison, *MDI,* 9.
19. Ibid., 9–11.
20. Ibid., 12.
21. Ibid., 12.
22. Ibid., xix.
23. *DSM-IV,* 328.
24. Kraepelin, Jaspers quoted in Goodwin and Jamison, *MDI,* 36, 32.
25. Bleuler, Kraepelin, Campbell in ibid., 33, 34–35.
26. Ibid., 37, 39, 37–38.
27. Ibid., 35.
28. Ibid., 38.
29. Ibid., 33, 36.
30. Ibid., 17.
31. Ibid., 17, 19.
32. Ibid., 23–24, xxii, 22, 44.

33. Ibid., 43–45.

34. Ibid., 45.

35. Ibid., 46–48, tables 2–4; 49.

36. Ibid., 49–52.

37. Ibid., 53.

38. Ibid., 53.

39. Ibid., 53.

40. Ibid., 57.

41. Ibid., 57.

42. Ibid., 57.

43. Ibid., 58–59, 66; see also 66–87 for clinical descriptions.

44. Ibid., 463.

45. Ibid., 413, 463.

46. Ibid., 411.

47. Ibid., 463, 589, 596, 601 (emphasis added).

48. Ibid., 411.

49. Ibid., 419; 411–414.

50. Ibid., 422, 549; 419 (emphasis added).

51. Ibid., 596.

52. Ibid., 597.

53. Ibid., 423, 426.

54. Ibid., 432–433.

55. Ibid., 595–596.

56. Ibid., 459 (emphasis added).

57. Ibid., 455, 457.

58. In a letter to the editor, Wenland et al. assert that the 5-HTTLPR polymorphism has been the subject of more than three hundred articles published in behavioral, pharmacologic and medical sciences. "Simultaneous genotyping of four functional loci of human *SLC6A4*, with a reappraisal of *5-HTTLPR* and rs25531," *Molecular Psychiatry* 11 (2006): 224–226.

59. Goodwin and Jamison, *MDI,* 443.

60. Ibid., 460–463.

61. Ibid., 598–599.

62. Ibid., 600.

63. Ibid., 626, 653.

64. Goodwin and Jamison, *MDI,* Chapter 15, "Neuroanatomy and Neuroimaging," 609—654.

65. Ibid., 653–654.

66. On methodological problems in epidemiological studies of manic-depressive illness see ibid., 157–158.

67. F. K. Goodwin and K. R. Jamison, *Manic-Depressive Illness* (New York: Oxford University Press, 1990), 167–168.

68. For methodological considerations, see R. C. Kessler and K. R. Merikangas.

"The National Comorbidity Survey Replication (NCS-R): Background and Aims," *International Journal of Methods in Psychiatric Research* 13 (2004): 60–68. For rates of prevalence among adolescents, see Merikingas et al. "Lifetime Prevalence of Mental Disorders in U.S. Adolescents: Results from the National Comorbidity Survey Replication–Adolescent Supplement (NCS-A)" *Journal of the American Academy of Child and Adolescent Psychiatry* 49 (2010): 980–989. For increase in rates from 1990–2003 see Kessler et al., "The Epidemiology of Major Depressive Disorder: Results From the National Comorbidity Survey Replication (NCS-R)," *JAMA* 289 (2003): 3095–3105.

69. Goodwin and Jamison, *MDI,* (1990), 174,175.
70. Goodwin and Jamison (2007), 182.
71. Ibid., 182.
72. Ibid., 182.
73. Ibid., 183.
74. Goodwin and Jamison, *MDI* (1990), 169.
75. Ibid., 169–172 (emphasis added).
76. Ibid., 170–172.
77. Low economic class is also shown to be a protective factor against suicide in Durkheim's classic study.
78. Goodwin and Jamison *MDI* (1990), 169
79. Ibid., 173 (emphasis added.)
80. Goodwin and Jamison, *MDI,* 182.
81. Goodwin and Jamison, *MDI* (1990), 180.
82. Ibid. 180; see Benjamin Malzberg, *The Mental Health of Jews in New York State* (Albany, NY: Research Foundation for Mental Hygiene, 1963); R. S. Cooklin, A. Ravindran, and M. W. Carney, "The Patterns of Mental Disorder in Jewish and Non-Jewish Admissions to a District General Hospital Psychiatric Unit: Is Manic Depressive Illness a Typically Jewish Disorder?" *Psychological Medicine* 13 (1983): 209–12.
83. See L Halpern, "Some Data of the Psychic Morbidity of Jews and Arabs in Palestine," *American Journal of Psychiatry* 94 (1938): 1215–1222; Jozef Hes, "Manic Depressive Illness in Israel," *American Journal of Psychiatry* 116 (1960): 1082–1086.
84. Hes, ibid. 1082, writes that the incidence of mdi in Israel in 1957 was 0.4 : 1000, whereas the incidence in the average population on the whole world is 3–4 : 1000.
85. Front and back covers, Kay R. Jamison, *An Unquiet Mind* (New York, NY: Vintage, 1996).
86. Ibid., 7.
87. Ibid., 58.
88. Ibid., 36–7.
89. Ibid., 58–59.
90. Ibid., 38–40.

91. Ibid., 42–47.
92. Ibid., 59.
93. Ibid., 67–68.
94. Ibid., 68.
95. Ibid., 69.
96. Ibid., 72–73.
97. Nasar, *Beautiful,* 320.
98. Ibid., 78–80.
99. Ibid., 76.
100. Ibid., 82–83.
101. Ibid., 6; 70; 144; 102.
102. Ibid., 12.
103. Ibid., 18.
104. Ibid., 29.
105. Ibid., 20–21.
106. Ibid., 27–28.
107. Ibid., 21–22.
108. Ibid., 31–33.
109. Ibid., 35–36.
110. Ibid., 41.
111. Ibid., 52.
112. Ibid., 56.
113. Ibid., 62–63.
114. Ibid., 86–87.
115. Ibid., 91–92.
116. Ibid., 77.
117. Ibid., 93–94.
118. Ibid., 97.
119. Ibid., 120–122.
120. Ibid., 122.

5. The Cradle of Madness

1. Thomas Elyot, *Dictionary* (1538), s.v. "man."
2. George Herbert, *Temple: Sacred Poems and Private Ejaculations* (London: Bell and Sons, 1904).
3. John Donne, "Sonnet 1 of The Westmoreland Sequence," *Part I The Holy Sonnets* in *The Varorium Edition of the Poetry of John Donne,* ed. Gary A. Stringer (Bloomington, IN: Indiana University Press, 2005), 11.
4. Shakespeare, Sonnets 9, 6, 18, 19, and 55, 60, 63, 65, 74, 81, 107, 108 in *The Norton Shakespeare Based on the Oxford Edition* eds. Stephen Greenblatt et al. (New York: W. W. Norton and Company, 1997).
5. Written either by Sir Edward Dyer or another Elizabethan courtier and poet Edward de Vere.

6. Shakespeare, *Troilus and Cressida* (Norton), 4.6.17. References are to act, scene, and line.

7. Shakespeare, *Twelfth Night* (Norton) 5.1.359; see also *OED* s.v. "achievement."

8. *OED* s.v. "ambition."

9. Shakespeare, *The Passionate Pilgrim*, (Norton), 6.

10. John Dowland, *Lachrimae pavane* (1596).

11. Shakespeare (Norton), Sonnet 29.

12. This holds true for legends of "romantic" love in other cultures. It was always *possible*, while being extremely *improbable*. After Shakespeare, it became most probable. See also William Jankowiak, ed., *Romantic Passion: A Universal Experience?* (New York: Columbia University Press, 1995); there Charles Lindholm "Love as an Experience of Transcendence"; also Lindholm "Love and Structure," *Theory, Culture and Society*, 15: 243–63.

13. Anders Nygren, *Agape and Eros: The Christian Idea of Love* (Chicago: University of Chicago Press, 1982); see also Alan Soble, ed., *Eros, Agape, and Philia: Readings in the Philosophy of Love* (St. Paul: Paragon House, 1989).

14. The concept "ideal type" is used here in the original Weberian sense of a cognitive construct developing the logical implications of a cultural phenomenon from its first premises.

15. Shakespeare (Norton), Sonnet 116.

16. Quoted from the Norton Edition.

17. For over four centuries after Shakespeare we have been taught the lesson of *Cosi fan tutte*—that true love is a chimera, that we are fools to pine for it, that we should reconcile to the fact and be satisfied with what there is, some sexual infatuation growing into habitual attachment under the protection of social norms. But, despite all the lessons, we continue to believe that—to quote that very famous distillation of Shakespeare's message put to music— "All you need is love. / All you need is love. / All you need is love, love. / Love is all you need." Lennon-McCartney, *All You Need Is Love*. Parlophone 7" Vinyl. Released July, 1967.

18. Shakespeare, Sonnet 129. I thank Sir Geoffrey Hill for turning my attention to it.

19. Katherine Philips, "To M. A. at Parting," *Poems: 1667*.

20. *OED* s.v. "pet."

21. *Jubilato Agno*, incidentally, was written in Bedlam.

22. These lines are dedicated, with gratitude and humility, to Billy.

23. That gentlemen were becoming "good cheap" was a sixteenth-century opinion; see Greenfeld, *Nationalism*, 49, for sources.

24. See, for example, Cotton Mather, *A Christian at His Calling*, Second Discourse ("Directing a Christian in his Personal Calling," 1701) in *Annals of America* 1, 1493–1754 (Chicago: Encyclopedia Britannica, 1976), 319–324.

25. Two of them are based on French literary sources: *Carmen* on Prosper Merimee's story, and *Manon* on Abbe Prevost's novel *Manon Lescaux*. In the "romans" of Mme de Lafayette, perhaps the first to treat the subject in

French literature, it is mostly women who are undone by love. From the start far more overtly sexual than in England, it seems to arrive in France as a passion more likely to destroy, than to constitute, one's happiness.

26. The authenticity of man's love is equal to the strength of his sexual desire for a particular woman, judged by what he is willing to sacrifice in order to satisfy it. The outstanding example of a man in love—a rare subject in Russian literature—is the hero of Kuprin's *The Duel,* who gratefully pays with his life for one night with his beloved, a married woman whose husband he must allow to kill him the morning after.

27. We would obviously tend to translate *chelovek* in this context as "human being," but Russian has an equivalent for the "human being"—*chelovecheskoe suschestvo*—meaning, literally, "a being of the kind of man," and in most contexts the "human being" translation of *chelovek* would significantly detract from the context; it must be translated as "man" and yet have no gender connotations whatsoever.

28. *N.B.* Psalm 23, "The Lord is my Shepherd," which in the Hebrew original contains words "Though I walk in the valley of deepest darkness, I fear no harm," but since Septuaginte is translated as "Though I walk through the valley of the shadow of Death, I will fear no evil."

29. See, for instance, Darrin M. McMahon, *Happiness: A History* (New York: Atlantic Monthly Press, 2006).

30. Thomas Elyot, *Dictionary* (1538), s.v. "fortuna."

31. Foucault, *La folie;* Thomas Szasz, *The Myth of Mental Illness: Foundations of a Theory of Personal Conduct* (New York: Hober-Harper, 1961.)

32. Gauchet and Swain, *Pratique,* i–xiii.

33. I am concerned here only with the medical concept of "pathology," and not at all with that of "pathology" as science of passions.

34. Regarding necessity of using language as an analytical tool see Bloch, *Craft,* 26 *ff.*

35. Thomas Vicary, "Chapter IV" *The Anatomie of the Body of Man* (London: Early English Text Society, 1888), 33.

36. Winfred Overholser, "Shakespeare's Psychiatry—And After," *Shakespeare's Quarterly* 10 (1959): 335–352; 337–338; the latter quotation is from Webster's *Duchess of Malfi.*

37. Act 33, Henry VIII, c. 20, "An Acte for the due Pces to be had in Highe Treason in Cases of Lunacye or Madnes," #1, in *Statutes of the Realm, Printed by command of His Majesty King George III in pursuance of an address of the House of Commons of Great Britain* (London, 1810–1821 reprinted in 1963 by Dawsons of Pall-Mall), 855.

38. Robert R. Reed, *Bedlam on the Jacobean Stage* (Cambridge: Harvard University Press, 1952), 16, 18, 20, 21.

39. According to Torrey, *Invisible Plague* (19, 337–344), the baseline rate of mental disease at any given time is reasonably estimated at one case per 1,000

adults or 0.5 per 1,000 total population, and rates higher than that should be taken as suggesting unusual conditions.

40. More on Bethlem from Reed, *Bedlam,* and Edward G. O'Donoghue, *The Story of Bethlehem Hospital from its Foundation in 1247* (London: T. Fisher Unwin, 1914).

41. William Carr, *The Dialect of Craven in the West Riding of the County of York: With a Copious Glossary, Illustrated by Authorities from Ancient English and Scottish Writers, and Exemplified by Two Familiar Dialogues.* 2 Vols. (London, 1828); also see *OED* s.v. "wood."

42. *Dictionnaire Littré,* s.v. "fou" and "folie"; the word "madness" derived from the Indogermanic verb *mei*—"to change," found in words for "changed," "adulterated," and "crippled," the word suggests something different from the norm, i.e., "abnormal." (*OED,* s.v. "madness.")

43. John Locke, "Chapter XI," in *An Essay Concerning Human Understanding* (London: Holt, 1690).

44. I was surprised to read in Carol Neely's informative feminist discussion of attitudes to mental disease in the Elizabethan period, *Distracted Subjects* (Cornell University Press, 2004), that "madness" was an old word, rarely used, and that mentally ill were most commonly referred to as "distracted." I fail to find support for this view in the texts. According to the *Concordance to Shakespeare,* for example, there are thirty-nine instances in total of "distracted" and derivatives, mostly used in comedies. In distinction, there are over 320 instances of "mad" and derivatives, used predominantly in tragedies and historical plays. Overholser, in "Shakespeare's Psychiatry," writes, "Various terms were applied to the victims of mental illness. They were referred to as maniacs, as melancholics, as suffering from phrenitis, frenzy, lunacy or demoniacal possession" (335), but does not mention "distracted."

45. *OED* s.v. "madness"; Bartholomaeus Anglicus *De Proprietatibus Rerum* (London: Berthelet, 1535) in Richard Hunter and Ida Macalpine *Three Hundred Years of Psychiatry 1535–1860: A History Presented in Selected English Texts* (London: Oxford, 1963), 1 (hereafter cited as *Three Hundred*).

46. Anglicus *De Proprietatibus Rerum,* 1–5.

47. Levinus Lemnius, *The Touchstone of Complexions,* 1576, in *Three Hundred,* 22–23

48. Lewes Lavaterus, Chapter 2, in *Of Ghosts and Spirits Walking by Night* (London: Benneyman, 1572).

49. Andrew Boorde *The Seconde Boke of the Breviary of Health, Named the Extravagantes* (London: Powell, 1552) in *Three Hundred,* 13–15.

50. The description of this case is based on Cynthia Chermely's "'Nawghtye Mallenchollye': Some Faces of Madness in Tudor England," *The Historian* 49 (1987): 309–328.

51. Richard Cosin *Conspiracie for Pretended Reformation: vix. Presbyteriall Discipline* (London: Barker, 1592) in *Three Hundred,* 43–45.

52. Hunter and Macalpine, *Three Hundred,* 7.

53. Thomas Elyot, "Of Affectes of the Mynde," Capitulo xi, "Of Dolour or Heuynesse of Mynde. Capitulo. xii." *The Castel of Healthe* (London: Berthelet, 1541), 62–68.

54. See "How Shall I Govern Me?" in Patterson, *The Life and Poems of William Dunbar* (Edinburgh: Nimmo, 1860), 222.

55. *Three Hundred*, 50–52.

56. "Throughout the sixteenth century, the term "melancholy" was used to designate a mild depression. . . . It also could, and frequently did, incorporate the most violent forms of madness." Chermely, "Nawghtye Mallenchollye," 311.

57. Christopher Langton *A very brefe treatise* . . . and *An introduction into phisycke* . . . (London: Whitchurch, 1547 and 1550) in *Three Hundred*, 10–11.

58. Overholser, "Shakespeare's Psychiatry," 345, quoting Timothy Bright, *Treatise of Melancholy* (1586) and T. Walkington, *The Optick Glasse of Humours* (1607), 343.

59. Philip Barrough, *The Methode of Phisicke*, . . . , *Three Hundred Years*, 24–28.

60. Thomas Cogan, *The Haven of Health*, 4th ed. (London: Griffin, 1636), 17.

61. Reginald Scot, *The Discoverie of Witchcraft*, 1584, in *Three Hundred Years*, 32–35, 33.

62. Hunter and Macalpine, *Three Hundred Years*, 36.

63. Timothy Bright, *A Treatise of Melancholie*, in ibid., 36–40. Reed writes, Bright "makes a clear-cut distinction between natural melancholy and the direct infliction of 'the heavy hande of God,' which he said might strike at the soul of human conscience regardless of pathological causes. . . . [he] accepted, although with one or two notable variations, the functional anatomy of Vicary and . . . expounded an almost purely psychological doctrine. . . . Bright's treatise constitutes the first substantial interpretation of the causes and symptoms of mental disease that was written by an Englishman; furthermore, in its scientific deductions, which were confined largely to contemporary medical interpretation, it was unquestionably a more concretely and professionally influential work than Burton's Anatomy of Melancholy, published 35 years later. Bright condensed the fragmentary knowledge of his times into a solid doctrine of humors; . . . [writing] a work that was, and still is, considered the most representative thesis upon melancholy and insanity of the Elizabethan period . . ." *Bedlam*, 68–69.

64. See Chermely, "Nawghtye Mallenchollye" and Overholser, "Shakespeare's Psychiatry," for different interpretations; I, obviously, believe the text supports me; more importantly, this interpretation is consistent with other changes of consciousness that happen at this time.

65. Bright, *A Treatise* in *Three Hundred* 38.

66. Shakespeare, *Love's Labors Lost* (Norton) 5.2,117; *The Taming of the Shrew* (Norton) Intro.i.133; *Twelfth Night* (Norton) 3.2,68.

67. See *Venus and Adonis* (1592) ln. 907; *Henry IV* 5.2, 19; *Taming of the Shrew* 3.2, 10; *Henry IV* 2.3, 81; *Romeo and Juliet* 3.1, 163; *King John* 2.1, 448; and ibid., 5.7, 50; *Richard III* 2.4, 64.

68. Bright, *A Treatise* in *Three Hundred*, 38.

69. Reed, *Bedlam*, 69.

70. Lawrence Babb, *Sanity in Bedlam: A Study of Robert Burton's Anatomy of Melancholy* (Lansing: MSU Press, 1959), 3; Vieda Skultans, *English Madness: Ideas on Insanity, 1580–1890* (New York: Routledge & Kegan Paul, 1979), 19; she also writes on page 18, "writers of the period distinguish so many subcategories of melancholy that it almost seems as though Renaissance psychopathology regards all mental abnormality as a species of melancholy. Roughly speaking, our term madness is synonymous with the Elizabethan term melancholy."

71. Lindsey Knights, *Drama and Society in the Age of Johnson* (London: Chatto, 1937), 324.

72. Reed, *Bedlam*, 71–72.

73. G. B. Harrison, in the introduction to Nicholas Breton's *Melancholike Humours*, 1929, 49.

74. Reed, *Bedlam*, 4, *passim*.

75. Ibid., 82–83.

76. Ibid., 71–74, 96.

77. According to the *OED*, only a dictionary definition preceded his employment of the concept in *Titus Andronicus*.

78. Amariah Brigham, "Insanity—Illustrated by Histories of Distinguished Men, and by the Writings of Poets and Novelists," *American Journal of Insanity* 1 (1844): 27.

79. Isaac Ray, "Shakespeare's Delineations of Insanity," *American Journal of Insanity* 3 (1847): 289–332, 325.

80. Brigham, "Insanity," 27–28; 40–41.

81. Ray, "Shakespeare's Delineations," 290–291.

82. Ibid., 319.

83. In what follows *King Lear* is quoted from the Norton edition.

84. Overholser, "Shakespeare's Psychiatry," 347.

85. The Fool plays a greater role than that, allowing us to see a part of Lear that is hidden behind his social self. All the other emotions we see Lear experience—rage, indignations, rashness, pride and humiliation, generosity and repentance—are moral sentiments tightly related to the ideas of duty and propriety. Only in regard to the Fool we see him simply affectionate. The very being of the Fool softens his heart. His utter dependency, utter lack of malice, and thus utter unfitness for the survival on his own in human society arouses in Lear the desire to protect him, an urge to indulge, to pet. In the very last scene of the play, when it seems the situation cannot be more tragic and one's sympathy is so fully engaged that to feel more appears impossible,

Shakespeare, with another master stroke, shocks us closer to the heart-breaking point when Lear, with dead Cordelia in his arms, suddenly exclaims, "And my poor fool is hang'd! No, no, no, life!" Three lines later he is dead.

86. In what follows *Hamlet* is quoted from the Norton edition.

87. Ray, "Shakespeare's Delineations,"; here and below 306–325.

88. Per the *OED,* the word, much in use in Shakespeare's time, does not carry the connotation of madness. It means "grotesque," or absurd, bizarre, and uncouthly ludicrous, in form or gesture.

89. The specific dating is unclear with 1602 being the latest that is estimated.

90. Brigham, "Insanity."

91. Reed, *Bedlam,* 4.

92. Robert Burton, *The Anatomy of Melancholy* (New York: NYRB Classics Complete Edition, 2001—following the 6th, 1639 edition), i, 172. At other places (e.g., 39) he says, "Folly, melancholy, madness, are but one disease, delirium is a common name to all."

93. Ibid., 71.

94. Ibid., 52–68, abridged in Robert Burton, *The Essential Anatomy of Melancholy* (Mineola, NY: Dover, 2002), 3–6.—first published as *Burton the Anatomist* (London: Methuen, 1924).

95. Burton, *Anatomy,* 38. There were other motives as well. The author himself was at one time "fatally driven upon this rock of melancholy," and thus wrote, "melancholy, by being busy to avoid melancholy," believing that "one must scratch where it itches." Having "felt and practiced" it himself and got his knowledge not like others, from books, but "by melancholizing," he "would help others out of a fellow-feeling." Ibid., 35, 20–22.

96. Ibid., 126–129.

97. Ibid., 264–268.

98. Ibid., iii, 40.

99. Ibid., 185–187.

6. Going International

1. Moore, *Backgrounds,* 180.

2. William Temple, "Of Poetry", *Essays on Ancient and Modern Learning* (Oxford: Clarendon Press, 1909), 75.

3. Torrey and Miller, *Invisible Plague,* 23–31.

4. Quoted in ibid., 31.

5. See A. M. Ludwig, *The Price of Greatness* (New York, N.Y.: Guilford Publications, 1995).

6. Philippe Pinel, Dora B. Weiner trans., "Memoir on Madness: A Contribution to the Natural History of Man," in "Philippe Pinel's 'Memoir on Madness' of December 11, 1794: A Fundamental Text of Modern Psychiatry," *The American Journal of Psychiatry,* 149 (June 1992): 725–732,

728; 1806 assertion and W. A. F. Browne's 1837 interpretation quoted in Torrey and Miller, *Invisible Plague,* 50.

7. An excerpt from a poem by John Clare (1793–1864), written in an asylum, quoted by Torrey, *Invisible Plague,* 66.

8. George Cheyne, *The English Malady (1733),* ed. Roy Porter (London: Routledge, 1991), ii.

9. That Cheyne was guilty on both counts is the opinion of Porter, ibid., ii.

10. Advertisements of Eastgate House in Lincolnshire and Dunnington House in Yorkshire, quoted in Torrey and Miller, *Invisible Plague,* 70. The number of private asylums grew from 72 to 149 between 1815 and 1849, while they also significantly increased in size.

11. Ibid., 32.

12. The Maudsley Hospital, a psychiatric institute, was established on the 30,000 pounds—a reflection of the fees he charged—he contributed for the purpose.

13. According to Denis Leigh, numbers of such books grew with the years, nine being published in the first quarter of the century, twenty-two in the second; twenty-nine in the third, and fifty-two in the last. Denis Leigh, *The Historical Development of British Psychiatry* (Oxford: Pergamon Press, 1961).

14. It was called, first, the Association of Medical Officers of Asylums and Hospitals for the Insane and later the Medico-Psychological Association.

15. Torrey and Miller, *Invisible Plague,* 49; 46–47.

16. Ibid., 125.

17. Ibid., 135–40; 125.

18. "Swift's asylum," write Torrey and Miller in ibid., "opened in 1757 as St. Patrick's Hospital, was the beginning of two hundred years of confinement of insane persons in Ireland on a scale unparalleled in the world." See also, "The Insanity of Dean Swift and his Hospital for the Insane," *American Journal of Insanity* 5 (1848): 214.

19. The publication of the Medico-Psychological Association, which started appearing in 1853.

20. Not according to the *American Journal of Insanity:* per figures it reported, Scotland led.

21. Torrey and Miller, *Invisible Plague,* 140–141; Hallaran, *Dublin Review* quoted ibid.

22. Andrew Scull's characterization in *The Most Solitary of Afflictions: Madness and Society in Britain, 1700 to 1900* (New Haven: Yale University Press, 1993), 182.

23. Torrey and Miller, *Invisible Plague,* 57–8; 80, 82.

24. "In the first years of the eighteenth-century, a great event happened in France: the discovery of England. Our seventeenth-century, monarchical, catholic, erudite and polite, had felt but an aversion mixed with a bit of pity for a country torn apart by civil and religious discords, and had no interest in ideas, mores or customs of a people that it imagined as drowned in absolute barbarity." René Doumic, "La Découverte de l'Angleterre au xviiie siècle,"

Études sur la littérature française, (Paris: Perrin et Cie, 1906), 5:71–85; also see Georges Ascoli, *La Grande-Bretagne devant l'opinion française au XVIIe siècle,* (Paris: Librarie Universitaire J. Gamber, 1930).

25. See Greenfeld, *Capitalism,* 125–127.

26. The description of foreign opinion is based on Moore, *Backgrounds,* 182–188.

27. George Cheyne, *The English Malady: Or a Treatise of Nervous Diseases of All Kinds* (London: Strahan, 1733), i–ii.

28. Joseph Spence, *Anecdotes Observations and Characters* (London: Carpenter, 1802), 251.

29. Beat L. Muralt, *Lettres sur les Anglois et les Francois et sur les voyages,* (1725) Lettre III, 88. (Translation from French is mine throughout.)

30. Thomas Arnold, *Observations on the Nature, Kinds, Causes and Prevention of Insanity* (London: Phillips, 1806), 18–24; also quoted in Torrey, *Invisible Plague,* 37.

31. Muralt, *Lettres,* Lettre III, 89–93.

32. William Temple, "«De la poésie»," in *Les Œuvres mêlées de Monsieur le Chevalier Temple,* seconde partie, (Utrecht:, Schouten, 1693),, p. 427.

33. *Dictionnaire de Trévoux* (Paris: Libraries Associés,1743), s.v. "rate."

34. F-M. A. Voltaire, "Du climat," in *Commentaire sur l'Esprit des lois,* 1777, XLVI, dans *Œuvres complètes,* (Paris: Garnier, 1880), t. 30, 442.

35. Voltaire, "Projet d'une letter sur les anglais," in *Lettres Philosophiques,* ed. Gustave Lanson (Paris: Librairie Marcel Didier, 1964), 2:261–263.

36. Some of the following discussion first appeared in Greenfeld, "E pluribus unum: L'émergence d'un mal-être modern et des mots pour le dire," in *Ennui,* eds. Nathalie Richard et al. (Paris: Presses Universitaires, 2012).

37. Jean Christophe Coffin, "L'ennui, antichambre de la decadence?" (lecture, Université Paris, November 30, 2007).

38. Moore, *Backgrounds,* 185.

39. Denis Diderot, Lettre à Sophie Voland, Au Grandval, 31 octobre 1760.

40. Baudelaire, "Spleen," *Les Fleurs du Mal* (Paris: Presses Universitaires de France, 1984).

41. Preface to the 1805 edition of *René* (1802) with extracts from *Genie du christianisme* (1802), in Francois Rene de Chateaubriand, *René* (Paris: Hatier, 2007), 9. (All translations from the text are mine.)

42. Chateaubriand's phrase is *à la souplesse de l'esprit,* which the editor of the text suggests should be understood as *opportunisme, arrivisme.* Ibid., 27.

43. Ibid., 30–33.

44. Ibid., 12, 11–14.

45. Christophe Bois, "Notes et dossier" to ibid., 62–63; Gautier, Baudelaire, Constant, Senancour quoted 68, 62, 71.

46. Gauchet and Swain, *Pratique.*

47. Quoted in René Semelaigne, *Les pionniers de la psychiatrie française avant et après Pinel* (Paris: Librairie J. -B. Bailliere et fils, 1930), 125.

48. The cases are described in ibid., 37–38; 43.
49. Michael H. Stone, *Healing the Mind: A History of Psychiatry from Antiquity to the Present,* (New York: Norton, 1997), 35–36.
50. Literary scholars Donald A. Beecher and Massimo Ciavolella have published an exhaustive critical edition of Ferrand's work in English (Jacques Ferrand, *A Treatise on Lovesickness.* (Syracuse, NY: Syracuse University Press, 1990). The discussion relies on the editors' critical introduction.
51. Semelaigne, *Pionniers,* 10.
52. For example, in Anne-Charles Lorry, *De melancholia et morbis melancholicis,* 1765, summarized in ibid., 70–73.
53. M. Pomme, Docteur en Médecine de l'Universite de Montpellier, Médecin consultant du Roi et de la Fauconnerie, *Traité des affections vaporeuses des deux sexes* (Lyon: Benoit Duplain, 1769), 1: 1–2.
54. Ibid., 2: 441.
55. Ibid., 2:440–446.
56. Ibid.,1:2–9.
57. Tenon quoted in Semelaigne, *Pionniers;* Pinel, *Memoir,* 731.
58. Semelaigne, *Pionniers,* 82; Daquin's *Philosophie de la folie* is discussed in ibid., 77–84.
59. Pinel, *Memoir,* 728.
60. Gauchet and Swain, *Pratique,* 41–42.
61. See ibid.
62. Pinel, *Memoir,* 728–730.
63. Semelaigne, *Pionniers,* 14.
64. Pinel, *Memoir,* 730.
65. In *Traité du délire appliqué à la médicine, à la morale et al la legislation* (Paris, 1817). "Néanmoins," writes Semelaigne (*Pionniers,* 101), "il emploie souvent, pour se conformer à l'usage . . . les mots folie et aliénation."
66. Fodéré's thought is discussed in ibid., 99–108.
67. Franz G. Alexander and S. T. Selesnick, *The History of Psychiatry: An Evaluation of Psychiatric Thought and Practice from Prehistoric Times to the Present* (New York: Harper and Row, 1966), 138.
68. The discussion of Esquirol is based on Semelaigne, *Pionniers,* 124–140.
69. Honore de Balzac, *Louis Lambert* (Paris: Dodo Press), 77; 32; 2–3.(My translation.)
70. Quoted in Yavorskaya, *Romantism i Realism vo Franzii v XIX veke* (Moscow,1938), 151.
71. Pierre Baillarger, "Introduction," in *Annales médico-psychologiques: journal de l'Anatomie, de la Physiologie et de la Pathologie du Système Nerveux, destiné particulièrement à recueillir tous les documents relatifs à la science des rapports du physique et du moral, à la pathologie mentale, à la médicine legale des aliénés, et à la clinique des névroses* 1 (January 1843), i–xxvii
72. Ibid., i–xxvii.

73. Ibid., i–xxvii.
74. Karl Marx to Arnold Ruge, September 1843; Karl Marx to his father, 10 November 1837 ; Heinrich Marx to Karl, 2 March 1837.
75. See my "Nationalism and Class Struggle: Two Forces or One?" *Survey: a Journal of East and West Studies* 29:3 (Autumn 1985): 153–174; for the original formulation of this interpretation of the two first essays of Karl Marx.
76. Karl Marx, "Economic and Philosophical Manuscripts of 1844," in *The Marx-Engels Reader,* ed. Robert C. Tucker, 2nd ed. (New York: Norton, 1972), 67, 115.
77. In the English translation used here (ibid.), the word *Entauesserung,* which literally means "objectification," is also translated as "alienation." This makes the interpretation of the text somewhat problematic and requires a more careful consideration of the immediate context in which "alienation" is used in each instance. Working with the original German version would eliminate this problem, but, since the discussion of Marx is an aside insofar as the argument of this book is concerned, I chose to rely on my old and shaggy *Marx-Engels Reader.* Hopefully, someone will find my interpretation interesting (or irritating) enough to check it further—and will use the German text.
78. Ibid., 78–81; 73; 84–87; 89–90.
79. The discussion of Griesinger and his views is based on Klaus Doerner, *Madmen and the Bourgeoisie: A Social History of Insanity and Psychiatry,* trans. Joachim Neugroschel and Jean Steinberg (Oxford: Basil Blackwell, 1981), 272–290; (first published in German in 1969);. Griesinger is quoted from ibid.
80. Otto M. Marx, "German Romantic Psychiatry, Part 1," in *History of Psychiatry* (1990), 351–381; 380.
81. See my "How Economics Became a Science: A Surprising Career of a Model Discipline," in *Disciplinarity at the Fin de Siècle,* eds. Amanda Anderson and J. Valente (Baltimore, MD: Johns Hopkins University Press, 2001), 87–125; and *Capitalism,* 162–171.
82. See Joseph Ben-David, "Science in a Small Country," in *The Ideals of Joseph Ben-David,* ed. Greenfeld (Piscataway, NJ: Transaction, 2012).
83. For a complete list, see Luc S. Cauwenbergh, "J. Chr. A. Heinroth (1773–1843): A Psychiatrist of the German Romantic Era," in *History of Psychiatry,* (1991), 2:365–383, 365.
84. Otto Marx, "GRP," 1:359.
85. Quoted in Doerner, *Madmen,* 227.
86. Otto Marx, "GRP," 1:360.
87. Schelling, *Von der Weltseele* (1798), quoted in Doerner, *Madmen,* 227–228.
88. For instance, Neugroschel and Steinberg, translators of Doerner, ibid.
89. Schelling, *Stuttgarter Privatvorlesungen* (1810), quoted in ibid., 230–233.
90. Otto Marx, "German Romantic Psychiatry, Part 2" in *History of Psychiatry* (1991), 2:1–25, 5.
91. Ibid., 25. The distinction between *psychici* and *somatici* was first made by J. B. Friedreich, a self-identified somatic, but, as Cauwenbergh ("Heinroth,"

373–4) also points out, it has been made "clear beyond doubt that the group of psychiatrists who lived and worked in the period between 1811 and 1842 . . . had much more in common than . . . Friedreich would like to believe."

92. Otto Marx, "GRP," 1:361.

93. Reil characterized and Arndt quoted in Doerner, *Madmen,* 198.

94. Even Father Jahn, apparently, tried his hand in theorizing about it in *Krankheit als Afterorganisationen* (Doerner, 234)

95. Doerner, *Madmen,* 200, 198; Otto Marx, "GRP," 1:362, 361.

96. Doerner, *Madmen,* 200; Reil, "Rhapsodies" quoted in ibid. 200.

97. Otto Marx, "GRP," 1:366, 363.

98. Ibid., 364, 365.

99. Henry C. Burdett, *Hospitals and Asylums of the World* (London: Churchill, 1891), 1:62.

100. Cauwenbergh, "Heinroth," 366, 374–375.

101. Otto Marx, "GRP," 1: 371, 373, 374–375.

102. Ibid., 372–3.

103. Doerner, *Madmen,* 215–216; Horn quoted in ibid., 216.

104. Otto Marx, "GRP," 2, 3, 6n.

105. Otto Marx, "GRP," 1, 372, 377, 373, 370; Doerner, *Madmen,* 334,199n. Otto Marx, ibid., 366.

106. *Die Tobsucht,* vol. 1, *Die Hauptformen der Seelenstoerungen in ihren Beziehungen zur Heilkunde nach der Beobachtung geschildert,* (Leipzig: Weidmann, 1844).

107. Otto Marx, "GRP," 2, 4–5.

108. Ibid., 5–6.

109. *Nationalism,* 293–358.

110. Martha Woodmansee, "The Genius and the Copyright: Economic and Legal Conditions of the Emergence of the 'Author,'" *Eighteenth-Century Studies,* 17:3 (Summer 1984), 425–448.

111. Wieland quoted in Henri Brunschwig, *Enlightenment and Romanticism in Eighteenth Century Prussia* (University Chicago Press, 1974), 140.

112. Quoted in ibid., 151.

113. Karl Philipp Moritz, *Anton Reiser: A Psychological Novel* trans. P. E. Matheson (Westport, CT: Hyperion Press, 1978), 329. Matheson translates this sentence as "humanity oppressed by its *social* conditions"; this does not, however, transmit the meaning of *bürgerliche,* with its emphasis on middle-class, plebeian reality.

114. Roy Pascal, *The German Sturm und Drang* (Manchester: Manchester University Press, 1967), 7.

115. Quoted in ibid., 9–10.

116. Goethe, *Truth and Fiction,* vol. 2, bk. IXX quoted in Henri Brunschwig *Enlightenment,* 214.

117. Pascal, Sturm and Drang, 12–19.

118. Ibid., 31–35.

119. David Phillips introduces his subject of copycat suicides by referencing what he calls 'the Werther effect' in "The Influence of Suggestion on Suicide: Substantive and Theoretical Implications of the Werther Effect," *American Sociological Review* 39 (1974): 340–354.

120. Brunschwig, *Enlightenment,* 220. Brunschwig also writes there: "Contemporaries had the impression that . . . the number of suicides was on the increase. One chronicler . . . found that 239 Berliners committed suicide between 1781 and 1786, accounting for 8 percent of all deaths. . . . The figures are probably not entirely reliable."

121. Quoted in *Nationalism,* 306–7, from K. P. Moritz, *Anton Reiser: A Psychological Novel* (1785), trans. P. E. Matheson (Oxford: Oxford University Press, Hyperion reprint, 1978), 237–238, 264.

122. Brunschwig, *Enlightenment,* 198; *Eumonia* (1801), 481–505, quoted in ibid., 197–8.

123. All the Romantics quoted in ibid., 198–204.

124. Doerner, *Madmen,* 284, 287.

125. For a detailed discussion of the psychological dynamics resulting in the formation of Russian national consciousness, see *Nationalism,* 189–274.

126. Grigory Chkhartishvili, *Pisatel' i Samoubiystvo* (Moscow: Zakharov, 1999; 2006), 201, 203, 207, 209–210. All translations from Russian, unless otherwise indicated, are mine.

127. Quoted from Lotman in ibid., 213–14.

128. See *Nationalism,* 230.

129. Alexandre Pushkin, *Evgeny Onegin,* stanzas xxxvi, xxxvii and xxxviii.

130. M. Yu. Lermontov, *Sobranie Sochineniy v 4kh Tomakh* (Moscow: Khudozhestvennaya Literatura, 1976); *Geroi Nashego Vremeni,* 4:7; "Net, ya ne Bayron, ya drugoi . . . ," 1:423.

131. Pushkin, "Ne dai mne bog soiti s uma . . . "

132. "Poprishschin," notably, can be translated as "belonging to a (social) place."

133. N. V. Gogol, "Diary of a Madman," in *The Mantle and Other* Stories, trans. Claud Field, (La Vergne, TN: Lighting Source, 2011).

134. G. P. Makogonenko, in *Russkie Poety: Antologia v 4kh Tomakh* (Moscow: Detskaya Literatura), 330.

135. According to the *Tenth Revision* (1858–1859).

136. Dostoyevsky's *Writer's Diary* is quoted in Chkhartishvili, *Pisatel',* 215, 214.

137. Perhaps, the trend continued after the Revolution, but so many other reasons for suicide were added, that trying to sort out the causes becomes futile, and I use 1917 as the cut-off point.

138. Chkhartishvili, "Encyclopedia of Literacide," app. 45–46.

139. Vsevolod Garshin, "The Red Flower," quoted from 1911 translation into English; "unknown translator at Brown Brothers."

140. A. M. Rote, "Ocherk istorii psychiatrii v Rossii i Pol'she," *Arkiv psychiatrii, neirologii i sudebnoy psychopatologii,* in three installments, 21:1–3; unfortu-

nately, the middle installment, probably addressing the development of the psychiatric profession in Russia, is lost.

141. "Editorial," *Arkhiv psychiatrii, neirologii i sudebnoy psychopatologii* 21 (1893): 1, Kharkov; from 1897, the journal was published in St. Petersburg.

142. Kovalevsky, *Arkhiv* 30 (1897): 1, 107.

143. Kovalevsky, *Nervnye bolesni nashego obscshestva* (1894) 55.

144. Kovalevsky, "Polozhenie dushevno-bol'nykh v Rossiyskoy Imperii," address read before the 2nd Congress of Russian Physicians in Moscow, Kharkov, (1887).

145. Kovalevsky, *Nervnye bolezni*, 19–20; 43; 58.

146. E.g., V. M. Bekhterev, "Oderzhimost' gadami," *Obozrenie Psychiatrii*, (May 1900) 330–332.

147. *Nervnye bolezni*, "Sifilitiki, ikh neschastie i spasenie", 61–88; *Arkhiv* 30: 1. (This throws a new light on the high society public at the balneological spas of the Caucases, described, for instance, by Lermontov. What cure did they seek there?)

7. Madder Than Them All

1. "Insanity Illustrated by Cases, and by the Conversation and Letters of the Insane" Case IV: Anonymous patient "Long Continued Mental Derangement, With Singular Pecularities," *American Journal of Insanity* 1 (July 1844): 60–61. It should be noted that the *American Journal of Insanity* contains an enormous wealth of information for the study of schizophrenia and manic-depressive illness before they were so distinguished and named, their early epidemiology, and the history of American psychiatry. In any of these areas, this exceptional resource has so far remained virtually untapped. At the time of my research only rare libraries contained the complete set (1844–1921) of the journal; in many issues of the set I used at the Widener Library pages were uncut, meaning that nobody had ever consulted them. (Now the journal archives have been digitized and are publicly available on the Internet.) A systematic examination of this remarkable resource would be very worthwhile, though impossible in any one chapter, and unnecessary in this particular one. I, therefore, limited such examination to the first decade of its publication, to provide the sharpest comparison with the materials pertaining to mental disease in the United States, reviewed in Chapters 3 and 4. It would be a great contribution to knowledge to publish a systematic compilation from the entire set, with chapters, for example, on poetry of the inmates; their letters and conversations; statistics of insanity; changing views on the subject among psychiatrists; their sources; views on and statistics of suicide; discussions of insanity legislation and of relation of insanity and violent crime; etc.

2. *American Journal of Insanity* 1 (January 1845): 288–289.

3. Amariah Brigham, "Definition of Insanity—the Nature of the Disease," *American Journal of Insanity* 1 (October 1844): 97.

4. Ibid., 99–106.

5. Ibid., 106.

6. Ibid., 106–107.

7. Ibid., 108–110.

8. Ibid., 110–111.

9. Ibid., 113.

10. Case IV: Anonymous patient "Long Continued Mental Derangement, With Singular Pecularities," *American Journal of Insanity* 1 (July 1844): 60–61.

11. It is notable that Bellow did not think that he was describing a schizophrenic.

12. Case II: Anonymous patient "Duration of Insanity Three Years—Complete Recovery," *American Journal of Insanity* 1 (July 1844): 56.

13. Case VI: Anonymous patient, *American Journal of Insanity* 1 (July 1844): 65.

14. Case VII: Anonymous patient, *American Journal of Insanity* 1 (July 1844): 67–69.

15. "Insanity Illustrated by Cases, and by the Conversation and Letters of the Insane" *American Journal of Insanity* 1 (July 1844): 52–71.

16. "An Account of Seven Months of Mental Depression, Occasioned by an Injury of the Head;—Furnished by the Patient himself, in a Letter to the Editor," *American Journal of Insanity* 5 (January 1849): 193–205. (E. B. was likely Massachusetts Congressman Ezekiel Bacon. I am grateful to David Phillippi for this information.)

17. *American Journal of Insanity* 1 (October 1844): 98–99.

18. Ibid., 85–86.

19. It moved to Belmont later and still exists, however pressed by new developments, in its luxurious park setting off Mill Street.

20. *American Journal of Insanity* 1 (July 1844): 81–88.

21. According to the numbers of 1840 census, reported in a comparative table by *London Medical Gazette* in April 1844 and reproduced in *American Journal of Insanity*, ibid., 89.

22. Benjamin Rush was certainly the most famous American who wrote on insanity in the early decades of the nineteenth century, but he was not the only one, and not even the first, to do so. In 1811, T. R. Beck published *Inaugural Dissertation on Insanity* in New York. *Statistical Notes of Some of the Lunatic Asylums in the United States* by the same author appeared in 1829. In 1817, George Parkman published in Boston *Management of Lunatics, with Illustrations of Insanity*. Also in Boston appeared in 1838 *Treatise on the Medical Jurisprudence of Insanity* by Dr. Ray, one of the thirteen founding superintendents, while another one of them, Dr. Pliny Earle, published *A Visit to Thirteen Asylums for the Insane in Europe, &c., &c., with an Essay on Insanity,* in Philadelphia in 1841.

23. *American Journal of Insanity* 4 (October 1847): 181.

24. Ronald Kessler, "The Epidemiology of Major Depressive Disorder," *JAMA* (June 18, 2003): 3095–3105. It should be noted that even in Kessler's own reports of the NCS-R data this number is rarely consistent, fluctuating between 16–16.7 percent, a difference of about two million Americans. For schizophrenia, see Regier et al. "The De Facto US Mental and Addictive Disorders Service System: Epidemiologic Catchment Area Prospective 1–Year Prevalence Rates of Disorders and Services," *Archives of General Psychiatry*, (February 1993): 85–94. For bipolar disorder, see Dunner, "Clinical Consequences of Under-recognized Bipolar Spectrum Disorder," *Bipolar Disorder* 5 (2003): 456–463.

25. Kessler quoted in Alex Barnum, "Mental Illness will hit half in U.S., study says/ Disorders often start in young people and go untreated for years—care usually poor," *San Francisco Chronicle*, June 7, 2005, http://www.sfgate.com/health/article/Mental-illness-will-hit-half-in-U-S-study-says-2629761.php#photo-2113043 (accessed June 26, 2012). And in William J. Cromie, "Half of us suffer from mental illness, survey finds," *Harvard Gazette*, June 16, 2005, http://www.news.harvard.edu/gazette/2005/06.16/05-suicide.html (accessed June 26, 2012).

26. NIMH public awareness campaign, BringChange2Mind, says on TV, one in six. http://www.youtube.com/watch?v=WUaXFlANojQ (accessed July 3, 2012).

27. See, for instance, Allan Horowitz and Jerome Wakefield, *The Loss of Sadness: How Psychiatry Transformed Normal Sorrow into Depressive Disorder* (New York: Oxford University Press, 2007); and Christopher Lane, *Shyness: How Normal Behavior Became a Sickness* (New Haven, CT: Yale University Press, 2008).

28. Torrey and Miller, *Plague*, 4–5.

29. Wu, et al. "The Economic Burden of Schizophrenia in the United States in 2002," *Journal of Clinical Psychiatry* 66 (September 2005): 1122–1129; Martin Knapp et al. ("The Global Costs of Schizophrenia, " *Schizophrenia Bulletin* 30, no. 2 (2004): 279–293) report regarding the United States: "[T]aking into account changes in the indexes . . . and the economic data, [t]otal costs of schizophrenia in 1990 were estimated to have risen by 43 percent in 5 years, to $32.5 billion . . . Wyatt et al. (1995) projected empirically obtained costs . . . to 1991, estimating the total economic burden of schizophrenia in the U.S. as $65 billion." (There were no studies estimating the cost of manic-depressive illness other than the ones carried out in 1990 and 1991 and quoted by Torrey, L. S. Kleinman et al., "Costs of Bipolar Disorder," *PharmacoEconomics* 21 (2003): 601–602.) Another telling comparison to costs of these diseases is provided by the 768 billion dollars held by China—the biggest foreign owner of US Treasury bonds—in treasuries as of March 2009 (Reuters, June 1, 2009).

30. These statistics are cited from the information presented by NIMH Director Thomas R. Insel during a lecture, "Translational Research: From Neurons to

Neighborhoods," delivered in April 2008 at Boston University's Medical School. For archived recording see http://www.bu.edu/phpbin/buniverse/videos/view/?id=223 (accessed June 26, 2012).

31. National Center for Injury Prevention and Control, "Suicide Facts at a Glance," Center for Disease Control and Prevention, Summer 2008, http://www.cdc.gov/ViolencePrevention/pdf/Suicide-DataSheet-a.pdf (accessed June 26, 2012).

32. E. Fuller Torrey and Michael Knable, *Surviving Manic Depression: A Manual on Bipolar Disorder for Patients, Families, and Providers* (New York, N.Y., Basic Books, 2005), 15–16.

33. Spain, 1:7180; Italy, 1:4876. Brigham, "Number of the Insane and Idiotic, with Brief Notices of the Lunatic Asylums in the United States," *American Journal of Insanity* 1 (1844).

34. E. K. Hunt, "Statistics of Suicide in the United States: Letter," *American Journal of Insanity* 1 (1844): 225–232.

35. A. Brigham, "Reply," ibid., 232–234.

36. C. H. Nichols, "Statistics of Suicides," *American Journal of Insanity* 4 (1847): 247–253.

37. Benedict Carey, "Study Ties Suicide Rate in Workforce to Economy" *The New York Times,* April 14, 2011, http://www.nytimes.com/2011/04/15/health/research/15suicide.html?_r=1 (Accessed June 28, 12)

38. George Cook, "Statistics of Suicides," *American Journal of Insanity* 5 (April 1849): 303–310.

39. Edward Jarvis, *The Autobiography of Edward Jarvis* (London, Wellcome Institute for the History of Medicine, 1992), 62–64.

40. Isaac Ray, "The Statistics of Insanity," *American Journal of Insanity* 6 (July 1849): 23–52.

41. Pliny Earle, "On the Causes of Insanity," *American Journal of Insanity* 4 (January 1848): 185–211.

42. "Miscellany," Ibid., 93.

43. *American Journal of Insanity* 1 (1844): 80.

44. For an early example, see "Institutions for the Insane in the United States," *American Journal of Insanity* 5 (July 1848): 53–62.

45. Edward Jarvis, "On the Supposed Increase of Insanity," *American Journal of Insanity* 8 (April 1852): 333–364.

46. Jarvis's explanation of the increase in the rates of insanity was rather common. For a particularly astute opinion see *American Journal of Insanity* 7 (October 1850): 189–191.

47. Edward Jarvis, *Diary,* 4, 9, 11, 12–13 (grammar and syntax of the original). The *Diary* is quoted from editor's notes to Jarvis's *Autobiography.*

48. Jarvis, *Diary,* 33.

49. Jarvis, *Autobiography,* 14.

50. Ibid., 16.

51. Ibid., 22–23.

52. Paul Starr, *The Social Transformation of American Medicine: The Rise of a Sovereign Profession and The Making of a Vast Industry* (New York: Basic Books, 1982).

53. Jarvis, *Autobiography,* 27–33.

54. Jarvis, *Diary,* 2, 71, 76, 78–79, quoted in the Introduction to *Autobiography,* xx.

55. *Autobiography,* 33–38.

56. Ibid., "Life in Kentucky," 39–55; quotations from, 55–58.

57. Ibid., 60.

58. Joseph Ben-David and R. Collins, "Social Factors in the Origin of a New Science: The Case of Psychology," *American Sociological Review* 31 (1966): 451–465.

59. So phrased in the famous 1871 lecture by Henry Maudsley, delivered to the British Medico-Psychological Association.

60. R. H. Chase, *The Ungeared Mind* (Philadelphia: F. A. Davis Co., 1919), 169.

61. Dr. L. S. Forbes Winslow (1843–1913) was an eminent British specialist on mental diseases and insanity legislation, the founder of the British Hospital for Mental Disorders, and the editor of *The Psychological Journal.* His father, Dr. Forbes B. Winslow, was one of the great alienists of the previous generation and in 1848 started the publication of the first British psychiatric periodical, *The Journal of Psychological Medicine and Mental Pathology.*

62. *American Journal of Insanity* 7 (July 1850): 75–77, and throughout.

63. See *American Journal of Insanity* 2 (1845): 56.

64. Sass quotes the medical historian Edward Hare who, after carrying out a meticulous examination of the evidence, concluded "not only that there was a significant rise in the incidence of insanity or lunacy in the nineteenth century but that this increase consisted largely of patients with the illness we now call schizophrenia (a condition that the president of the Medico-Psychological Association of Great Britain and Ireland described in 1906 as 'then apparently so rare, but now so common.')." *Madness,* 365–366.

65. See Griesinger, W. "German Psychiatrie," *American Journal of Insanity* 21 (1865): 353–380.

66. Torrey and Miller, *Plague,* 274–297.

67. Torrey and Knable, *Surviving Manic Depression* (the authors compared two well-regarded studies from 1880 and early 1980s), 13–14.

68. Ibid.

69. Ibid., 14–15. Sass, *Madness,* 366.

70. I have quoted this in the Introduction and do so twice not because there is nothing else to quote (there is clearly more than enough), but because of its biographical significance.

71. E. H. Van Deusen, "Observations on a Form of Nervous Prostration, (Neurasthenia,) Culminating in Insanity," *American Journal of Insanity* 25 (April 1869): 445–461. Sinclair Lewis, *Main Street* (New York: Penguin Classics, 1995).

72. G. Beard, "Neurasthenia, or nervous exhaustion," *The Boston Medical and Surgical Journal* 3 (1869): 217–221.

73. Annie Payson Call, *Power Through Repose* (Boston: Little, Brown and Co., 1922), 13. Thanks to David Phillippi for drawing my attention to this and the next quoted texts.

74. George Miller Beard, *American Nervousness: Its Causes and Consequences; A Supplement to Nervous Exhaustion (Neurasthenia)* (New York: Putnam, 1881), vii.

75. *American Journal of Insanity* 1(1844): 249–252.

76. It was to this "neurotic" condition that Dr. Kovalevsky in Russia referred in the 1880s, claiming that "the American disease" was more common in his unhappy country than in America itself.

77. *American Journal of Insanity* 3–4 provides scores of fascinating examples. See, for instance, the issue for January 1847.

78. A. Brigham, editorial preface to "Money-Making Mania," *American Journal of Insanity* 4 (1847): 327–328.

79. "Selections—A new form of Insanity," *American Journal of Insanity* 9 (October 1851): 195 cites the University of Berlin's refusal of proposed thesis by doctoral student M. Groddeck entitled *De morbo democratico, nova insaniae forma.* Upon appeal from M. Groddeck, the University Senate reversed their decision and the thesis was accepted.

80. Rick Weiss, "Study: U.S. Leads in Mental Illness, Lags in Treatment," *Washington Post,* June 7, 2005.

Afterword

1. Consider, for instance, Jared Loughner's poems, Martin Kaste, "Suspect a Puzzle, Even Before Arizona Shooting," *National Public Radio* January, 12, 2011, http://www.npr.org/2011/01/12/132869053/Who-Is-Jared-Loughner (accessed October, 12, 2012).

2. As is emphasized, indeed, by the original title of Brunschwig's classic *Enlightenment and Romanticism*: La Crise de l'État prussien à la fin du XVIIIe siècle et la genèse de la mentalité romantique, (Paris: PUF, 1947).

3. See Greenfeld, *Nationalism,* 383–395 and *Capitalism,* 199–214.

4. In Germany *Allgemeine Zeitschrift für Psychiatrie und Psychisch-Gerichtliche Medizin,* which started publication in 1845.

5. *American Journal of Insanity* 3 1847: 281–285.

Index

5

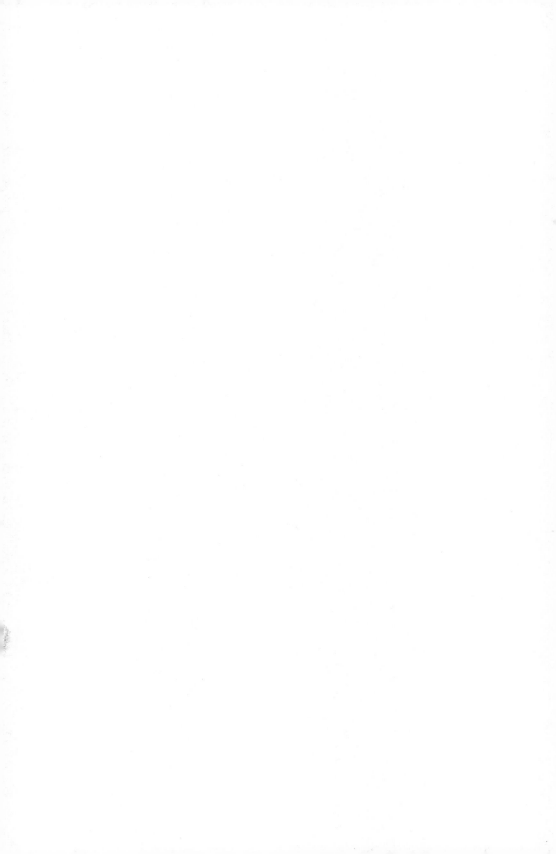